Musculoskeletal Imaging THE REQUISITES

SERIES EDITOR **James H. Thrall, MD**
Radiologist-in-Chief
Massachusetts General Hospital
Juan M. Taveras Professor of Radiology
Harvard Medical School
Boston, Massachusetts

OTHER VOLUMES IN
THE REQUISITES IN RADIOLOGY SERIES

Breast Imaging

Cardiac Imaging

Gastrointestinal Imaging

Genitourinary Radiology

Neuroradiology

Nuclear Medicine

Pediatric Radiology

Ultrasound

Thoracic Radiology

Vascular & Interventional Radiology

Musculoskeletal Imaging

THE REQUISITES

Third Edition

B.J. Manaster, MD, PhD, FACR
Professor and Vice Chairman
Department of Radiology
University of Colorado Health Sciences Center
Denver, Colorado

David A. May, MD
Radiology Associates of Richmond
Associate Clinical Professor
Department of Radiology
Medical College of Virginia
Virginia Commonwealth University
Richmond, Virginia

David G. Disler, MD, FACR
Associate Clinical Professor
Department of Radiology
Medical College of Virginia
Virginia Commonwealth University
Commonwealth Radiology
Richmond, Virginia

Artist:
James F. Snyder, MD

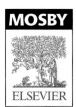

MOSBY

ELSEVIER

MOSBY
ELSEVIER

1600 John F. Kennedy Boulevard
Suite 1800
Philadelphia, PA 19103-2899

THE REQUISITES ™
THE REQUISITES
THE REQUISITES
THE REQUISITES
THE REQUISITES

THE REQUISITES is a proprietary trademark
of Mosby, Inc.

MUSCULOSKELETAL IMAGING: ISBN-13: 978-0-323-04361-8
THE REQUISITES IN RADIOLOGY   ISBN-10: 0-323-04361-5
Copyright © 2007, 2002, 1996 by Mosby, Inc., an affiliate of Elsevier Inc.

Notice

Knowledge and best practice in this field are constantly changing. As new research and experience broaden our knowledge, changes in practice, treatment and drug therapy may become necessary or appropriate. Readers are advised to check the most current information provided (i) on procedures featured or (ii) by the manufacturer of each product to be administered, to verify the recommended dose or formula, the method and duration of administration, and contraindications. It is the responsibility of the practitioner, relying on his or her own experience and knowledge of the patient, to make diagnoses, to determine dosages and the best treatment for each individual patient, and to take all appropriate safety precautions. To the fullest extent of the law, neither the Publisher nor the Authors assumes any liability for any injury and/or damage to persons or property arising out or related to any use of the material contained in this book.

Library of Congress Cataloging-in-Publication Data

Manaster, B.J.
    Musculoskeletal imaging.–3rd ed. / B.J. Manaster, David A. May, David G. Disler; artist, James F. Snyder.
        p. ; cm.– (The requisites)
    Includes bibliographical references and index.
    ISBN 0-323-04361-5
    1. Musculoskeletal system–Imaging. I. May, David A. II. Disler, David G. III. Title. IV. Series: Requisites series.
    [DNLM: 1. Musculoskeletal Diseases–diagnosis. 2. Musculoskeletal System–radiography. WE 141 M267m 2007]
    RC925.7.M35 2007
    616.7'0754–dc22

                                                                    2006046666

Acquisitions Editor: Maria Lorusso
Developmental Editor: Martha Limbach
Project Manager: Bryan Hayward

Printed in the United States of America.

Last digit is the print number: 9   8   7   6   5   4   3   2   1

With love to
Steve, Tracy Joy, and Katy Rose
Robin, Mathew Joseph, and Emily Rose
Julie, Daniel Alden, and Kathryn Whitney
With deep gratitude to our many teachers and mentors

Preface

The Requisites series is pleased to present the third edition of Musculoskeletal Imaging. This version builds upon the second edition. The authors have reorganized the text into smaller chapters, which are arranged so the reader can complete a chapter in a single sitting—making this edition ideal for studying for Boards or for a radiology practitioner reviewing a single topic. With an additional 300 images (primarily MR, but CT and US as well), the topics are much more richly illustrated. There are also easily accessed practical hints. For example, the suggested injection sites for joints are illustrated inside the front cover, with easy references to text descriptions. The "Key Concepts" boxes have been both streamlined and increased in number, making quick reference to the key elements of the most common entities. Boxes describing "What the Clinician Needs to Know" have been added. More expanded discussion is readily available in the text, which has been updated and is both straightforward and practical.

The authors feel comfortable that this text is a complete source for both an introduction to musculoskeletal radiology and for musculoskeletal board review for radiologists. Orthopedic residents, as well as clinicians in rheumatology and rehabilitative medicine, will find pertinent information relating to their interests. We hope that this is a welcome new edition to the Requisites series.

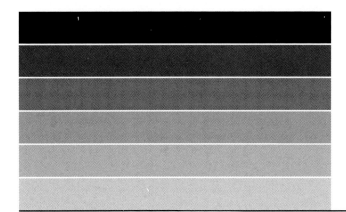

Acknowledgments

This new edition adds artistic contributions by Diagnostic Radiologist James Snyder, MD, of Richmond, Virginia, in addition to artwork from Laurie Persson (carried over from the second edition). As always, we thank our many colleagues who contributed cases and the technologists who skillfully obtained these studies. Trevor MacDougall at SPi helped guide this new edition through the editing and layout process.

Contents

PART 1   INTRODUCTION TO IMAGING OF MUSCULOSKELETAL INJURY

1   Introduction to Imaging of Musculoskeletal Injury: Bones   3

2   Introduction to Imaging of Musculoskeletal Injury: Joints and Soft Tissues   26

3   Special Considerations in Imaging of Musculoskeletal Injury in Children   49

PART 2   UPPER EXTREMITY AND SPINE

4   Shoulder 1: Anatomy and Fractures   67

5   Shoulder 2: Soft Tissues   88

6   Elbow   112

7   Wrist   134

8   Hand   159

9   Spine Trauma   164

PART 3   LOWER EXTREMITY

10   Pelvis   183

11   Hip and Femur   194

12   Knee 1: Fractures and Dislocations   209

13   Knee 2: Soft Tissues   224

14   Ankle   249

15   Foot   271

PART 4   ARTHRITIS

16   Introduction to Arthritis   285

17   Rheumatoid Arthritis and Juvenile Rheumatoid Arthritis   290

18   Productive Arthritis   304

19   Mixed Productive and Erosive Arthritis   318

20   Connective Tissue Disorders   328

21   Arthritis Due to Biochemical Disorders and Depositional Disease   335

22   Avascular Necrosis   346

23   Miscellaneous Joint Disorders   355

24   Joint Arthroplasty   360

PART 5   METABOLIC BONE DISEASE

25   Disorders of Calcium Homeostasis   373

26   Miscellaneous Metabolic Bone Diseases   386

27   Osteoporosis   391

28   Paget's Disease   397

PART 6   TUMORS

29   Introduction to Musculoskeletal Tumor Imaging   407

30   Bone-Forming Tumors: Benign   419

31   Bone-Forming Tumors: Malignant (Osteosarcoma)   429

32   Cartilage-Forming Tumors   442

33   Fibrous Tumors and Tumor-Like Conditions   460

34   Fatty and Vascular Tumors   475

35   Marrow Tumors and Metastatic Disease of Bone   489

36   Neural and Synovial Tumors   500

37   Miscellaneous Tumors and Tumor-Like Lesions   509

38   Musculoskeletal Tumor Staging, Biopsy, and Follow-Up   530

PART 7   MARROW, INFECTION, AND HEMATOLOGIC IMAGING

39   Bone Marrow   539

40   Musculoskeletal Infection   545

41   Hematologic Disorders   565

PART 8   CONGENITAL AND DEVELOPMENTAL CONDITIONS

42   **Introduction to Congenital and Developmental Skeletal Conditions**   577

43   **Spine Disorders**   582

44   **Congenital and Developmental Hip Disorders**   597

45   **Common Congenital Foot Deformities and Tarsal Coalitions**   610

46   **Skeletal Dysplasias**   622

47   **Miscellaneous Congenital and Developmental Conditions**   643

PART 9   TECHNIQUES

48   **Arthrography**   657

49   **Bone Biopsy**   664

50   **Ultrasonography of the Infant Hip: Technique**   666

Index   671

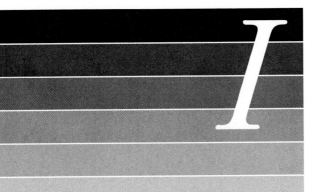

I

INTRODUCTION TO IMAGING OF MUSCULOSKELETAL INJURY

Introduction to Imaging of Musculoskeletal Injury: Bones

BASIC BONE ANATOMY
BONE BIOMECHANICS
FRACTURE DESCRIPTION TERMINOLOGY
    Open Versus Closed Fracture
    Complete Versus Incomplete Fractures
    Fracture Location, Position, and Alignment
STRESS FRACTURES
FRACTURE REDUCTION AND HEALING
COMPLICATIONS OF FRACTURES AND FRACTURE HEALING

Most musculoskeletal imaging is performed to investigate bone and soft tissue injury. This and the following two chapters provide an introduction to imaging of musculoskeletal injury. Chapters 4 to 9 review upper-extremity and spine conditions, and Chapters 10 to 15 review lower-extremity conditions; both sets of chapters emphasize traumatic injury.

BASIC BONE ANATOMY

Mature bone is composed of calcium hydroxyapatite deposited on a matrix made of collagen and other proteins. Bone is organized into a relatively thick outer cortex that surrounds an inner network of cancellous (trabecular) bone. Both cortex and trabeculae are composed of lamellar bone, and both contribute to bone strength. Long bones have epiphyses at the ends, a diaphysis (shaft) in the middle, and metaphyses in between. The long bones of growing children also have one or two physes, or growth plates, composed primarily of cartilage, between metaphysis and epiphysis. The anatomy of the physis is discussed in Chapter 42. The marrow cavity contains trabecular bone and varying amounts of cellular and fatty marrow. Periosteum covers the bone surface, except at the joints, where cartilage, the joint capsule, and ligaments usually cover the bone surface. Periosteum is a thin, tough tissue that contributes to bone production and remodeling, especially during growth and fracture healing.

Normal adult bone undergoes constant turnover in a balanced process of bone resorption by osteoclasts and bone pro-

duction by osteoblasts. This process maintains bone strength by continuously replacing aging bone, which may contain microfractures, with new bone. An increase in bone stress shifts this balance toward greater bone production. This observation is known as *Wolff's law*. In contrast, decreased bone loading and certain hormonal and metabolic states cause bone resorption to exceed bone production. If unchecked, this leads to osteoporosis.

BONE BIOMECHANICS

A basic knowledge of bone biomechanics is helpful to understand how and why bone fractures. The three primary forces of trauma are compression, tension, and shear. Compression is force that pushes two portions of a bone together. Tension is the opposite: it is force that pulls two portions of a bone apart. Shear is force that slides two portions of a bone past one another. These forces act on both gross and microscopic levels. Any material—be it metal, wood, or bone—has a unique threshold at which it will fail (fracture) with each of these forces. Bones and joints are *anisotropic* (i.e., not the same in each direction). Specifically, bones are stronger in compression, and weaker in tension and shear.

Key Concepts	Fractures Reflect Bone Biomechanics

- The three primary forces of trauma are compression, tension, and shear
- Rotation and bending are combinations of these forces
- Bones are most resistant to compression
- The bones of children can bend or buckle without breaking into separate fragments

Normal mature bone is strong and rigid. If enough force is applied, a normal adult bone will break rather than permanently deform. Children's bones, and to a lesser degree adult bones weakened by certain disease states such as osteomalacia or osteoporosis, are "softer," and can permanently deform without breaking into two separate fragments. (Actually, such deformities represent numerous microscopic fractures.)

A fracture can be caused by just one of the three basic mechanical forces, or by a combination. An example of a fracture due to isolated *tension* is the transverse fracture of the patella, in which violent contraction of the extensor mechanism of the thigh places the patella under extreme tension. If the patella fails, the resulting fracture will be transverse (Fig. 1-1). This example illustrates the general rule that fracture lines resulting from tension occur perpendicular to the direction of the applied force. The common avulsion fracture is another example of a tension fracture. Isolated *compression* force in a long bone usually produces an oblique fracture (Fig. 1-2), and in the spine produces a vertebral body compression or burst fracture (Fig. 1-3). *Shear* forces tend to create fracture lines oblique to the line of force. Shear forces are present on a microscopic level in most fractures because the multidirectional bone trabeculae are placed under shear stress regardless of whether the primary force is compression or tension.

Many fractures are caused by a combination of the three basic mechanical forces. One such example is bending. If a bone is bent, tension forces develop along the convex portion of the curve while compressive forces develop along the concave portion of the curve. Bone is better able to withstand compression forces than tension forces, so the convex margin will fail first. Examples of bending-type fractures are a childhood pure plastic bowing fracture (Fig. 1-4A), childhood greenstick fracture (Fig. 1-4B), and butterfly-shaped comminuted fracture in adults (Fig. 1-5). Another combination force

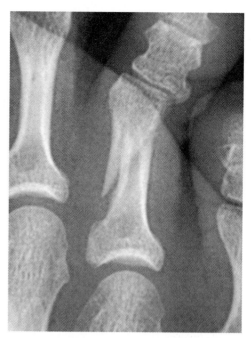

Figure 1-2 Oblique fracture of the fourth toe proximal phalanx.

is a twisting or rotational injury in which rotational force is applied around the circumference of a bone. This mechanism combines compression, tension, and shear, resulting in a spiral fracture (Fig. 1-6).

Another important biomechanical property of bone is that the fracture threshold is inversely related to the rate at which a load is applied. In other words, bone is more resistant to a slowly increasing force than to a rapidly increasing force.

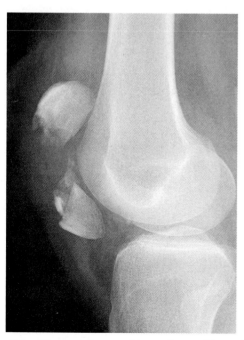

Figure 1-1 Transverse fracture of the patella caused by tension failure during extreme quadriceps contraction.

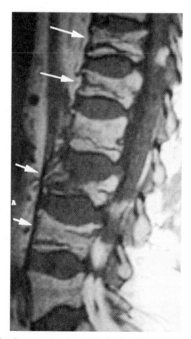

Figure 1-3 Multiple compressions of the lumbar vertebral bodies *(arrows)* in a patient with osteoporosis (sagittal T1-weighted MR image). The irregular low signal lines within the vertebral bodies are fracture lines.

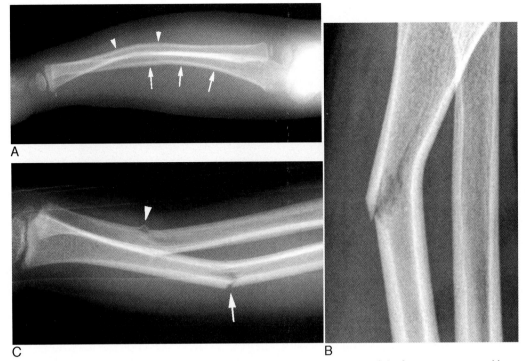

Figure 1-4   Bowing fractures in children. **A,** Pure plastic bowing fracture of the forearm in a 5-year-old. The ulna is laterally bowed *(arrows)* and the radius is dorsally bowed *(arrowheads).* These bones are normally mildly bowed in these directions, but the degree of bowing, combined with a history of fall and forearm pain, establishes the diagnosis. **B,** Greenstick fracture of the distal radius. **C,** Greenstick fracture in a different patient. Note the distraction on the convex side of the radius fracture *(arrows)* and the buckle fracture on the concave (compression) side of the ulna *(arrowhead).*

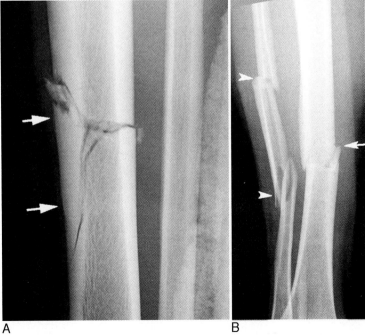

Figure 1-5   Comminuted fractures. **A,** Adult equivalent of bowing fracture: butterfly comminution fracture. The *arrows* point to the butterfly fragment in a tibial fracture. **B,** Segmental fracture. Lateral view of the leg shows two fracture sites in the fibula *(arrowheads)* separated by a segment of normal bone. The tibia fracture *(arrows)* is nearly transverse, reflecting a high-force injury.

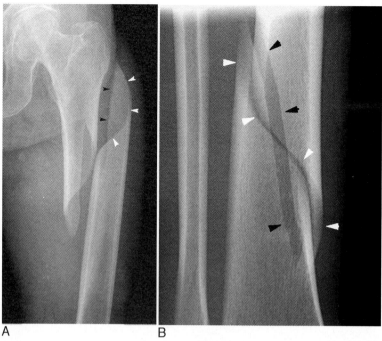

Figure 1-6   Spiral fractures. **A and B,** Laterally displaced (A) and mildly displaced (B) fractures. Note the typical combination of a spiral component *(white arrowheads)* and a straight, longitudinal component *(black arrowheads).*

A rapidly delivered, sharp impact such as from a bullet or a direct blow to a bone is more likely to cause a fracture than is a greater force that builds slowly. However, even a slowly increasing force can eventually exceed a bone's fracture threshold, often with severe damage to the bone, if a great deal of force is present. In the soft tissues, a rapidly applied force also is more likely to cause tissue failure. This is why a high-velocity injury such as a gunshot wound can cause so much damage to the soft tissues.

A small defect in a bone, such as an orthopedic screw tract or a foramen where a blood vessel enters a bone, can allow force to be concentrated at a single point termed a *stress riser*. A stress riser can significantly lower the fracture threshold of a long bone shaft, and many fractures begin at a stress riser.

The first and often the best imaging examination with which to evaluate suspected bone trauma (or bone pathologic abnormalities of any kind) is radiography. Computed tomography (CT), magnetic resonance imaging (MRI), and radionuclide scanning can be important adjuncts. Magnetic resonance imaging is especially sensitive for detection of an acute nondisplaced fracture. Fluid-sensitive sequences, such as inversion recovery or fat-suppressed T2-weighted images, demonstrate marrow edema. The fracture line often is best seen on T1-weighted images as a low signal line (Fig. 1-7).

FRACTURE DESCRIPTION TERMINOLOGY

When reading a radiograph of an injured bone or joint, imagine that you are talking on the phone to the orthopedic surgeon who will treat the patient. Accurate description of a fracture is extremely important and requires conventional language to facilitate communication of the findings. There are scores of eponyms and classification systems for specific fractures, some of which are reviewed in later sections of this book. These have the potential advantage of quickly communicating essential features of a fracture that an orthopedic surgeon needs to know. However, many of these fracture classification systems are imperfect or not widely used. In contrast, the descriptive terminology that follows is universally used and understood.

WHAT THE CLINICIAN WANTS TO KNOW: FRACTURE DESCRIPTION TERMINOLOGY

Consistent use of precise language required
Always describe: fracture location, position, alignment
Alignment: displacement, angulation, distraction, fragment overlap, rotation
Always describe if present:
    Comminution
    Joint involvement
    Evidence of open fracture, such as gas in soft tissues
    Foreign body
    Evidence of pre-existing lesion (pathologic fracture)

Open Versus Closed Fracture

In a *closed fracture,* osseous fragments do not breach the skin surface. In contrast, an *open fracture* is associated with

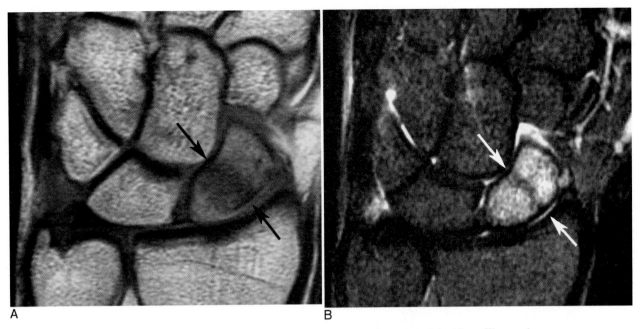

Figure 1-7   MR image of radiographically occult fracture. **A and B,** Young adult with snuff box tenderness and normal radiographs. Coronal T1 (A) and inversion recovery (B) images show a scaphoid waist fracture *(arrows).* Note the diffuse marrow edema in part B.

skin disruption and exposure of a bone fragment (Fig. 1-8). This substantially increases the risk for infection and is considered an emergent situation for surgical reduction and lavage of the fracture site. Wound contamination also increases the risk for infection.

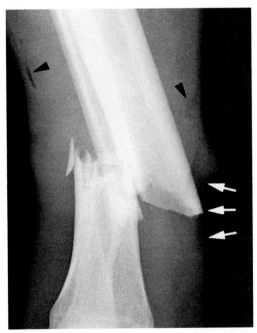

Figure 1-8   Open fracture of the tibia. Note bone fragment projecting through skin wound *(white arrows).* Also note the subcutaneous gas *(black arrowheads)* that can be an important telltale sign of skin disruption in subtler cases of open fracture.

Complete Versus Incomplete Fractures

Complete fractures result in two or more separate bone fragments. Complete fractures are described as *transverse, oblique,* or *spiral.*

Incomplete fractures are those in which the cortex is only partially interrupted. Such fractures occur most often in children because bone in children has different mechanical properties than in adults, as noted previously. Most incomplete fractures in children involve some deformity of the bone, with the notable exception of the toddler's fracture (Fig. 1-9). Three major types of displaced incomplete fractures in children are buckle, greenstick, and plastic bowing deformity. *A buckle fracture* is focal compression of cortex due to an axial load (Fig. 1-10, see Fig. 1-4B). A torus fracture is a complete (circumferential) type of buckle fracture, but these terms are often used interchangeably. A *greenstick fracture* results from bending force with distraction of cortex fragments on the convex side of the bone (see Fig. 1-4B). A *pure plastic bowing deformity,* also termed a *plastic deformation,* is a bending of bone without a discrete fracture line (see Fig. 1-4A). This injury represents innumerable microfractures of a long segment of bone. Incomplete fractures in adults are less common and usually nondisplaced. Such fractures may have unusual mechanisms, or occur in bone weakened by disease such as osteomalacia (Fig. 1-11).

Comminution indicates that the bone is fractured into more than two fragments. A *segmental comminuted fracture* is one in which the same bone is fractured in two separate sites, with an intact segment of bone between the fracture sites (see Fig.

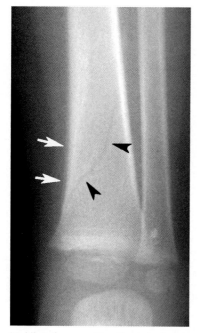

Figure 1-9 Toddler's fracture. AP radiograph shows an oblique fracture of the distal tibia *(arrowheads)*. Note the periosteal reaction on the medial tibial cortex *(arrows)* indicating that this is not an acute fracture. These nondisplaced fractures of the lower extremities of toddlers are always subtle, and often are only detected on follow-up radiographs. Most toddler's fractures occur in the tibia.

1-5B). *A butterfly-comminuted fracture* is one in which a wedge-shaped "butterfly" fragment of intervening bone is present (see Fig. 1-5A). This fracture often requires internal or external fixation.

Fracture Location, Position, and Alignment

The radiologist's report must describe the location of the fracture and the relative position and alignment of the bone fragments. It is useful to localize a long bone fracture by dividing the length of the bone into thirds. Thus, a fracture can be located in the proximal third, the junction of the proximal and middle thirds, the middle third, the junction of the middle and distal thirds, or the distal third. A long bone fracture can also be described as being epiphyseal, metaphyseal, metadiaphyseal, or diaphyseal. It is important to describe whether a fracture extends to a joint surface because such fractures are more likely to need surgical intervention and less likely to have an optimal outcome (Fig. 1-12). In skeletally immature patients, it is important to describe whether a fracture extends to or through a physis, because such fractures increase the likelihood of growth plate arrest, which can result in limb-length discrepancy and angular deformity. Physeal fractures and their classification system are discussed in Chapter 3.

Once the exact location of the fracture fragments has been identified, it is important to describe deformities of *position and alignment*. It is unusual for a fracture to present in anatomic (normal) position and alignment. More commonly, fractures are displaced. By convention, *displacement* is

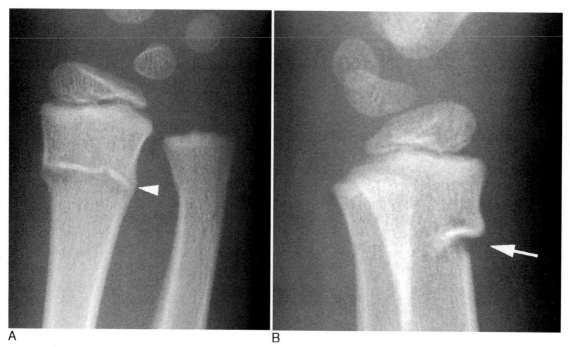

A   B

Figure 1-10 Childhood buckle fracture. **A and B,** PA (A) and lateral (B) views show a dorsal distal radial metaphyseal buckle fracture *(arrows)*.

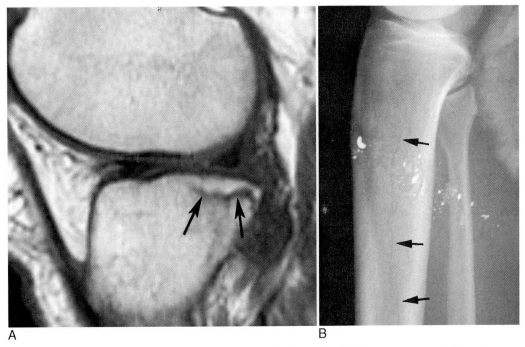

A   B

Figure 1-11 Incomplete fractures in adults. **A,** Sagittal T1-weighted MR image shows irregular linear low signal in the lateral posterior tibia *(arrows)* representing a nondisplaced, incomplete trabecular fracture, in this case caused by impaction. **B,** Incomplete tibial fracture in an adult *(black arrows)* due to a gunshot wound. Note the metal fragments that mark the bullet tract.

described by the position of the more distal fragment relative to the more proximal fragment. Displacement can occur in any direction, and the amount of displacement should be described. Again by convention, the amount of transverse displacement of a long bone shaft fracture is described as a per-

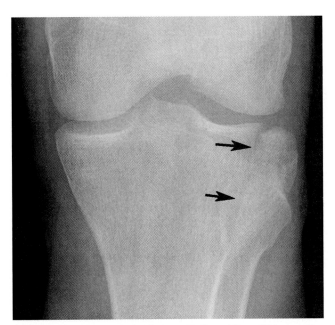

Figure 1-12 Intra-articular fracture. Shallow oblique AP knee radiograph shows a lateral tibial plateau fracture *(arrows)* with mild diastasis and depression of the lateral fragment.

centage of the cross-sectional diameter of the dominant osseous fragment. If displacement is greater than 100% of the shaft diameter, muscle pull can cause the fracture fragments to slide past one another. Such overlap of the fragments is sometimes termed *overriding* or *bayonet apposition*. In contrast, *distraction* is longitudinal separation of the fracture fragments along the long axis of the bone. Distraction of fracture fragments may be due to muscle pull or to interposed soft tissue. The length of any fragment overlap or distraction should be included in the report.

Fracture alignment, also termed *angular deformity,* refers to a directional change of the fracture fragments relative to the long axis of the fractured bone. This is usually described in one of two ways: by the direction of the apex of the angle formed by the fracture fragments or by the orientation of the distal fracture fragment relative to the proximal fragment. Orthopedic surgeons often use the latter system. For example, *medial angulation* or *varus* means that the distal fracture fragment is pointing relatively more toward the midline of the body when compared with the proximal fragment. *Lateral angulation* or *valgus* is the opposite, that is, the distal fracture fragment is pointing relatively more away from the midline of the body than is the proximal fragment. Anterior and posterior angulation are similar. Note that "apex anterior" is the same as "posterior" angulation. Because of this potential for confusion, one should describe the angular deformity by using either the term "apex" angulation or specify "angulation of the distal fragment."

Rotation, or *torsion,* refers to twisting of one fracture fragment relative to another around the long axis of a bone. Rotational deformity is important but can be difficult to determine with radiographs. It is necessary to image the entire length of a fractured bone as well as the joint at either end. Clinical evaluation is usually adequate, but CT can be helpful in difficult cases.

Key Concepts	CT with Reformats

CT with Reformats Is Particularly Useful for Fractures of:
  Pelvis
  Knee (tibial plateau)
  Ankle (pilon)
  Calcaneus
  Glenoid
  Proximal humerus
  Elbow
  Wrist (distal radius or scaphoid for evaluation of healing)

It is important to estimate the amount of displacement, angulation, or rotation. Different amounts may be more or less acceptable in different fractures. This often relates to the type of adjacent joint. Thus, malrotation or abnormal angulation may be acceptable in a humeral fracture since the shoulder joint is a ball-and-socket type and thus can compensate for malalignment. On the other hand, little if any varus or valgus malalignment or rotation is acceptable in a tibial fracture because both the ankle and knee are hinge joints and cannot compensate.

Avulsion fractures are caused by tension (traction) by a tendon or ligament (Fig 1-13). The term *chip fracture* is often used to describe any small cortical fragment, but is more precisely limited to fractures caused by focal impaction or shearing rather than avulsion. Avulsion fractures are more significant because they may be associated with joint laxity. Knowledge of the normal sites of ligament attachment can be helpful in distinguishing avulsion fractures from the less significant chip fractures.

An *intra-articular fracture,* or more precisely an articular fracture, extends through an articular surface (see Fig. 1-12). Intra-articular fractures can be surprisingly subtle on routine radiographs, requiring special views or sometimes CT or MRI for diagnosis. One potential telltale sign of an intra-articular fracture is the finding of a joint effusion with a fluid-fluid level on a horizontal beam radiograph. This finding is caused by a hemarthrosis, due to settling of the cellular components of blood, with serum on top. A *fat-fluid level* is caused by escape of marrow fat into a joint space, and is much more specific for an intra-articular fracture, but is less commonly seen. Sometimes three levels are seen, with the fat on top and the cellular layer on the bottom (Fig. 1-14). Regardless, detection of any fluid-fluid level in a traumatized joint warrants close inspection for an intra-articular fracture. A *die punch fragment* is an articular surface fragment that is driven into the epiphysis. The fragment may be rotated or driven straight into the trabecular bone of the epiphysis or metaphysis. Die punch frag-

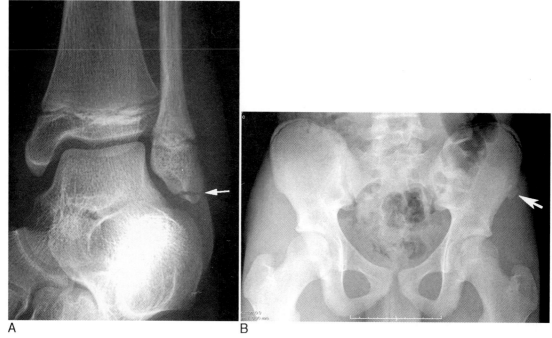

A   B

Figure 1-13 Avulsion fracture. **A,** Avulsion fracture tip of lateral malleolus *(arrow)* following a supination ankle injury. **B,** Avulsion of the anterior superior iliac spine *(arrow)* due to sartorius origin avulsion.

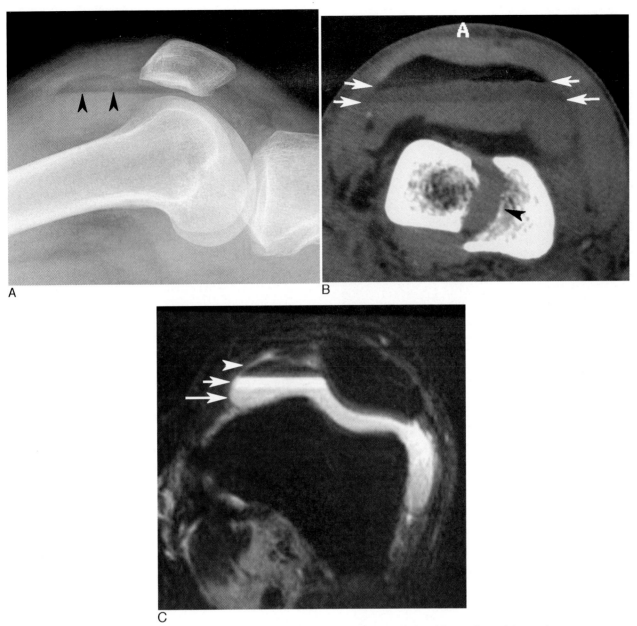

Figure 1-14   Traumatic joint effusions with fluid levels. **A,** Cross-table lateral knee radiograph in a patient with a tibial plateau fracture. Note the fat-fluid level *(arrowheads)* with low-attenuation fat layer on top and the dependent blood below. **B,** Axial CT image in a different patient with an intra-articular distal femur fracture *(arrowhead)* shows three layers, with fat on top, a dense serum layer in the middle (between the *white arrowheads),* and a slightly denser layer containing serum and blood cells at the bottom *(arrows).* **C,** Lipohemarthrosis. Axial fat-suppressed T2-weighted MR image in the knee of a patient with a tibial plateau fracture shows layering identical to that seen in part B. The fat layer has low signal intensity because of fat suppression. If this image had been obtained without fat suppression, the fat would be bright. The cellular (most dependent) layer is slightly darker than the serum (middle) layer because of susceptibility artifact due to intracellular hemoglobin. See also Figures 12-6 and 12-7.

ments occur most commonly in tibial plateau fractures (Fig 1-15). An *osteochondral* fracture is a compression or shear fracture of the subchondral bone and overlying cartilage confined to the peripheral portion of an epiphysis. An osteochondral fracture caused by compression may displace by impaction, and a fracture caused by shear may result in displacement of an osteochondral fragment into the joint (Fig 1-16).

One of the most important complications of an intra-articular fracture is post-traumatic osteoarthritis. Attention to fragment position and alignment along the articular surface is important, as a step-off or a gap of more than 2 mm in a small joint such as the wrist is associated with a significantly increased rate of development of post-traumatic osteoarthritis. Surgical reduction and fixation is usually necessary for these fractures.

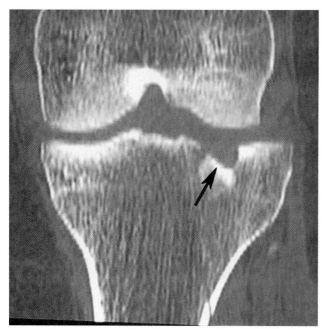

Figure 1-15   Die punch fragment. Coronal CT reconstruction of a tibial plateau fracture shows depressed lateral plateau fragment *(arrow)*.

STRESS FRACTURES

In precise usage, a *stress fracture* occurs as either a fatigue fracture or an insufficiency fracture, but the terms *stress fracture* and *fatigue fracture* are often used interchangeably. A *fatigue fracture* occurs when abnormal stresses are placed on normal

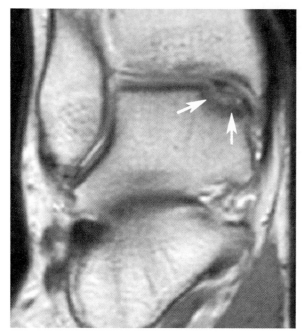

Figure 1-16   Osteochondral fracture. Coronal T2-weighted MR image shows medial talar dome osteochondral fracture *(arrows)*. Note high T2 signal between the fragment and the talus.

bone, usually in the form of multiple and frequent repetition of otherwise normal stress. Several factors contribute to the development of a fatigue-type stress fracture. First, the muscles, tendons, and ligaments normally help to redistribute forces applied to the bones and joints. However, muscle fatigue during prolonged exercise results in less protection of the bones and joints. Second, increased bone loading stimulates a normal adaptive process that leads to new bone formation. As noted previously, this is Wolff's law. The mechanism of this phenomenon is not completely understood but on a microscopic level appears to be stimulated by microfractures. New bone formation requires the activity of both osteoblasts and osteoclasts, as the weaker or injured old bone is replaced with stronger new bone. Unfortunately, the osteoclasts begin first; thus, paradoxically, an increase in bone stress such as increased physical activity first results in the bones becoming weaker for a few weeks before ultimately becoming stronger. This creates a window of vulnerability during which the microfractures can coalesce into a discrete fracture.

Stress fractures evolve over time. Early stress injuries tend to be distributed along a long segment of the cortex. Radiographs at this stage are usually normal, but faint cortical resorption or periosteal reaction may be seen. This stage is sometimes termed a *stress reaction* or, in the tibia, a *shin splint,* but the terminology is not standardized. With ongoing microfractures, a focal segment within the stress reaction may weaken more rapidly. This weaker segment becomes a focal point for bone deformation during repeated loading (that is, a stress riser) because it is less able to resist deformation than is the remainder of the bone. This concentration of microscopic bone deformation at the focally weakened segment has two important consequences. First, the stresses applied to the remainder of the bone are partially relieved, allowing it to heal. Second, the microfractures in the weakened segment are subject to greater deformation, so they are more likely to progress. In any terminology, this is a true stress fracture (Figs. 1-17, 1-18). Bone scanning at this stage will show intense tracer uptake confined to one portion of the cortex. Radionuclide bone scanning has high sensitivity and negative predictive value in that a negative finding nearly excludes the possibility of a stress fracture. Radiography is more specific than radionuclide scanning because it may reveal focal periosteal reaction or fuzzy sclerosis at or near the weakened segment, but it is much less sensitive than bone scanning. Linear sclerosis, often perpendicular to major trabecular lines, is due to attempted healing. Magnetic resonance imaging is the most sensitive test for stress injury because of the associated marrow edema; it is highly specific when a fracture line is shown (see Fig. 1-18). This test also may demonstrate an injury in an adjacent tissue, such as a muscle strain that clinically simulates a bone stress injury.

If untreated, a stress fracture can progress to a complete fracture. Stress fractures can occur in almost any weight-bearing bone. Classic locations are the femoral neck and tibial shaft in runners and the metatarsals of new military recruits (*march fracture,* see Fig. 1-17D). Lumbar spondylolysis, discussed in Chapter 43, is also a form of stress fracture.

Treatment of a stress fracture requires rest and, in more advanced cases, immobilization. Successful treatment also requires the cooperation of the patient. Many stress fractures are self-inflicted overuse injuries, in which patients ignore the warning signs because of their passion for the injurious activity. Knowledge that earlier intervention results in more rapid healing may help to persuade the injured patient to allow the fracture to heal.

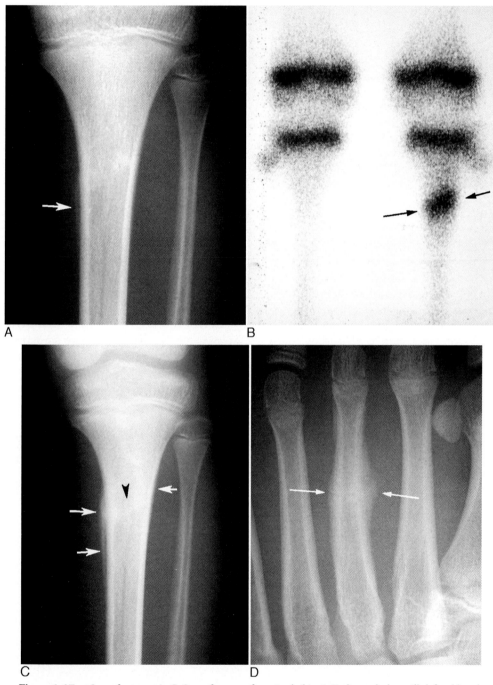

Figure 1-17   Stress fractures. **A–C,** Stress fracture of proximal tibia. **A,** Radiograph shows ill-defined lamellar periosteal bone formation in proximal medial tibial diaphysis *(arrow).* **B,** Bone scan shows oblique transverse stress fracture in the proximal tibia *(arrows).* **C,** Frontal tibial radiograph obtained 3 weeks later demonstrates progressive formation of periosteal new bone formation *(arrows)* and appearance of subtle linear sclerosis at the stress fracture site *(arrowhead).* **D,** March fracture in a different patient. Note the periosteal new bone formation in the metatarsal shaft *(arrows)* and the subtle sclerosis caused by healing response to the metatarsal fracture.

(Continued)

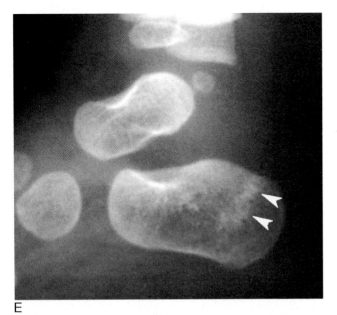

Figure 1-17—(Cont'd)   E, Calcaneus stress fracture in a young child. Note the sclerotic zone in the posterior calcaneus *(arrowhead)*. Some authors consider this to be a type of toddler's fracture.

An *insufficiency fracture* occurs when normal stresses are placed on bone that is demineralized, typically by osteoporosis or metabolic bone disease. The multiple osteoporotic compressions in Figure 1-3 are examples of insufficiency fracture. Like a fatigue-type stress fracture, an insufficiency fracture can often be diagnosed by clinical history, but imaging is helpful for con-

firmation. Detection of a nondisplaced insufficiency fracture on radiographs can be quite difficult because of osteopenia. Initial films are negative about 80% of the time. Bone scanning is sensitive but nonspecific unless a specific pattern of tracer uptake can be identified, such as the H-shaped pattern of activity in a sacral insufficiency fracture (Fig 1-19). Magnetic resonance imaging is highly sensitive to the presence of a fracture and is more specific than radionuclide imaging because it usually can depict a fracture line (see Fig. 1-3). Although less sensitive than MRI, CT can also be helpful, especially if MR images are dominated by extensive edema that obscures a fracture line. In this setting, CT often shows a lucent fracture line and evidence of early bone healing, which are specific for the presence of fracture.

The more general term *pathologic fracture* includes any fracture that occurs with normal stresses in an abnormal bone. Technically speaking, an insufficiency fracture is a type of pathologic fracture. However, the term "pathologic" is usually reserved to describe a fracture through bone weakened by a tumor (Fig. 1-20).

FRACTURE REDUCTION AND HEALING

Fracture reduction is restoration of anatomic (normal) alignment. *Closed reduction* is achieved by manipulation of the fractured extremity and casting. *Open reduction* involves operative access to the injured bone, often for the purpose of applying fixating hardware or assessment of the alignment of intra-articular

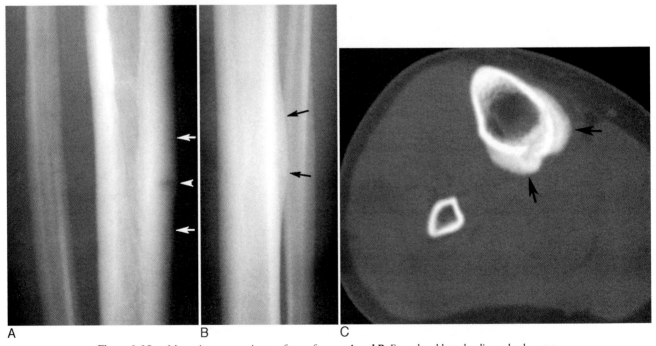

Figure 1-18   Magnetic resonance image of stress fracture. **A and B,** Frontal and lateral radiographs show typical posteromedial location of a midtibial stress fracture as indicated by fracture line *(arrowhead)* and periosteal new bone formation *(arrows)*. **C,** Axial CT image also shows prominent posteromedial solid periosteal new bone formation *(arrows)*.

(Continued)

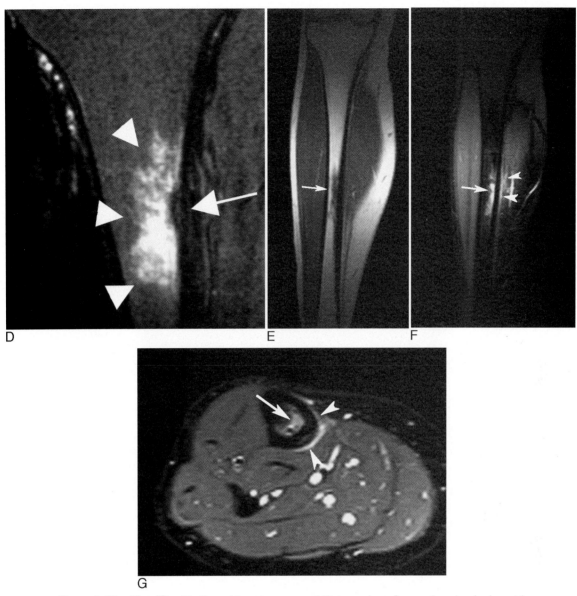

Figure 1-18—(Cont'd) **D,** Coronal inversion recovery MR image shows fracture *(arrow)* and substantial surrounding bone marrow edema *(arrowheads)*. **E–G,** Different patient with a midtibial stress fracture. Coronal T1 (E) and inversion recovery (F) and axial inversion recovery (G) show marrow edema *(arrows)* and periosteal edema *(arrowheads* in parts F and G). See also Figure 11-17.

fragments. *Internal fixation* is usually achieved by placement of a cortical plate fixed with transverse screws on the surface of the bone, pin or screw placement across the fracture, or rod or nail within the medullary space along the long axis of the bone (Figs. 1-21, 1-22, 1-23). External fixation is achieved by pins placed through the skin into the bone remote from the fracture site. The pins are fixed to one another externally (Fig. 1-24). *External fixation* is often used when the fracture site may be infected or for fractures near the end of a bone. Regardless of the method of reduction and immobilization, the main bone fragments must be in contact to allow healing. Compression across the fracture improves contact between the fragments and reduces the risk for nonunion. A variety of techniques may be used to achieve such compression (see Fig. 1-22). On the other

hand, compression must sometimes be limited, for example in comminuted long bone fractures that would telescope and shorten if compressed. The length of the bone can be controlled by fixation with a cortical plate or an intramedullary nail (rod) with proximal and distal interlocking screws (see Fig 1-23).

Dynamic fixation means that fragment motion is allowed in one direction but is constrained in all others. Examples are a dynamic hip screw (discussed further in Chapter 11) and "dynamizing" an intramedullary nail. In the latter, after a fracture has partially healed and gained a degree of stability, bone apposition may be improved by removal of the interlocking screws at one end of the nail. This allows the fragments to slide along the nail and impact against one another (Fig. 1-25), thereby improving bone apposition and healing.

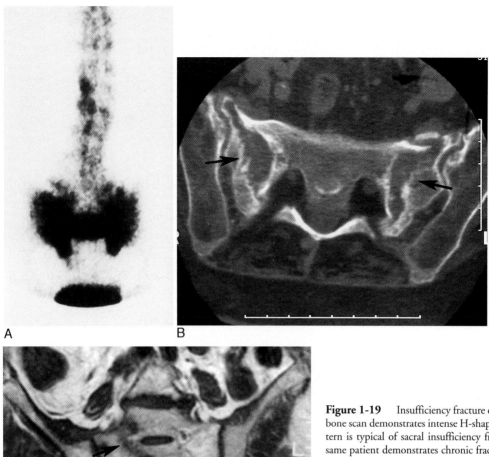

Figure 1-19   Insufficiency fracture of the sacrum. **A,** Radionuclide bone scan demonstrates intense H-shaped uptake in sacrum. This pattern is typical of sacral insufficiency fracture. **B,** Axial CT image of same patient demonstrates chronic fracture lines in both sacral wings *(arrows)*. Sclerotic opposing margins indicate chronic nature of insufficiency fracture. **C,** Oblique coronal T1-weighted spin-echo image in a different patient demonstrates low signal insufficiency fracture line in right sacral wing *(arrows)*.

When reducing a fracture, the orthopedic surgeon *reverses* the forces that caused the fracture. For example, a Colles fracture is caused by compression of the dorsal aspect of the distal radius. When reducing a Colles fracture, the surgeon must distract the dorsal radius, which is accomplished by distraction and palmar flexion of the wrist. Although the goal of fracture reduction is restoration of anatomic alignment, compromises must often be made to achieve the best possible outcome. A host of factors determine the desired fragment positions after reduction, including maximizing the likelihood of healing or minimizing the risk for complications. Maintaining function of nearby joints is one of the most important goals. Angulation of a long bone shaft fracture is generally undesirable but may be tolerated if it is in the same plane as the motion of an adjacent joint. An intra-articular fracture with a stepoff or diastasis of greater than 2 to 3 mm has significantly increased risk for developing post-traumatic

osteoarthritis, so great effort is often made to restore, or nearly restore, the normal articular surface contour.

After the initial reduction, the purpose of subsequent imaging is to assess for the presence of healing and the occurrence of complications. Normal fracture healing is a predictable process, although it is affected by several factors, including the age of the patient; the degree of local bone and soft tissue devitalization; the location of the fracture; the degree of immobilization and apposition of bone fragments after reduction; and the presence of complicating factors such as including infection, tumor at the site of fracture, bone necrosis, and systemic factors (e.g., nutritional status, cigarette smoking, and corticosteroid treatment).

In the earliest phases of healing, a hematoma forms at the fracture site and induces a healing response associated with the release of growth factors and neovascularization. This initially results in localized bone demineralization around the fracture site. In addition, the bone at the margins of the frac-

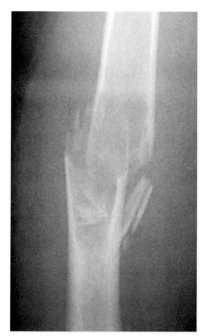

Figure 1-20 Pathologic fracture through a unicameral bone cyst in the humerus of a child.

ture is necrotic and is removed by osteoclasts. These changes cause blurring of the fracture margins as one of the first radiographic findings in fracture healing. Subsequently, immature (woven) bone called *callus* is formed within the hematoma, and between the apposing margins of the fracture fragments.

Over time, the callus is remodeled into mature lamellar bone and biomechanical stability is restored (Fig. 1-26).

COMPLICATIONS OF FRACTURES AND FRACTURE HEALING

The rate of fracture healing depends on several variables. Healing is generally slower in elderly persons, malnourished individuals, and cigarette smokers. Corticosteroid treatment and, to a lesser degree, nonsteroidal anti-inflammatory drugs retard fracture healing. Microscopic motion at the fracture site stimulates healing. Extremely rigid fixation with orthopedic hardware can slow the rate of healing by removing this stimulus. However, inadequate fixation causes abundant callus formation, but the callus cannot mature into biomechanically stable bone.

WHAT THE CLINICIAN WANTS TO KNOW: FRACTURE FOLLOW-UP RADIOGRAPHS

1. Fragment position and alignment: change or no change. If changed, describe.
2. Assess maturity of fracture healing
   Earliest: softened fracture lines
   Callus
   Maturing callus
   Late: remodeling
3. Complications of fracture healing or hardware

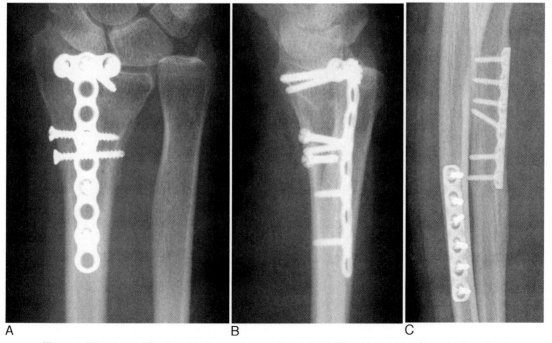

A   B   C

Figure 1-21 Internal fixation with plates and screws. **A and B,** AP (A) and lateral (B) radiographs show dorsal T-plate fixation of distal radius fracture. Also note the two lateromedial transverse screws. **C,** Forearm fractures in adult bones fixed with cortical compression plates. The slots for the screw heads are designed to force the fragments toward the center of the plate. Such compression increases apposition of bone fragments and thus speeds healing.

(Continued)

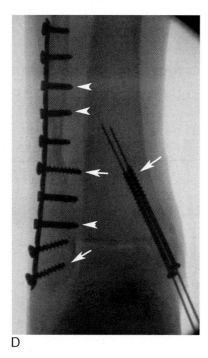

D

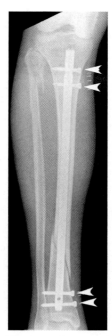

Figure 1-21—(Cont'd)   D, Screw types. Screws designed to gain purchase in cortex have fine threads *(arrowheads)*. Screws designed to gain purchase in softer trabecular bone have wider threads *(arrows)*. The medial malleolus screws are lag screws. The gap (lag) between the threads and the head allows compression as the screw is tightened.

Figure 1-23   Internal fixation with intramedullary nail. Frontal radiograph of the tibia demonstrates intramedullary rod with interlocking screws *(arrowheads)*, which prevent rotation and shortening after reduction.

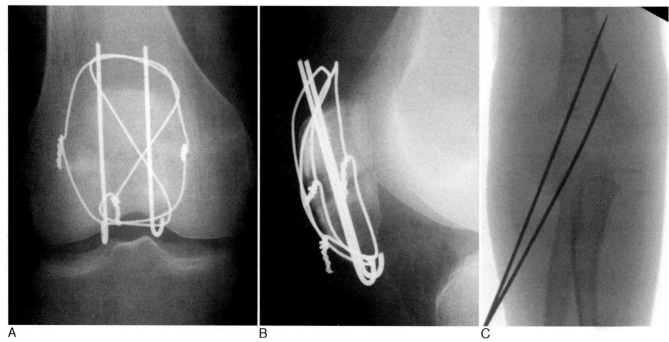

A   B   C

Figure 1-22   Internal fixation with cerclage wires and pins. **A,** AP radiograph and **B,** lateral radiograph of compression wiring fixation of patellar fracture. Same patient as in Figure 1-1. **C,** Kirschner wires, more often termed *K wires,* for fixation of a distal humeral condylar fracture in a child. These small wires allow stabilization with minimal trauma to the physis. The excess wire will be trimmed and the elbow casted. The wires will be removed as the fracture heals.

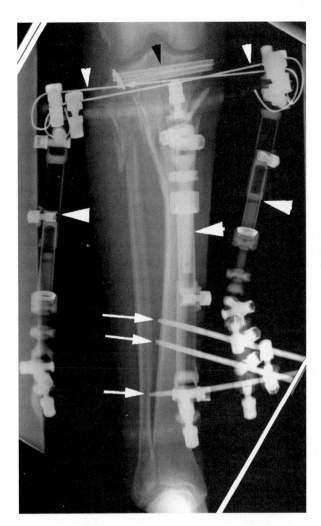

Figure 1-24   External fixation. Note the fixation of the main proximal tibial fragment with crossing wires *(small white arrowheads)*, the main distal fragment with pins *(white arrows)*, and the adjustable external frame *(large white arrowheads)*. This patient also has a tibial plateau fracture that is fixed with two transverse screws *(black arrowhead)*.

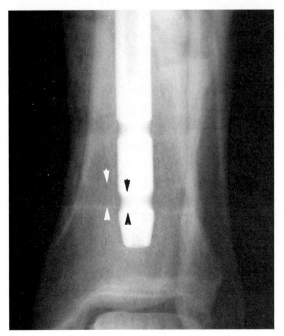

Figure 1-25   Dynamized intramedullary nail. This distal tibial fracture is in the late stages of healing. The fracture was initially fixed with an intramedullary nail with proximal and distal interlocking screws. After the healing process had begun and partial fracture stability was achieved, the distal interlocking screws were removed. This allowed the distal fragment to slide proximally along the nail until fully impacted against the proximal fragment, causing the old screw tracts *(white arrowheads)* to shift proximally relative to the screw holes in the nail *(black arrowheads)*.

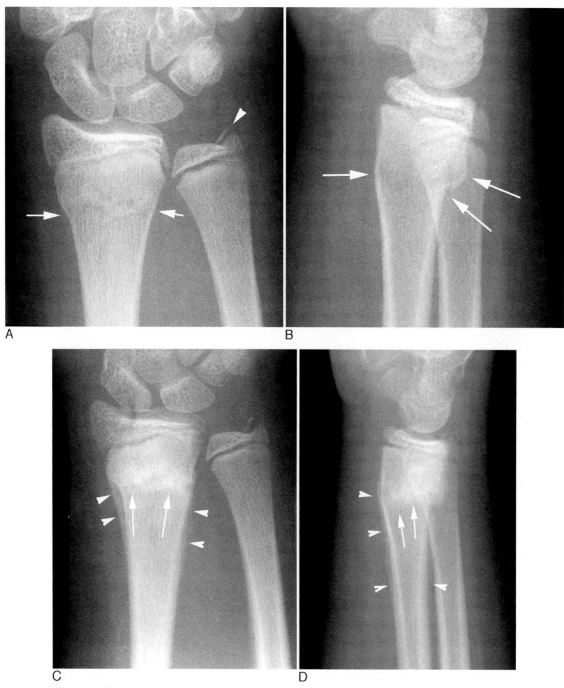

Figure 1-26   Fracture healing in a child. **A and B,** PA (A) and lateral (B) views show an acute distal radius buckle fracture *(arrows)*. Also note the ulnar styloid avulsion (*arrowhead* in part A). **C and D,** Follow-up views obtained 3 weeks later show trabecular healing seen as increased density along the fracture line *(arrows)*. Also note the periosteal new bone formation *(arrowheads)*. The periosteum is loosely adherent to the underlying bone in children, except at the physis, where it is tightly attached. Childhood fractures often result in periosteal elevation due to hematoma associated with the fracture. The elevated periosteum begins to form new bone soon after the fracture.

(Continued)

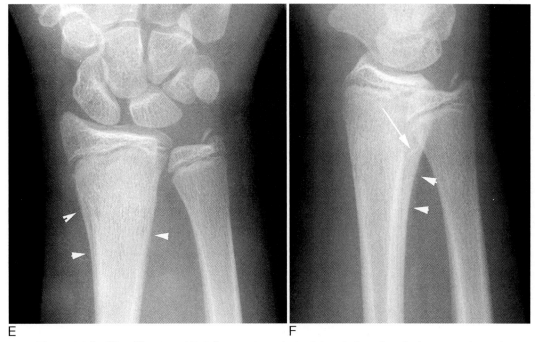

Figure 1-26—(Cont'd)   **E and F,** Follow-up views obtained 5 weeks later show further maturation and remodeling of the periosteal new bone and remodeling of the old fractured cortex (*arrow* in part F). On subsequent radiographs (not shown), the bone remodeled to anatomic alignment with no evidence that the fracture had ever occurred.

The site of the fracture also affects the rate of healing. The tibia normally takes months to heal, in contrast to 6 to 8 weeks in most other bones. The term *delayed union* should be used with caution by a radiologist because it may be incorrectly applied to a fracture that is healing slowly but satisfactorily. *Nonunion,* however, is a radiographic diagnosis in which no evidence of bridging bone is seen (Fig. 1-27). Nonunion may be *hypertrophic,* that is, sclerotic and associated with excessive bone deposition, or *atrophic,* that is, associated with demineralization. Computed tomography can be a useful adjunct to radiography in assessing osseous union (Fig. 1-28). Surgeons sometimes place autologous or donor bone graft, hydroxyapatite paste, pulverized coral, or similar biomaterial around an acute fracture at risk for poor healing, or during surgical treatment of a nonacute fracture that has failed to heal properly. Each of these materials is radiodense. Methacrylate beads or similar material impregnated with antibiotics may be placed around an infected bone and might be confused with bone

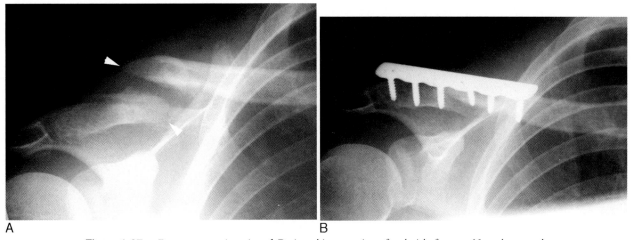

Figure 1-27   Fracture nonunion. **A and B,** Atrophic nonunion of a clavicle fracture. Note the smooth, tapering margins of the fragments (*arrowheads* in part A). Surgical fixation was elected (B).

(Continued)

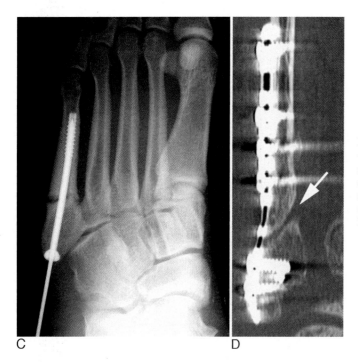

C   D

Figure 1-27—(Cont'd) **C,** Nonunion of fracture of the fifth meta-tarsal proximal shaft. Note the smooth, sclerotic fracture margins. This radiograph also illustrates the technique of placement of a cannulated lag screw. The guide pin is placed under fluoroscopic observation, then the screw is placed over the pin. Because only the tip of the screw is threaded ("lag" screw), tightening the screw compresses the fragments together. **D,** Nonunion in an internally fixed distal fibular fracture *(arrow).*

augmentation biomaterials on a radiograph. These beads are usually much larger and are typically used after infected hardware is removed (Fig. 1-29).

Key Concepts	Delayed Union Versus Nonunion

Delayed union is a clinical diagnosis, with time to union affected by any number of issues that are not evident on the radiograph. These may include:
  Nutritional status
  Alcohol use
  Steroids
  Smoking
  Patient age
  Metabolic state
  Soft tissue damage
  Devascularization
  Particular bone involved
Nonunion is a radiographic diagnosis, with signs of:
  Absence of bone crossing the fracture
  Sclerosis at the fracture margins
  Rounding of the fracture edges

Malunion is fracture healing with angular or positional deformity. Malunion can result in a limb-length discrepancy or limb deformity that may limit function or cause pain. Not all malunion is equally disabling. The patient is more likely to tolerate some angular deformity if it is in the plane of motion of adjacent joints. For example, anterior angulation of a tibial fracture can be compensated at the knee and ankle. Anterior or posterior angular deformities in children may be corrected over time by the normal remodeling of ongoing bone growth. However, varus or valgus angular deformity in children tends to remodel less well, and rotational deformity very little.

Avascular necrosis occasionally occurs after a fracture and is more common in bones or portions of bones with tenuous blood supply. Examples include the proximal pole of the scaphoid, the talar dome, and the head of the femur. These bones have in common an extensive covering by articular cartilage, which limits the available sites for a blood vessel to enter the bone. If a bone's vascular supply is disrupted by a fracture, the affected bone does not develop the expected finding of demineralization related to hyperemia around the fracture site. The necrotic fragment remains dense while the vascularized surrounding bone becomes osteopenic (Fig 1-30). Although increased density is generally a sign of avascular necrosis, mild sclerosis of the proximal pole of the scaphoid can be a benign finding in a healing scaphoid fracture. Fractures complicated by avascular necrosis may require grafting or surgical removal for treatment. Avascular necrosis is discussed further in Chapter 22.

Key Concepts	Trauma Complications

Delayed union
Nonunion
Malunion
Avascular necrosis (AVN)
Soft tissue injury
Infection (open fracture, open reduction, orthopedic hardware)
Hardware failure
Reflex sympathetic dystrophy (RSD)
Myositis ossificans, heterotopic ossification

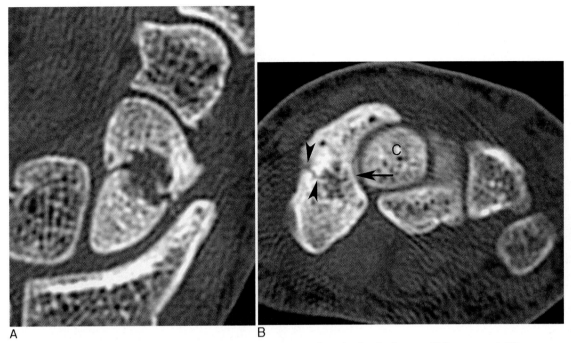

Figure 1-28 CT for assessing fracture union. **A,** Ununited scaphoid waist fracture. Oblique coronal CT reconstruction in a patient who sustained a scaphoid waist fracture 10 weeks previously. No bridging bone was present on this image, nor on any other. **B,** Partial union of a scaphoid waist fracture. Axial CT image in a different patient obtained several weeks after a scaphoid waist fracture shows partial union, with bridging bone along the medial cortex *(arrow)*, but most of the fracture line is still visible *(arrowheads)*. C, capitate.

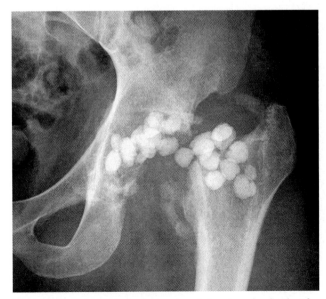

Figure 1-29 Antibiotic-impregnated methyl methacrylate beads. After the patient underwent a total hip arthroplasty, the hardware became infected and was removed. The hip is allowed to "float" during long-term antibiotic therapy before a new arthroplasty is performed. The beads theoretically create high local antibiotic concentration.

Osteomyelitis is a potential complication of an open fracture or orthopedic hardware placement. Open fractures are at especially high risk for infection and should be followed carefully for the development of soft tissue gas or other radiographic signs of osteomyelitis. Osteomyelitis can be related to percutaneous pin placement and is usually manifested radiographically as an area of osteolysis surrounding the pin or tract enlargement on follow-up imaging after removal of a pin (Fig. 1-31). Osteomyelitis is discussed more thoroughly in Chapter 40.

Orthopedic hardware failure can occur in three settings. The first setting occurs with inadequate fracture reduction, which results in undue strain on applied hardware. The second setting is inadequate hardware. The third setting occurs in patients who place excessive loads on their reduced fractures and hardware before the bone can heal (Fig. 1-32). Unless the bone heals, even the strongest hardware may eventually fail.

Reflex sympathetic dystrophy, also known as Sudeck's atrophy, is caused by a poorly understood alteration in the sympathetic nervous system that causes regional hyperemia, pain, osteoporosis, soft tissue trophic changes, and alteration in temperature control. Reflex sympathetic dystrophy is discussed further in Chapter 27.

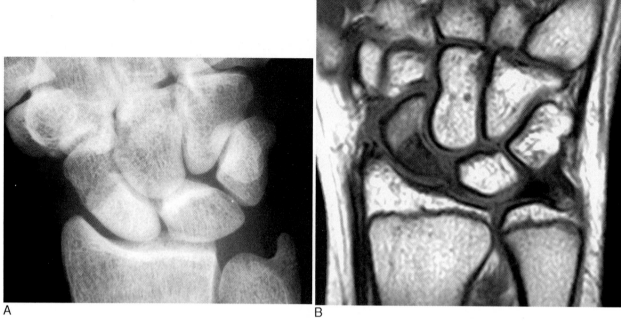

A B

Figure 1-30 Post-traumatic avascular necrosis. **A,** AP wrist radiograph obtained after a nondisplaced scaphoid fracture shows dense proximal pole due to lack of hyperemic healing response. **B,** Coronal T1-weighted MR image in a different patient shows lack of normal fat signal in the proximal pole due to avascular necrosis.

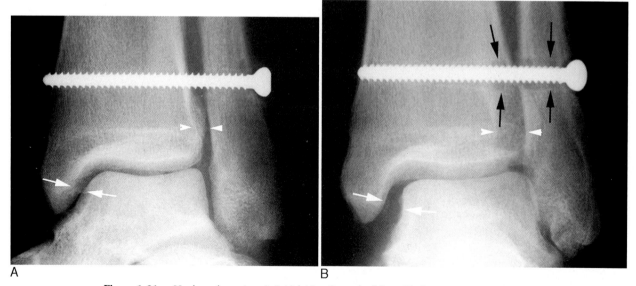

A B

Figure 1-31 Hardware loosening. **A,** Initial AP radiograph of the ankle shows an intact syndesmotic screw fixing a distal tibiofibular diastasis injury. Note the normal alignment of the distal tibiofibular joint *(arrowheads)* and the medial ankle mortise *(arrows)*. **B,** Radiography repeated several weeks later shows bone resorption seen as lucency around the lateral aspect of the screw, especially in the fibula and lateral tibia *(black arrows)*. Note the widening of the distal tibiofibular joint *(arrowheads)* and the medial mortise *(white arrows)*. Infection or mechanical loosening could cause this appearance.

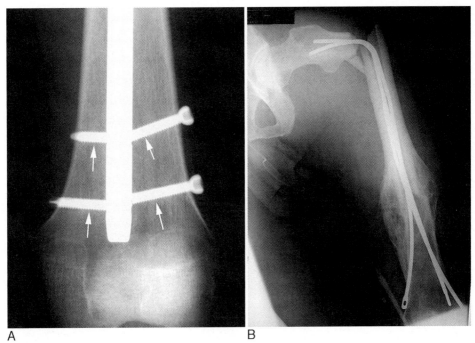

A   B

Figure 1-32   Hardware failure. **A,** AP radiograph in a patient with a femoral shaft fracture that was fixed with an interlocking intramedullary nail. He resumed weight bearing earlier than advised, which placed shearing force on the interlocking screws. The distal screws failed *(arrows)*. **B,** Failed fixation of proximal femur fracture with Steinman pins. Fixation was revised to an intramedullary nail.

Soft tissue injury invariably occurs with a fracture, particularly if there is significant fragment displacement or associated dislocation. Suspected arterial injury is an indication for emergent angiography. Nerve or ligament injury can result in poor limb function despite satisfactory fracture healing. Additional forms of post-traumatic soft tissue injury are discussed in Chapter 2.

Introduction to Imaging of Musculoskeletal Injury: Joints and Soft Tissues

JOINT AND LIGAMENT BASICS
TENDON BASICS
MUSCLE BASICS
ARTICULAR CARTILAGE BASICS
NERVE BASICS
FOREIGN BODY IMAGING

This chapter provides an overview of imaging findings in normal and injured musculoskeletal soft tissues. Many of the generalizations and specific injuries introduced in this chapter are discussed in greater detail in later chapters.

JOINT AND LIGAMENT BASICS

Joints are the structures that connect adjacent bones. There are three types of joints: synovial, cartilaginous, and fibrous. A *synovial joint,* also termed a diarthrosis, is a freely mobile joint with a wide range of motion. It has hyaline articular cartilage covering the ends of the bones; a flexible, synovium-lined fibrous joint capsule; and stabilizing ligaments. The articular cartilage cushions the bones and allows for nearly frictionless joint motion. The synovium produces synovial fluid that lubricates and nourishes the articular cartilage. Most of the joints of the extremities, the facet joints of the spine, and the inferior portion of the sacroiliac joints are synovial joints. A *cartilaginous joint* is a joint with limited range of motion in which the articulating bones are covered with fibrocartilage. This type of joint has no synovial lining, and is usually invested with a central disc. Examples of cartilaginous articulations are the intervertebral discs of the spine and the symphysis pubis. A *fibrous joint* is the strongest type of joint; it allows almost no motion because it has only fibrous tissue between the bones. The cranial sutures and superior portions of the sacroiliac joints are fibrous joints.

Ligaments are strong, flexible bands or cords of fibrous tissue composed of highly ordered collagen fibers. Ligaments provide joint stability by resisting tension. Most ligaments are

Key Concepts	Joint Alignment Terminology

Valgus: Distal bone is oriented more lateral than normal
Varus: Distal bone is oriented more medial than normal
Subluxation: Partial loss of contract between joint surfaces
Dislocation: Complete loss of contract between joint surfaces
Diastasis: Separation of a normally minimally mobile joint

contiguous with the joint capsule. Notable exceptions include the anterior and posterior cruciate ligaments of the knee, which are located inside the joint capsule (although they are technically extra-articular because they are separated at the joint compartment by synovium). The site of attachment of a ligament (or a tendon) to a bone is an *enthesis. Sharpey's fibers* form the intraosseous root of an enthesis.

Forces applied across a joint may injure or completely disrupt a ligament, or avulse a small bone fragment from the ligamentous attachment (*avulsion fracture,* see Fig. 1-13). A ligamentous injury less severe than complete disruption is a *sprain.* The terminology is imprecise because some authors consider complete ligament tears to be high-grade sprains. Mild sprains show edema on magnetic resonance imaging (MRI), with intact fibers (Fig. 2-1). Partial tears may show some of the ligament fibers to be lax or wavy. Complete ligament tears may show obvious interruption, or edema with laxity of all fibers. An avulsion fracture of a ligament insertion may mimic a complete tear on MR images. Bone edema at the avulsion site is usually minimal, in contrast to the intense and extensive edema associated with bone bruises due to impaction. Careful review of the MR images and radiographs for an avulsion fragment is always a good idea. Knowledge of the sites of ligament attachments to bone can help to distinguish an avulsion fracture from a less important small cortical "chip" fracture. Ligament sprains may be graded according to features on MRI, but the gold standard evaluation is clinical examination, which is based on pain and stability.

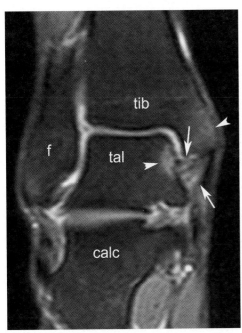

Figure 2-1 Ankle ligament sprain. Coronal fat-suppressed T2-weighted MR image of the right ankle in a 30-year-old woman who sustained an ankle inversion injury shows edema in the deltoid ligament (between *arrows*). Also note bone marrow edema in the medial malleolus and talus at the ligament insertions *(arrowheads)*. calc, calcaneus; f, fibula; tal, talus; tib, tibia.

Sprains are more common than fractures during adolescence through middle age, whereas fractures are more frequent in the very young and the elderly. In these latter groups, the bones are frequently weaker than the ligaments, a characteristic that probably accounts for this distribution.

Subluxation is partial loss of contact between the articular surfaces. Causes of subluxation include acute or chronic ligamentous injury (Fig. 2-2), laxity due to a generalized process such as Ehlers-Danlos syndrome (discussed in Chapter 47), or articular cartilage thinning in the setting of arthritis. *Dislocation* ("luxation") is complete loss of contact between the articular surfaces. *Diastasis* is separation or widening of a slightly mobile joint, such as the acromioclavicular joint or the symphysis pubis. The term "diastasis" is also used to describe gaps between articular surface fragments of an intra-articular fracture. A complete ligament tear or avulsion often occurs with transient joint subluxation or dislocation. Traumatic dislocation and diastasis generally imply the presence of significant ligamentous injury and the potential for chronic joint instability.

Intra-articular bodies can cause joint pain and locking (Fig. 2-3). A common source is displaced articular cartilage fragments and, in the knee, a displaced meniscal fragment. Not all bodies are loose bodies; many intra-articular bodies are fixed to the synovium. The bone portion of an osteochondral fragment or a displaced cartilage fragment that has calcified or has undergone metaplasia and ossified may be seen with radiography or unenhanced computed tomography (CT). Magnetic resonance imaging or CT arthrography is more sensitive for detection of noncalcified bodies.

Impingement is abnormal tissue compression. It is a common reason for a patient's presenting to a sports medicine clinic. The term is most often applied to pathologic compression of soft tissues in or near a joint that has the potential to cause pain and lead to more serious injury. For example, the supraspinatus tendon of the shoulder is vulnerable to impingement between the humeral head and the acromion, especially

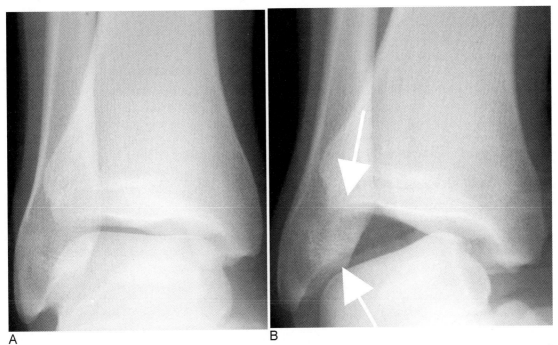

A   B

Figure 2-2 Instability of the ankle related to chronic lateral collateral ligament tears. **A,** Frontal radiograph is normal. **B,** With varus stress applied at the calcaneus, the lateral ankle mortise is substantially widened *(arrows)*.

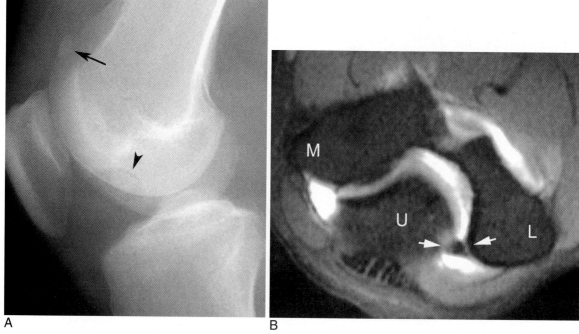

Figure 2-3   Intra-articular loose bodies. **A,** Lateral knee radiograph shows a small bone fragment in the superior joint recess *(arrow).* Also note the donor site of this osteochondritis dissecans fragment on the medial femoral condyle defect *(arrowhead).* **B,** Elbow intra-articular body diagnosed by use of MR arthrography. Axial fat-suppressed T1-weighted MR arthrogram shows a small filling defect *(between arrows)* between the ulna and humerus in the lateral aspect of the olecranon fossa. This body caused pain upon elbow extension and therefore was removed. L, lateral epicondyle; M, medial epicondyle; U, ulna.

during overhead activities such as throwing a ball. Impingement is diagnosed clinically. Imaging studies may not directly demonstrate impingement that occurs transiently during joint motion; instead, we search for associated anatomic features and tissue injury patterns.

A *bursa* is a synovium-lined potential space that allows reduced friction so that adjacent extra-articular tissues such as ligaments or tendons can slide easily past one another or an adjacent bone. *Bursitis* (i.e., inflammation of a bursa) can be due to trauma, calcium salt deposition *(calcific bursitis),* infection, and causes of generalized synovial inflammation such as rheumatoid arthritis. Normal bursae are nearly invisible on imaging studies, but an inflamed bursa is readily apparent because of the presence of fluid and synovial thickening (Fig. 2-4).

Ligaments and tendons can be directly imaged with MRI and, if accessible to a transducer, ultrasonography (US). Ligaments are indirectly imaged with arthrography and stress radiography (see Fig. 2-2). The synovial membrane is not normally visible unless thickened by synovitis (Fig. 2-5). Use of light T2 weighting with an echo time (TE) of about 35 to 45 msec maximizes contrast between joint fluid and synovitis. Because inflamed synovium enhances intensely, T1-weighted images obtained with intravenous injection of gadolinium can also can be used to distinguish synovitis from joint effusion. Bursae are only faintly visible on imaging studies unless dis-

tended by fluid, thickened by synovitis, or surrounded by inflammation (see Fig. 2-4). Calcific tendinitis and calcific bursitis are often well seen on radiographs. The numerous causes of soft tissue calcification are listed in Table 2-1 and are discussed throughout this book.

TENDON BASICS

A tendon connects a muscle to a bone. Tendons are structurally and biomechanically nearly identical to ligaments. Surgeons routinely exploit this similarity by using tendon to replace a damaged ligament.

Normal tendons and ligaments are dark on all MRI sequences because of their highly ordered, anisotropic ultrastructure (Fig. 2-6). As noted in Chapter 1, *anisotropic* means "not the same in either direction." In simple terms, this property allows MR energy to dissipate within a ligament or tendon, markedly diminishing its signal intensity. Thus, intermediate or high signal intensity in a tendon or ligament usually indicates an abnormality. However, there are important exceptions to this general rule. First, some tendons normally have intermediate signal at or near the insertion or origin, or at sites where the tendon normally fans out or merges with other tendons. The tendon fibers at these sites are less anisotropic. An example is the distal quadriceps tendon, which

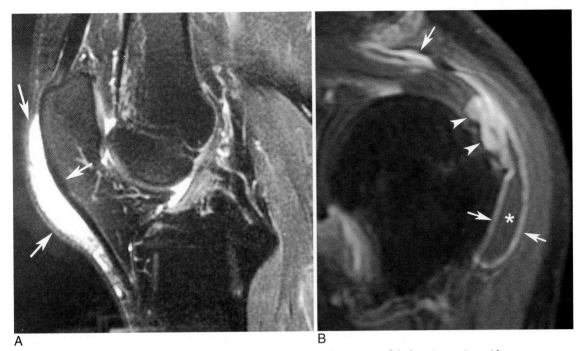

A   B

Figure 2-4   Bursitis. **A,** Sagittal fat-suppressed T2-weighted MR image of the knee in a patient with anterior knee pain and swelling shows fluid distention of the prepatellar bursa *(arrows)*. **B,** Sagittal fat-suppressed T1-weighted MR image with intravenous gadolinium of the left shoulder shows synovial enhancement of subacromial subdeltoid bursa *(arrows)* in this patient with bursitis. The bursal fluid *(asterisk)* does not enhance. Also note enhancement of granulation tissue *(arrowheads)* in a supraspinatus tendon tear.

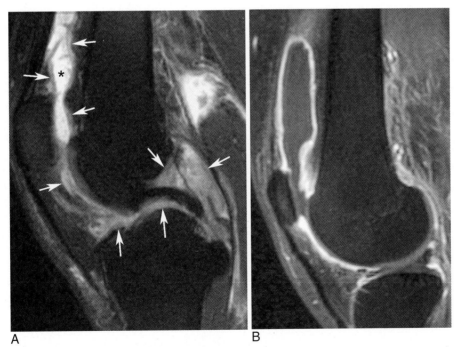

A   B

Figure 2-5   Synovitis. **A,** Sagittal fat-suppressed T2-weighted MR image of the knee in a patient with new onset of inflammatory arthritis shows extensive synovial hypertrophy. The thickened synovium is seen as intermediate signal intensity *(arrows)*, compared to the higher signal intensity of joint fluid *(asterisk)*. **B,** Sagittal fat-suppressed gadolinium enhanced T1-weighted image of the knee in a different patient with a septic knee shows uniform, intense synovial enhancement. The synovitis is not as bulky as in the case shown in part A.

Table 2-1   Soft Tissue Calcification

1. Trauma
   a. Myositis ossificans: Characteristic timing and maturation with peripheral calcification
   b. Burns: Often associated with contractures and acro-osteolysis
   c. Frostbite: Thumb is often spared; acro-osteolysis
   d. Head injury
   e. Paraplegia or quadriplegia: Especially about the hips
2. Tumor: Any soft tissue tumor may have dystrophic calcification
   a. Synovial cell sarcoma
   b. Liposarcoma
   c. Fibrosarcoma/MFH (malignant fibrous histiocytoma)
   d. Soft tissue osteosarcoma
   e. Phleboliths in vascular tumors
3. Collagen vascular diseases
   a. Scleroderma: Usually subcutaneous, with other changes including acro-osteolysis
   b. Dermatomyositis: Sheet-like in muscle or fascial planes, but other calcification patterns are also seen
   c. SLE (systemic lupus erythematosus): Calcification is uncommon, but may occur, especially in lower extremities; consider when AVN (avascular necrosis) is also seen
   d. CREST syndrome: Calcinosis cutis, Raynaud's phenomenon, scleroderma, telangiectasias
   e. Calcinosis cutis
4. Arthritis
   a. CPPD (calcium pyrophosphate deposition) arthropathy: TFCC (triangular fibrocartilage complex), menisci, pubic symphysis, hyaline cartilage
   b. HADD (hydroxyapatite deposition disease): Especially calcific bursitis, tendonitis, juxta-articular
   c. Gout: Tophus is usually juxta-articular
   d. Synovial chondromatosis: Intra-articular
5. Congenital
   a. Tumoral calcinosis: Periarticular
   b. Myositis ossificans progressiva: Usually axial, bridging between bones of the thorax
   c. Pseudohypoparathyroidism, pseudo-pseudohypoparathyroidism
   d. Progeria
   e. Ehlers-Danlos disease
6. Metabolic disorders
   a. Hyperparathyroidism (primary or secondary)
   b. Hypoparathyroidism
   c. Renal dialysis sequela: Periarticular
7. Infectious disorders
   a. Granulomatous: Tuberculosis, brucellosis, coccidioidomycosis
   b. Dystrophic calcification in abscesses
   c. Leprosy: Linear calcification in digital nerves
   d. Cysticercosis: Small calcified oval bodies in muscle
   e. *Echinococcus* infection: Usually liver or bone, but occasionally in soft tissue
8. Drugs
   a. Hypervitaminosis D
   b. Milk-alkali syndrome

Key Concepts   Normal Tendon

Ultrasonography: Echogenic, uniform pattern of parallel fibers
Magnetic resonance imaging: Normally dark on all sequences.
   Exceptions:
1. Specific areas of normal variation, often where tendons fan out or merge.
2. Magic angle. Solution: Evaluate tendons with T2-weighted images.

---

magic angle effect or *phenomenon* (Fig. 2-7). Magic angle effect occurs in the ankle tendons as they curve around the malleoli and in the supraspinatus tendon as it curves over the humeral head. Because magic angle effect occurs only with short-TE sequences, a sequence with a longer TE such as a T2-weighted sequence can be used to avoid this potential pitfall. The sequence need not be heavily T2-weighted. We routinely use a fat-suppressed fast spin-echo T2-weighted sequence with a TE of about 60 msec. This sequence provides excellent visualization of marrow, ligaments, tendons, articular cartilage, and other soft tissues and is not affected by the magic angle phenomenon.

Images on US readily display the parallel tendon fibers of a normal tendon. Tendon echogenicity depends on the angle of the transducer. If the transducer is held exactly perpendicular to a normal tendon, the tendon appears fairly hyperechoic because of specular reflections from the parallel tendon fibers (Fig. 2-8). Inability to induce these specular echoes can indicate tendon abnormality.

Many tendons—notably most tendons of the wrists, hands, feet, and ankles—course within a synovium-lined tendon sheath that allows the tendon to glide without friction within narrow spaces, such as the carpal tunnel, or around bony prominences, such as the malleoli of the ankles. *Tenosynovitis* is inflammation of a tendon sheath (Fig. 2-9). Stenosing tenosynovitis is scarring of the tendon with adhesion to the tendon sheath.

Tendons can be injured by acute or chronic overloading, extrinsic compression such as impingement, tenosynovitis, infection, crystal deposition, and tumors. Tendons have a poor blood supply, so an injured tendon tends to heal poorly. Injured tendon fibers may be replaced by mucoid degeneration or fibrosis, and the tendon may become thicker or thinner. Microscopic injuries accumulate over many years, with associated gradual tendon weakening. Thus, tendon injuries in patients in their 20s and 30s tend to be associated with a high-force acute injury, whereas tendon injuries in older patients often occur after minimal trauma or overuse (Table 2-2).

Tendon abnormality as depicted on imaging studies can be roughly categorized as complete tear, partial tear, tendinosis, subluxation, calcific tendinitis, and tenosynovitis. A completely

has a striated appearance on sagittal images. Second, because of a quirk in MR physics, a normal ligament or tendon will have intermediate or bright signal when oriented 55 degrees relative to the bore of the magnet (β_0) on short-TE sequences such as gradient echo, T1, or proton density. This is known as the

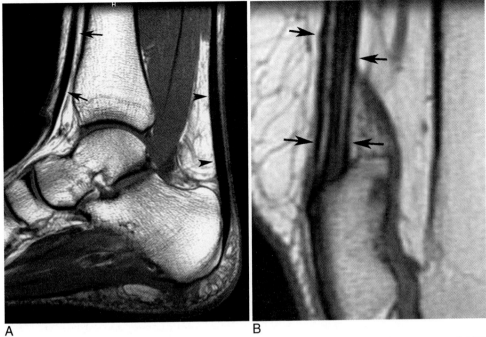

Figure 2-6   Normal tendons on MR imaging. **A,** Normal tendons have low signal intensity on all MRI sequences, with a few specific exceptions. Sagittal T1-weighted MR image of the ankle and hindfoot shows normal Achilles *(arrowheads)* and tibialis anterior *(arrows)* tendons. **B,** As shown in this sagittal T1-weighted MR image, one exception is the distal quadriceps tendon, which is formed from four muscles in three layers *(arrows)*.

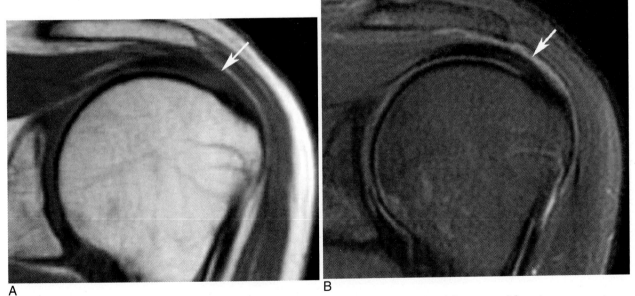

Figure 2-7   Magic angle effect. **A and B,** Oblique coronal T1-weighted (A) and fat-suppressed fast spin-echo T2-weighted (B) (echo time effective, 60 msec) MR images show the normal curved course of the supraspinatus tendon over the humeral head. Images were obtained in a high field magnet with β_0 oriented head to toe. Note increased tendon signal in part A but normal low signal in part B, where the tendon is oriented about 55 degrees away from β_0 *(arrow)*.

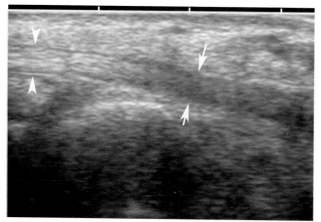

Figure 2-8   Normal tendon on US. Normal flexor hallucis longus tendon in the foot. Note the normal high echogenicity of normal tendon that is perpendicular to the transducer (between *arrowheads*), and lower echogenicity of tendon that is not perpendicular to the transducer (between *arrows*).

interrupted tendon usually has fluid or granulation tissue between the torn fragments that is evident on MRI as a very bright T2 signal, or on US as very low echogenicity (Figs. 2-10, 2-11). Partial tendon tears may be similarly visualized on imaging examinations as a focal defect or tendon thinning, but experience has shown that not all partial tears are readily demonstrated. Some chronic tears are manifest only as tendon thickening or thinning. An *intrasubstance tear* does not extend to a tendon surface. Related terms include *interstitial tear* (a tear that is longitudinally oriented along the course of the ten-

don) and *laminar* or *cleavage tear* (a sheet-like interstitial tear in a flat tendon such as the rotator cuff).

Tendinosis is an umbrella term for chronic tendon tearing and repair. Histologically, there is replacement of normal collagen fibers with mucoid tissue, granulation, or fibrosis, and the tendon may be thinned or thickened. Imaging studies show a thickened or occasionally a thinned tendon, usually with increased but not very bright T1 and T2 signal on MRI, or decreased tendon echogenicity on US (see Fig. 2-11). The term "tendinosis" is deliberately vague because of the overlap in appearance of these varied pathologic states on imaging studies. In general, a thickened tendon results from multiple repetitive microtears and repairs. Tendon signal may be homogeneously diminished signal on T1-weighted and T2-weighted images if repair predominates over injury, or it may be heterogeneous if mucoid degeneration or interstitial tendon tears are present. An abnormally thin tendon is probably partially ruptured and often functionally elongated. Some authors include complete tendon rupture under the term "tendinosis."

Additional forms of tendon abnormality include *subluxation, calcific tendinitis,* and *tenosynovitis.* Many tendons, as they curve around osseous structures at a joint, are held in position by a groove in adjacent bones and an overlying retinaculum. If the bony groove is malformed, or the retinaculum is lax or deficient, the tendon may sublux from its normal position, either transiently or continuously. The tendons most prone to subluxation are the extensor carpi ulnaris at the ulnar styloid, the peroneus longus and brevis at the lateral malleolus, and the tibialis posterior at the medial malleolus (Fig. 2-12). The long head tendon of the biceps may chronically sublux in the setting

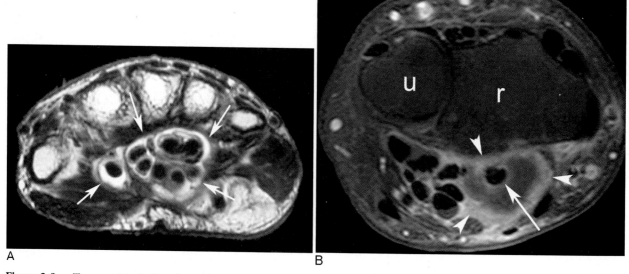

A   **B**

Figure 2-9   Tenosynovitis. **A,** Carpal tunnel tenosynovitis due to overuse. Axial T2-weighted fast spin-echo image shows fluid distention of the carpal tunnel tendon sheaths *(arrows).* **B,** Infectious tenosynovitis. Axial fat-suppressed contrast-enhanced T1-weighted MR image through the distal forearm at the distal radioulnar joint shows distended, enhancing tendon sheath *(arrowheads)* and low-signal-intensity fluid surrounding the flexor pollicis longus tendon *(arrow).* The nonenhancing fluid in the tendon sheath in this case was pus related to *Staphylococcus aureus* infection. r, radius; u, ulna.

Table 2-2   Tendon Injury Patterns

Complete tear:
  MRI
    Tendon interruption visible
    Bright T2 signal (fluid or granulation) fills the gap between torn
      tendon fragments
    Retraction may or may not be present
    Chronic tear: Fatty muscle atrophy
  US
    Tendon interruption visible
    Anechoic or hypoechoic fluid may fill gap between tendon
      fragments
    Fragments move separately
    Retraction may or may not be present
Partial tear: Similar to complete tear, but tendon partially intact
Chronic partial tear: Tendon may be too thick or thin, with normal
  signal
Tendinosis: Spectrum of abnormal findings due to degeneration,
  tendonitis, or partial tears
  Too thick
  Too thin
  Abnormal signal/echogenicity
Tenosynovitis: Increased fluid in tendon sheath
Stenosing tenosynovitis: Difficult to diagnose with imaging studies
  MRI
    Tendon sheath fluid may be in pockets or absent
    Fibrosis may be visible around sheath
  US
    May show fluid pockets, tendon tethering due to fibrosis
Calcific tendinitis:
  Plain radiography: Amorphous calcification
  MRI: Low signal on all sequences
  US: Hyperechoic with shadowing

of a subscapularis tendon tear. Recurrent subluxation may cause tendon degeneration, dysfunction, and pain. *Tendinitis* is a clinical term for a tender, painful tendon. Tendinitis is usually associated with imaging findings in the tendinosis spectrum discussed in the preceding paragraph. *Calcific tendonitis* is a special case. A calcium deposit within a tendon usually has uniform density on radiographs (see Fig. 2-12), has low signal intensity on all MRI sequences, and is hyperechoic with posterior acoustic shadowing on US. Calcific tendonitis is discussed further in Chapter 5, as the rotator cuff is the prototypic site for this condition. *Tenosynovitis,* as noted previously, is inflammation of a tendon sheath. Tenosynovitis is detected on imaging studies by an abnormal amount of fluid within a tendon sheath. Tenosynovitis may result from more generalized synovitis (e.g., rheumatoid arthritis) or may be localized because of tendon degeneration, inflammation, tear, overuse, or tendon sheath trauma or infection. *Stenosing tenosynovitis* is adhesion of the tendon to the tendon sheath. Magnetic resonance imaging may show irregular, low signal fibrosis around the tendon sheath. Ultrasonography can show the fixation of the tendon to the sheath in some cases. Either modality may show tendon sheath fluid loculated in pockets.

MUSCLE BASICS

A skeletal muscle is composed of ordered bundles of muscle fibers and an investing fascial sheath. It attaches to bone by a tendon and is supplied by blood vessels, lymphatics, and nerves. The tendons usually extend far into the muscle belly. Normal muscle has intermediate signal on T1-weighted images and low to intermediate signal intensity on T2-weighted images (Fig. 2-13). Fat may be found between the muscle fibers, especially in obese patients or in chronically injured muscle. Magnetic resonance imaging is the most sensitive modality for evaluating most types of muscle injuries. Inversion recovery or fat-suppressed T2-weighted images may reveal edema, masses, and fluid collections. T1-weighted images may reveal severe fatty infiltration, a finding that indicates chronic and generally irreversible muscle injury, or the high signal intensity of methemoglobin in a subacute hematoma. An older hematoma is likely to contain hemosiderin in macrophages at its margins, which results in marked signal loss on all MRI sequences, especially gradient echo images. Radiography and CT can display intramuscular calcification that can be a subacute or late finding after many types of muscle injury. These modalities also allow assessment of the pattern of calcification, as in the peripheral calcification of myositis ossificans or the streaky, sheet-like pattern of polymyositis.

Key Concepts	Magnetic Resonance Imaging to Evaluate Unknown Muscle Abnormality

Axial T1 is used to assess for fatty infiltration (which
  indicates nonspecific end stage).
Axial "fluid-sensitive" sequence (T2 with fat suppression or
  inversion recovery) is used to assess for edema.
Including both sides for comparison can be helpful.
Use gadolinium enhancement if necrosis or abscess is suspected.
Edema without fatty infiltration indicates good site for biopsy.

Traumatic muscle injury may be produced by an extrinsic force, such as blunt trauma or a knife wound, or by intrinsic force generated by the muscle itself. The classic intrinsic muscle injury is the *muscle strain* (Figs. 2-14, 2-15). A strain begins as microscopic muscle fiber tearing at the musculotendinous junction that is caused by forceful contraction while under load. Strains are most common in muscles that elongate while they contract, such as the hamstrings and the biceps. Sprains may be classified on the basis of MRI findings as mild, moderate, or severe, or as grades 1 to 3 if you prefer numbers. The MR images of a mild (grade 1) muscle strain show edema between the muscle fibers, usually centered along the

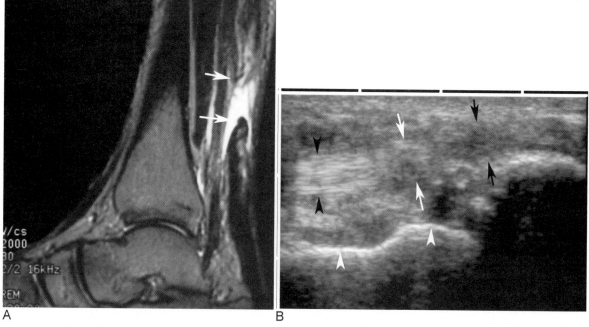

Figure 2-10   Complete tendon tears. **A,** MR image of Achilles tendon rupture. Sagittal T2-weighted spin-echo image shows complete tear at the musculotendinous junction of the Achilles. Note wide, fluid-filled gap due to retraction of the distal muscle fibers *(arrows)*. **B,** Ultrasonogram of complete tear of the posterior tibial tendon in the foot. Note normal tendon proximally *(black arrowheads, at the left side of the image),* but low echogenicity at the torn tendon margin *(white arrows),* and empty tendon sheath more distally *(black arrows).* Also note medial cortex of talus *(white arrowheads).*

musculotendinous junction (see Fig. 2-15). Moderate (grade 2) strains have more extensive edema and fluid collections. Severe (grade 3) strains involve disruption of the musculotendinous junction with loss of muscle function. Both MR and US images reveal the musculotendinous disrup-

tion, as well as fluid collections and extensive regional edema (Table 2-3).

Extrinsic muscle injuries caused by blunt trauma include contusion, intramuscular hematoma, and myositis ossificans.

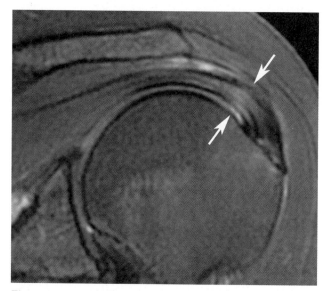

Figure 2-11   Tendinosis. Compare with Fig. 2-7B. Coronal fat-suppressed T2-weighted fast spin-echo MR image shows increased signal intensity in the rotator cuff (between *arrows*). This is an example of mild tendinosis. More severe cases might show tendon thickening or thinning.

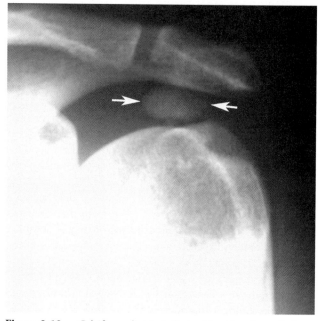

Figure 2-12   Calcific tendinitis. Left shoulder AP radiograph shows typical uniform calcification *(arrows)* of calcific tendonitis of the rotator cuff.

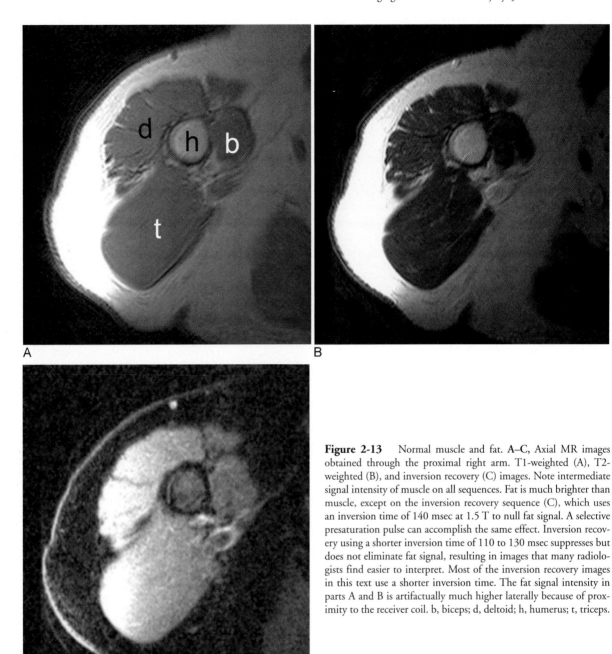

Figure 2-13 Normal muscle and fat. **A–C,** Axial MR images obtained through the proximal right arm. T1-weighted (A), T2-weighted (B), and inversion recovery (C) images. Note intermediate signal intensity of muscle on all sequences. Fat is much brighter than muscle, except on the inversion recovery sequence (C), which uses an inversion time of 140 msec at 1.5 T to null fat signal. A selective presaturation pulse can accomplish the same effect. Inversion recovery using a shorter inversion time of 110 to 130 msec suppresses but does not eliminate fat signal, resulting in images that many radiologists find easier to interpret. Most of the inversion recovery images in this text use a shorter inversion time. The fat signal intensity in parts A and B is artifactually much higher laterally because of proximity to the receiver coil. b, biceps; d, deltoid; h, humerus; t, triceps.

A muscle contusion produces intramuscular edema and small fluid collections, usually centered at the site of injury. An intramuscular hematoma may contain a fluid-fluid level and have high signal on T1-weighted images because of the presence of methemoglobin (Fig. 2-16). An older hematoma may have a low signal intensity rim resulting from the presence of hemosiderin.

Myositis ossificans is a poorly understood potential complication of blunt muscle trauma (Fig. 2-17). It consists of immature granulation tissue that may ossify after several weeks. Early myositis ossificans presents as a mass-like intramuscular lesion that can be confused at imaging and at biopsy with an aggressive sarcoma. There may be adjacent periosteal reaction, but no bone destruction is seen. After about 8 weeks, initially amorphous soft tissue calcification evolves into characteristic maturing *peripheral* ossification that reveals the true, benign nature of this process. Over weeks to months, the new bone may resolve or diminish, migrate toward and ultimately merge with the adjacent bone, or remain unchanged. Careful evaluation, including patient history, may mitigate potentially confusing biopsy findings. Myositis ossificans is discussed in greater detail in Chapter 37.

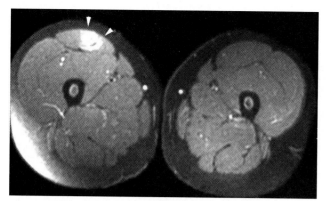

Figure 2-14 Muscle strain. Axial fat-suppressed T2-weighted MR image shows high signal intensity along the musculotendinous junction of the right rectus femoris muscle *(arrowheads).* (Reprinted with permission from May DA, Disler DG, Jones EA, et al: Abnormal signal within skeletal muscle in magnetic resonance imaging: Patterns, pearls, and pitfalls. Radiographics 20:S295–S315, 2000.)

Heterotopic ossification is *any* extraskeletal ossification, including myositis ossificans. Heterotopic ossification is especially common around the hip joint after hip arthroplasty or placement of an intramedullary nail in the femur (Fig. 2-18). The heterotopic bone can limit the range of motion of an adjacent joint, and in extreme cases effectively fuse the joint. Heterotopic ossification can also occur when joint motion is profoundly reduced, as for example in patients paralyzed by a spinal cord injury.

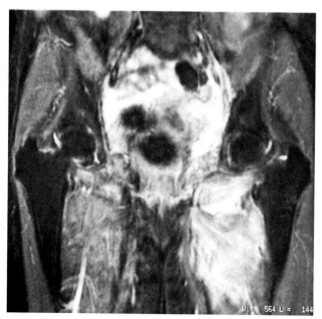

Figure 2-15 Muscle strain in elderly patient who fell. Coronal inversion recovery MR image shows high signal intensity *(arrows)* in the left hip adductors. (Reprinted with permission from May DA, Disler DG, Jones EA, et al: Abnormal signal within skeletal muscle in magnetic resonance imaging: Patterns, pearls, and pitfalls. Radiographics 20:S295–S315, 2000.)

Table 2-3 Muscle Injury Patterns
Localized fluid collection:
At musculotendinous junction: Strain
Anywhere:
Hematoma
Abscess
Myonecrosis
Myonecrosis causes:
Severe trauma
Compartment syndrome
Infection
Autoimmune disorders
Diabetes mellitus
Edema without fluid collection:
Diffuse:
Overuse (delayed-onset muscle soreness [DOMS])
Subacute denervation (after 2 to 4 weeks)
Radiation therapy
Focal:
At musculotendinous junction:
Strain
Anywhere:
Trauma
Early myonecrosis
Infection without abscess
Tumor
Atrophy with fatty infiltration:
Paralysis, chronic denervation
Chronic tendon tear
End-stage autoimmune disease
Muscular dystrophy
Chronic corticosteroid use
Muscle calcification:
Mass with peripheral calcification: Myositis ossificans
Sheet-like: Autoimmune disorder
Small nodules: Parasites
Tumors: Various patterns

Muscle deprived of normal innervation undergoes degeneration and atrophy. Magnetic resonance imaging is highly sensitive to muscle injury due to denervation and can provide prognostic information (Figs. 2-19, 2-20). During the first 2 to 4 weeks after denervation, muscle signal is normal. After about 2 to 4 weeks, the denervated muscle becomes diffusely edematous, with high signal on inversion recovery and fat-suppressed T2-weighted images. If normal innervation is restored within a few weeks, the muscle returns to normal both clinically and on MR images. However, denervation that persists for several weeks to months results in irreversible muscle wasting, manifesting as fatty atrophy. T1-weighted images show markedly decreased muscle bulk with increased signal intensity. A chronic complete tendon tear results in a similar appearance on MR images and may also show muscle and tendon retraction. Long-term high-dose corticosteroid use can cause fatty atrophy, especially of trunk and proximal extremity muscles.

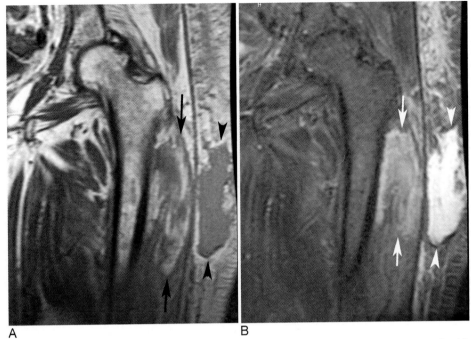

Figure 2-16   Intramuscular contusion and hematoma. **A and B**, MR images in elderly patient who fell. Coronal T1-weighted (A) and inversion recovery (B) images show hematomas in the vastus lateralis *(arrows)* and subcutaneous fat *(arrowheads)*. Note the complex signal intensity in the intramuscular hematoma *(arrows)*, with areas of very high signal intensity in part A due to methemoglobin.

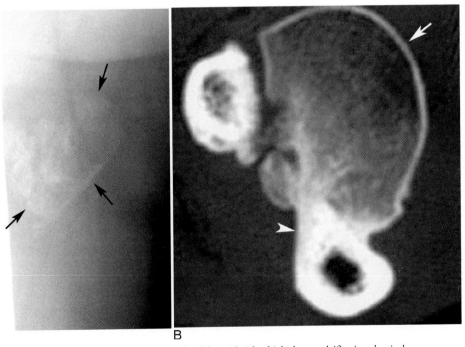

Figure 2-17   Myositis ossificans. **A**, AP radiograph of the mid-right thigh shows calcification that is densest at the periphery *(arrows)*. **B**, Axial CT image in a different patient with myositis ossificans in the forearm shows mature ossification with cortex and trabeculae *(arrow)* that is fusing with the ulna *(arrowheads)*. (Part A reprinted with permission from May DA, Disler DG, Jones EA, et al: Abnormal signal within skeletal muscle in magnetic resonance imaging: Patterns, pearls, and pitfalls. Radiographics 20:S295–S315, 2000. Part B courtesy of William Pommersheim, MD.)

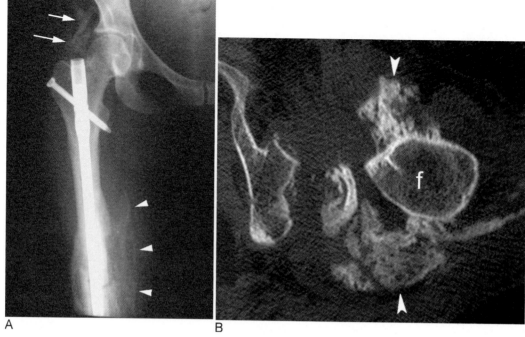

Figure 2-18 Post-traumatic heterotopic ossification. **A,** AP radiograph of the right thigh and hip shows mature bone above the femoral neck *(arrows)* and medial thigh *(arrowheads)*. **B,** Heterotopic ossification *(arrowheads)* surrounding chronically dislocated left hip. f, proximal femur.

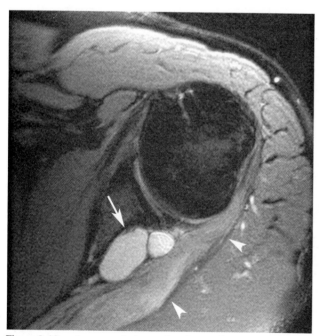

Figure 2-19 Acute muscle denervation. Acute infraspinatus denervation caused by nerve compression. Axial fat-suppressed T2-weighted MR image shows diffusely increased signal intensity in the infraspinatus muscle *(arrowheads)* caused by compression of the suprascapular nerve in the scapular spinoglenoid notch by a large paralabral cyst *(arrow)*. T1-weighted images (not shown) showed no fatty infiltration, indicating that the muscle injury is reversible.

Degenerative neuromuscular conditions (e.g., muscular dystrophy) and autoimmune inflammatory conditions (e.g., dermatomyositis or polymyositis) may also progress from edema during the active phase of the disease to end-stage irreversible fatty atrophy. These processes may be patchy or irregular in distribution. Magnetic resonance imaging is useful in guiding a biopsy when these conditions are suspected because an optimal biopsy site should not show nonspecific end-stage fatty atrophy but rather edema related to active inflammatory cell infiltration. Late-stage dermatomyositis or polymyositis may show streaky or sheet-like calcifications. These conditions are illustrated and discussed further in Chapter 20.

Muscle infection may cause diffuse or focal edema. Infectious myositis due to pyogenic organisms can result in formation of an intramuscular abscess (Fig. 2-21). This condition is well known in the tropics but also occurs in temperate climates. Patients with immune dysfunction are the most vulnerable. An intramuscular abscess is similar in appearance to an abscess elsewhere in the body, with central fluid surrounded by an enhancing margin. Intramuscular gas bubbles suggest infection with a highly aggressive organism such as a *Clostridium* species; this condition is a surgical emergency requiring prompt debridement.

Diabetic myonecrosis is an incompletely understood condition that resembles severe infectious myositis, with a complex

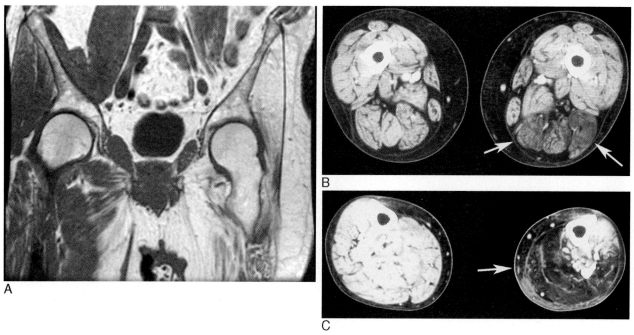

Figure 2-20   Chronic muscle denervation. **A,** Coronal T1-weighted MR image in an adult who had polio as a child shows profound fatty atrophy of left pelvic and thigh musculature. **B and C,** Sciatic nerve injury. Axial CT images in the thighs (B) and calves (C) show fatty atrophy *(arrows)* of the hamstrings in part B and ankle flexors in part C. Fatty atrophy indicates irreversible muscle injury

appearance on imaging studies (Fig. 2-22). However, diabetic myonecrosis is not due to infection and does not require aspiration, antibiotics, or surgical drainage. This condition is extremely painful. Additional clues to the diagnosis are a history of poorly controlled diabetes mellitus and a normal or near-normal leukocyte count.

Radiation therapy produces long-lasting soft tissue edema throughout the radiation field. Magnetic resonance images often show a sharp, straight margin between the edematous radiated tissue and the normal adjacent tissue (Fig. 2-23). This finding helps to distinguish incidental radiation therapy–induced edema from other causes of muscle and soft tissue edema.

Muscles of the leg and volar forearm are invested in indistensible superficial fascia and hence are vulnerable to *acute compartment syndrome*. Fracture, blunt or sharp trauma, or a surgical procedure can cause muscle swelling or hemorrhage that leads to a vicious cycle of increasing intracompartmental pressure, ischemia, more edema and swelling, further increased pressure, and ultimately tissue necrosis. If undetected, the compartment contents atrophy and scar, with contracture

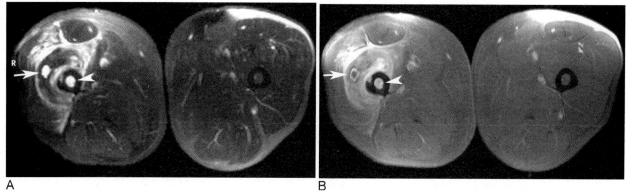

Figure 2-21   Infectious myositis, intramuscular abscess, and osteomyelitis. **A and B,** Axial fat-suppressed T2-weighted (A) and contrast-enhanced fat-suppressed T1-weighted (B) MR images show small abscess in the right vastus intermedius *(arrow)* with surrounding muscle edema and enhancement, and femur midshaft marrow edema and enhancement *(arrowheads)* due to *Staphylococcus aureus* infection. (Reprinted with permission from May DA, Disler DG, Jones EA, et al: Abnormal signal within skeletal muscle in magnetic resonance imaging: Patterns, pearls, and pitfalls. Radiographics 20:S295–S315, 2000.)

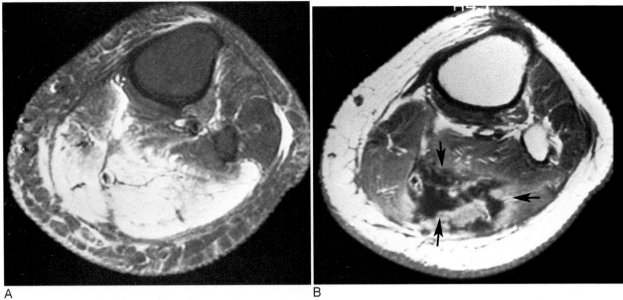

A   B

Figure 2-22   Diabetic myonecrosis. **A and B,** Axial fat-suppressed T2-weighted (A) and contrast-enhanced T1-weighted (B) MR images show intense edema in the left soleus in part A and heterogeneous enhancement and an irregularly shaped muscle infarct (*arrows* in part B). (Reprinted with permission from May DA, Disler DG, Jones EA, et al: Abnormal signal within skeletal muscle in magnetic resonance imaging: Patterns, pearls, and pitfalls. Radiographics 20:S295–S315, 2000.)

and irreversible complete loss of function. Early detection is imperative to avoid this devastating outcome. Acute compartment syndrome is treated by decompression with fasciotomy. When acute compartment syndrome is suspected, direct measurement of intracompartmental pressure is the appropriate test. This should not be delayed to perform MRI or other imaging study. A tight cast can contribute to a similar syndrome. The treatment for cast-related compression symptoms is usually simple: the cast is revised or simply divided longitudinally into two pieces ("bivalve" cast, like a clam's shell) and

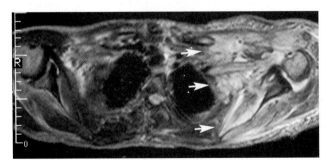

Figure 2-23   Radiation therapy. Axial T2-weighted MR image of the upper chest in a patient previously treated with radiation therapy to the left shoulder and axilla region shows diffuse edema in the radiated soft tissues. Note sharp, straight margin between the radiated and normal tissues *(arrows)*. (Reprinted with permission from May DA, Disler DG, Jones EA, et al: Abnormal signal within skeletal muscle in magnetic resonance imaging: Patterns, pearls, and pitfalls. Radiographics 20:S295–S315, 2000.)

wrapped with elastic wrap. This allows the soft tissues to swell without necessitating replacement of the cast. *Exertional compartment syndrome* is an intermittent form of compartment syndrome, with reproducible pain during exercise. This condition can be detected with MRI. The symptomatic extremity can be scanned during or immediately after the offending activity. Muscle edema, often subtle, develops in the affected muscle.

A *myofascial defect* presents as a bump or protrusion along the surface of a muscle, often in the calf. The bump is caused by muscle bulging through a defect in the muscle fascia (Fig. 2-24). These defects are often incidental but may cause concern for a neoplasm, and in some cases are symptomatic during exercise. Because some of these lesions can be reproduced with muscle contraction, US or rapid MRI with the muscle relaxed and contracted may show the muscle bulging through the defect, or may show nothing at all. The absence of a mass and edema are key findings in an incidental myofascial defect.

ARTICULAR CARTILAGE BASICS

The ultrastructure and imaging features of articular cartilage are under intense study as drugs are being developed that can modify joint diseases, and surgical therapies for articular cartilage are becoming more widely used. Articular cartilage is composed of a complex matrix of collagen and large proteo-

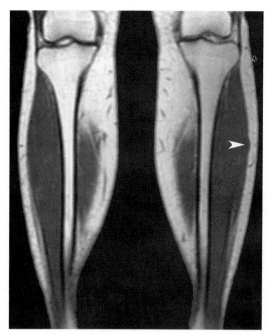

Figure 2-24   Myofascial defect. Coronal T1-weighted MR image in a 20-year-old patient with a palpable lump in the lateral left calf shows subtle lateral muscle protrusion *(arrowhead)*.

glycan molecules, chondrocytes, and water bound by hydrogen bonds (Fig. 2-25). A simplified model of articular cartilage anatomy consists of three layers, distinguished by the orientation of the collagen fibers. In the deepest layer, the collagen fibers are oriented radially, that is, mostly perpendicular to the subchondral bone. In the middle layer, collagen fiber orientation is overall relatively random as the fibers transition from perpendicular to parallel to the cartilage surface. In the most superficial layer, which is very thin, the fibers are generally parallel to the cartilage surface. The result is a tissue that permits a uniform distribution of loads to the subchondral bone, and

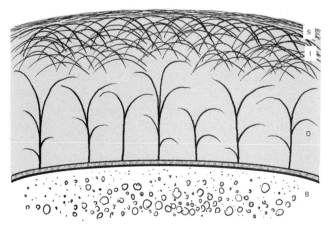

Figure 2-25   Articular cartilage. Diagram shows the predominant orientation of collagen and proteoglycan fibers in the superficial, intermediate, and deep layers. This diagram exaggerates the thickness of the superficial layer, which is actually very thin. B, subchondral bone; D, deep; I, intermediate; S, superficial.

an extremely low coefficient of friction for smooth gliding. Articular cartilage is avascular tissue that relies on the diffusion of nutrients from synovial fluid and, to a lesser extent, the extracellular space of subchondral bone. Thus, joint motion with normal loading nourishes the cartilage by driving in nutrients from the synovial fluid.

Articular cartilage is one of the few tissues of the musculoskeletal system that is incapable of regeneration. Limited repair of tissue occurs only if subchondral bone is breached by injury or by a surgeon to induce a repair response. Surgical techniques are abrasion, microfracture, or drilling of small shallow holes in the exposed subchondral cortical bone. This allows the subchondral blood supply to elicit a cytokine-generated repair response that produces fibrocartilage rather than hyaline cartilage. The eventual response of articular cartilage injury is osteoarthritis. Osteoarthritis is the most common disability in the United States and is associated with enormous direct and indirect costs to society, not only from a treatment standpoint but also from economic loss of productivity.

WHAT THE CLINICIAN WANTS TO KNOW:
ARTICULAR CARTILAGE DEFECTS

Defect size, grade, location
Underlying subchondral bone: edema, sclerosis, cysts
Associated lesions such as synovitis, meniscal tears

Cartilage defects are frequently associated with joint pain. Articular cartilage contains no neural tissue, so the pain must originate from other tissues. Defects in articular cartilage are often associated with joint effusion and synovial inflammatory changes, which can be painful and probably account for much of the pain associated with early osteoarthritis. Damaged cartilage inadequately cushions the subjacent subchondral bone, which may result in painful trabecular microinjury. Over time, the increased stress results in adaptive changes in the subchondral bone, including osteophyte formation and subchondral fibrosis and sclerosis, which may also be painful.

Radiographs have a limited role in assessment of articular cartilage injury. The radiolucent "cartilage space" or "joint space" narrows with gross cartilage loss. By the time such changes are visible on radiographs, cartilage loss is often extensive. Magnetic resonance imaging with optimized sequences can detect and be used to stage articular cartilage defects earlier and with much greater accuracy than can radiography. At the present time, the sequence most commonly used to assess articular cartilage is probably intermediate-weighted fast spin-echo. An optimal TE is about 45 msec. Normal articular cartilage has low to intermediate signal intensity on this sequence (Fig. 2-26). The deep cartilage layer may display slightly lower signal intensity because of its anisotropic ultrastructure. A cartilage defect may be seen as a region of increased signal intensity or decreased cartilage thickness. Fat suppression may accentuate subtle cartilage defects as it increases the dynamic range of signal changes in cartilage. Either MR arthrography

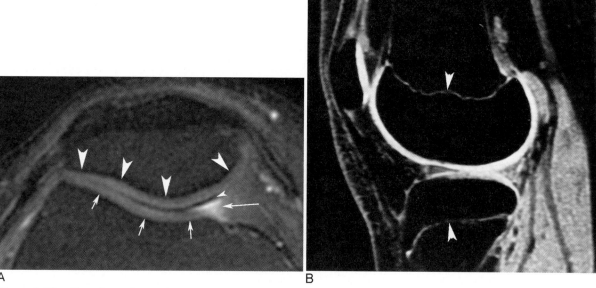

A   B

Figure 2-26   Normal articular cartilage. **A,** Axial fat-suppressed T2-weighted fast spin-echo (echo time, 45 msec) MR image obtained through the patella shows patellar *(large arrowheads)* and femoral trochlea *(short arrows)* cartilage. Careful observation shows slightly higher signal intensity in the intermediate layer (due to lack of anisotropy in this layer). The dark line between the patellar and trochlear cartilage *(small arrowhead)* is due to susceptibility artifact. Contrast the overall intermediate signal intensity of the normal articular cartilage with the high signal intensity of joint fluid *(long arrow)*. Cartilage defects are seen as high signal regions. **B,** Sagittal fat-suppressed three-dimensional spoiled gradient echo MR image (repetition time, 60 msec; echo time, 5 msec; flip angle, 40 degrees) shows normal articular cartilage of the knee. Also note similar, normal signal of distal femoral and proximal tibial growth plates *(arrowheads)*. Hyaline cartilage is bright on this imaging sequence. Cartilage defects are seen as low signal regions.

or CT arthrography can also be used to evaluate articular cartilage, with excellent spatial resolution. Fat-suppressed three-dimensional spoiled gradient echo sequence is used to evaluate articular cartilage because this sequence provides higher spatial resolution than does a fast spin-echo sequence. Normal cartilage is bright on this sequence (see Fig. 2-26). However, in contrast to fast spin-echo sequences, this sequence does not help in assessing other tissues and displays only cartilage morphology. Thus, it is not widely used. Both CT and MR arthrography can depict cartilage surface defects with greater contrast than can T2 fast spin-echo images. Conventional spin-echo MRI sequences do not allow reliable assessment of articular cartilage.

Key Concepts	Articular Cartilage Imaging

Radiographs provide only crude estimate of cartilage loss
Best imaging studies:
   Fast spin-echo intermediate-T2 (normal cartilage has
     intermediate signal)
   Fat-suppressed spoiled three-dimensional gradient echo
     (normal cartilage has bright signal)
   Magnetic resonance imaging or CT arthrography

The current gold standard for articular cartilage assessment is arthroscopy. Arthroscopic evaluation involves a search for visually apparent morphologic defects as well as palpable defects. Articular cartilage is normally smooth, firm, and glistening. The earliest surgically detectable form of cartilage derangement is softness to a metal probe at arthroscopy. More severe defects extend deeper into the cartilage; the most severe is complete cartilage loss with exposed subchondral bone. Magnetic resonance imaging grading of articular cartilage defects is modeled on arthroscopic grading systems and is based on cartilage signal intensity, defect depth, and signal change in the underlying bone (Table 2-4, Figs. 2-27–2-29). There are two popular arthroscopic grading systems, a four-grade system (Outerbridge) and a three-grade system (Noyes). The MRI modification of the four-grade system is probably the most widely used by musculoskeletal radiologists (Table 2-4). A grade 1 defect is most often due to degradation of the articular cartilage surface or microscopic disruption of the cartilage matrix deep to the cartilage surface. In either case, the damaged cartilage may imbibe (literally, "to drink") free water from the joint fluid, resulting in increased T2 signal, or the MRI findings may be normal. Evaluation of grade 2 to 4 defects is based on the depth of the defect, as described previously. Grade 2 defects affect less than 50% thickness of articular cartilage or consist of localized areas of swelling of

Table 2-4 Articular Cartilage Defects

Grade 1: Soft at arthroscopy
  MRI: May be normal, or may show mild increased T2 signal
  MRI or CT arthrography: May show contrast absorption into
    cartilage surface
Grade 2: Defect less than 50% thickness
Grade 3: Defect greater than 50%, less than full thickness
Grade 4: Full thickness, often with underlying bone sclerosis or edema

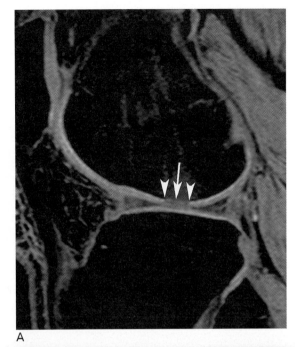
A

articular cartilage. Grade 3 defects affect greater than 50% thickness. Grade 4 defects are full-thickness abnormalities; they often have associated underlying bone sclerosis or fibrosis and edema. Some authors consider any defect with an associated subchondral cyst or edema to be a grade 4 defect, regardless of the apparent depth of the defect on MRI. Some authors have created MRI modifications of the three-grade arthroscopic system by lumping together grades 1 and 2 or

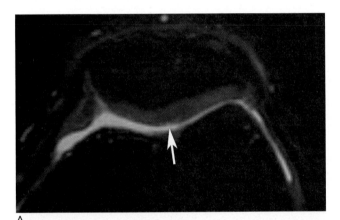
A

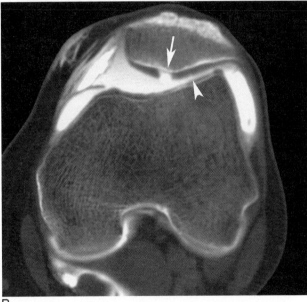
B

Figure 2-28 Articular cartilage defects. **A,** Sagittal fat-suppressed spoiled gradient echo MR image shows grade 4 defect of the lateral femoral condyle *(arrow).* The arrowheads mark the margins of this sharply marginated cartilage defect. **B,** Axial CT arthrogram of the left knee shows grade 4 defect of the medial patellar facet *(arrow).* Also note small, grade 1 defect of the lateral patellar facet *(arrowhead).*

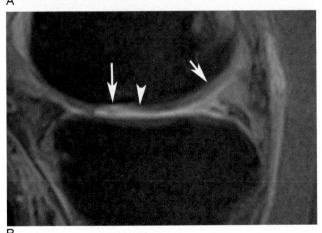
B

Figure 2-27 Articular cartilage defects. **A,** Axial fat-suppressed spin-echo T2-weighted MR image (echo time [TE], 42 msec) shows grade 1 or shallow grade 2 defect of the median ridge of the patella *(arrow).* **B,** Sagittal fat-suppressed fast spin-echo T2-weighted MR image (TE, 60 msec) of the knee shows grade 4 *(long arrow)* and grade 2 *(arrowhead)* defects of the lateral femoral condyle. Contrast with the normal cartilage more posteriorly *(short arrow).*

grades 2 and 3 into a single grade, with a grade 3 being a full-thickness defect in these systems, and grades 1 and 2 being something less.

Additional patterns of cartilage injury include fissure and delamination. A *fissure* is a crack in the cartilage surface of variable depth. *Delamination* is separation of the cartilage from the subchondral bone. Magnetic resonance imaging shows fluid

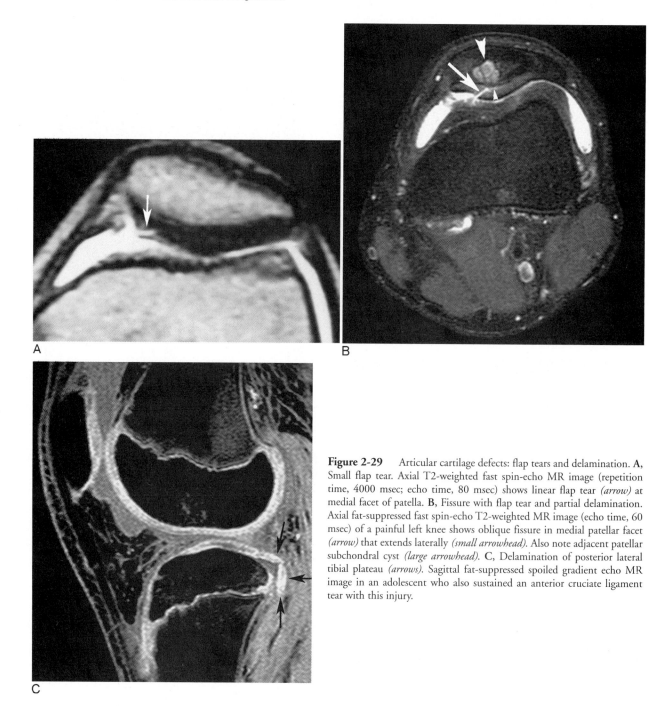

Figure 2-29   Articular cartilage defects: flap tears and delamination. **A,** Small flap tear. Axial T2-weighted fast spin-echo MR image (repetition time, 4000 msec; echo time, 80 msec) shows linear flap tear *(arrow)* at medial facet of patella. **B,** Fissure with flap tear and partial delamination. Axial fat-suppressed fast spin-echo T2-weighted MR image (echo time, 60 msec) of a painful left knee shows oblique fissure in medial patellar facet *(arrow)* that extends laterally *(small arrowhead)*. Also note adjacent patellar subchondral cyst *(large arrowhead)*. **C,** Delamination of posterior lateral tibial plateau *(arrows)*. Sagittal fat-suppressed spoiled gradient echo MR image in an adolescent who also sustained an anterior cruciate ligament tear with this injury.

signal intensity in the defect (see Fig. 2-29). If the delaminated cartilage is partially disrupted, the cartilage may form a *flap tear*. If the cartilage surface is intact, a delamination defect may falsely appear to the surgeon as a comparatively benign grade 1 defect. Delamination injuries are sometimes successfully reattached to the subchondral bone. However, they often eventually break away or are resected when diagnosed, resulting in a grade 4 defect. An *osteochondral* fragment (i.e., a fragment that includes both cartilage and subchondral bone), has a higher likelihood of successful reattachment (Fig. 2-30)

because bone heals to bone better than cartilage. Acute and chronic articular cartilage injuries can be associated with a spectrum of subchondral bone injuries, including osteochondral fracture, marrow edema, and osteochondritis dissecans (see Chapter 3). Magnetic resonance imaging is excellent in evaluating these conditions. *Chondromalacia* literally means "soft cartilage." However, this term has been used so variably that many authors believe is it has lost its usefulness.

Cartilage defects can theoretically be evaluated in any joint. However, lesions can be subtle because of the thinness of artic-

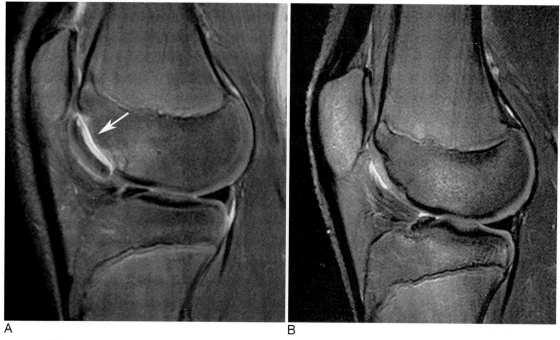

A   B

Figure 2-30 Osteochondral defect with successful repair. **A,** Sagittal fat-suppressed lightly T2-weighted fast spin-echo MR image (echo time, approximately 45 msec) shows detached lateral femoral trochlea osteochondral defect *(arrow)*. **B,** Follow-up MR study performed several months after surgical fragment reattachment shows successful repair, with healing of the bone fragments and smooth articular cartilage contour.

ular cartilage, especially in joints other than the knee. The thickest cartilage is in the knee, up to 5 mm thick in the patella. In contrast, cartilage at the ankle joint, for example, is only about 1.5 mm on each surface. Thus, it is no surprise that MRI has been most successful in evaluation of cartilage defects in the knee.

With the advent of new surgeries aimed at restoring articular surfaces, restoring articular congruence of focal chondral defects may be possible. One such treatment is osteochondral autologous transplantation (also known as OATS, mosaicplasty, or autologous osteochondral transplantation [AOTS]), in which osteochondral plugs from non–weight-bearing parts of the joint are transplanted to the site of a chondral or osteochondral defect. At present, this technique is limited to lesions that are about 2 cm² or less in size, although some surgeons use this approach for larger lesions. An alternative technique for larger defects is to replace the abnormal articular surface with a cadaver osteochondral allograft. These grafts are prone to poor incorporation and immune rejection. Another method of treatment is with autologous chondrocyte implantation, in which cartilage tissue is harvested and chondrocytes from this tissue grown *ex vivo,* after which a second surgery is performed and the new cells are implanted into a site of articular defect under a periosteal flap (Fig. 2-31). A simpler, popular approach to surgical management of high-grade chondral defects is a variety of methods of disruption of exposed subchondral bone with small drill holes, abrasion, or minute local

fractures ("microfracture technique"). As noted previously, these intentional injuries induce fibrocartilage production in the defect. The resulting fibrocartilage repair tissue is inferior to normal articular cartilage but is much better than bare bone. Patients can increase their activity level with less pain.

Acute chondrolysis is the sudden diffuse uniform loss of articular cartilage. This rare condition typically occurs after trauma or surgical intervention, most frequently in the hip joint. Acute chondrolysis may also be seen idiopathically

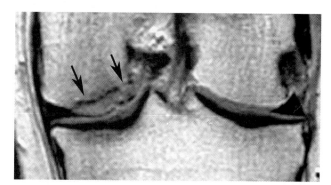

Figure 2-31 Autologous chondrocyte transplantation (ACI). Coronal proton density fast spin-echo MR image shows successful repair of a medial femoral condyle osteochondral defect. Note the intermediate-signal-intensity new cartilage *(arrows)* filling the defect. The mildly irregular and raised articular surface is considered to be an acceptable finding.

among immobilized individuals. The cause for such sudden loss of articular cartilage is unclear. It may relate to changes to cyclic load bearing at the joint because such bearing is essential for diffusion of nutrients across the cartilage tissue. As noted previously, articular cartilage is avascular and depends on joint fluid for its nutrition. Interference with nutrient diffusion will result in cell death. The appearance of acute chondrolysis can be confused with infection, which is identical in uniform, rapid articular cartilage thinning and joint space narrowing.

Chondrocalcinosis is calcification of cartilage. Articular cartilage calcification can be seen in association with crystal deposition arthropathies (in particular calcium pyrophosphate deposition) and hemochromatosis, as well as in elderly persons as a degenerative finding.

NERVE BASICS

The peripheral nerves are composed of bundles of nerve fibers termed *fascicles*. The myelin within the nerve sheaths has imaging features similar to fat. Thus, nerves have lower attenuation than muscle or water on CT images, and greater signal intensity on T1- and T2-weighted MR images without fat suppression. Nerve signal intensity drops considerably on fat-suppressed or inversion recovery MR images. High-resolution MRI and US demonstrate the individual fascicles within a peripheral nerve. Many of the major nerves of the extremities are part of a *neurovascular bundle* of a nerve, artery, and vein.

Peripheral nerves are vulnerable to injury by direct trauma, compression, tension, tumor, autoimmune conditions, infection, radiation, and hereditary neuropathies such as Charcot-Marie-Tooth disease (slow progressive distal peripheral sensomotor neuropathy that classically presents with peroneal weakness and atrophy). Direct trauma can be caused by an external source such as a knife wound, or by a bone fragment following a fracture. For example, the radial nerve of the arm is vulnerable to laceration or displacement by a humeral shaft fracture because it courses along the posterior margin of this bone. Surgeons often choose not to attempt to reduce a humeral fracture to avoid the risk of injuring this nerve while manipulating the fracture fragments. *Peripheral nerve entrapment syndrome* refers to a variety of clinical nerve dysfunction syndromes caused by nerve compression in relatively narrow anatomic spaces (Table 2-5; see Fig. 2-19). The most common example is carpal tunnel syndrome, in which the median nerve is compressed within the carpal tunnel by a mass or mass effect (e.g., tendon sheaths enlarged by rheumatoid arthritis) (Fig. 2-32). Any tumor may displace a nerve, and nerve encasement indicates an aggressive tumor. Careful attention to the status of nerves near a tumor is an essential part of evaluating surgical options for tumor treatment. Nerve and nerve sheath tumors are discussed in Chapter 36. Neuritis may be caused by peripheral nerve infection, notably by viral agents, or immune-mediated inflammation, often following a systemic viral infection.

Table 2-5 Peripheral Nerve Entrapment Syndromes
Median nerve
Wrist: Carpal tunnel syndrome
Causes: Congenitally narrow tunnel, overuse, synovitis (e.g., rheumatoid arthritis), mass, hypothyroidism, fracture, idiopathic
Proximal forearm: Pronator syndrome
Cause: Compression within pronator teres
Distal arm: Ligament of Struthers
Cause: Anatomic variant, avian spur
Radial nerve
Proximal forearm: Posterior interosseous nerve syndrome
Cause: Compression of deep branch within supinator muscle
Mid-arm: Compression or injury by humerus shaft fracture
Axilla: Sleep palsy
Cause: Compression while sleeping on side
Ulnar nerve
Elbow: Cubital tunnel syndrome
Cause: Nerve subluxation, mass, trauma, inflammation
Wrist: Guyon's canal syndrome
Cause: Mass, trauma, inflammation
Axillary nerve
Quadrilateral space syndrome
Cause: Fibrotic bands, mass
Suprascapular nerve
Suprascapular notch syndrome
Cause: Mass or inflammation in spinoglenoid or suprascapular notch
Posterior tibial nerve
Tarsal tunnel syndrome
Cause: Nerve subluxation, mass, trauma, inflammation
Sciatic nerve
Piriformis syndrome
Lateral femoral cutaneous nerve
Meralgia paresthetica
Cause: Compression as nerve courses over inguinal ligament adjacent to anterior superior iliac spine

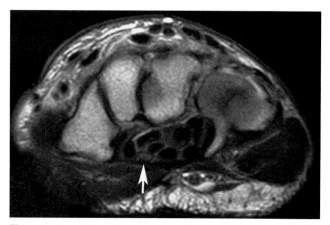

Figure 2-32 Normal nerve. Axial T2-weighted fast spin-echo MR image obtained through the wrist shows the intermediate-signal-intensity median nerve *(arrow)* in the carpal tunnel. Contrast with the low signal of the carpal tunnel tendons.

An injured or inflamed nerve may be associated with edema, enhancement, or swelling. Muscle innervated by an injured motor nerve may show MRI findings of denervation (see Figs. 2-19, 2-20). Electromyelography is generally superior to imaging studies for assessing nerve injury or dysfunction. However, imaging studies can be useful when an intrinsic mass such a neurofibroma or schwannoma or an extrinsic mass that compresses the nerve is suspected to be the cause of nerve dysfunction.

FOREIGN BODY IMAGING

The term "foreign body" includes surgical implants as well as unwanted objects, such as metal or wood splinters, that are usually introduced by direct penetration. Sufficiently radiodense foreign bodies may be detected with radiographs (Fig. 2-33). A skin marker at the penetration site is useful for localization. Ultrasonography is helpful for localization of superficial foreign bodies (Fig. 2-34). The MRI appearance of foreign bodies varies widely depending on their composition. Microscopic metallic fragments are common after arthroscopy, and can be numerous if a drill or burr was used. These small fragments are too small to be seen with radiography or CT. However, they cause susceptibility artifact and local field inhomogeneities that can be conspicuous on MR images, especially on gradient echo images, where they are seen as small areas of low signal

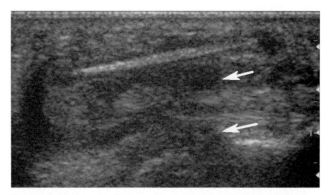

Figure 2-34 Foreign body seen at US. Image of the foot shows an echogenic needle fragment. Note the posterior acoustic shadowing *(arrows)*.

intensity. This artifact can be minimized by using fast spin-echo sequences. Wood splinters are often simply invisible on MR images. When visible, they usually have low signal intensity on all sequences (Fig. 2-35). Foreign bodies may develop a surrounding rim of granulation, sterile fluid, or

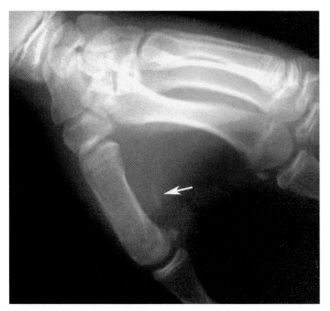

Figure 2-33 Foreign body seen at radiography. Oblique hand radiograph shows a linear foreign body in the soft tissues medial to the thumb *(arrow)*. This was the graphite core of a pencil.

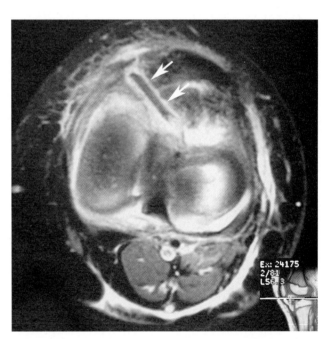

Figure 2-35 Foreign body seen at MR imaging (MRI). Axial T2-weighted MR image of the knee in a child who sustained an anterior left knee puncture wound by a tree branch 2 weeks previously shows a linear low-signal-intensity splinter with surrounding high-signal-intensity granulation tissue *(arrows)* at the level of the knee joint (note the localizer image at the lower right corner of the image). MRI is insensitive to small nonmetallic foreign bodies. However, reaction to the foreign body may include edema and granulation that can be detected with MRI.

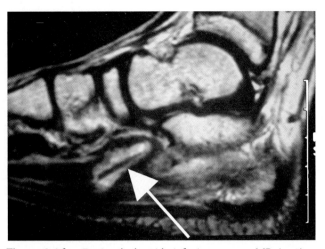

Figure 2-36   Foreign body with infection seen at MR imaging. Sagittal T2-weighted spin-echo MR image of the foot in a child with a clinically evident plantar soft tissue infection demonstrates a long, thin low-signal foreign body surrounded by high signal *(arrow)*. The foreign body proved to be a toothpick that the child was unaware he had stepped on. (Courtesy of Carol Andrews, MD.)

pus with high T2 signal intensity and low echogenicity on US (Fig. 2-36; also see Figs. 2-34, 2-35).

APPENDIX: MRI TECHNIQUES TO MINIMIZE METAL ARTIFACT

Increase receiver bandwidth.
Use fast spin-echo rather than conventional spin-echo.
Do not use gradient echo.
Increase matrix.
Do not use chemical fat suppression.
Orient frequency encoding direction parallel to long axis of the metal object.
Use low field strength magnet.

Note: The amount of metal artifact is greatly influenced by the type of metal alloy. Cobalt chromium steel alloys tend to cause much greater metal artifact than titanium and zirconium oxide alloys.

CHILDHOOD FRACTURES
OSTEOCHONDRITIS DISSECANS
CHILD ABUSE

CHILDHOOD FRACTURES

Children's bones are different from those of adults. First, the biomechanical properties of children's bones are different than those of the adult. As noted in Chapter 1, children's bones can permanently deform without fracturing into separate fragments. This plasticity decreases with age. Consider the analogy of an aging bagel, provided by the late pediatric radiologist Robert Wilkinson, MD. The bones of a newborn are like a fresh bagel, soft and easily bent with only minimal disruption of the outer "cortex." As a child grows, the bones become progressively stronger and stiffer, like a bagel that has been left out on the kitchen counter for a few days. The bagel is stiffer yet can still be bent, but with multiple cracks and circumferential disruption of the outer "cortex." Adult bones are like a bagel that has been left out on the kitchen counter for weeks. The bagel is strong enough to support a stack of cookbooks, but it cannot bend, at least not perceptibly. If enough bending force is applied, the bagel, like an adult bone, will break into separate fragments rather than permanently bend.

A second important difference between the bones of children and adults is that fractures in the growing skeleton have potential for remodeling during later growth (see Fig 1-26). Remodeling potential after a fracture depends on the age of the child (younger is better), the location (metaphyseal is best), and, when present, the orientation of any angular deformity. Angular deformity in the same plane of motion of adjacent joints remodels better than angular deformity perpendicular to the plane of motion of adjacent joints. For example, a tibial shaft fracture with angular deformity in the coronal plane (valgus or varus) tends to remodel less than a fracture with angular deformity in the sagittal plane (apex anterior or posterior). This is unfortunate, as the knee and ankle can partially com-

pensate for angular deformity in the sagittal plane but not in the coronal plane.

Third, the periosteum of children's bones is loosely attached to the underlying bone, except at the physis, where it is very tightly attached. This allows blood, pus, or tumor to accumulate between the cortex and the periosteum, without extension into adjacent soft tissues. The periosteum contributes to bone healing and remodeling. Early new bone that is created by a displaced periosteum can be seen on radiographs as a thin line or arc of calcification roughly parallel to the shaft (see Fig. 1-26D).

A fourth important difference between the bones of children and adults is the presence of a cartilaginous *physis (growth plate, epiphyseal growth plate)* near the ends of the long bones and at the apophyses. The physis contributes to bone growth as part of a process termed *enchondral ossification*. Bone growth and development are discussed in greater detail in Chapter 42, but enchondral ossification is briefly introduced here because it is pertinent to trauma. Enchondral ossification produces new bone in a two-step process: the physis produces a cartilage model, then osteoblasts replace the cartilage with bone. The physis is weaker than adjacent bone in resistance to shearing and torsional forces, but it is not weaker in resistance to compression. Fractures that cross or extend along a physis account for 15% of all pediatric fractures. The percentage is not higher because most pediatric fractures are caused by compression resulting from a fall.

Physeal fractures are classified by the Salter-Harris system (Fig. 3-1). A Salter-Harris I fracture involves only the physis, with displacement of the epiphysis relative to the metaphysis. If the fracture also extends through a portion of the metaphysis, it is classified as Salter-Harris II. This is the most frequent pattern, accounting for about 85% of physeal fractures. Salter-Harris III fractures involve the physis and epiphysis. A Salter-Harris IV fracture extends through the epiphysis, physis, and metaphysis. The rare Salter-Harris V fracture is a compression injury of the physis, which may be missed or confused with a Salter-Harris I fracture. Some authors extend the Salter-

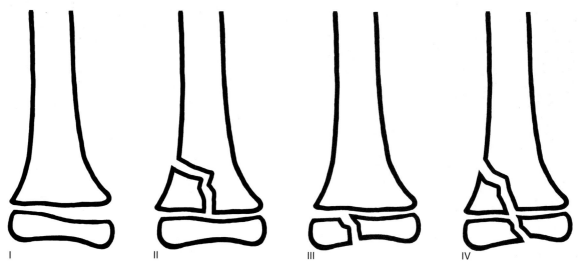

Figure 3-1   Salter-Harris classification system of pediatric fractures that involve the physis. Salter-Harris V is a crush injury of the physis.

Harris system with a variety of pure metaphyseal and epiphyseal injuries because such injuries can interrupt the physeal blood supply and hence indirectly injure the physis. These additional Salter-Harris categories are not widely used.

Physeal fractures are usually first detected on physical examination and radiography. Ultrasonography (US) and magnetic resonance imaging (MRI) can be useful in infants because they provide excellent visualization of the unossified epiphyseal cartilage. Radionuclide bone scanning is hampered by normal intense tracer uptake at the physes. Pinhole imaging and careful comparison with the contralateral side improve the accuracy of bone scintigraphy, but this modality is inferior to MRI and US.

The feared complication of a physeal injury is growth arrest due to formation of a bone bridge across the physis (Figs. 3-2–3-5). The main risk factors for growth arrest are fracture orientation, fracture site, and the child's age. A Salter-Harris IV fracture in which a single fracture line extends longitudinally through the metaphysis and epiphysis, sometimes termed a "vertical fracture," can allow a metaphyseal fragment to abut and heal directly to an epiphyseal fragment with only slight longitudinal displacement. The distal tibia and femur are the most common sites of growth arrest. The physes at these sites have an undulating contour, which allows slight fracture displacement to appose metaphyseal and epiphyseal bone. Other mechanisms of bone bridge formation include traumatic or ischemic injury to the physeal chondrocytes, the latter caused by interruption of the epiphyseal blood supply that nourishes the physeal chondrocytes.

Growth arrest can be trivial in a teenager in whom the physis is about to close but devastating in a younger child with several years of potential growth. Thus, radiographs are obtained frequently after a high-risk injury to assess for fracture healing and evidence of a developing bone bridge with growth disturbance. A bone bridge in the center of the physis will cause growth arrest without an angular deformity but may cause a ball-in-cup appearance. A more peripheral bone bridge results in angular deformity as the uninjured portion of the physis continues to grow (see Fig. 3-5). One must pay close attention to growth recovery lines. The line initiated by the fracture should uniformly separate from the growth plate on subsequent radiographs. If focal physeal tethering is present, the growth recovery line may merge with the bone bridge (see Fig. 3-5). Magnetic resonance imaging can be used to confirm or exclude a bone bridge when this condition is suspected on radiographs. Continuous marrow fat signal across the physis is pathognomonic but not always present. Fat-suppressed three-dimensional (3D) spoiled gradient echo, the same sequence used for articular cartilage imaging, is excellent for detection of a bone bar, which is seen as interruption of the bright signal of the normal physis (see Figs. 3-2, 3-3).

The goal of management of a bone bridge is to prevent the development of deformity. If the damaged physis is close to completion of growth, it can be surgically fused (epiphysiodesis) to prevent development of angulation. In a younger child, physeal growth may be salvaged by resection of the bone bridge with a drill using an oblique approach through the

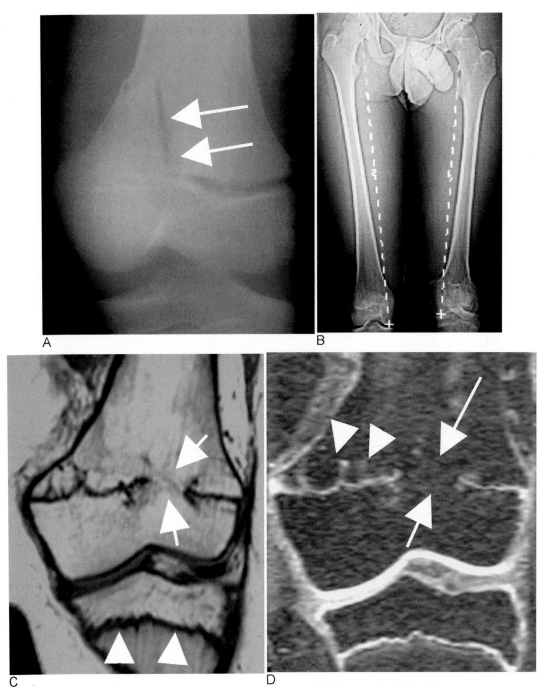

Figure 3-2   Growth plate arrest after distal femur physeal fracture. **A,** Frontal radiograph obtained at the time of injury shows Salter-Harris II fracture of the distal left femur *(arrows)*. **B,** CT scanogram obtained 3 years later demonstrates shortening of left femur, the site of previous fracture. Dashed lines of each femur indicate degree of left-sided shortening. **C,** Coronal T1-weighted MR image shows substantial irregularity of distal femoral physis and focal absence of growth plate *(arrows)*. Note smooth contour of proximal tibial physis *(arrowheads)*. **D,** Coronal fat-suppressed three-dimensional spoiled gradient echo MR image (repetition time, 60 msec; echo time, 5 msec; flip angle, 40 degrees) shows cartilaginous irregularities of medial aspect of distal femoral physis *(arrowheads)* and focal absence of growth plate cartilage *(arrows)*. Note smooth contour of proximal tibial physis. (Part D adapted and reproduced, with permission, from Disler DG: Fat-suppressed three-dimensional spoiled gradient-recalled MR imaging: Assessment of articular and physeal hyaline cartilage. AJR 169:1117–1123, 1997.)

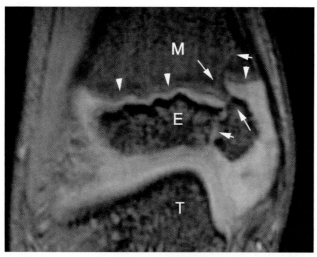

Figure 3-3   Growth arrest after distal tibial physeal injury. Coronal fat-suppressed spoiled gradient echo MR image shows the bony bridge *(long arrows)*, old Salter-Harris IV fracture line *(short arrows)*, and the physis *(arrowheads)*. E, epiphysis; M, metaphysis; T, talus.

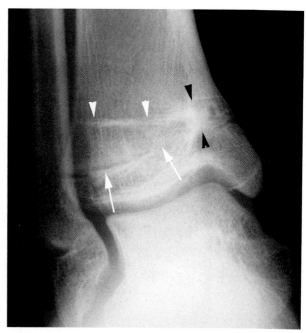

Figure 3-5   Growth deformity after a distal tibial physeal injury. This AP view was obtained several months after a distal tibia fracture that healed with casting. Note the osseous healing across the medial physis, forming a continuous bony bridge between the metaphysis and epiphysis *(black arrowheads)*. Also note the growth recovery line in the distal tibial metaphysis that was formed as a result of the fracture *(white arrowheads)*. Since the fracture, there have been normal growth laterally but absent growth medially due to physeal tethering by the bony bridge. As a result, the growth recovery line is seen to merge with the physis *(white arrows)* at the bony bridge.

metaphysis. Preoperative MRI with fat-suppressed 3D spoiled gradient echo can be helpful in planning this procedure because it allows precise localization of the bridge (see Fig. 3-2, 3-3). For an excellent discussion of MRI for preoperative planning of growth plate injuries, see Ecklund and Jaramillo, 2002. If the bone bridge has replaced more than 50% of the physis, it is unlikely to be successfully salvaged. In this instance, the surgeon may choose to fuse the contralateral physis in an older child to prevent development of leg-length discrepancy. A leg-length discrepancy caused by early closure

of a physis can be salvaged by performing an osteotomy with a leg-lengthening procedure. This is discussed further in Chapter 43.

Growth arrest may also occur after extreme vascular insult, such as disseminated intravascular coagulation (e.g., as may result from meningococcemia) (Fig. 3-6). Limb amputation is a common sequela of meningococcemia, but if the child survives with the limbs intact, growth deformities become apparent over subsequent months. The growth arrest often begins at the central portion of each physis, probably because of greater vulnerability of the blood supply, resulting in a cupped shape of the physes.

The growth plate is also prone to stress injury. This can be considered a chronic Salter-Harris I injury and can be recognized on radiographs by widening and irregularity of the growth plate. These injuries occur as overuse injuries in high-performance child and adolescent athletes. They tend to arise in the distal radius and ulna of gymnasts (Fig. 3-7), the proximal humerus of baseball pitchers, and the lower extremities of runners. These injuries usually resolve with conservative therapy.

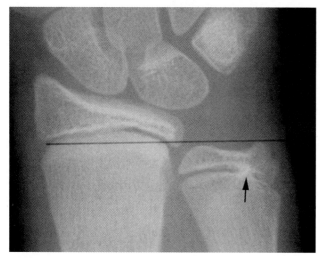

Figure 3-4   Ulnar shortening without other deformity due to a bony bridge *(arrow)*.

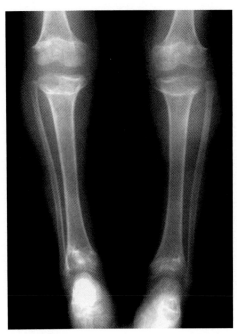

Figure 3-6 Growth arrest after meningococcemia. Radiograph shows irregular, premature fusion of all physes.

OSTEOCHONDRITIS DISSECANS

Osteochondritis dissecans (OCD) is a distinctive type of osteochondral injury that occurs in children and teenagers. The cause is not certain but is most likely a chronic shear stress injury that begins within subchondral bone and extends to the overlying articular cartilage. Patients present with joint pain, swelling, clicking, and locking. Pathologically, OCD is a spectrum disorder ranging from subchondral bone edema to subchondral fractures and fragmentation with displacement of an osteochondral fragment (Figs. 3-8–3-16). The knee is by far the most common site for OCD, especially at the lateral aspect of the medial femoral condyle (mnemonic: LAME, for Lateral Aspect of the Medial femoral [Epi]condyle). Other sites are listed in Table 3-1.

Key Concepts	Osteochondritis Dissecans (OCD)

Distinctive form of osteochondral injury of older children and adolescents
Subchondral stress injury
May heal or result in a fragment that is loose *in situ* or displaced into the joint

The disease process and imaging findings in OCD are probably similar at all sites, but most literature has focused on the knee. The disorder begins as a subchondral trabecular stress

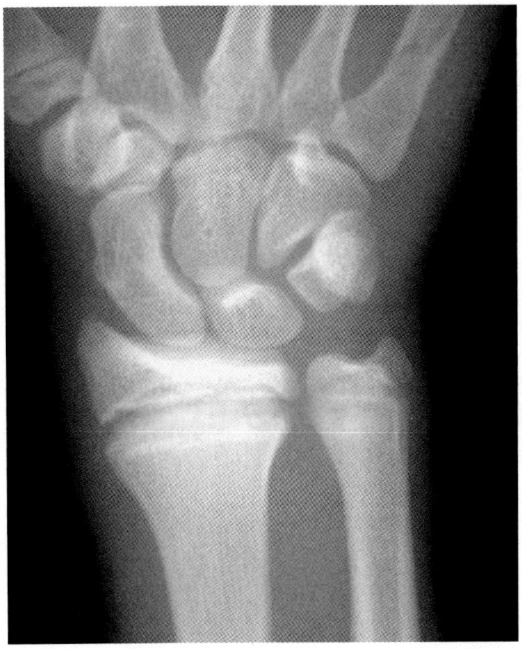

Figure 3-7 Chronic Salter-Harris I injury of the distal radius in a young female gymnast. Note the sclerosis and irregularity around the physis.

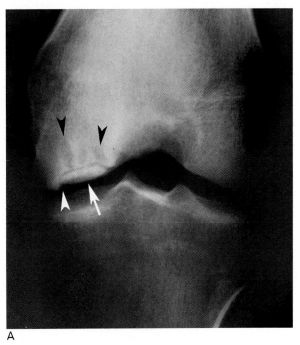

A

Figure 3-8 Osteochondritis dissecans (OCD), knee. **A and B,** Classic radiographic appearance. AP (A) and

(Continued)

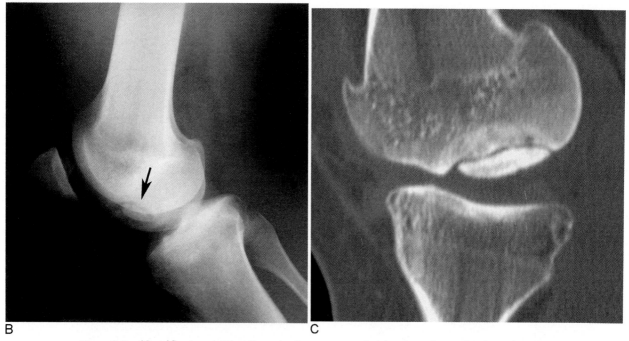

Figure 3-8—(Cont'd) lateral (B) radiographs demonstrate typical location of osteochondritis dissecans along lateral aspect of medial femoral condyle. Note osteochondral fragment *(arrows)* and linear lucency separating fragment from underlying bone. Note also adjacent cyst-like bone lucencies *(black arrowheads* in part A), which suggest instability of bone fragments. Incongruence of osteochondral fragment and underlying bone *(white arrowhead* in part A) also suggests instability of fragment. **C,** Sagittal CT reformat in a different patient shows similar findings, sclerotic OCD fragment separated from the host femur by soft tissue attenuation that could be fluid, granulation tissue, or fibrous or cartilaginous connective tissue.

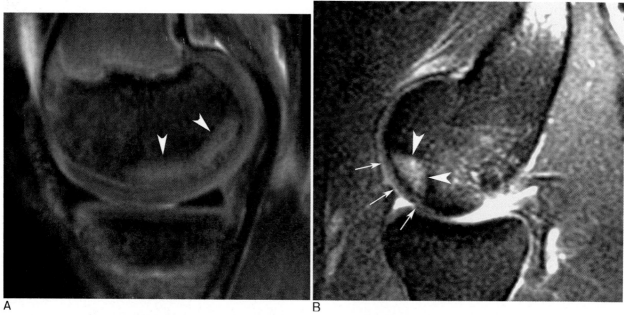

Figure 3-9 Early osteochondritis dissecans (OCD). **A,** Very early OCD. Sagittal fat-suppressed T2-weighted MR image shows subchondral marrow edema in the medial femoral condyle *(arrowheads).* This edema is not specific and may resolve. In this child, painful subchondral fragmentation typical of OCD subsequently developed. **B,** Early OCD of the humeral capitellum (Panner's disease). Sagittal fat-suppressed T1-weighted MR image obtained after administration of intravenous contrast medium and elbow exercise shows enhancement of the OCD lesion *(arrowheads),* which indicates an intact blood supply, with good potential for resolution without further progression. Note the intact overlying cartilage *(small arrows).* This image also illustrates the technique of indirect arthrography, which delivers gadolinium to the joint via diffusion through the synovium.

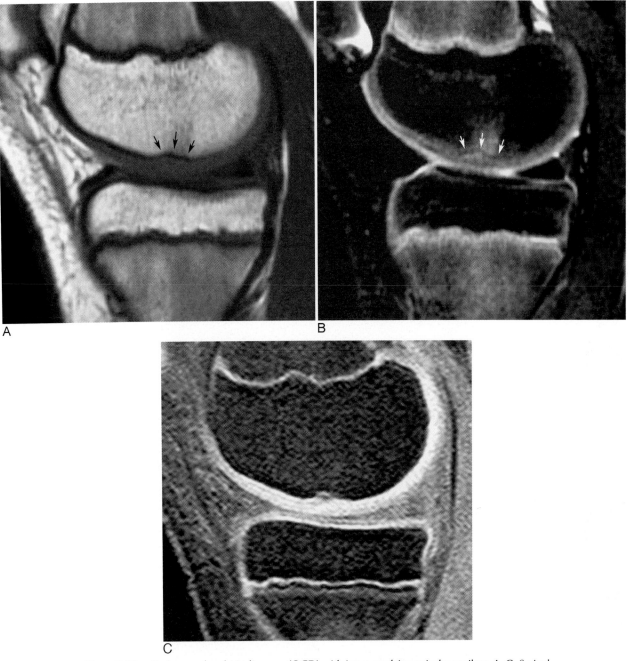

Figure 3-10   Early osteochondritis dissecans (OCD) with intact overlying articular cartilage. **A–C,** Sagittal T1-weighted (A), fat-suppressed T2-weighted (B), and sagittal fat-suppressed spoiled gradient echo MR images show subchondral irregular low signal line *(small arrows)* with adjacent marrow edema. Note intact overlying articular cartilage, best seen in part C, with normal signal intensity. This could be a subchondral impaction fracture as well as early OCD.

reaction with intact overlying articular cartilage. At this stage, MRI shows only subchondral marrow edema (see Fig. 3-9). Contrast enhancement of the fragment in early lesions implies intact blood supply, but the process can still progress. Next, subchondral trabecular microfractures coalesce into a fracture line that is roughly parallel to the subchondral cortex, with intact overlying articular cartilage (see Fig. 3-10). The fracture line can subsequently extend to and through the subchondral cortex, interrupting the blood supply to the osteochondral fragment; however, partially intact cartilage keeps the fragment from displacing away from the epiphysis (see Figs. 3-11, 3-12, 3-15). If OCD reaches this stage, the fragment is now likely to

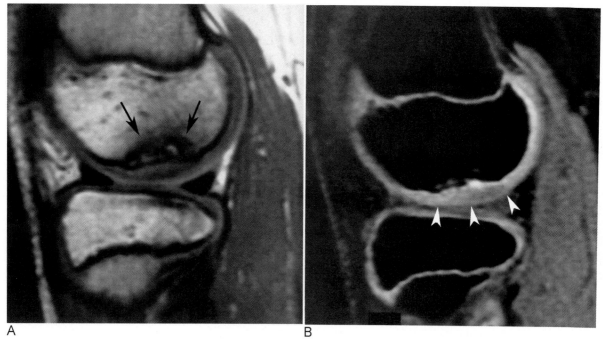

A   B

Figure 3-11   Osteochondritis dissecans with intact overlying articular cartilage. **A and B,** Sagittal T1-weighted (A) and fat-suppressed spoiled gradient echo (B) MR images show the osteochondral fracture lines (*arrows* in part A). Note how the overlying articular cartilage is intact (*arrowheads* in part B).

progress to an *in situ* loose body with complete disruption of overlying articular cartilage (see Figs 3-13, 3-14). The osteochondral fragment may subsequently displace into the joint (see Fig. 3-16).

WHAT THE CLINICIAN WANTS TO KNOW:
OSTEOCHONDRITIS DISSECANS AND
OSTEOCHONDRAL DEFECTS

Lesion size and location
Stable, partially loose or loose *in situ*, or displaced
Condition of overlying cartilage
Fragment osteonecrosis

Table 3-1   Osteochondritis Dissecans: Sites

Knee (most common site):
   Lateral aspect of medial femoral condyle (mnemonic: LAME)
   Less common: patella, any surface of the femoral condyles
Elbow: Distal capitellum
Shoulder: Humeral head
Ankle: Talar dome, most often medial
Useful MRI sequences:
   Sagittal and coronal fat-suppressed T2
   Cartilage-specific fat-suppressed SPGR
     Fat suppressed 3D SPGR (General Electric) or Flash 3D
     (Siemens) with fat suppression or water excitation
   MR arthrography may depict a loose *in situ* lesion better than
     T2-weighted MRI

SPGR, spoiled gradient echo sequence.

The main goal of MRI for OCD is to evaluate the stability of the osteochondral fragment. Fragment enhancement with intravenous injection of contrast medium early in the process suggests better potential for healing, but the signal intensity of the fragment may vary and does not predict the stability of the fragment in more advanced OCD. Rather, it is the findings at the fragment margins that correlate with fragment stability. Linear or cyst-like high T2 signal intensity at the margin of the OCD fragment and the adjacent epiphysis indicates an unstable or potentially unstable fragment. The bright T2 signal may be due to granulation, edematous fibrous tissue, or fluid, but the distinction is not

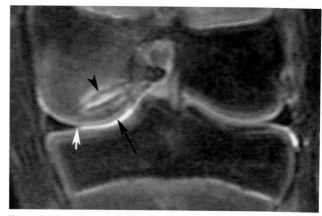

Figure 3-12   Osteochondritis dissecans (OCD). Loose *in situ* fragment medial condyle with partially intact overlying cartilage. Coronal fat-suppressed proton density MR image of the left knee shows medial femoral condyle OCD fragment (*long arrow*), high T2 signal between the fragment and the host femur (*arrowhead*) indicating that the fragment is loose, and intact medial articular cartilage (*short white arrow*).

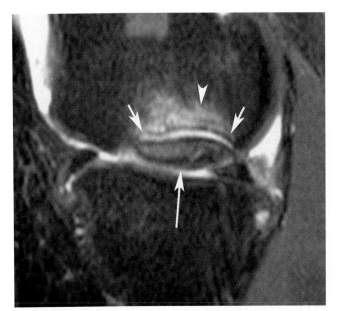

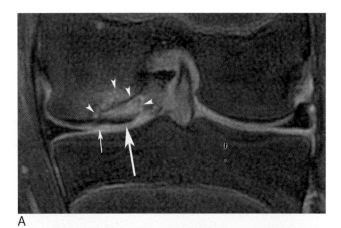

A

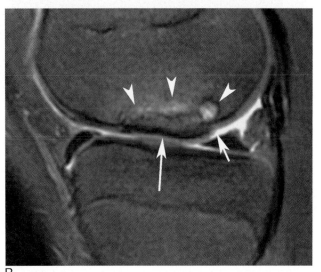

B

Figure 3-13 Osteochondritis dissecans (OCD) with loose *in situ* fragment. Sagittal fat-suppressed T2-weighted MR image shows medial femoral condyle OCD fragment *(long arrow)* with uniform high signal intensity consistent with fluid *(short arrows)* surrounding the fragment. Also note the intense marrow edema in the adjacent femur *(arrowhead)*. Same patient as shown in Figure 3-8C.

important. If most or all of the interface between the OCD fragment and the parent bone has high T2 signal, the lesion is considered to be unstable by MRI and thus at risk for displacement. Extensive edema in the adjacent epiphysis is also concerning. These lesions can be especially challenging for the radiologist if the overlying cartilage is intact because the surgeon sees intact cartilage at arthroscopy and therefore may doubt the severity of the MRI findings. If high signal outlines the entire fragment margin, the fragment is an *in situ* displaceable loose body. The signal intensity of the osseous portion of the OCD fragment varies. It may have normal marrow fat signal (i.e., high T1 signal intensity and low signal on fluid sensitive sequences). Frequently, the fragment is osteonecrotic or densely sclerotic on radiographs, with low T1 signal. Magnetic resonance imaging arthrography or high-resolution CT arthrography is occasionally requested. Joint contrast that surrounds part or all of the fragment indicates an unstable fragment.

Management of OCD is based on the stability of the OCD lesion. Stable lesions are treated with non–weight-bearing and have a good prognosis. Unstable lesions require surgery. Lesions that are partially displaceable at arthroscopy are treated with subchondral pin fixation. Loose *in situ* fragments may be treated with pin fixation if the overlying articular cartilage is largely intact, but usually removal of the fragment with debridement of the crater is required. Management of lesions that are partially loose by MRI but are not displaceable at arthroscopy varies, depending on clinical features and the surgeon's preferences. Newer surgical techniques, such as osteochondral transplant discussed in Chapter 2, may also be applied to OCD, but these techniques are usually reserved for skeletally mature individuals.

Figure 3-14 Osteochondritis dissecans (OCD) with loose *in situ* fragment. The MR imaging findings in a loose fragment are not always as unambiguous as seen in Fig. 3-13. **A and B**, Coronal fat-suppressed proton density (A) and sagittal fat-suppressed T2-weighted (B) MR images of the left knee show medial femoral condyle OCD fragment *(large arrow)*, with surrounding high signal, small cyst-like lesions, and marrow edema at the margin of the fragment and the host bone *(arrowheads)*. Also note the small articular stepoff posteriorly *(short arrows)*. These findings are highly suggestive of a loose fragment, but a fragment that is healing in place could have a similar appearance. Arthroscopy was needed to confirm that this fragment was loose *in situ*.

Normal variation in epiphyseal ossification can overlap the imaging appearance of osteochondritis dissecans (Fig. 3-17). Radiographs frequently show irregularity of the margin of the condylar ossification centers in 3- to 6-year-olds. Magnetic resonance images often show *mildly* greater T2 signal in the unossified growth cartilage in the posterior femoral condyles of younger children. Among 10- to 13-year-olds, fragmentation of the posterior portion of the femoral condyles may be seen as a normal variant. Incidental cases usually are bilaterally symmetric and asymptomatic, with intact overlying cartilage on imaging studies. However, this normal variant occasionally progresses to OCD, especially if the fragmentation is extensive, the joint is painful, and the child maintains a high level of

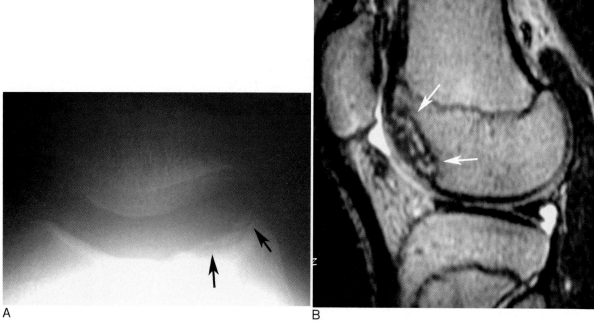

A   B

Figure 3-15   Osteochondritis dissecans (OCD) in the femoral trochlea. MR arthrogram obtained to exclude loose fragment. **A,** Sunrise view of the left knee shows subchondral bone fragmentation of the lateral trochlea *(arrows)*. The usual location of OCD in the knee is demonstrated on the previous figures in this chapter. However, occasionally OCD is found in other locations, either at various sites of the femoral condyles or the patella. **B,** Sagittal T2-weighted spin-echo MR image obtained after intra-articular saline injection shows heterogeneous signal at the OCD fragment margins *(arrows)*; however, there is no separation of the fragments from the underlying bone, and no fluid from the joint extends between the fragments and host bone. These findings are compatible with fragments that are healing in.

activity. In unclear cases, MRI provides the answer by demonstrating normal bone marrow and articular cartilage signal in incidental cases, versus edema and epiphyseal bone and chondral fragmentation in the pathologic variant.

CHILD ABUSE

Knowledge of the radiologic findings in child abuse (inflicted or nonaccidental trauma, battered child syndrome, shaken baby syndrome, trauma X) is essential for any radiologist who interprets pediatric images. This discussion briefly reviews the skeletal findings that are most specific for child abuse. Other organ systems, notably the central nervous system, may also sustain injuries that are fairly specific for child abuse.

Proper radiographic assessment of a possibly abused infant or young child includes a complete set of high-quality radiographs of the entire body (Table 3-2). As recommended by Paul Kleinmann, MD, we prefer to obtain the views of each extremity separately, which results in a total of 19 images. Obtaining these radiographs is time-consuming and requires a highly skilled and diplomatic technologist. In children younger than 2 years of age, a repeat examination after 2 weeks is helpful to detect healing fractures that were originally occult. Bone scintigraphy becomes useful by age 2 years, either as a

primary screening method or as an adjunct to the radiographic series. The examination can be tailored in many older children who can communicate "where it hurts," but some sort of whole-body screening may still be appropriate. Computed tomography may improve detection of subtle rib fractures not visible on chest radiographs, but it requires additional radiation and is not widely used at present. Magnetic resonance imaging can be helpful in detecting marrow and subperiosteal edema. Both MRI and US can detect fractures of unossified epiphyseal cartilage that are not visible on radiographs.

Skeletal findings associated with child abuse have been thoroughly described by Paul Kleinmann, MD, in his textbook *Diagnostic Imaging of Child Abuse* and are summarized

Table 3-2 Radiographic Series for Suspected Child Abuse	
AP skull	AP humeri
Lateral skull	AP forearms
Lateral cervical spine	Oblique hands
AP thorax	AP femora
Lateral thorax	AP tibias
AP pelvis	AP feet
Lateral lumbar spine	

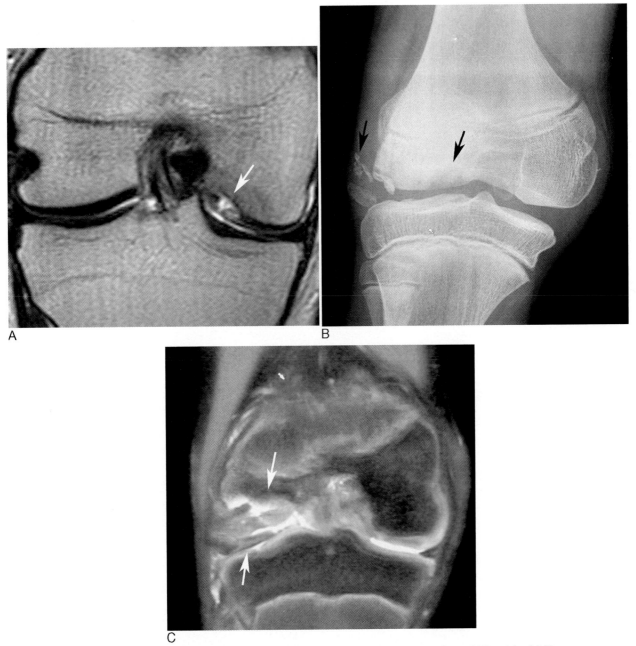

Figure 3-16   Osteochondritis dissecans (OCD) with displaced fragments. **A,** Coronal T2-weighted MR image of the right knee shows fluid filling medial femoral condyle OCD defect *(arrow).* The fragment was displaced into the joint. (Same patient as shown in Fig. 2-3A). **B and C,** AP radiograph (B) and coronal fat-suppressed proton density MR image (C) in a different patient show severe fragmentation of the medial femoral condyle *(arrows).*

in Table 3-3. The *classic metaphyseal lesion* is also known as the metaphyseal corner fracture and the bucket handle fracture. These actually are the same injury, seen from different perspectives (Fig. 3-18A, B). The classic metaphyseal lesion is radiographically similar to a Salter-Harris II fracture, but the transverse component extends through the immature

bone of the distal metaphysis rather than through the cartilaginous physis as in a true Salter-Harris II fracture. The mechanism is a combination of twisting and tension, as can occur when a child is violently shaken or when an extremity is violently pulled and twisted. Fractures around the infant thorax, especially the posterior ribs, result from forceful squeezing of the thorax by adult hands (Fig. 3-18C). Cardiopulmonary resuscitation of infants does not cause posterior rib fractures. Birth injury, often associated with shoulder dystocia or breach vaginal delivery, can cause clavicle and rib fractures and the classic metaphyseal lesion in the extremities. Review of the birth history and clinical follow-up are usually adequate to exclude abuse. Vigorous physical therapy in disabled children or children with rickets can cause fractures, including the classic metaphyseal lesion. Other types of fractures are frequently seen in child abuse, but are less specific (see Table 3-3, Fig. 3-18D).

Radiologists are often asked to date healing fractures. Callus first usually appears within 7 to 14 days but can be seen as early as 4 days. Most other generalizations are not reliably applied to an individual fracture, especially a fracture that has not been treated with immobilization. Therefore, the following should be considered only as vague generalizations. Immature endosteal callus develops along the fracture, resulting in increased density within 10 to 14 days and is maximal at 2 to 3 weeks. The endosteal callus matures and is subsequently removed by remod-

Table 3-3	Specificity of Radiologic Findings for Child Abuse
High specificity	
Classic metaphyseal lesions	
Rib fractures, especially posterior	
Scapular fractures	
Spinous process fractures	
Sternal fractures	
Moderate specificity	
Multiple fractures, especially bilateral	
Fractures of different ages	
Epiphyseal separations	
Vertebral body fractures and subluxations	
Digital fractures	
Complex skull fractures	
Common but low specificity	
Subperiosteal new bone formation	
Clavicular fractures	
Long bone shaft fractures	
Linear skull fractures	

Source: Kleinman P: Diagnostic Imaging of Child Abuse. St. Louis, Mosby, 1998.

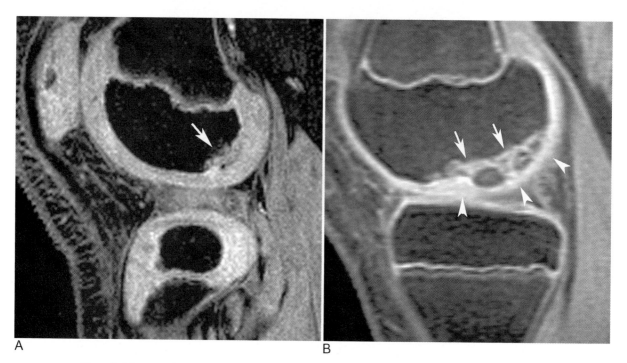

A   B

Figure 3-17 Disorders that mimic osteochondritis dissecans (OCD). Subchondral bone irregularity or fragmentation is a frequent finding in the posterior femoral condyles of children. **A,** Sagittal fat-suppressed spoiled gradient echo MR image shows corresponding finding of subchondral irregularity, with cartilage filling the defect. Note the normal contour of overlying articular cartilage. Also, fluid sensitive sequences showed no marrow edema, which is another clue to a benign process. **B,** More extensive fragmentation *(arrows)* in a different child, in this case with potential to progress to OCD. Note the intact overlying cartilage *(arrowheads)*. Other sequences showed normal marrow signal, and the child had only minimal symptoms. These rather extreme findings resolved with restriction of the child's activities.

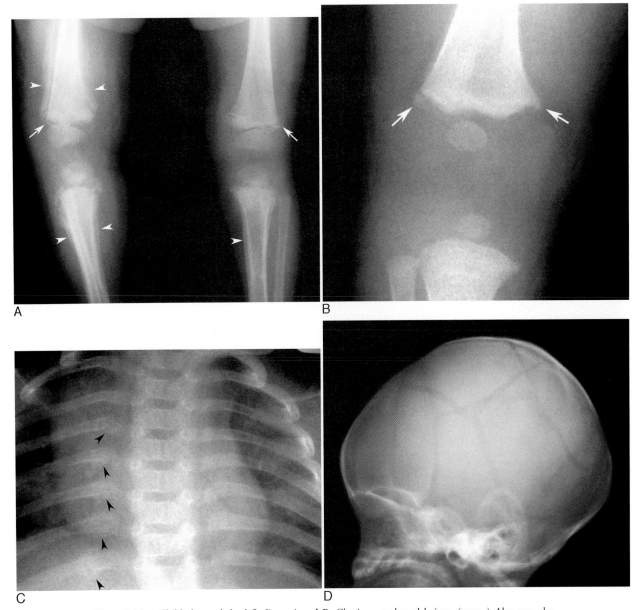

Figure 3-18 Child abuse, skeletal findings. **A and B,** Classic metaphyseal lesions *(arrows)*. Also note the extensive periosteal new bone formation of varying maturity in part A *(arrowheads)*, reflecting fractures of different ages. **C,** Posterior rib fractures. The fracture lines are not visible, but the callus formation indicates their presence *(arrowheads)*. These can be undetectable at the time of injury, illustrating the usefulness of follow-up radiographs. Even on delayed radiographs, subtle fractures of child abuse may remain nearly occult and must be carefully sought. **D,** Multiple skull fractures. This finding is less specific for child abuse than the classic metaphyseal lesion and posterior rib fractures.

eling by 7 to 13 weeks after the fracture. Remodeling of a deformity begins by 3 months and can take up to 2 years. Repeated injury can prolong all of these time periods.

The main differential diagnosis of radiographic evidence of child abuse is osteogenesis imperfecta (OI), discussed in

Chapter 46. Most children with OI have blue sclerae. About 5% have type 4 OI, without blue sclerae. Other exceedingly rare syndromes also may produce findings suggestive of child abuse in the absence of true abuse. Examples of such conditions include Schmid type metaphyseal chondrodysplasia, Langer type spondyloepiphyseal dysplasia, Caffey's disease (discussed in Chapter 46), Menkes syndrome (abnormal copper metabolism leading to weak bones), and congenital indifference to pain. Causes of periosteal elevation in children are numerous (Table 3-4). Congenital infection (e.g., due to syphilis), scurvy, and rickets also may produce features suggestive of child abuse. The clinical and laboratory work-up and follow-up skeletal surveys are usually adequate to diagnose or exclude all of these conditions.

Table 3-4 Periosteal New Bone Formation in Children
Infection/inflammation
Healing fracture
Metabolic (scurvy, hypervitaminosis A and D, Gaucher's disease, others)
Physiologic (during rapid growth)
Solid tumors (often aggressive periosteal reaction)
Leukemia
Premature birth (prostaglandin E, physiologic, metabolic disease of prematurity)
Melorheostosis

Part I Sources and Suggested Readings

Beaman FD, Bancroft LW, Peterson JF, et al: Imaging characteristics of bone graft materials. RadioGraphics 26:373–388, 2006.

Chew FS: Skeletal Radiology: The Bare Bones, ed 2. Baltimore, Williams & Wilkins, 1997.

Chem RK, Cardinal E, eds: Guidelines and Gamuts in Musculoskeletal Ultrasound. New York, Wiley-Liss, 1999.

Ecklund K, Jaramillo D: Patterns of premature physeal arrest: MR imaging of 111 children. AJR 178:967–972, 2002.

Greenspan A: Orthopedic Radiology: A Practical Approach, ed 3. Philadelphia, Lippincott Williams & Wilkins, 2000.

Kleinmann P: Diagnostic Imaging of Child Abuse. St. Louis, Mosby, 1998.

Lonergan GJ, Baker AM, Morey MK, Boos SC: From the archives of the AFIP. Child abuse: Radiologic-pathologic correlation. Radiographics 23:811–845, 2003.

Manaster BJ: Handbook of Skeletal Radiology, ed 2. St. Louis, Mosby, 1997.

Manaster BJ, Johnson T, Narahari U: Imaging of joint cartilage in the athlete. Clin Sports Med. 24:13–38, 2005.

May DA, Disler DG, Jones EA, et al: Abnormal signal within skeletal muscle in magnetic resonance imaging: Patterns, pearls, and pitfalls. Radiographics 20:S295–S315, 2000.

McCarthy EF, Sundaram M: Heterotopic ossification: A review. Skel Radiol 34:609–619, 2005.

Recht MP, Goodwin DW, Winalski CS, White LM: MRI of articular cartilage: Revisiting current status and future directions. AJR 185:899–914, 2005.

Resnick D: Diagnosis of Bone and Joint Disorders, ed 4. Philadelphia, Saunders, 2002.

Resnick D, Kransdorf M: Bone and Joint Imaging, ed 3. Philadelphia, Elsevier/Saunders, 2004.

Rockwood CH, Green DP, Bucholz RW, Heckman JD, eds: Fractures in Adults, ed 4. Philadelphia, Lippincott-Raven, 1996.

Rockwood CH, Wilkins KE, Beaty JH, eds: Fractures in Children, ed 4. Philadelphia, Lippincott-Raven, 1996.

Rogers LF: Radiology of Skeletal Trauma, ed 3. New York, Churchill Livingstone, 2002.

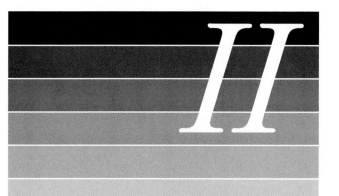

UPPER EXTREMITY AND SPINE

CHAPTER 4

Shoulder 1: Anatomy and Fractures

IMAGING TECHNIQUES

ANATOMY

    Clavicle

    Proximal Humerus and Humeral Shaft

    Scapula

    Sternoclavicular Joint

    Acromioclavicular Joint

    Glenohumeral Joint

    Coracoacromial Arch

    Quadrilateral Space

IMAGING TECHNIQUES

Dozens of radiographic projections of the shoulder have been described. Routine radiographic positions often include anteroposterior (AP) in internal and external rotation, axillary, trans-scapular Y, and Grashey (true AP) views, discussed in this chapter. Radiographs identify dislocations, most fractures, many of the osseous findings associated with rotator cuff impingement, and tell-tale signs of a previous dislocation such as Hill-Sachs and Bankart fractures.

Conventional arthrography allows demonstration of a complete rotator cuff tear and of partial-thickness inferior surface tears. The technique of shoulder arthrography is discussed in Chapter 48. Computed tomography (CT) is useful in characterizing fractures, dislocations, glenoid and humeral head morphology, and soft tissue calcifications such as calcific tendinitis. Computed tomography performed after arthrography (CT arthrography) allows evaluation of the anterior and posterior labrum, joint capsule, most articular cartilage defects, and rotator cuff tears. Use of CT arthrography with the latest-generation multislice scanners, when used with multidirectional reformations, demonstrates the entire labrum in most patients and therefore is a useful alternative to magnetic resonance imaging (MRI).

Ultrasonography (US) can be reliably used to diagnose joint effusions, many rotator cuff tears, and tears and dislocations of the biceps long head tendons. Ultrasonography of the shoulder requires a high degree of operator experience and requires more physician time than does MRI. Many patients prefer US to MRI. Shoulder US is gradually increasing in popularity, although it is not yet widely used.

Magnetic resonance imaging of the shoulder is accomplished in planes parallel to the rotator cuff and parallel to the articular surface of the glenoid, that is, oblique coronal and oblique sagittal planes, respectively, as well as in the axial plane. Sequence selection is largely a matter of personal preference and the capabilities of the available MRI scanner. Every examination should include a long echo time (TE) sequence in the oblique coronal and sagittal planes to assess for abnormal signal within the rotator cuff tendons. We always include a T1-weighted sequence to assess marrow signal and include fat-suppressed T2-weighted fast spin-echo sequences in all three planes to assess rotator cuff signal. As noted in Chapter 2, a moderate TE of 50 to 60 msec is long enough to avoid magic angle effect and also allows assessment of articular cartilage defects. Fat suppression enhances detection of marrow and rotator cuff edema.

Magnetic resonance imaging performed after arthrography (MR arthrography) is the gold standard radiologic examination of the labrum. Depending on whether gadolinium or saline is injected, T1-weighted or T2-weighted imaging is emphasized, respectively. Indirect MR arthrography can be accomplished by intravenous injection of gadolinium, followed by exercise and a delay of 15 to 20 minutes before imaging to allow the gadolinium to diffuse across the synovium into the joint. Indirect arthrography is less invasive than direct arthrography, but is less reliable in delivering contrast into the joint, and does not distend the joint. This limits its usefulness in assessing the joint capsule and glenohumeral ligaments.

ANATOMY

The shoulder girdle is composed of the scapula, the proximal humerus, the lateral clavicle, and related muscles and connective tissues. Joints of the shoulder girdle include the glenohumeral, acromioclavicular, and scapulothoracic joints. The sternoclavicular joint is also included in this discussion. Reference to an anatomy atlas may be helpful as you read this section.

Clavicle

The clavicle is S-shaped, with an anterior convex margin along its medial half. The clavicle articulates with the manubrium medially and with the acromion process of the scapula laterally. The *rhomboid fossa* is a variable, frequently irregular concavity in the undersurface of the medial clavicle above the costal cartilage of the first rib, more common in males (Fig. 4-1). This normal variant should not be mistaken for a lytic or erosive process. In both children and adults, most clavicle fractures are caused by a fall on an outstretched hand, and most fractures occur through the middle third. The fracture fragments are frequently displaced because the sternocleidomastoid muscle pulls the medial fragment superiorly and the weight of the arm, transmitted through the acromioclavicular and coracoclavicular ligaments, pulls the distal fragment inferiorly (Fig. 4-2). In addition, the muscles that attach the shoulder to the chest wall, such as the pectoralis major and latissimus dorsi, often medially displace the distal fragment, causing the fragments to override. Despite

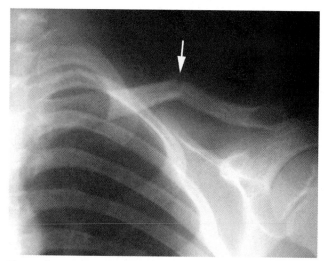

Figure 4-2   Clavicle fracture in a child *(arrow)*. As in an adult, the sternocleidomastoid muscle pulls the proximal fragment superiorly.

such displacement, most clavicle fractures heal rapidly, without complication, and with minimal immobilization required. Childhood clavicle fractures may be incomplete (see Fig. 4-2). Surgical fixation of clavicle fractures is usually reserved for open fractures, fractures in high-level athletes, cases of delayed union or nonunion (see Fig. 1-27), and distal fractures associated with acromioclavicular or coracoclavicular ligament disruption.

Proximal Humerus and Humeral Shaft

The proximal humerus is composed of the articular surface or head (which is bordered by the anatomic neck), the lesser and greater tuberosities, and the vertically oriented intertubercular or bicipital groove between the tuberosities. The surgical neck is the ill-defined, transverse junction of the humeral shaft with the tuberosities and head. Radiographic anatomy of the shoulder depends on the projection. Anteroposterior radiographs in external rotation profile the greater tuberosity laterally and the articular surface medially, with the lesser tuberosity projecting over the center of the humeral head. Internal rotation projects the greater tuberosity over the head, resulting in a rounded contour (Fig. 4-3). A true AP or *Grashey view* is obtained at a 40-degree mediolateral angle. This view profiles the glenohumeral joint (Fig. 4-4A). An axillary view is obtained with the x-ray beam passing caudocranially with the arm abducted (Fig. 4-4B). If normally located, the humeral head aligns with the glenoid on this view. A *trans-scapular Y view* is obtained by angling the x-ray beam parallel to the scapula (Fig. 4-4C). This view superimposes a normally located humeral head and the glenoid. The Y is formed by the scapular spine superiorly and posteriorly, the coracoid superiorly and anteriorly, and the scapular body inferiorly. Unlike the axillary view, the Y view does not require manipulation of

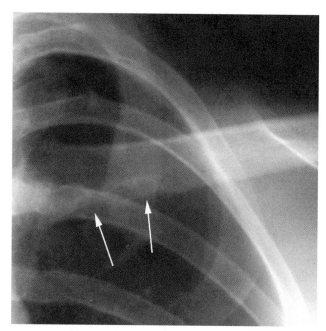

Figure 4-1   Rhomboid fossa. Note the irregular defect in the inferior medial clavicle adjacent to the first rib *(arrows)*.

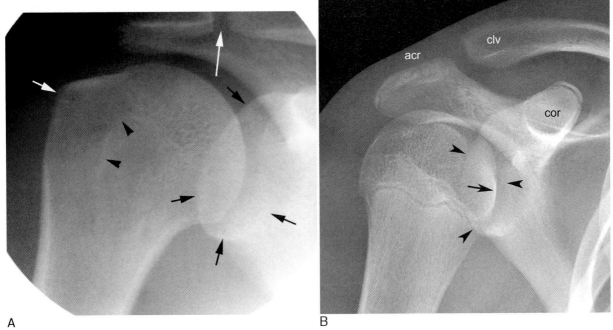

Figure 4-3 Normal shoulder anatomy on radiography. **A,** AP view in external rotation in an adult shows the greater tuberosity *(short white arrow)*, glenoid rim *(short black arrows)*, bicipital groove *(black arrowheads)*, and acromioclavicular joint *(long white arrow)*. **B,** AP view in internal rotation in a child shows glenoid rim *(arrowheads)*, lesser tuberosity *(arrow)*, and acromion (acr), distal clavicle (clv), and coracoid process (cor).

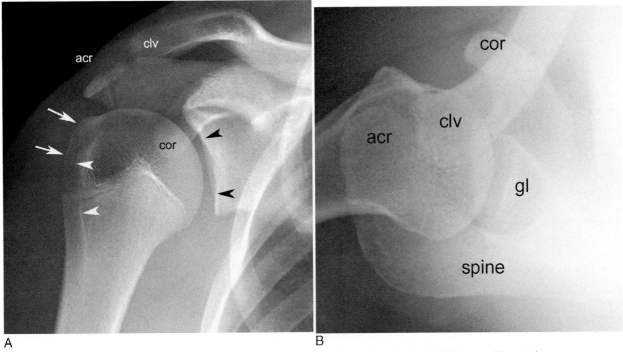

Figure 4-4 Shoulder anatomy on radiography. **A,** Grashey (true AP) view is obtained 40 degrees oblique in the horizontal plane to align the x-ray beam with the glenoid *(black arrowheads)*. Note that the radiolucent glenohumeral joint space is visible. The humerus is in external rotation in this example. Note acromion, clavicle, tip of coracoid process, and the greater *(arrows)* and lesser *(white arrowheads)* tuberosities. The bicipital groove is between these tuberosities. **B,** Axillary view is obtained with the arm abducted and the beam passing vertically through the shoulder. Note the normal alignment of the humeral head with the glenoid. Also note the distal clavicle, coracoid process tip, scapular spine, and acromion. acr, acromion; clv, clavicle; cor, coracoid; gl, glenoid; sp, scapula spine.

(Continued)

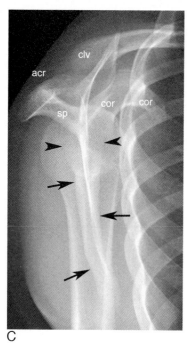

C

Figure 4-4—(Cont'd)   C, Transscapular Y view is obtained with the patient turned approximately 45 degrees oblique to the x-ray beam with patient's hand resting on the opposite shoulder to align the beam with the scapula. The Y is formed by the spine of the scapula spine posteriorly, the coracoid process anteriorly, and the body or blade of the scapula *(arrows)*. Note that the humeral head is centered normally over the glenoid *(black arrowheads)* at the center of the Y. Also note the acromion process and distal clavicle. acr, acromion; clv, clavicle; cor, coracoid; gl, glenoid; sp, scapula spine.

the shoulder. The *outlet view* is a modified Y view with the beam angled 10 degrees caudad (assuming the film cassette is placed against the lateral shoulder), parallel to the supraspinatus tendon as it curves over the humeral head. This view optimally profiles the acromion process undersurface and is therefore useful in evaluating rotator cuff impingement. Many other specialized views have been described.

A widely used classification of proximal humeral fractures in adults was described by the orthopedic surgeon Neer. The *Neer system* provides prognostic information and aids in treatment planning. This system is based on recognition of four potential fracture sites: the anatomic neck, the lesser tuberosity, the greater tuberosity, and the surgical neck. Each of the four fracture sites results in a potential fragment, or "part." A fracture fragment is not considered to be a separate part in the Neer system unless it is displaced by more than 1 cm or rotated by more than 45 degrees. Thus, a single fracture line could result in a one-part fracture or a two-part fracture, depending on the degree of fragment displacement or angular deformity. A comminuted proximal humerus fracture could range from a one-part fracture to a four-part fracture, again depending on the degree of fragment displacement or angulation. Fractures of the surgical neck are the most common proximal humeral fracture in adults, especially frequent in older

patients with osteoporosis (Fig. 4-5A). Surgical neck fracture has a good prognosis because the blood supply to the humeral head is preserved. Anatomic neck fracture is rare and has a poor prognosis because the blood supply to the head is completely disrupted, causing poor healing, humeral head avascular necrosis, and secondary osteoarthritis. Fractures of the proximal humerus, glenoid, or acromion may have associated inferior and lateral subluxation of the humeral head because of transient reflexive regional muscle atony or a hemarthrosis.

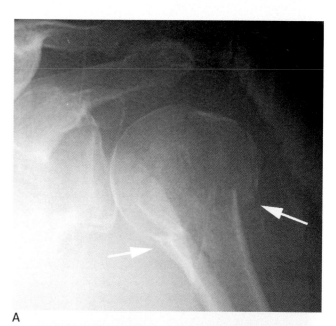

A

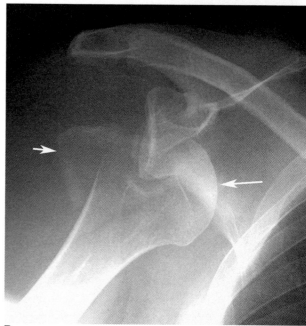

B

Figure 4-5   Proximal humerus fractures in adults. **A,** Surgical neck fracture *(arrows)*. **B,** Fracture dislocation. The humeral head *(long arrow)* is anteriorly dislocated. The greater tuberosity *(short arrow)* was sheared off and is laterally displaced from the remainder of the proximal humerus by greater than 1 cm, making this a Neer 2 fracture.

Proximal humeral fractures are much less common in children than adults. Buckle or torus fractures of the surgical neck and proximal shaft region are most common (Fig. 4-6). The head and greater tuberosity are formed from separate ossification centers that unite during childhood, resulting in an inverted V shape of the combined physis that may simulate a fracture on radiographs, depending on the rotation of the humerus (see Fig. 4-6). True Salter-Harris fractures are most frequently type I fractures in preschoolers up to about 5 years of age (Fig. 4-7) or type II fractures in preteens.

The humeral shaft includes the broad deltoid tuberosity on its proximal lateral surface. The ulnar, median, musculocutaneous, and radial nerves course through the arm. When a percutaneous biopsy of the humerus is performed, these nerves may be avoided by choosing an anterolateral approach (Fig. 4-8).

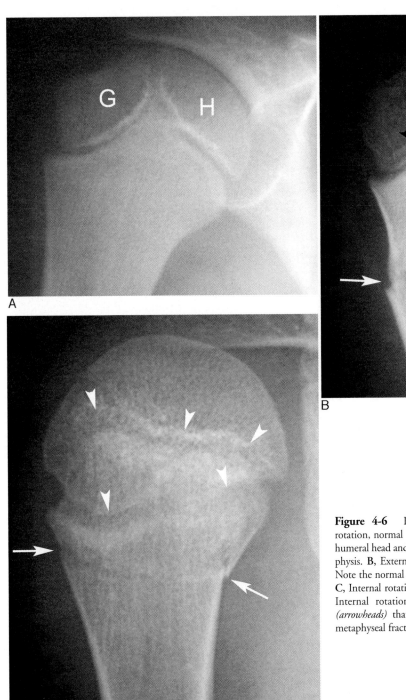

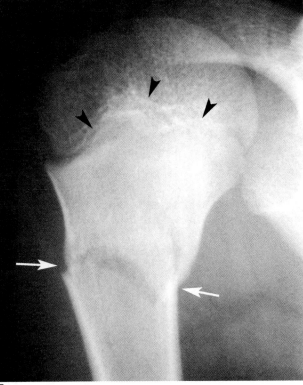

Figure 4-6   Proximal humerus fractures in children. **A,** External rotation, normal appearance. Note the separate ossification centers for the humeral head and the greater tuberosity result in an inverted V shape of the physis. **B,** External rotation view in a child with a metaphyseal fracture. Note the normal physis *(arrowheads)* and the more distal fracture *(arrows).* **C,** Internal rotation view in a different child with a metaphyseal fracture. Internal rotation causes the physis to have a complex appearance *(arrowheads)* that should not be confused with a fracture. Note the metaphyseal fracture *(arrows).* G, greater tuberosity; H, humeral head.

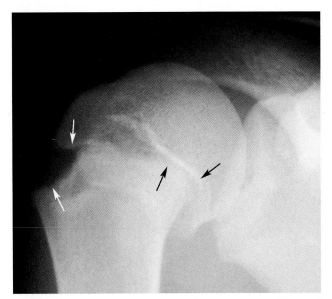

Figure 4-7 Salter-Harris I proximal humerus fracture. The distal fragment is displaced laterally with varus alignment. The white and black pairs of *arrows* show the displacement.

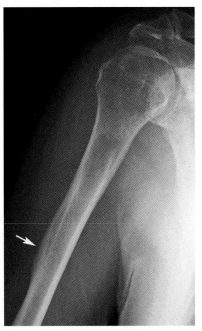

Figure 4-8 Normal deltoid tuberosity *(arrow).*

Fractures of the humeral shaft are predictably displaced by traction by the muscles that insert at different locations on the humerus (Fig. 4-9). As noted previously, the surgical neck is the most frequent site of a humerus fracture in adults. Surgical neck fractures can result in abduction of the proximal frag-

ment by the rotator cuff. Fractures between the pectoralis major and deltoid insertions result in adduction of the proximal fragment by the pectoralis. Fractures distal to the deltoid insertion result in abduction of the proximal fragment by the deltoid (see Figs. 4-9, 4-10). Humeral fractures, or attempts at

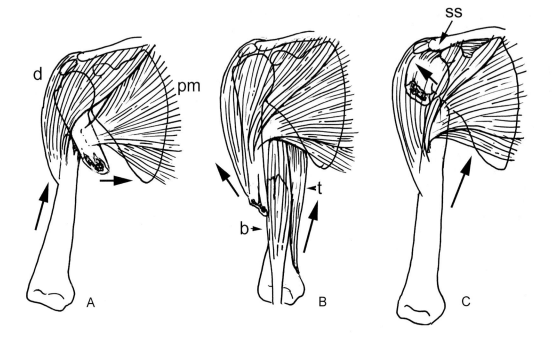

Figure 4-9 Displacement of humeral fractures. **A,** Fractures between the pectoralis major and deltoid insertions result in adduction of the proximal fragment by the pectoralis. **B,** Fractures distal to the deltoid insertion result in abduction of the proximal fragment by the deltoid (see also Figure 4-10). The fragments may override, as shown in the diagram. The distal fragment is pulled proximally by the biceps and triceps muscles and medially by the pectoralis major muscle. **C,** Displaced surgical neck fractures can result in abduction of the proximal fragment by the supraspinatus muscle as well as proximal displacement of the distal fragment, similar to part B. b, biceps; d, deltoid; pm, pectoralis major; ss, supraspinatus muscle; t, triceps.

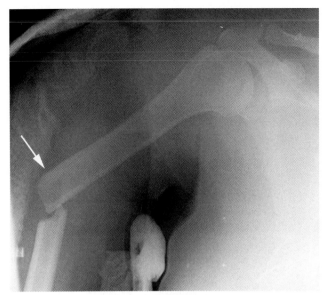

Figure 4-10   Humeral fracture distal to the deltoid tuberosity *(arrow)* results in abduction of the proximal fragment.

closed reduction of a humeral fracture, may injure the radial nerve as it courses posterior to the shaft. Humeral shaft fractures are usually treated by placement of a hanging cast, which immobilizes the elbow and extends part way up the arm. Most patients tolerate less than anatomic alignment quite well because the highly mobile shoulder joint can compensate for some rotational and angular deformity. Internal fixation is usually reserved for severe or complex fractures, such as segmental or intra-articular fractures, or for cases with associated neurovascular injury.

Scapula

The scapula consists of the body, spine, acromion process, scapular neck, glenoid, and coracoid process. Two important landmarks adjacent to the scapular neck are the spinoglenoid notch posteriorly and the suprascapular notch superiorly. The neurovascular supply to the supraspinatus and infraspinatus muscles passes through these notches. A mass lesion, such as a ganglion cyst, or a displaced fracture fragment in this region can compress this neurovascular bundle, causing muscle weakness that can simulate rotator cuff pathology. This is discussed further in Chapter 5.

Fractures of the scapula are rare in children. In both children and adults, scapular fractures are usually the result of direct blunt trauma. Scapula fractures can be a challenge to identify on radiographs obtained in the acute trauma setting owing to overlapping anatomy and support equipment, as well as the frequent presence of other fractures. Knowledge of the mechanism of injury and careful scrutiny of the scapula is needed (Fig. 4-11). Scapular body fractures are usually treated with immobilization. Fractures of the glenoid, scapular neck, and coracoid process are often treated with surgical reduction

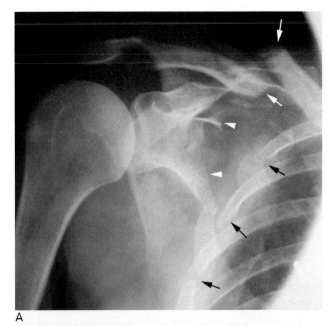

A

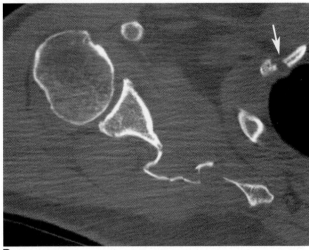

B

Figure 4-11   Scapula fracture. **A,** Radiograph shows scapular fracture *(white arrowheads)*. Also note the rib fractures *(black arrows)* and the clavicle fracture *(white arrows)*. **B,** Axial computed tomography in a different patient shows typical comminution of the scapular blade. Also note superior rib fracture *(arrow)*. Scapular fractures often occur in high-force injuries such as motor vehicle accident ejections, with frequent associated fractures.

and fixation. Computed tomography can be helpful in detecting and characterizing these fractures. When a scapular body fracture is detected with radiographs, CT is also useful for identifying or excluding extension to the glenoid articular surface.

The normal development of the scapula from numerous separate ossification centers can simulate a fracture in children, adolescents, and young adults. Separate ossifications centers form the tip of the coracoid process, the acromion process, the glenoid rim, the inferior angle of the scapular body, and the vertebral border of the scapular body. Failure of fusion of the acromial ossification center results in the normal variant *os acromiale*. Although os acromiale is a normal variant, it is associated with rotator cuff impingement and therefore should be noted when observed on imaging studies. Os acromiale is most readily identified on axillary shoulder radiographs and axial CT or MR images, where it is seen as a coronally oriented linear defect traversing the acromion. Os acromiale may be distinguished from an acromial fracture by

its smooth, straight, and frequently uniformly sclerotic margins (Fig. 4-12). Os acromiale is present in 2% to 3% of the population and is bilateral in 60% of cases.

Another normal variant of the scapula that may simulate a lytic process is a *scapular foramen*. A scapular foramen is a well-circumscribed "hole" in the center of the scapular body. A similar finding occasionally occurs in the iliac wings. This normal variant occurs in flat bones that have strong opposing muscles on each side of the bone.

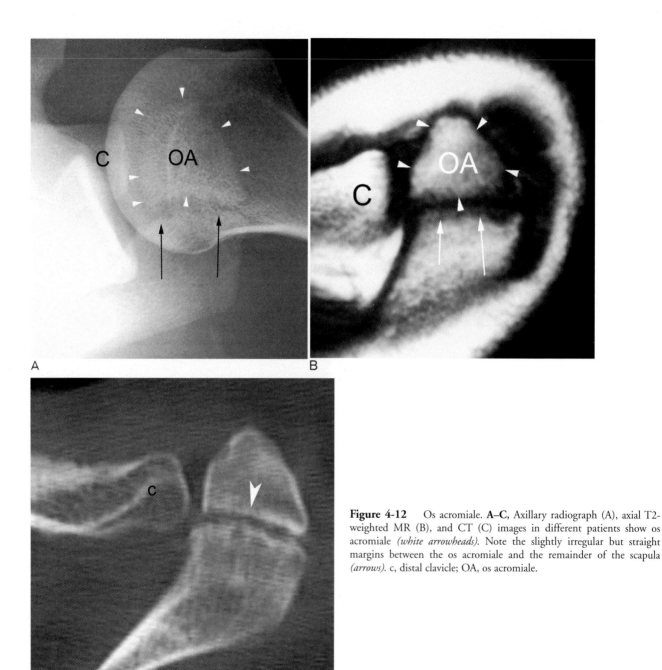

Figure 4-12   Os acromiale. **A–C,** Axillary radiograph (A), axial T2-weighted MR (B), and CT (C) images in different patients show os acromiale *(white arrowheads)*. Note the slightly irregular but straight margins between the os acromiale and the remainder of the scapula *(arrows).* c, distal clavicle; OA, os acromiale.

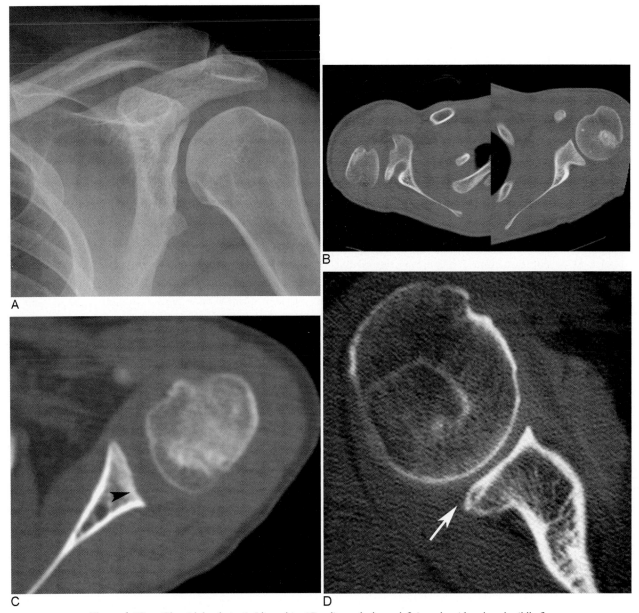

Figure 4-13   Glenoid dysplasia. **A,** Idiopathic. AP radiograph shows deficient glenoid neck and mildly flat humeral head. The right shoulder had the same appearance. **B,** Composite CT image of a young adult with right Erb's palsy shows small, dysplastic humeral head and glenoid related to disuse since birth. **C,** CT image of less severe dysplasia in a child with Erb's palsy shows deficient posterior glenoid *(arrowhead)*. **D,** Mild dysplasia. CT image shows medial slope of the posterior glenoid *(arrow)*, considered by many authors to be glenoid dysplasia. This mild dysplasia may be associated with posterior instability and posterior labral tear.

Glenoid dysplasia is a spectrum of developmental deformity of the scapular neck and glenoid. In the most severe cases, also termed *glenoid hypoplasia*, or *scapular neck dysplasia*, the scapular neck is deficient (small or absent) and the glenoid is wide and medially positioned. There may be associated acromial or humeral head deformity (Fig. 4-13). Causes include absence of the glenoid neck ossification center or a childhood neuromuscular condition such as Erb's palsy. There may be associated gross shoulder instability. A much milder form of glenoid dysplasia is deficiency of the posterior glenoid. This defect may be associated with posterior shoulder instability and posterior labral tears. Axial CT or MRI is needed to detect this condition.

Sternoclavicular Joint

The *sternoclavicular* (SC) *joint* is the articulation of the medial-inferior clavicle with the superior-lateral manubrium. The SC joint is lined with fibrocartilage and contains a small fibrocartilage disc. The SC joint is difficult to evaluate with radiographs owing to overlapping spine, ribs, and mediastinum. The AP and lordotic views can be helpful, but thin-section CT or MRI is usually superior. Ideally, CT or MRI is obtained with the patient prone because this position immobilizes the sternum.

The most frequent pathologic conditions of the SC joint are degeneration, dislocation, and infection. Degenerative arthrosis of the SC joint is fairly common in older individuals. It usually is incidental. Prominent osteophytes may simulate a mass. The strong SC joint can be dislocated in a high-speed motor vehicle crash or similarly violent injury (Fig. 4-14). The medial clavicle can dislocate in any direction. Superior dislocation may be detected with radiographs, but posterior dislocation, which can result in compression of the great vessels or trachea, usually requires CT for diagnosis. An important potential pitfall is distinguishing a SC dislocation from a fracture of the medial clavicle in a young adult. The last epiphysis to ossify, the medial clavicular epiphysis does not begin to ossify until 18 to 20 years of age and does not fuse with the remainder of the clavicle until about 25 years of age. Because SC dislocations occur most frequently in this age range, Salter-Harris I or II fractures may be misinterpreted as SC dislocations or vice versa. Careful attention to the CT images for a smoothly marginated, calcified epiphysis or an irregularly marginated fracture fragment can avoid this pitfall.

Infection of the SC joint occurs most frequently in intravenous drug users and elderly patients. Such infection may clinically simulate a traumatic injury because both result in joint pain, tenderness, and soft tissue swelling. Computed tomography or MRI of an infected SC joint may reveal cortical destruction. If infection is suspected, aspiration of the joint is the best diagnostic test.

Acromioclavicular Joint

The *acromioclavicular* (AC) *joint* is tightly invested with connective tissue, resulting in a strong joint with limited mobility. The nearby, strong coracoclavicular ligaments add to the stability of the AC joint. The AC joint is a synovial joint, and like any other synovial joint is vulnerable to osteoarthritis. Osteophytes projecting inferiorly from the AC joint can narrow the subacromial space and cause rotator cuff abnormality, discussed in Chapter 5. Traumatic injury to the AC joint is graded by clinical and radiographic findings.

Radiographs of a normal AC joint show the inferior margins of the acromion and clavicle forming a continuous line or arc across the joint, with a symmetric appearance of the right and left AC joints. Traumatic injury disrupts the relatively weaker AC ligaments before the relatively stronger coracoclavicular ligaments, resulting in a predictable pattern of injury that is described by a three-stage grading system (Fig. 4-15). A grade 1 AC injury is an AC joint sprain without gross disruption of the AC joint. The AC joint is painful and tender. Radiographs may be normal or may show mild AC joint laxity with minimal subluxation or widening. A grade 2 AC injury or separation consists of complete disruption of the AC ligaments with intact coracoclavicular ligaments. Radiographs reveal discontinuity or widening of the AC joint, but a normal coracoclavicular distance. A grade 3 AC injury or separation consists of complete disruption of both the AC and coracoclavicular ligaments. Passive inferior traction on the arm, usually accomplished by attaching a weight to the wrist, about 7.5 kg in an adult male, may reveal or help upgrade an AC injury that is not apparent without traction. Useful rules of thumb are that the AC joint space is usually no more than 5 mm wide, with right and left differing by no more that 2 to 3 mm. The coracoclavicular distance is usually no wider than 11 to 13 mm, with right and left differing by no more that 5 mm. Although these numbers are worth remembering as useful guidelines, clinical findings and comparison with the uninjured side may reveal a ligament injury despite "normal" measurements or, conversely, may reveal intact ligaments despite measurements that exceed the "normal" range. A 50% difference between the two sides is considered significant. Thus, radiography of both the injured and uninjured sides can be helpful because normal variation may simulate or mask an injury.

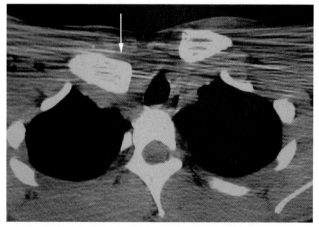

Figure 4-14   Sternoclavicular joint posterior dislocation *(arrow)*. Axial CT shows the left medial clavicle to be in normal position.

Key Concepts	Acromioclavicular (AC) Joint Injuries
Grade 1: AC ligament sprain Grade 2: AC ligament rupture, intact coracoclavicular ligaments Grade 3: AC and coracoclavicular ligaments rupture Grade 4: Clavicle dislocated posteriorly; axillary view or computed tomography needed	

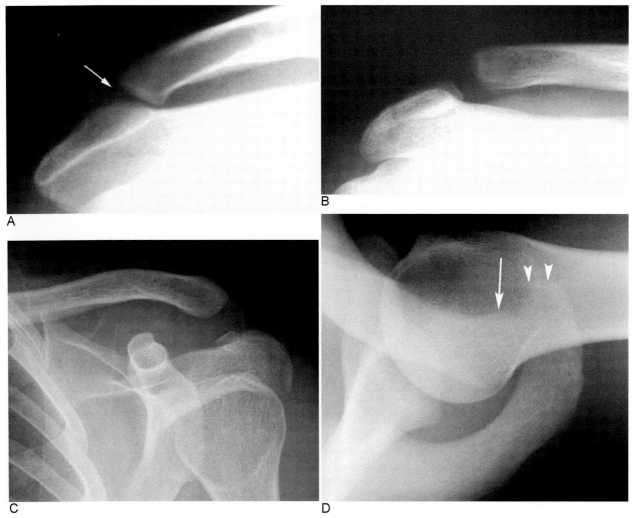

Figure 4-15   Acromioclavicular joint injury. **A and B**, Grade 2 acromioclavicular (AC) sprain. AP radiograph without (A) and with (B) distraction of the AC joint (*arrow* in part A) shows widening in part B. **C**, Grade 3 AC sprain. The coracoclavicular distance was much greater than the contralateral shoulder and widened with traction. **D**, Grade 4 AC separation. AP view (not shown) showed no definite abnormalities. Axillary view shows that the distal clavicle *(arrow)* is displaced posteriorly relative to the acromion *(arrowheads)*.

The distal clavicle also may dislocate posteriorly relative to the acromion into or through the trapezius muscle, sometimes described as a grade 4 AC injury (see Fig. 4-15C). The posteriorly displaced clavicle can compress the supraspinatus muscle against the scapula, causing pain and dysfunction. Surgical correction is required. Radiographic diagnosis of posterior dislocation requires axillary radiography, and CT may be needed for precise determination of the clavicle position and identification of possible associated fractures. An unusual form of AC separation is inferior dislocation of the distal clavicle below the coracoid process and posterior to the biceps short head tendon. This injury also requires surgical correction.

Old AC injuries may heal with persistently abnormal alignment. The injured ligaments may calcify or ossify.

Finally, the AC joint may appear widened by erosion of the distal clavicle because of rheumatoid arthritis, hyper-parathyroidism, infection, and traumatic osteolysis. Cleidocranial dysplasia also may cause a wide AC joint with varying degrees of clavicular hypoplasia. Clinical correlation and careful inspection of the distal clavicle for erosion, irregularity, or absence of the subchondral cortex usually leads to the correct diagnosis, as will comparison with the contralateral side.

Glenohumeral Joint

The glenohumeral joint is the most mobile, least stable major joint in the body, and consequently is a frequent site of pain and dysfunction. Despite having a fairly simple appearance on radiographs, the articulation of the humerus and the scapula is remarkably complex because of numerous supporting soft tissue structures.

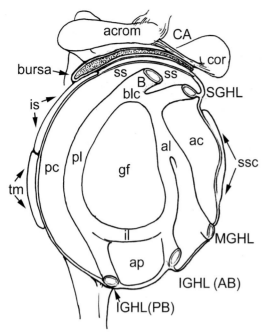

Figure 4-16   Glenohumeral joint anatomy. This diagram views the glenoid fossa *en face* with the humeral head removed. Anterior is to the viewer's right, by a convention used by orthopedic surgeons. The MR images in this chapter display anterior to the viewer's left, by a convention often used by radiologists.*

Figures 4-16–4-18 review the normal anatomy of the glenohumeral joint. The glenohumeral joint is a ball and socket joint. The osseous glenoid is oval in shape, with its long axis oriented in a roughly superior-inferior direction. The subchondral bone of the glenoid is nearly flat, with a shallow central depression. The overlying glenoid articular cartilage is thinnest at its central portion, slightly enhancing the concavity of the glenoid fossa. The fibrocartilaginous glenoid labrum forms a rim around the glenoid that contributes about 3 mm of additional depth to the glenoid fossa and increases the joint contact area. This anatomy results in a shallow socket that allows for extraordinary mobility but poor intrinsic stability.

When viewed *en face* with anterior to the viewer's right, the glenoid fossa may be compared to the face of a clock. Thus, the superior glenoid is at 12 o'clock, the inferior glenoid is at 6

*Key to Figures 4-16–4-18: *Bones:* acrom, acromial arch; cl, clv, clavicle; cor, coracoid process; gt, greater tuberosity; lt, lesser tuberosity; sgn, spinoglenoid notch (posterior scapular neck); sp, spine of scapula; ssn, suprascapular notch (superior scapular neck). *Muscles and tendons:* B, biceps long head; is, infraspinatus; ri, rotator interval; ss, supraspinatus; ssc, subscapularis; tm, teres minor. *Ligaments:* CA, coracoacromial ligament; IGHL, inferior glenohumeral ligament; IGHL (AB), inferior glenohumeral ligament anterior band; IGHL (PB), inferior glenohumeral ligament posterior band; MGHL, middle glenohumeral ligament; SGHL, superior glenohumeral ligament. *Capsule:* ac, anterior capsule; ap, axillary pouch; pc, posterior capsule; scr, subscapular recess or bursa (subcoracoid recess). *Labrum:* al, anterior labrum; blc, biceps labral complex; il, inferior labrum; pl, posterior labrum. bursa: subacromial subdeltoid bursa; gf, glenoid fossa.

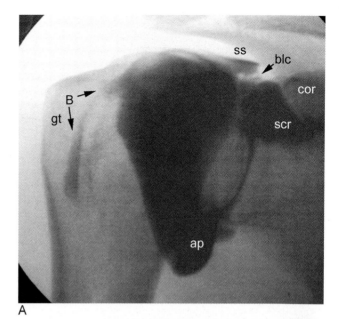

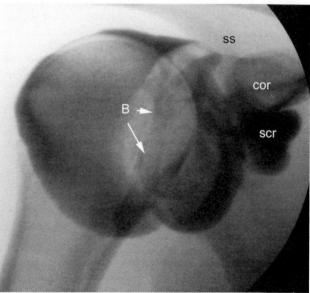

Figure 4-17   Glenohumeral joint: normal arthrographic anatomy. **A,** AP external rotation. **B,** AP internal rotation.*

o'clock, the anterior glenoid is at 3 o'clock, and the posterior glenoid is at 9 o'clock (see Fig. 4-16). This orientation is used in the orthopedic literature and is recommended for reporting imaging findings such as the location of a labral tear.

The muscles of the *rotator cuff* originate from the medial scapula and insert on the proximal humerus. The rotator cuff tendons are broad and sheet-like at their humeral insertions. The *supraspinatus* muscle is located above the scapular spine and superior to the humeral head. The *infraspinatus* muscle is located below the scapular spine and superior-posterior to the humeral head. The *teres minor* muscle is located inferoposteriorly, below the infraspinatus.

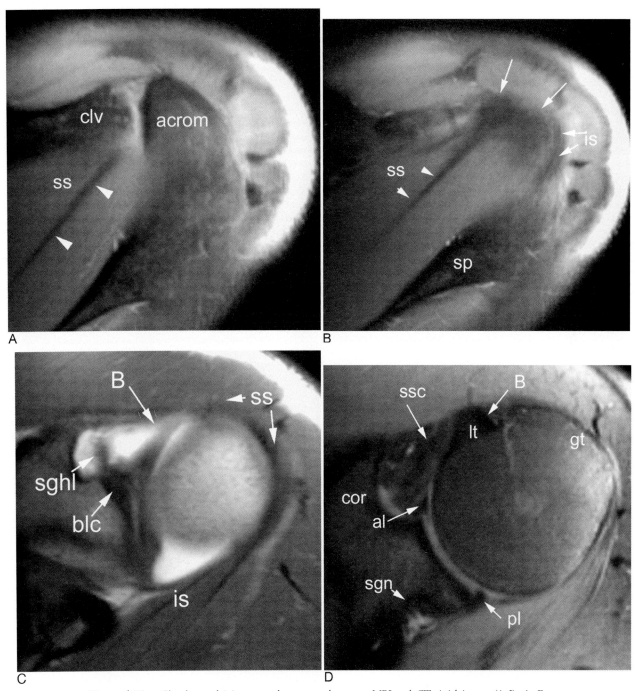

Figure 4-18   Glenohumeral joint: normal anatomy shown on MRI and CT. Axial images (A–I). **A,** Fat-suppressed proton density image obtained through the acromioclavicular joint. The most superior image should include this joint to assess for os acromiale and anterior spurs. Note the central slip of the supraspinatus tendon *(arrowheads).* The oblique coronal scans should be aligned with this portion of the tendon. **B,** Image obtained just below A, same study. Note how the supraspinatus tendon becomes broad distally, like a cuff *(long arrows).* **C,** MR arthrogram obtained through the top of the humeral head is perpendicular to the supraspinatus tendon as it curves over the head toward its insertion onto the greater tuberosity. For this reason, distal supraspinatus tears may be best seen on axial images. **D,** Fat-suppressed proton density image at the level of the base of the coracoid. (See key in footnote on p 78.)

(Continued)

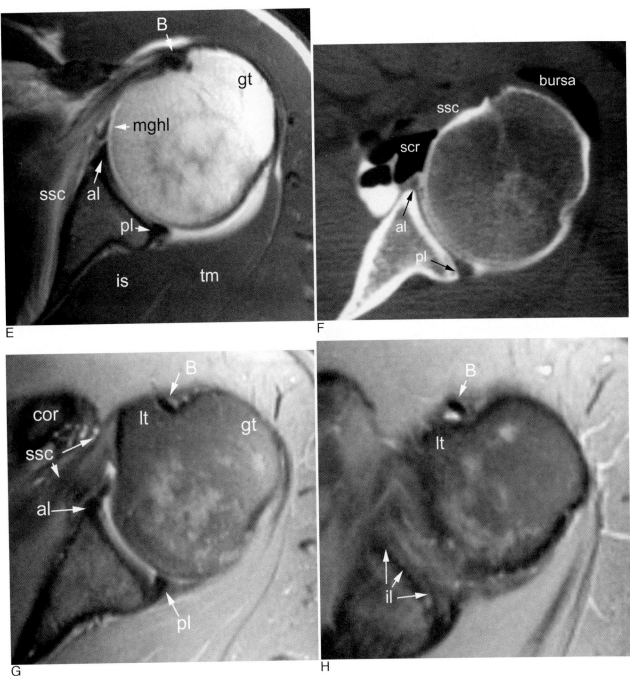

Figure 4-18—(Cont'd) E, T1-weighted MR arthrogram obtained at approximately the 9 and 3 o'clock level. The increased signal intensity in the subscapularis tendon and muscle was due to a combination of harmless contrast extravasation from the joint and direct injection during needle placement. F, CT air contrast arthrogram in a different patient performed at approximately the same level as the image in part E. The gas in the subdeltoid bursa was due to a rotator cuff tear (not shown). G, Fat-suppressed proton density image at approximately the 4 o'clock to 8 o'clock level. H, Fat-suppressed proton density image obtained through the inferior glenoid. (See key in footnote on p 78.)

(Continued)

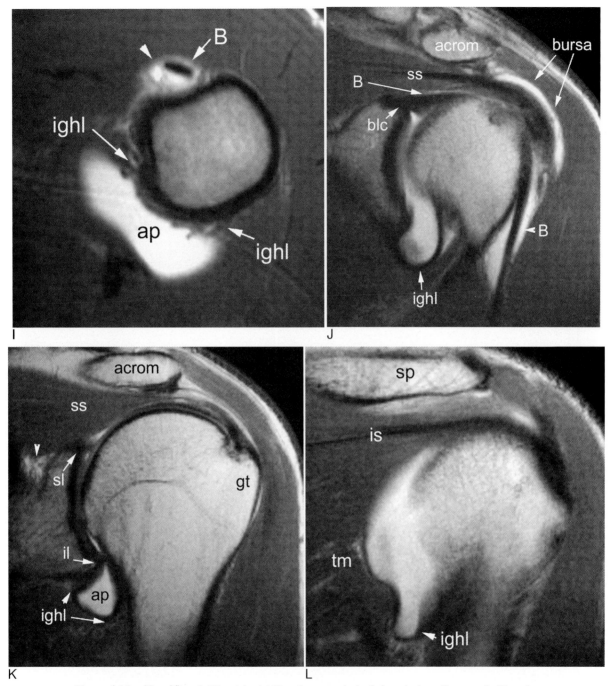

Figure 4-18—(Cont'd)   I, T1-weighted MR arthrogram obtained through the axillary pouch. Note that contrast fills the biceps tendon sheath *(arrowhead),* a normal finding. Oblique coronal images (J–L). **J–L,** All images are T2-weighted arthrograms obtained from the same study. **J,** Anterior image. **K,** Central image. Note the suprascapular notch *(arrowhead)* that contains the suprascapular nerve that innervates the supraspinatus and infraspinatus muscle. **L,** Posterior image. (See key in footnote on p 78.)

(Continued)

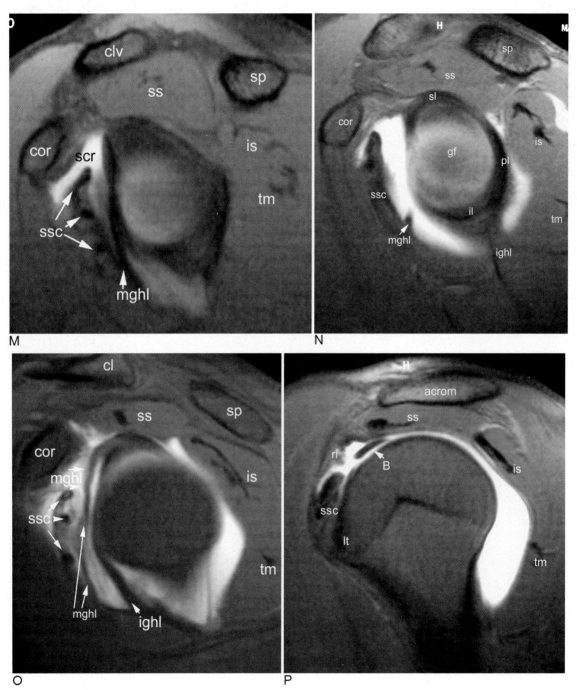

Figure 4-18—(Cont'd) Oblique sagittal images. **M–P,** All images are T1-weighted MR arthrograms but were not obtained from the same study. **M,** Slightly medial to the glenoid fossa. **N,** At the glenoid fossa. **O,** Lateral to the glenoid fossa. **P,** Through the center of the humeral head. (See key in footnote on p 78.)

The supraspinatus, infraspinatus, and teres minor muscles insert onto the greater tuberosity. The *subscapularis* muscle is the only rotator cuff muscle located anterior to the scapula, and it alone inserts onto the lesser tuberosity. Subscapularis fibers extend beyond the lesser tuberosity, across the intertubercular groove to the greater tuberosity. In many patients, fixation of subscapular tendon fibers to the greater tuberosity may be stronger than fixation to the lesser tuberosity. The fibers that traverse the groove are also known as the *transverse humeral ligament.* These fibers contain the biceps long head tendon within the intertubercular groove; thus, dislocation of the biceps tendon indicates a tear. The subscapularis is the largest rotator cuff muscle, about as large as the infraspinatus and teres minor muscles combined.

The biceps muscle has two heads. The biceps short head originates at the coracoid process. The biceps long head tendon originates at the supraglenoid tubercle and the superior glenoid labrum at the 1 o'clock position within the joint capsule, arches over the humeral head within the joint capsule, then courses inferiorly in the intertubercular groove. This anatomy allows the biceps long head tendon to resist anterior and superior humeral head subluxation and thus contributes to glenohumeral joint stability. The synovial sheath of the biceps long head tendon in the intertubercular groove communicates with the glenohumeral joint. The biceps long head may originate entirely from the labrum, entirely from the scapula, or some combination. Because the biceps origin often includes the labrum, it is termed the *biceps labral complex.*

The supraspinatus and subscapularis tendons divide as they pass around the base of the coracoid process. The gap between these tendons lateral to the coracoid is the *rotator interval.* The rotator interval contains the sheet-like *coracohumeral ligament,* which traverses the entire rotator interval, the superior glenohumeral ligament that is further discussed later in this chapter, and the biceps long head tendon.

The rotator cuff muscles and the biceps individually contribute to shoulder motion. The subscapularis internally rotates the shoulder, the teres minor and infraspinatus externally rotate the shoulder, and the supraspinatus abducts the shoulder. The biceps long head contributes to shoulder flexion. However, the primary function of the rotator cuff is to act as a *dynamic stabilizer* of the glenohumeral joint, that is, to resist glenohumeral subluxation during shoulder motion. To understand the importance of the rotator cuff in maintaining glenohumeral stability, consider the effect of contraction of the powerful deltoid muscle during shoulder abduction. Deltoid contraction applies a superior subluxation force to the humeral head, which, if not counterbalanced, would result in impingement of the supraspinatus and infraspinatus tendons between the humeral head and the coracoacromial arch. The muscles of the rotator cuff, operating as a unit and assisted by the biceps long head tendon, apply compressive force across the

glenohumeral joint that maintains normal glenohumeral joint alignment.

The normal labrum varies in terms of shape as well as fixation to the glenoid. The labrum is most frequently triangular in cross-section, but the posterior labrum often has a rounded lateral contour. Small articular surface irregularities such as small clefts may occur as a normal variant. The peripheral margin of the labrum is fixed to the glenoid periosteum, and usually to the joint capsule and underlying glenoid articular cartilage as well. However, several patterns of normal variation of labral fixation occur fairly commonly. A *sublabral foramen* is absent fixation of the labrum between 1 and 3 o'clock (Fig. 4-19). If the biceps long head tendon originates both

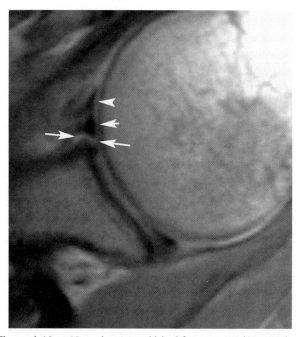

Figure 4-19   Normal variant sublabral foramen. Axial T2-weighted MR arthrogram shows contrast medium *(long arrows)* passing between the anterior labrum *(short arrow)* and the glenoid. This finding is a normal variant only between 1 o'clock and 3 o'clock. Also note the middle glenohumeral ligament *(arrowhead)*. Contrast between this ligament and the labrum should not be mistaken for a labral tear.

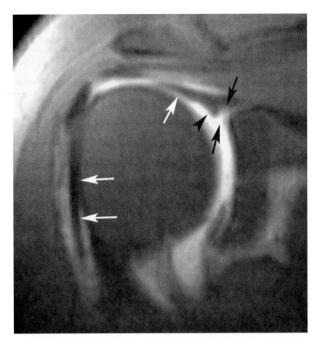

Figure 4-20   Sublabral sulcus *(black arrows)*. Note the biceps long head tendon *(white arrows)* and the meniscus-like superior labrum *(black arrowhead)*.

from the osseous glenoid and the labrum, the superior labrum may be fixed to the biceps tendon and the glenoid periosteum superiorly, but not to the glenoid articular cartilage medially. A *sublabral recess* or *sulcus* is a cleft between the *superior* labrum and the glenoid (Fig. 4-20). This normal variant can imitate a superior labral (SLAP) tear. The less common *Buford complex* is an absent anterior superior labrum and a thickened, cord-like middle glenohumeral ligament that may simulate a

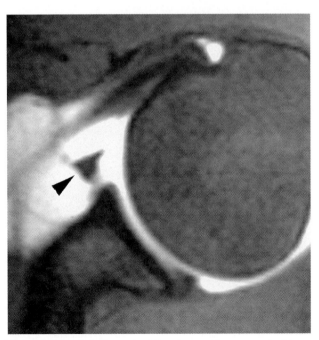

Figure 4-21   Buford complex. Note absence of anterosuperior labrum and thick middle glenohumeral ligament *(arrowhead)*.

labral detachment (Fig. 4-21). Note that complete absence of labral fixation below 3 o'clock or posterior to about 12 o'clock generally indicates labral abnormality, especially in young adults. However, minimal partial detachments may be seen as an age-related finding in older individuals.

The *glenohumeral joint capsule* is difficult to assess on imaging studies unless the capsule is distended by a joint effusion or by direct arthrography. The capsular anatomy is fairly simple and constant posteriorly. The posterior joint capsule is attached to the glenoid labrum and adjacent glenoid periosteum, and is bounded by the rotator cuff. In contrast, the anterior labrum is quite complicated and variable. The medial anterior capsule may attach to the glenoid rim, or may insert onto the scapula medial to the labrum. A classification system is sometimes used to describe this variation (Fig. 4-22), although some authors discount the usefulness of such classification. A type 1 anterior capsular insertion is attachment of the anterior joint capsule to the lateral glenoid, type 2 is up to 1 cm medial to the labrum, and type 3 is attachment of the capsule more than 1 cm medial to the labrum. Some authors believe that type 2 and especially type 3 anterior capsular insertions are associated with a greater risk of anterior shoulder instability in some patients, but this is controversial. Such medial attachment may occur as a normal variant or a consequence of a previous anterior shoulder dislocation that stripped the capsule and periosteum off of the glenoid. The latter condition may be associated with other evidence of a prior shoulder dislocation and is further discussed in Chapter 5.

The glenohumeral joint capsule also varies in terms of the redundancy of its tissues. Some capsular redundancy is required to allow for a normal range of motion. Excessive redundancy may predispose the shoulder to instability, dislocation, rotator cuff degeneration and tears, and labral tears. Conversely, an overly tight joint capsule, as can occur after inflammatory processes ("adhesive capsulitis," Fig. 4-23) or surgical "tightening" procedures performed to correct shoulder instability, can cause pain and reduced shoulder mobility. Estimation of capsular laxity on imaging studies is subjective and arguably should be avoided unless the findings are extreme. Normal synovial recesses, or pouches, extending from the glenohumeral synovial compartment include the *subscapularis bursa (or subcoracoid recess)* anteromedially and the *axillary pouch or recess* inferiorly (see Figs. 4-17, 4-18). These recesses are nearly always distended during shoulder arthrography and should not be confused with capsular defects or excessive laxity or redundancy.

The three glenohumeral ligaments (GHLs) are thick fibrous bands within the anterior portion of the joint. The GHLs are important contributors to anterior shoulder stability. The thickest and most important is the inferior glenohumeral ligament (IGHL), which extends from the inferior glenoid labrum to the proximal humeral shaft in a sling-like arrangement of thick anterior and posterior bands connected by a thin membrane. The IGHL is lax and redundant when the arm is adducted, contributing to the normal axillary pouch (see Figs. 4-17, 4-18). However, when the arm is abducted 90 degrees, the IGHL tightens and becomes the primary stabilizer

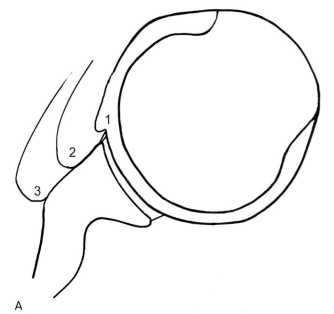

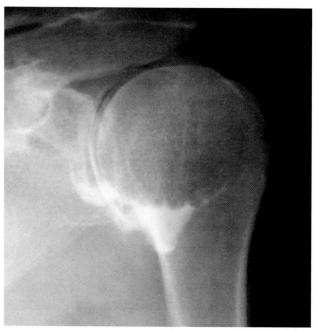

Figure 4-23 Adhesive capsulitis. Arthrogram shows a very-low-capacity joint capsule.

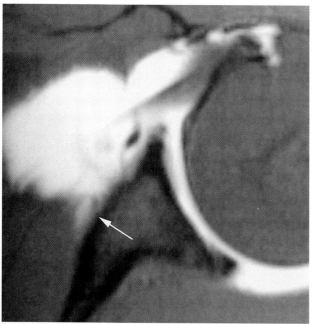

Figure 4-22 Anterior capsule insertion variation. **A,** Classification—type 1: capsule attached to anterior labrum; type 2: capsule attached to scapula up to 1 cm medial to anterior labrum; type 3: capsule attached to scapula more than 1 cm medial to anterior labrum. (From Massengill AD, Seeger LL, Yao L, et al: Labrocapuslar ligamentous complex of the shoulder: Normal anatomy, anatomic variation, and pitfalls of MR imaging and MR arthrography. Radiographics 14:1211–1223, 1994.) **B,** Axial T1-weighted fat-suppressed MR arthrogram shows a type 3 anterior capsular insertion *(arrow).*

of the glenohumeral joint. The highly variable middle glenohumeral ligament (MGHL) originates at the superior portion of the anterior labrum or adjacent glenoid neck, and attaches to the base of the lesser tuberosity of the humerus with the subscapularis muscle. The MGHL is absent in about one fourth of patients. When present, the MGHL may be of variable thickness and is occasionally duplicated. The normal variant Buford complex of an absent anterior-superior labrum and thick MGHL was noted previously (see Fig. 4-21). The superior glenohumeral ligament (SGHL) originates from the superior-anterior labrum, MGHL, or the biceps long head tendon, and attaches distally to the superior aspect of the lesser tuberosity. The middle and superior glenohumeral ligaments contribute to anterior glenohumeral stability, but are not as critical as the IGHL. The GHLs are best demonstrated on imaging studies with distension of the joint capsule using CT or MR arthrography.

Coracoacromial Arch

The acromion process and the coracoacromial ligament form the *coracoacromial arch* (Fig. 4-24). The contour of the acromial undersurface is important to note because it can contribute to rotator cuff impingement (Table 4-1). This can be determined by an outlet radiograph or on sagittal oblique MR images

Table 4-1	Bigliani Classification of Acromial Undersurface Morphology
Type 1: Flat	
Type 2: Concave	
Type 3: Anterior hook	
Evaluation with MRI: Use only the two most lateral images from oblique sagittal sequence	

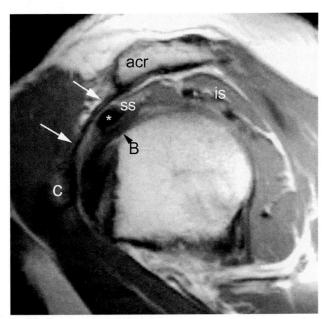

Figure 4-24   Coracoacromial arch. Oblique sagittal MR image happens to include the entire coracoacromial ligament on one image *(arrows)*. Note that the supraspinatus tendon is deep to the coracoacromial ligament, which is often a factor in supraspinatus impingement. In this case, the supraspinatus tendon is focally thickened with low signal intensity *(asterisk)* because of a calcium deposit. Also note the infraspinatus tendon and biceps long head tendon. acr, acromion; c, coracoid; is, infraspinatus tendon; ss, supraspinatus tendon.

(Fig. 4-25). The *Bigliani classification* describes the acromial undersurface as flat (type 1), concave, without focal subacromial space narrowing (type 2), or with an acute anterior downslope ("hooked") with associated narrowing of the subacromial space (type 3). Type 3 morphology is strongly associated with rotator cuff impingement. The reader is cautioned that the apparent contour on sagittal oblique MRI images is somewhat dependent on the orientation of the images, as well as which image is selected. Relatively medial images (adjacent to the AC joint) may suggest an anterior hook when none is present.

The coracoacromial ligament varies in thickness, ranging from about 2 to 5 mm. It is seen on MR images as a low-signal-intensity structure that can be traced between the anterior acromion process and the coracoid on sequential images. The *subacromial space* is the space between the humeral head and the coracoacromial arch. Important contents of the subacromial space, from superior to inferior, are the subacromial bursa, the supraspinatus and infraspinatus tendons, and the joint capsule. The subacromial bursa communicates with the more lateral subdeltoid bursa, and for practical purposes, they may be considered as a single bursa (subacromial subdeltoid bursa). This bursa allows the rotator cuff to glide beneath the coracoacromial arch and the deltoid muscle. The coracoacromial arch contributes to shoulder stability by limiting superior subluxation of the humeral head. This anatomy also makes the coracoacromial arch a major factor in rotator cuff impingement. Any process that narrows the subacromial space has the potential to compress the rotator cuff and other soft tissues in the subacromial space. This is discussed further in Chapter 5.

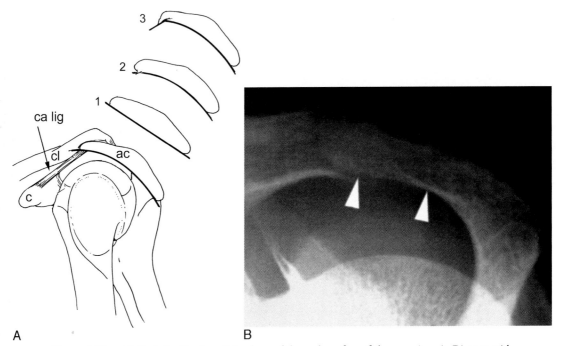

Figure 4-25   Bigliani classification of the shape of the undersurface of the acromion. **A,** Diagram with anterior to the viewer's left shows the contour of type 1 (flat), type 2 (concave), and type 3 (anterior hook). ac, acromion; c, coracoid process; ca lig, coracoacromial ligament; cl, clavicle. **B,** Type 1. Outlet view shows a flat acromial undersurface *(arrowheads)*.

(Continued)

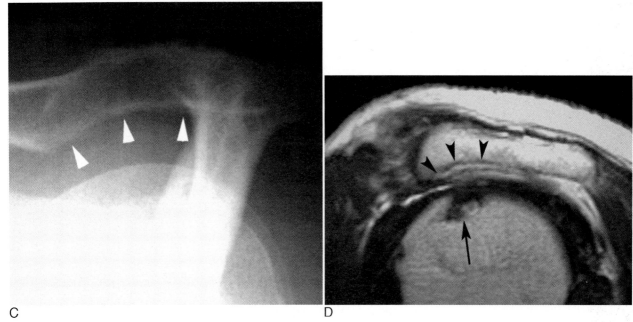

C

D

Figure 4-25—(Cont'd) C, Type 2. Outlet view shows a concave acromial undersurface *(arrowheads)*. **D,** Type 3. Oblique sagittal T2-weighted MR image shows anterior hook *(arrowheads)*. Also note the signal changes in the humeral head marrow *(arrow)* caused by chronic impingement. The subacromial space is narrow because there is a complete rotator cuff tear with retraction (not shown).

Quadrilateral Space

The quadrilateral space is formed by the teres minor muscle superiorly, the teres major muscle inferiorly, the humerus laterally, and the triceps muscle medially. The axillary nerve courses through the quadrilateral space, where it is vulnerable to entrapment due to fibrous bands, mass lesions, fracture, or abduction of the arm. Such entrapment may cause denervation of the posterior deltoid and teres minor muscles that may become evident as atrophy and weakness of these muscles. Imaging studies may show evidence of deltoid and teres minor denervation (edema, fatty infiltration, atrophy), and can reveal a mass when present. Most cases are due to fibrous bands that can be difficult or impossible to see with imaging studies. Low-signal strands may be seen on T1-weighted images.

ROTATOR CUFF IMPINGEMENT
ROTATOR CUFF DEGENERATION AND TEAR
BICEPS TENDON PATHOLOGY
CLINICAL MIMICKERS OF ROTATOR CUFF PATHOLOGY
GLENOHUMERAL DISLOCATION, INSTABILITY, AND LABRAL
  TEARS
    Dislocation
    Shoulder Instability
    Labral Tears
POSTOPERATIVE SHOULDER
MISCELLANEOUS SHOULDER CONDITIONS

ROTATOR CUFF IMPINGEMENT

Most rotator cuff pain is related to impingement (compression) of the rotator cuff, the biceps long head tendon, and the subacromial bursa between the humeral head and the coracoacromial arch. Rotator cuff impingement syndrome occurs in both young and old patients. A cardinal feature of rotator cuff impingement is reproducible pain with overhead maneuvers. Not surprisingly, impingement occurs more frequently in individuals who perform repetitive overhead activities, such as throwing athletes or certain workers. Although rotator cuff impingement syndrome is a clinical diagnosis, many of the anatomic factors that contribute to rotator cuff impingement may be seen on imaging studies, which can assist in the diagnosis.

Most rotator cuff tendon tears are the result of chronic impingement and thus usually occur in older individuals. Chronic impingement causes tendon degeneration and weakening, leading to tendon disruption after seemingly trivial trauma. The supraspinatus tendon is the most vulnerable of the rotator cuff tendons to impingement, degeneration, and tear because of its anatomic location at the most frequent site of impingement between the anterior acromion and the humeral head. Impingement also may occur anteriorly between the proximal humerus and the coracoid process, which is most likely to injure the subscapularis. Another form of rotator cuff impingement

that is seen in throwing athletes, especially baseball pitchers, is posterior-superior glenoid impingement, also termed *internal impingement*. The extreme abduction and external rotation that occurs during the "cocking" phase of throwing—when the elbow is most posterior, just before forward motion of the arm begins—causes compression of the posterior and superior soft tissues. In this position, the glenoid rim can impinge upon the infraspinatus and supraspinatus tendon insertions. The superior labrum, rotator cuff, inferior glenohumeral ligament, humeral greater tuberosity, and glenoid may be injured by such impingement. Internal impingement in skeletally immature baseball pitchers can result in irregularity and sclerosis of the posterior aspect of the proximal humeral physis.

Several anatomic and dynamic factors contribute to rotator cuff impingement. At least one, and often several, is present in a patient who develops a rotator cuff tear. The shape of the acromion process is often the single most important anatomic factor in most cases of impingement. Acromial features associated with impingement include anterior and lateral spurs, a hooked anterior undersurface of the acromion process (Bigliani type 3, see Fig. 4-25), acromioclavicular joint osteophytes (Fig. 5-1) or capsule hypertrophy, and lateral or anterior downsloping of the acromion. An anterior acromial spur is a traction spur (enthesophyte) at or adjacent to the acromial attachment of the coracoacromial ligament. This spur may be seen on anteroposterior (AP), Y, axillary, or outlet radiographs or an AP radiograph angled 30 degrees caudally. It extends anteriorly, medially, and inferiorly from the anterior acromion process (Fig. 5-2A). Acromial spurs at the attachment of the coracoacromial ligament can be distinguished from the ligament on sagittal oblique magnetic resonance imaging (MRI) because they contain marrow fat (Fig. 5-2B). Degeneration of AC joints, with associated inferiorly oriented osteophytes, callus, or capsule hypertrophy, can markedly narrow the subacromial space (see Fig. 5-1). The developmental variant, *os acromiale* (see Fig. 4-12), discussed earlier in this book, is associated with rotator cuff impingement, but is relatively uncommon and is less significant than acromial and AC joint spurs.

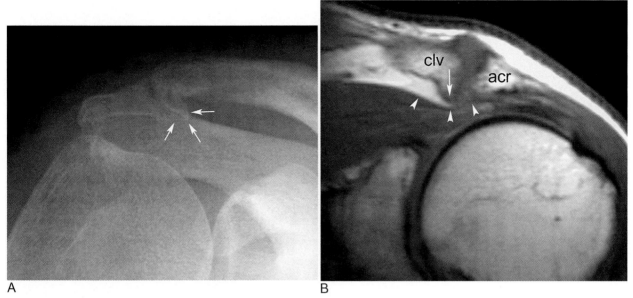

A   B

Figure 5-1   Acromioclavicular osteophytes. **A and B,** AP radiograph (A) and oblique coronal T1-weighted MR image in a different patient (B) show spurs protruding inferiorly from the acromioclavicular joint *(arrows),* with deformation of the supraspinatus tendon in part B *(arrowheads).* acr, acromion; clv, clavicle.

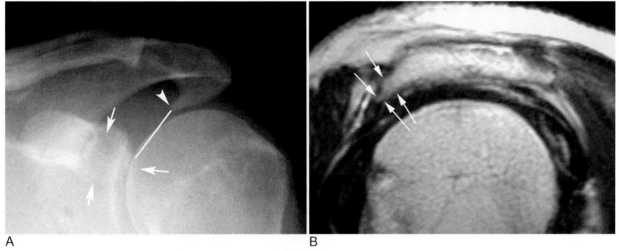

A   B

Figure 5-2   Anterior acromial spur. **A,** AP radiograph shows an unusually long anterior enthesophyte (spur, *arrowhead*) originating from the anterior acromion. The line marks the location of the coracoacromial ligament. *Arrows* mark the coracoid, which is superimposed on the glenoid. **B,** Oblique sagittal T2-weighted MR image shows a spur *(arrows)* at the attachment of the coracoacromial ligament. Note that the spur contains marrow, which allows it to be distinguished on MR images from the coracoacromial ligament, which has low signal intensity on all sequences.

A previous humeral head fracture that heals with deformity may cause rotator cuff impingement. In addition to these anatomic features, superior or multidirectional glenohumeral instability can contribute to rotator cuff impingement, and is often a major factor in younger individuals.

Chronic or repetitive impingement can cause secondary changes in the acromion and humeral head. The cortex of the anterior acromion and the superior aspect of the greater tuberosity may become irregular, vaguely suggestive of erosive disease.

Small "cysts," best appreciated on MRI, may develop in the greater tuberosity near the rotator cuff insertion, in the anterior and posterior humeral head, and in the acromion (Fig. 5-3). The acromial undersurface may become sclerotic and acquire a concave contour that matches the contour of the humeral head. This finding suggests that a chronic large rotator cuff tear is present.

Subacromial bursitis is associated with rotator cuff impingement, both as a cause and an effect. An example of the former is bursal enlargement due to rheumatoid arthritis that reduces the

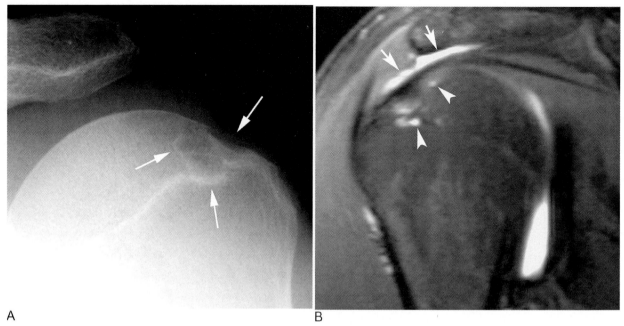

A   B

Figure 5-3   Chronic rotator cuff impingement. **A,** AP radiograph in internal rotation shows cyst-like lucencies in the posterior-superior humeral head and adjacent greater tuberosity. **B,** Oblique coronal fat-suppressed T2-weighted MR arthrogram shows tiny cyst-like lesion in the posterior-superior lateral humeral head *(arrowheads)*. The patient also has a rotator cuff tear (not shown) that has resulted in contrast medium entering the subacromial bursa *(arrows)*.

subacromial space available for the rotator cuff tendons. Bursitis also may occur as a direct consequence of impingement. Images on MRI and ultrasonography (US) reveal increased fluid in the bursa, a nonspecific finding that may also be seen in the presence of a full-thickness rotator cuff tear (Fig. 5-4).

Special mention of *calcific bursitis* and *calcific tendinitis* must be made. Although the two conditions are not necessarily related, bursitis often follows tendinitis as part of an interesting progression (Fig. 5-5). Initially, small asymptomatic calcium deposits, usually calcium hydroxyapatite, form in injured portions of the rotator cuff tendons ("silent phase"). Such clinically silent calcium deposition is surprisingly common. However, if the calcium deposits enlarge, an associated mass effect effectively narrows the subacromial space, and impingement symptoms of variable degrees develop ("mechanical phase"). The calcium deposits may subsequently erupt from the tendon into the joint space, the subacromial bursa, the greater tuberosity, or periarticular tissues. Intrabursal rupture causes a clinical syndrome of acute bursitis. Eruptions of calcific deposits from the tendon may occur repeatedly until the tendon is cleared of such deposits. Bursal fibrosis can occur as a late-stage complication. Calcific tendinitis and bursitis is usually diagnosed with radiographs (see Fig. 5-5A). Magnetic resonance images may reveal low signal intensity on all imaging sequences (see Fig. 5-5B). Calcium deposits can be treated with surgical enucleation or with fluoroscopy- or US-guided

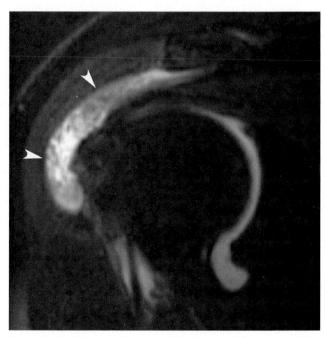

Figure 5-4   Subacromial bursitis. Oblique coronal fat-suppressed T2-weighted MR arthrogram shows distension of the subacromial subdeltoid bursa with fluid and synovitis *(arrowheads)*. T1-weighted images showed no gadolinium in the bursa. Thus, there is no communication between the joint and the bursa, indicating that the cause of the bursal fluid is bursitis rather than rotator cuff tear.

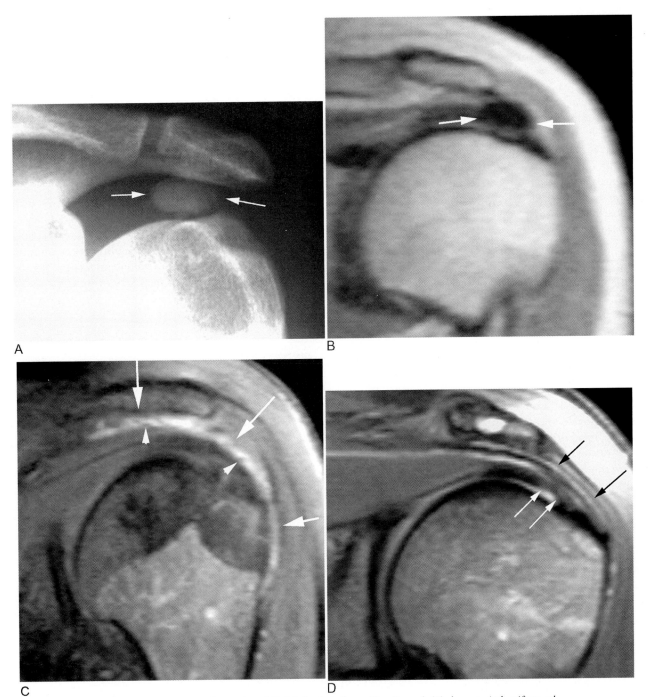

Figure 5-5   Calcific tendinitis. **A and B,** Mechanical phase. AP radiograph (A) shows typical uniform calcification of in expected position of the supraspinatus tendon *(between arrows).* Oblique coronal proton density-weighted MR image obtained in a low-field magnet (B) shows supraspinatus tendon thickening and very low signal intensity in the region of mineralization *(between arrows).* Tendon calcium deposits have similar low signal on all MR sequences. The patient subsequently underwent surgical debridement of the calcific tendinitis with significant symptomatic improvement. **C,** Follow-up oblique coronal fat-suppressed T2-weighted MR image obtained 4 months later shows a more normal appearance of the rotator cuff tendons *(arrowheads).* Radiographs (not shown) also showed resolution of the calcium deposit. However, now note the bursal fluid *(arrows)* with tiny, low-signal-intensity filling defects, thought to represent residual hydroxyapatite crystals and other debris. The patient was only mildly symptomatic. **D,** Oblique coronal fat-suppressed T2-weighted MR image obtained 2 months later shows only a trace amount of fluid in the subacromial bursa *(black arrows)* and mild findings of supraspinatus tendinosis *(white arrows).* Bursal fibrosis is a potential late-stage complication of calcific tendinitis, but this patient clinically did not have such fibrosis.

percutaneous aspiration and lidocaine lavage using an 18-gauge needle. Some operators follow this lavage with a corticosteroid injection.

Surgical treatment of rotator cuff impingement usually is accomplished by acromioplasty (i.e., surgical decompression of the subacromial space) (Fig. 5-6). Acromioplasty is frequently performed during rotator cuff repair surgery to correct the cause of the rotator cuff tear. The inferior surface of the acromion is resected, along with any associated acromial and AC spurs, and the coracoacromial ligament is released at its attachment to the acromion. Current surgical technique favors performing this procedure through an arthroscope placed in the subacromial bursa, termed *arthroscopic subacromial decompression.*

ROTATOR CUFF DEGENERATION AND TEAR

Recurrent impingement causes tendon edema and hemorrhage, and can lead to tendinitis, fibrosis, and degeneration. "Tendinitis" is a bit of a misnomer, as inflammatory cellular infiltrates in the symptomatic tendon are usually not a prominent feature. The alternative umbrella terms "tendinopathy" or "tendinosis" are preferable, as they do not attempt to distinguish tendonitis, fibrosis, and degeneration. However, the term "tendinitis" remains popular because the acuity of clinical features in some patients suggests an acute inflammatory process. Regardless, all these changes result in an increase in free water within the tendon that is seen on MRI

as increased signal intensity on both T1- and T2-weighted sequences (see Fig. 5-6). Healing is possible but is limited by poor tendon blood supply, which consists primarily of tiny vessels that extend from the muscle belly and the humerus. Ongoing tendon impingement in the presence of one or more of the anatomic factors discussed earlier can result in a partial-thickness tendon tear. A partial-thickness tear may occur in the bursal or articular surface, within the substance of the tendon (intrasubstance tear), or as a combination. A partial-thickness tear may have an MRI appearance similar to that of tendinosis (Fig. 5-7) or may be seen as a discrete defect on the bursal or articular surface, usually with higher signal intensity than seen with tendon degeneration (Figs. 5-8, 5-9). Some partial-thickness tears are intrasubstance and extend along the length of the tendon, with or without extension to the tendon surface (see Fig. 5-9). Fluid-filled cysts within the muscle belly are associated with such tears.

Key Concepts	Rotator Cuff Tear

Most frequent cause: Chronic impingement.
Other causes: Rheumatoid arthritis (pannus), acute injury.
Most frequent site: Supraspinatus anterior insertion.
Less frequent: Infraspinatus, subscapularis.
Confusing terminology: "Complete tear" means rupture of entire tendon to some but only a probe-patent perforation to others. Suggestion: Use "full-thickness" to describe a perforation that extends from bursal to articular surfaces and use "complete" to describe interruption of the entire tendon.
Full-thickness tear: Bright T2 signal/low echogenicity across full thickness of tendon. Increased fluid in subacromial bursa. Look for tendon retraction.
Chronic complete tear: Retraction, muscle atrophy.
Partial tear: Bright T2 signal/low echogenicity in tendon does not cross full thickness of tendon. May be upper (bursal), lower (humeral or articular), or intrasubstance.

The terminology to distinguish a perforating tear that does not involve the entire tendon from complete tendon failure can be somewhat confusing. We suggest using the term "full thickness" for an tear that includes tendon perforation, but with some of the tendon intact, and "complete" for complete tendon interruption. A full-thickness tear is fairly reliably detected on arthrography as contrast medium passes through the defect into the subacromial subdeltoid bursa. Also reliable is MRI, which shows the tear as a fluid-signal filled defect in the tendon. The tear fills with joint fluid or granulation tissue, both of which have high signal intensity on T2-weighted images (Fig. 5-10, 5-11). Increased fluid in the subacromial bursa is frequently an

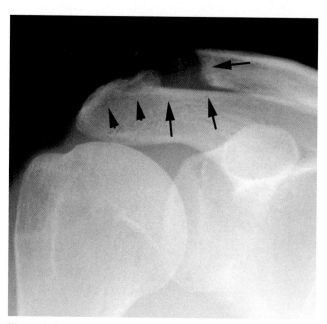

Figure 5-6 Acromioplasty. The acromial undersurface *(arrowheads)* and the distal clavicle and acromioclavicular joint *(arrows)* and accompanying spurs were resected to relieve rotator cuff impingement.

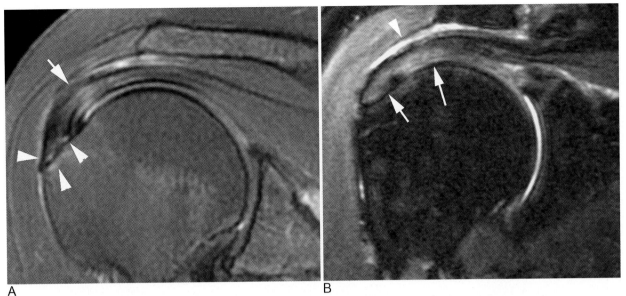

Figure 5-7   Rotator cuff tendinosis (tendinopathy). **A,** Mild. Oblique coronal T2-weighted MR arthrogram with fat suppression shows increased signal in the rotator cuff tendons *(arrows)*, but no areas of very high signal intensity to indicate tear. Also note areas of intrasubstance high signal intensity and mild marrow edema at the insertion *(arrowheads)*. Arthroscopy showed no tear, and the signal changes are probably due to tendon degeneration. **B,** Severe. Sagittal fat-suppressed T2-weighted MR image shows thick, edematous supraspinatus tendon *(arrows)* that at arthroscopy was shown to be extensive degeneration and undersurface fraying. Fluid in the subacromial bursa *(arrowhead)* was due to a full-thickness tear at a different site (not shown).

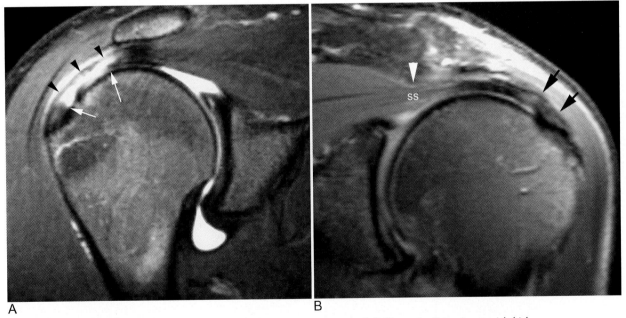

Figure 5-8   Rotator cuff partial-thickness tear: spectrum of findings. **A,** Extensive partial-thickness supraspinatus undersurface tear *(arrows)*. Coronal T2-weighted saline MR arthrogram shows only a thin layer of intact tendon *(arrowheads)*. The subacromial bursal fluid was due to a minute perforation of the infraspinatus (not shown). **B,** Partial-thickness tear resembling tendinosis. Oblique coronal fat-suppressed T2-weighted MR image shows supraspinatus tendon thickening with moderately increased signal intensity that is greatest along the bursal (superior) surface *(arrows)*. No high-signal defect is seen, but this was a bursal surface partial-thickness tear at arthroscopy. Note the acromioclavicular osteophytes *(white arrowhead)* that deflect the supraspinatus musculotendinous junction. When the arm is abducted, these spurs compress the distal supraspinatus tendon. (This is the same study as shown in Fig. 5-1B.) ss, supraspinatus musculotendinous junction.

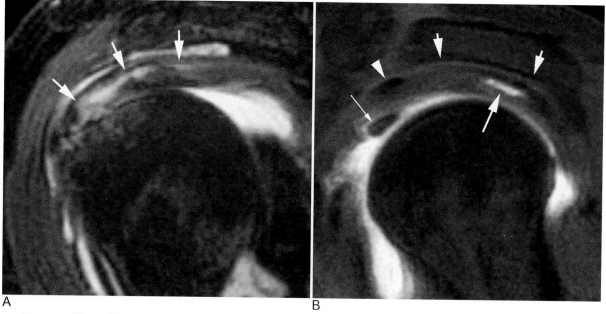

Figure 5-9   Partial-thickness tear: laminar interstitial tears. **A,** Oblique coronal fat-suppressed T2-weighted MR image shows intrasubstance high signal within the supraspinatus tendon *(arrows)*. Another term for this type of tear is "interstitial delamination." **B,** Oblique sagittal fat-suppressed T1-weighted MR arthrogram in a different patient shows contrast medium within the infraspinatus tendon *(long arrow)* that entered the tendon from a distal undersurface tear. For orientation, note the acromial undersurface *(short arrows)*, supraspinatus tendon *(arrowhead)*, and biceps long head tendon *(small arrow)*.

associated finding. Careful attention to window and level settings and correlation of the oblique coronal images with the oblique sagittal and axial images are often helpful in confirming a subtle partial- or full-thickness tear. A large full-thickness tear and a complete tear allow for varying degrees of tendon retraction; this finding should be noted in the report because retraction in excess of 3 to 4 cm has reduced potential for successful surgical repair (Fig. 5-12). A chronic tear may have associated fatty atrophy of the muscle belly, which is unlikely to benefit from surgical repair.

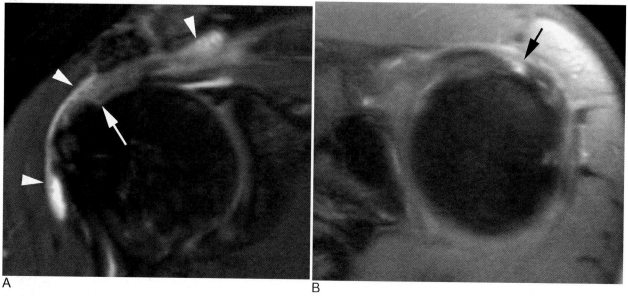

Figure 5-10   Supraspinatus full-thickness tears. **A,** Coronal fat-suppressed T2-weighted MR image shows a small, subtle full-thickness tear *(arrow)* surrounded by extensive tendinosis. The fluid within the subacromial subdeltoid bursa *(arrowheads)* helps to confirm that the rotator cuff is perforated. **B,** Axial fat-suppressed T2-weighted MR image shows a small tear at the anterior supraspinatus insertion *(arrow)*.

(Continued)

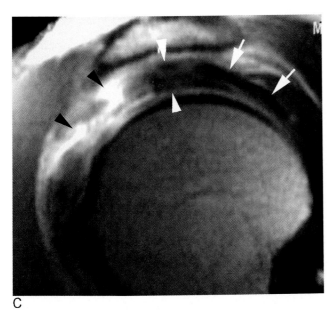

C

Figure 5-10—(Cont'd)   C, Large tear. Oblique sagittal fat-suppressed T1-weighted MR arthrogram in a different patient shows anterior supraspinatus tear *(black arrowheads)* with intact posterior tendon *(white arrowheads)* and intact infraspinatus *(white arrows).*

**WHAT THE CLINICIAN WANTS TO KNOW:
ROTATOR CUFF TEAR**

Tear: Present or absent
If tear is present: Partial or full thickness
Tear size
Retraction
Muscle belly atrophy
Acromiohumeral outlet findings:
    Bigliani classification
    Acromial or acromioclavicular (AC) spurs
    Os acromiale
    Bursal effusion

Most rotator cuff tears occur in the supraspinatus tendon, often at its anterior insertion onto the greater tuberosity. Some authors describe insertion tears as "rim rent" or "footprint." Rotator cuff tears can and do occur in other locations. The *critical zone,* approximately 1 cm proximal to the distal insertion, is the watershed between the humeral and muscular blood supplies and is most vulnerable to degeneration and tearing because of its poor blood supply. Massive tears involving more than one tendon most frequently begin in the anterior supraspinatus tendon and extend posteriorly into the infraspinatus tendon and anteroinferiorly through the rotator interval into the subscapularis tendon. A chronic massive rotator cuff tear with retracted tendons results in a chronically high-riding humeral head (see Fig. 5-11). Radiographs may reveal the subacromial space to be obviously narrowed (6 mm or less), and may reveal remodeling of the acromial undersurface into a concave contour that

matches the contour of the humeral head due to chronic impaction and mechanical erosion.

    Ultrasonography can also depict rotator cuff tears (Fig. 5-13). Conventional arthrography is extremely accurate in showing

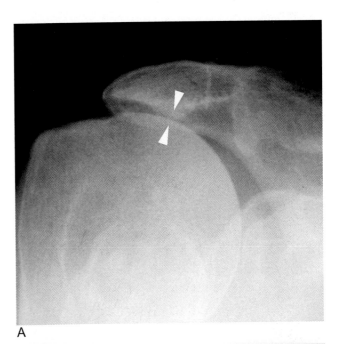

A

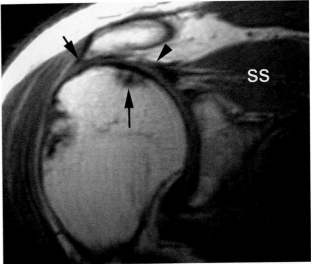

B

Figure 5-11   Complete supraspinatus tears with retraction. **A,** AP radiograph in a patient with a retracted complete rotator cuff tear shows narrow subacromial space *(arrowheads).* No additional imaging study is needed to diagnose the tear. Note the sclerosis of the acromial undersurface due to chronic impaction by the humeral head. **B,** Oblique coronal T1-weighted MR arthrogram in a different patient also shows a complete tear with retraction, but no supraspinatus muscle atrophy. Note the retracted tendon margin *(arrowhead),* signal changes in the superior humeral head due to impaction against the acromion *(long arrow),* and lateral acromial spur *(short arrow).* This patient's tear was successfully repaired. ss, supraspinatus muscle.

(Continued)

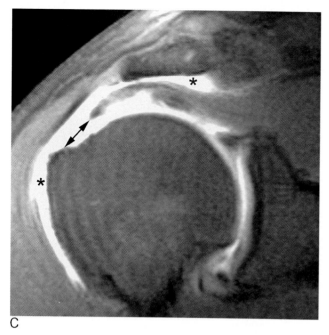

Figure 5-11—(Cont'd) **C,** MR arthrogram in a different patient shows milder retraction *(arrows)*. Note contrast medium filling the subacromial subdeltoid bursa *(asterisks)*.

full-thickness tears. Contrast medium injected into the glenohumeral joint flows through the tear into the subacromial bursa (Fig. 5-14).

BICEPS TENDON PATHOLOGY

The biceps long head tendon originates at the biceps labral complex at the 12 o'clock to 1 o'clock position (usually 1 o'clock) of the superior-anterior glenoid. Superior labral tears (discussed later in this chapter) can involve the biceps tendon. The intra-articular portion of the biceps tendon is vulnerable to impingement, degeneration, and tearing by the same mechanism as the rotator cuff impingement (Fig. 5-15). Biceps tendon dislocation or subluxation from the intertubercular groove indicates interruption of the transverse ligament. Because the transverse ligament receives fibers from the subscapularis tendon and coracohumeral ligament, biceps subluxation is associated with injury to these structures (see Fig. 5-12). An empty intertubercular groove, containing only joint fluid, may indicate biceps long head dislocation or complete tendon rupture with retraction. Tenosynovitis also causes the tendon sheath to fill with fluid. However, this is nonspecific because the tendon sheath usually communicates with the glenohumeral joint; a finding of tendon sheath fluid thus may be secondary to a joint effusion.

CLINICAL MIMICKERS OF ROTATOR CUFF PATHOLOGY

Numerous conditions share clinical features with rotator cuff impingement and tear. Imaging studies in these patients can exclude rotator cuff disease and frequently can help identify the

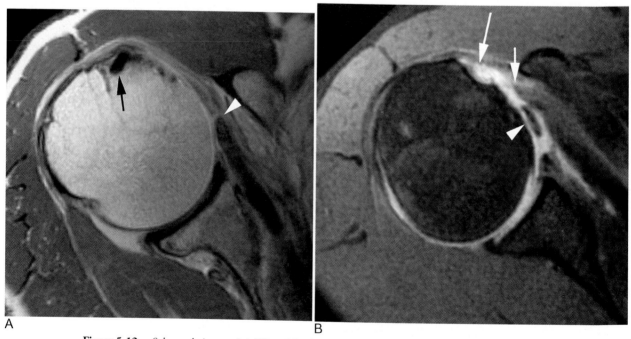

Figure 5-12 Subscapularis tears. Axial T1-weighted MR arthrograms in two different patients. **A,** Tear with retraction. Note torn tendon *(arrowhead)*. The biceps long head tendon is normally positioned *(arrow)*. **B,** Complete tear with retraction *(short arrow)*. Also note medial biceps dislocation *(arrowhead)* and empty bicipital groove *(long arrow)*.

(Continued)

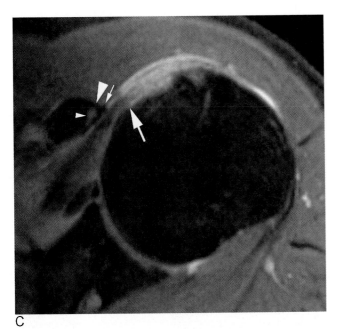

C

Figure 5-12—(Cont'd) **C,** Coracohumeral impingement with subscapularis tear with retraction *(arrow)*. Note the narrow space between the coracoid process tip *(arrowhead)* and the humerus. Also note the small spur *(small arrow)* and adjacent cyst *(small arrowhead)* in the coracoid tip caused by mechanical impingement against the humerus.

true cause of the symptoms. A fall in a patient with healthy rotator cuff tendons can result in a nondisplaced avulsion fracture of the greater tuberosity. Such a fracture can be imperceptible on radiographs. Magnetic resonance imaging is diagnostic (Fig. 5-16). Suprascapular nerve dysfunction can cause a syndrome of

Key Concepts	Rotator Cuff Tear: Clinical Mimics

Suprascapular nerve injury or neuritis (MRI shows muscle signal changes of denervation, may show cause)
Nondisplaced greater tuberosity avulsion fracture (MRI shows the fracture)
Bursitis (MRI shows bursal fluid, intact rotator cuff)

supraspinatus and infraspinatus denervation that clinically mimics a rotator cuff tear. Denervation results in diffuse muscle edema beginning about 2 to 4 weeks after the initial insult (see Figs. 2-19, 5-17). Chronic denervation causes irreversible fatty infiltration and atrophy. The suprascapular nerve may be injured by traction, neuritis, and compression. The suprascapular nerve is vulnerable to entrapment in the spinoglenoid notch and the adjacent suprascapular notch. A mass or displaced fracture fragment may cause such compression. Special mention must be made of a paralabral cyst (i.e., a ganglion or synovial cyst adjacent to the glenoid labrum) as a potential cause of suprascapular nerve entrapment. Such cysts are frequently a consequence of a labral tear. In this situation, the labral tear functions as a one-way valve, allowing joint fluid to pass through the tear and out of the joint but not back in, thereby permitting the formation of a fluid-filled cystic mass. A paralabral cyst can progressively enlarge into the spinoglenoid notch or the suprascapular notch (see Fig. 2-19). Brachial neuritis, also known as *Parsonage-Turner syndrome,* can cause selective suprascapular nerve dysfunction (see Fig. 5-17). Parsonage-Turner syndrome is an idiopathic, possibly postviral

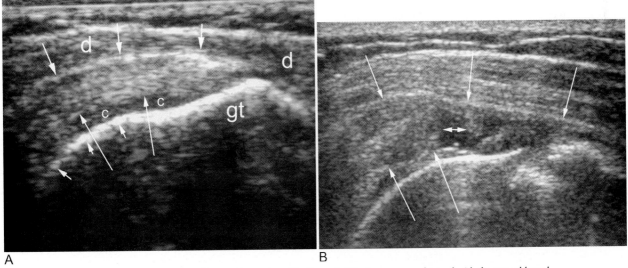

A　　　　　　　　　　　　　　　　　　　**B**

Figure 5-13 Rotator cuff tears: ultrasonographic diagnosis. The images were obtained with the arm adducted and internally rotated. This position moves the distal supraspinatus tendon out from under from the acromion, allowing it to be imaged with ultrasound. **A,** Normal supraspinatus tendon *(long arrows)*. Also note the greater tuberosity, deltoid muscle, subchondral cortex of the humeral head *(short arrows)*, and articular cartilage. c, cartilage; d, deltoid muscle; gt, greater tuberosity. **B,** Partial-thickness undersurface tear *(double arrow)* seen as hypoechoic defect within the supraspinatus tendon *(arrows)*.

(Continued)

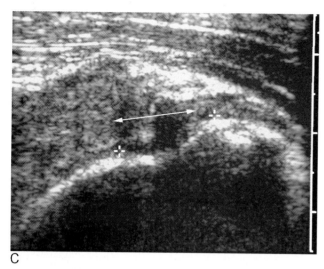

C

Figure 5-13—(Cont'd) **C,** Complete tear *(double arrow)* (Courtesy of Doohi Lee, MD.)

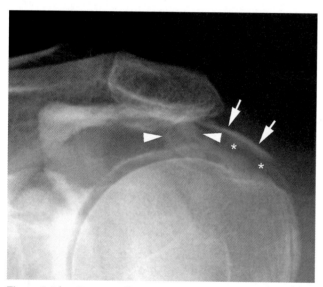

Figure 5-14 Rotator cuff tear: arthrography diagnosis. AP spot view shows contrast medium passing through a supraspinatus tear *(between arrowheads)* into the subacromial subdeltoid bursa *(arrows)*. Note the "filling defect" of the distal supraspinatus tendon *(asterisks)*.

condition that occurs most frequently in young men. Most cases spontaneously resolve after several months. Traction nerve injury may result in an identical MRI appearance and, in our experience, is more frequent.

GLENOHUMERAL DISLOCATION, INSTABILITY, AND LABRAL TEARS

Dislocation

The shoulder is the most frequently dislocated major joint. Glenohumeral dislocation may occur in almost any direction, but most (95%) dislocations are anterior. The most frequent mecha-

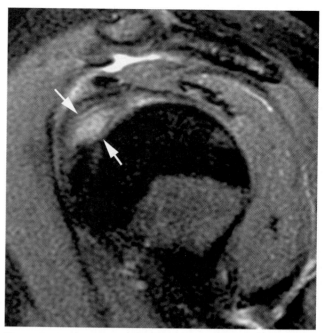

Figure 5-15 Biceps long head tendinosis. Oblique sagittal fat-suppressed T2-weighted MR image shows thick, edematous biceps tendon *(arrows)*.

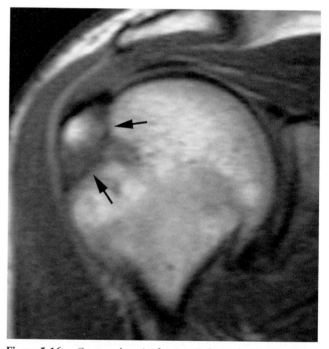

Figure 5-16 Greater tuberosity fracture. Radiographs (not shown) did not reveal a fracture. Oblique coronal T1-weighted MR image shows a nondisplaced fracture, seen as a low signal line *(arrows)*. The rotator cuff was intact.

nism of anterior shoulder dislocation is forced extension, abduction, and external rotation of the arm. A direct blow to the posterior shoulder or anterior distraction also can result in anterior dislocation. Radiographs are diagnostic (Fig. 5-18). A transscapular Y, axillary, or transthoracic view is necessary in any

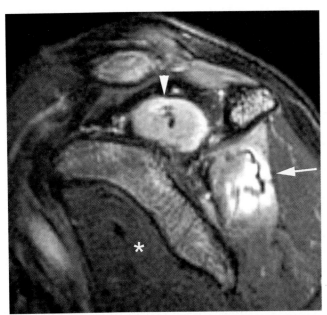

Figure 5-17   Parsonage-Turner syndrome. Oblique sagittal fat-suppressed T2-weighted MR image shows edema in the supraspinatous *(arrowhead)* and infraspinatous *(arrow)* muscles. Contrast this finding with the normal signal intensity of the adjacent muscles, such as the subscapularis *(asterisk)*. The patient had recently experienced a viral illness, no mass was found, and there was no history of trauma.

traumatized patient because these views reliably demonstrate or exclude a dislocation. Radiographs of anterior shoulder dislocation reveal the humeral head to be positioned anterior, medial, and slightly inferior to the glenoid fossa. Once dislocated, the superior-

posterior humeral head is in contact with the anterior inferior glenoid rim. This may result in a wedge-shaped posterior superior humeral head impaction fracture, termed a *Hill-Sachs lesion*. A Hill-Sachs lesion may be apparent only on radiographs obtained after the dislocation is reduced, and even then may be quite subtle. Radiographs obtained in internal rotation are more sensitive than those obtained in external rotation because the lesion is located posterolaterally. Both CT and MR images are highly sensitive in depicting Hill-Sachs lesions. These modalities reveal a wedge-shaped defect in the posterolateral superior humeral head at or just above the level of the coracoid process (Fig. 5-19). Magnetic resonance images of fractures less than 6 to 8 weeks old also typically reveal adjacent humeral marrow edema. The size of a Hill-Sachs lesion should be noted because larger lesions are more strongly associated with subsequent anterior glenohumeral instability.

Key Concepts	Glenohumeral Joint Instability

Anterior instability. Look for evidence of prior anterior dislocation: Bankart lesion, Hill-Sachs lesion, torn glenohumeral ligaments, anterior capsular stripping.
Posterior instability. Look for evidence of prior posterior dislocation: Reverse Bankart fracture and Hill-Sachs lesion, posterior capsular stripping, posterior labral tear.
Multidirectional instability. Capsular laxity, dyscoordination of rotator cuff muscles. Clinical diagnosis.

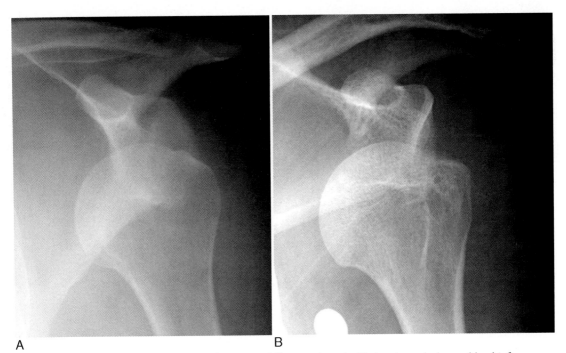

Figure 5-18   Anterior shoulder dislocation in different patients **A,** AP view shows the humeral head inferior to the coracoid. **B,** Grashey (true AP) view in a different patient also shows the subcoracoid and medial position of the humeral head

(Continued)

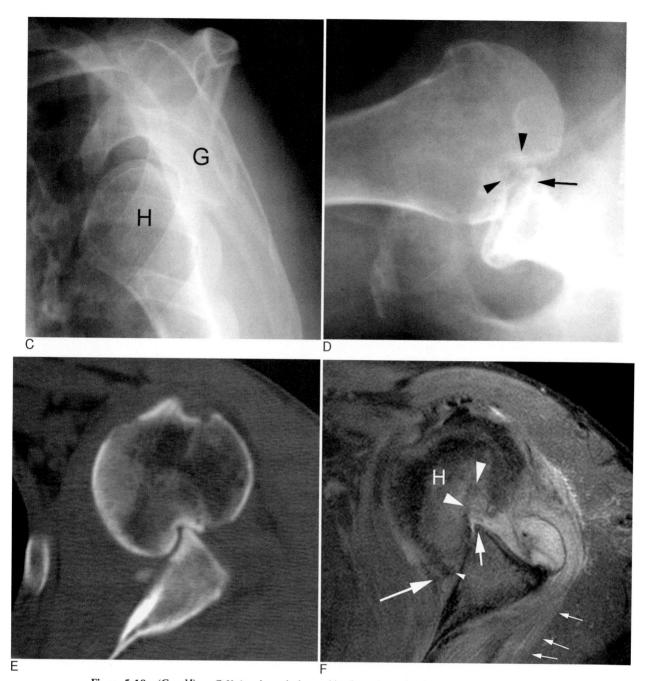

Figure 5-18—(Cont'd)   **C,** Y view shows the humeral head anterior to the glenoid. **D,** Axillary view shows a Hill-Sachs fracture *(arrowheads)* caused by impaction against the anterior labrum *(arrow)*. **E,** Axial CT scan shows similar findings. **F,** Axial fat-suppressed proton density MR image shows anteriorly dislocated humeral head impacted against the anterior labrum *(short arrow)* and a Hill-Sachs fracture *(arrowheads)*. The anterior labrum is displaced medially *(small arrowhead)*. Also note stripped anterior capsule *(long arrow)* and edema in the infraspinatus and teres minor muscle bellies *(small arrows)* due to muscle strains. G, glenoid; H, humeral head.

Anterior dislocation also injures the anterior soft tissue structures of the shoulder. The *Bankart lesion* is a tear or separation of the anterior inferior glenoid labrum, classically, but not necessarily, with a chip fracture from the glenoid rim (Figs. 5-20, 5-21). A variety of patterns of anterior labral tear may be seen (see Fig. 5-21). Associated soft tissue injuries include glenohumeral ligament (GHL) tears, coracohumeral ligament tear or avulsion, subscapularis tears with possible subluxation of the biceps long head tendon or avulsion fracture of the lesser tuberosity, and stripping of the anterior joint capsule from its glenoid attachment. The inferior GHL may tear away from its labral origin or, rarely, from its humeral attachment, in which case it is termed the *HAGL lesion* (humeral avulsion of the inferior glenohumeral ligament) (Fig. 5-22B). The presence of

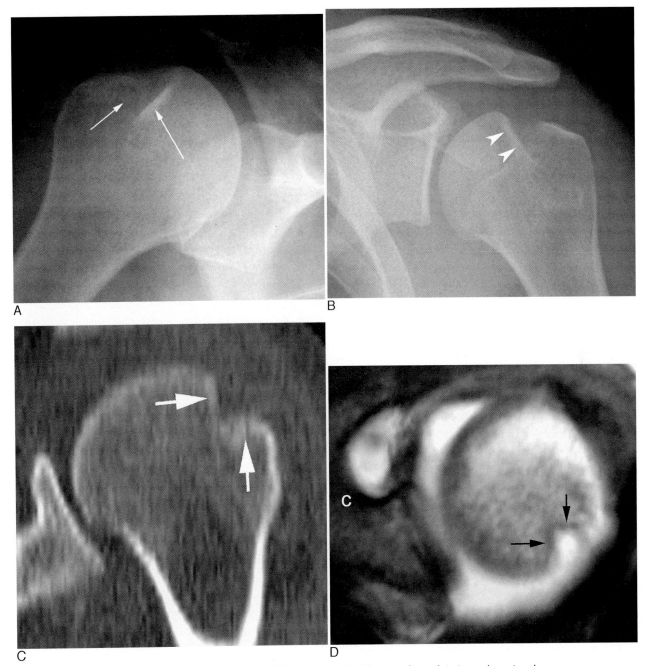

Figure 5-19   Hill-Sachs fractures in different patients. **A,** AP view radiograph in internal rotation shows a notch-like defect in the superoposterior humeral head *(arrows)*. **B,** Grashey view radiograph shows a larger fracture *(arrowheads)*. **C,** Coronal computed tomography reformat shows similar defect *(arrows)*. **D,** Axial T1-weighted MR arthrogram also shows notch-like defect. Note that the Hill-Sachs fracture is seen at the level of the base of the coracoid process. A Hill-Sachs fracture generally does not occur below this level, although it often occurs above. C, coracoid process.

glenoid marrow edema indicates that a Bankart lesion is likely to be acute. A Bankart fracture may be a subtle finding on radiographs but is more easily identified with CT (see Fig. 5-20B).

Bankart lesions and related soft tissue injuries are the most important sequelae of an anterior shoulder dislocation because they damage the anterior glenohumeral stabilizers, with result-

ing anterior glenohumeral instability and the potential for recurrent anterior dislocations. Anterior dislocation in a teenager or young adult is particularly likely to result in extensive anterior soft tissue injury and chronic anterior instability. These soft tissue injuries are difficult to detect on routine MR images unless the joint capsule is distended by an effusion or after arthrography. Careful scrutiny of the anterior joint structures is required. Findings to look for include tears or fraying of the glenohumeral ligaments and anterior inferior labrum, subscapularis tendon tear or muscle atrophy, subluxation of the biceps long head tendon, anterior capsular stripping, subluxation of the humeral head, and Hill-Sachs and Bankart fractures.

Several potential pitfalls may falsely suggest anterior capsular injury on MR arthrograms. Differentiation of traumatic capsular stripping from atraumatic, normal variant medial capsular attachment can be difficult. The appearance of the joint capsule on imaging studies depends on the amount of fluid in the joint and the position of the humerus. If the joint is distended with fluid, a previously stripped joint capsule may be seen to join the scapula at a shallow angle (see Figs. 5-20C,

5-22A), whereas an atraumatic, normal variant medial capsular attachment often forms an obtuse angle (see Fig. 5-21A). Alternatively, injected contrast medium may "extravasate" along the anterior-medial scapula, simulating capsular stripping. Such extravasated contrast often dissects into the subscapularis muscle, resulting in a distinctive pattern that may be distinguished from the more homogeneous signal intensity of intracapsular contrast (see Fig. 4-18E). Normal subcoracoid and axillary recesses should not be mistaken for a pathologically redundant capsule. Small clefts in the anterior labrum are a frequent normal variant that may simulate a labral tear. Similarly, the anterior superior labrum may not be attached to the glenoid (sublabral foramen), or may be entirely absent as part of the Buford complex (see Fig. 4-21). The superior GHL and espe-

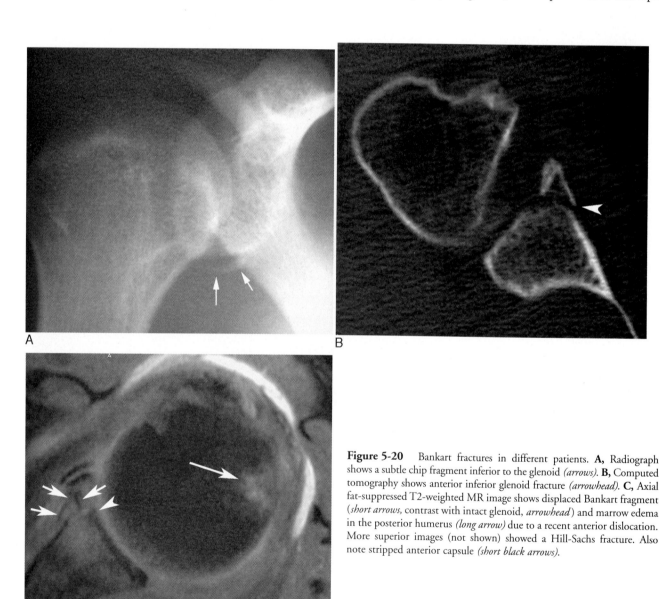

Figure 5-20 Bankart fractures in different patients. **A,** Radiograph shows a subtle chip fragment inferior to the glenoid *(arrows).* **B,** Computed tomography shows anterior inferior glenoid fracture *(arrowhead).* **C,** Axial fat-suppressed T2-weighted MR image shows displaced Bankart fragment *(short arrows,* contrast with intact glenoid, *arrowhead)* and marrow edema in the posterior humerus *(long arrow)* due to a recent anterior dislocation. More superior images (not shown) showed a Hill-Sachs fracture. Also note stripped anterior capsule *(short black arrows).*

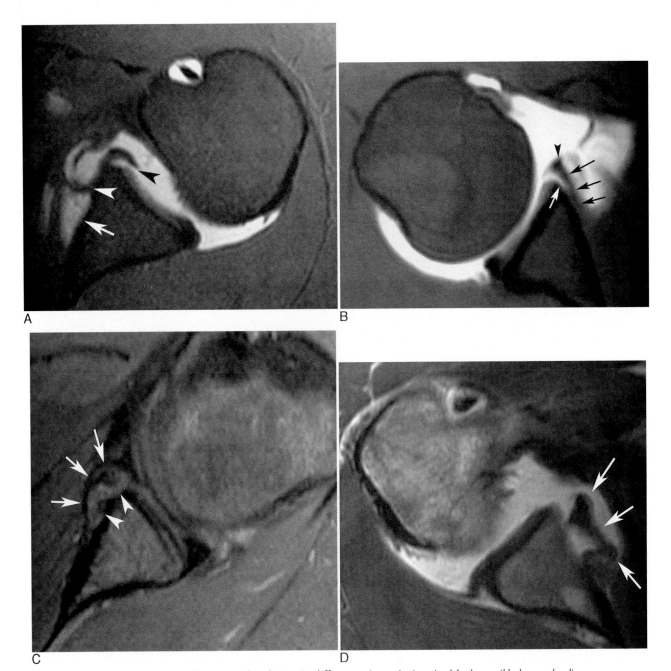

Figure 5-21   Soft tissue Bankart lesions in different patients. **A,** Anterior labral tear *(black arrowhead)* shown on fat-suppressed T1-weighted MR arthrogram. Note the normal attachment of the anterior capsule *(white arrowhead)* and incidental medially extravasated contrast *(arrow)* that simulates anterior capsule stripping. In contrast with the following cases, this was a simple lesion in a stable shoulder. **B,** Perthes lesion. Axial T1-weighted axial MR arthrogram shows that the anteroinferior labrum *(arrowhead)* is torn away from the glenoid. In this variant, the labrum remains attached to the periosteum *(arrows)*, which is partially stripped off of the anterior glenoid. Note high signal intensity of contrast medium between the stripped periosteum and the labrum *(white arrow)*. **C,** Another Perthes lesion, shown on plain MR imaging (MRI). Axial fat-suppressed T2-weighted image shows the stripped capsule and labrum *(arrows)*, separated from the scapula by intermediate-signal material *(arrowheads)* that was granulation tissue and hemorrhage at arthroscopy. **D,** ALPSA lesion (anterior labral periosteal sleeve avulsion, *arrows*). This lesion may be considered a medially displaced Perthes lesion. The labrum, inferior glenohumeral ligament anterior band, and associated stripped periosteum have displaced medially. This Bankart variant has a high association with anterior instability and recurrent shoulder dislocation.

(Continued)

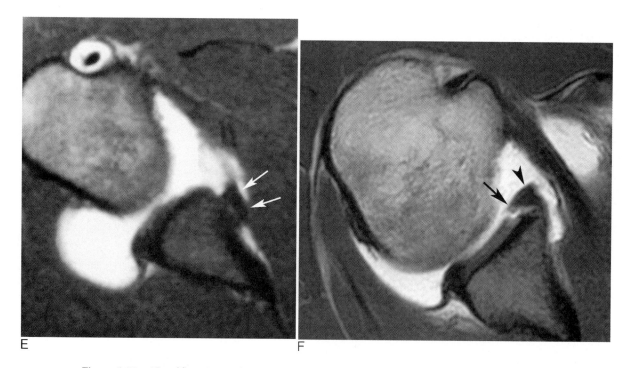

Figure 5-21—(Cont'd) **E,** Another ALPSA lesion, which healed in this abnormal location *(arrows).* **F,** Glenolabral articular disruption (GLAD lesion). The anteroinferior labrum *(arrowhead)* and a fragment of underlying cartilage *(arrow)* have stripped away from the glenoid as a unit.

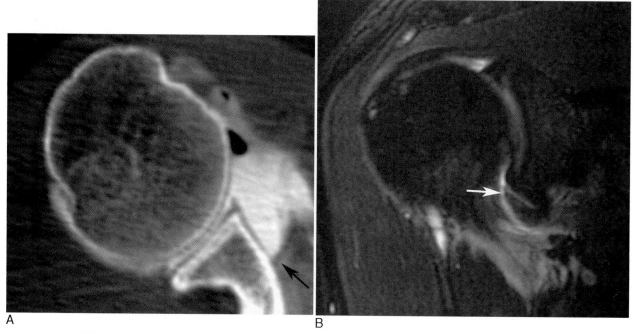

Figure 5-22 Additional anterior soft tissue injuries following anterior shoulder dislocation. **A,** Anterior capsular stripping. CT arthrogram shows acute angle formed by the anterior capsule and the scapula *(arrow).* Contrast this finding with the obtuse angle in Fig. 5-21A. **B,** Humeral avulsion of the inferior glenohumeral ligament (HAGL) lesion. Note interrupted lateral inferior glenohumeral ligament (GHL) *(arrow),* which is curved into a J shape. Tears of the GHLs are common after dislocation, and tears of the inferior GHL are the most significant.

cially the middle GHL are variable in their size and course, and may be absent in normal individuals. The inferior GHL is more constant, with the anterior band usually thicker than the posterior band. However, this situation may be reversed, with the posterior band being thicker. The posterior-lateral humeral head has a normal indentation above the surgical neck, potentially simulating a Hill-Sachs fracture. This indentation occurs below the level of the coracoid process, whereas Hill-Sachs fractures are seen at or above the level of the coracoid process. Normal synovial folds or inadvertently injected air bubbles may simulate an intra-articular loose body. Shoulder surgery can leave extensive metal artifact in and around the shoulder, especially if metallic suture anchors were placed.

Posterior glenohumeral dislocation is much less common than anterior dislocation. Posterior dislocation is caused by forceful muscle contraction (seizure or electrocution, potentially resulting in bilateral dislocations), or may be caused by a fall on a flexed and adducted arm. The humeral head usually dislocates directly posteriorly and is locked in internal rotation. Anteroposterior radiographs may be misleading because the posteriorly dislocated humeral head can project over its normal position in this projection. A trans-scapular Y or axillary view is diagnostic (Fig. 5-23). A Y view must be perfectly positioned for reliable detection of a posterior dislocation. For this reason, some orthopedic surgeons prefer the axillary view, which can be obtained with the film cassette on top of the shoulder and the x-ray tube by the patient's side, with only minimal abduction of the shoulder.

Associated osseous and soft tissue injuries mirror those of anterior dislocation. The posterior joint capsule is stripped off of the glenoid and the posterior labrum is often torn or separated from the glenoid, resulting in posterior glenohumeral instability and leaving the patient vulnerable to recurrent posterior dislocations. The anterior humeral head impacts against the posterior glenoid rim and a humeral head fracture (reverse Hill-Sachs fracture), posterior labral tear, or a posterior glenoid rim chip fracture (reverse Bankart chip fracture, Fig. 5-23C) may result. A reverse Hill-Sachs fracture may be appreciated on an AP radiograph as a vertically oriented linear impression (*trough sign;* Figs. 5-23A and C, 5-24).

Shoulder dislocation in other directions is unusual. A distinctive form of inferior dislocation termed *luxatio erecti* results in fixed abduction of the arm (Fig. 5-25). Inferior humeral head subluxation is a frequent finding after a stroke or fracture around the shoulder due to reflex muscle atony. This phenomenon has been misnamed "pseudosubluxation," but it is true subluxation.

Shoulder Instability

Glenohumeral joint stability depends on a combination of static and dynamic mechanisms. Static mechanisms include the labrum, capsule and glenohumeral ligaments, and negative pressure at the area of contact of the articular surfaces. This last mechanism is due to complex osmotic effects within the joint that may be likened to a suction cup applied to a pane of glass.

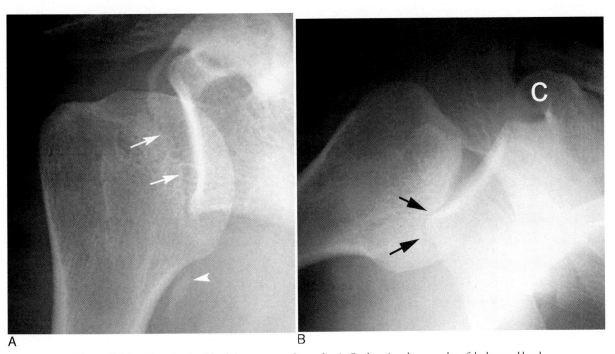

Figure 5-23   Posterior shoulder dislocation on radiography. **A,** Grashey view shows overlap of the humeral head and glenoid, indicating that a dislocation is present. Note the subtle humeral head impaction fracture *(arrows),* called the "trough sign," and the small reverse Bankart chip fracture *(arrowhead).* **B,** Oblique axillary view shows reverse Hill-Sachs impaction fracture *(arrows).* Note that the dislocation is opposite from the coracoid process. C, coracoid process.

(Continued)

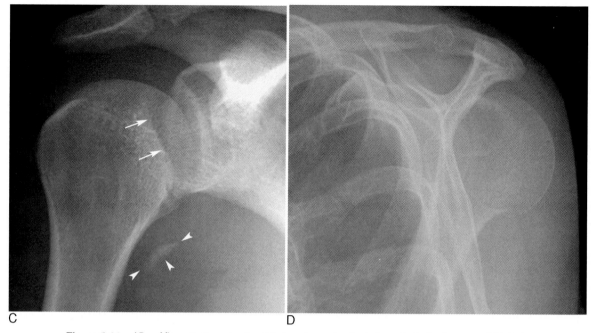

Figure 5-23—(Cont'd) **C,** Postreduction AP view shows the classic "trough sign" of a reverse Hill-Sachs fracture *(arrows).* Also note the reverse Bankart chip fracture fragment *(arrowhead).* **D,** Y view in a different patient with posterior dislocation.

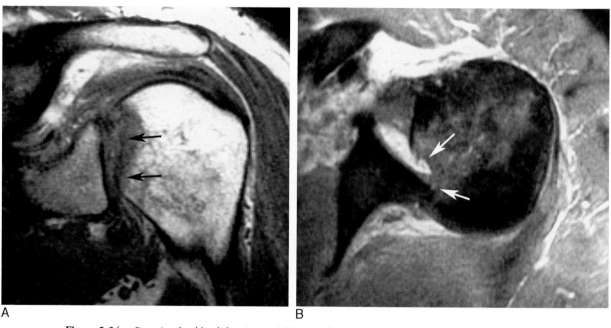

Figure 5-24 Posterior shoulder dislocation on MRI. **A and B,** Coronal T1-weighted (A) and axial fat-suppressed T2-weighted (B) MR images show posterior dislocation with impaction fracture *(arrows)* and adjacent marrow edema.

The coracohumeral arch also limits superior humeral head subluxation. Dynamic mechanisms include compressive force applied by the rotator cuff and biceps long head tendons.

Shoulder instability, or more precisely glenohumeral instability, is a tendency of the humeral head to sublux or dislocate. Glenohumeral instability can occur in any direction, but the most common pattern is anterior instability. *Anterior instability* is usually the consequence of prior anterior shoulder dislocation, with disruption of the anterior shoulder stabilizers, as discussed previously. Recurrent anterior dislocations are a classic feature of anterior instability. However, a history of dislocation is not present in all individuals with anterior instability.

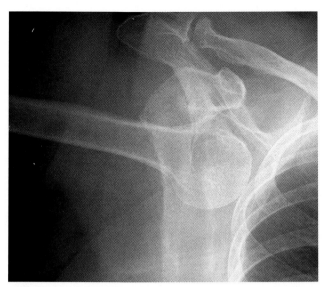

Figure 5-25 Luxatio erecti. The humeral head is dislocated inferiorly with the humerus locked in abduction.

Treatment of anterior instability is usually surgical. The goal is to restore normal anatomy by repairing the damaged structures. If this is not possible, or if the original anatomy was not sufficiently stable, the orthopedic surgeon may choose from a variety of procedures that enhance shoulder stability by tightening the joint capsule or shortening the subscapularis muscle.

Posterior instability, like posterior dislocation that may precede it, is relatively rare. MR findings include disruption of the posterior labrum, lax posterior joint capsule, and interruption of the posterior band of the inferior GHL (reverse Bankart lesion). Treatment is also surgical. The *Bennett lesion* is a rim of calcification immediately posterior to the posterior osseous glenoid rim that is associated with posterior labral injuries and posterior rotator cuff injuries. The calcification, best demonstrated by CT, is thought to represent an enthesophyte in the posterior band of the inferior GHL.

Multidirectional instability is glenohumeral joint laxity due to a lax joint capsule, often exacerbated by poorly coordinated action of the rotator cuff muscles. This condition is frequently bilateral, and most patients are young. Generalized joint laxity throughout the body may be present. Humeral head subluxation can result in pain, labral injuries, and rotator cuff impingement. Imaging findings are often absent, although the labrum may be small and the capsule lax and redundant. Treatment consists of rotator cuff strengthening exercises. Surgical tightening of the joint capsule is sometimes needed.

Labral Tears

Discussion of labral tears is included with the discussion of shoulder dislocation and instability because most labral tears occur in association with these conditions. Anterior labral tears associated with anterior dislocation were discussed previously. The Bankart lesion is the classic example of a labral tear caused by shoulder dislocation. However, labral tears can occur in the absence of shoulder instability. For example, only about 20% of superior labral anterior and posterior (SLAP) tears are associated with shoulder instability.

Key Concepts	Labral Tear

MR or CT arthrography
Contrast in tear
Pitfalls:
    Normal variants: Sublabral foramen between 1 o'clock and
      3 o'clock; sublabral sulcus in superior labrum; Buford
      complex; irregular labral margins
    Normal finding of articular cartilage between labrum and
      glenoid
    Magic angle effect
    Partial labral detachments may be incidental in older
      individuals

Imaging diagnosis of labral tears is complicated by the normal variation of labral shape and fixation to the glenoid, particularly the anterior-superior labrum as discussed previously. The normal labrum has low signal intensity on all MRI sequences. Magic angle effect results in increased signal intensity on short TE sequences in portions of the labrum oriented 55 degrees from the bore of the magnet. Linear or amorphous high signal intensity suggests a labral tear. Direct CT and MR arthrography are superior to conventional MRI in revealing a labral tear because contrast flows into the tear, increasing its conspicuity. Both CT and MR arthrography also are the best imaging studies to demonstrate a labral detachment. Detection of an anterior labral tear is slightly improved by placing the arm in the "ABER" position (ABduction and External Rotation), by placing the patient's forearm behind his or her head. This position pushes the humeral head against the anterior labrum, which can "pry open" an anterior labral tear (Fig. 5-26).

WHAT THE CLINICIAN WANTS TO KNOW:
LABRAL TEAR
Location (clock face with anterior at 3 o'clock, also relative
  to biceps tendon)
Displacement

SLAP tears are tears of the biceps labral complex (Fig. 5-27). The superior labrum, proximal biceps tendon, and biceps attachment to the labrum are variably involved. Many SLAP

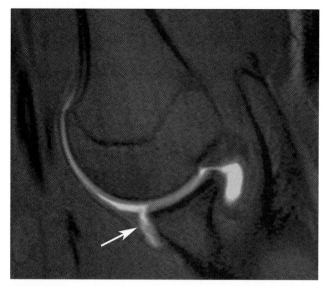

Figure 5-26 Abduction and external rotation (ABER) position to enhance detection of anterior labral tear. MR arthrogram obtained with the arm in ABER position shows an anterior tear *(arrow)*.

following classification system is used: Type 1 SLAP tears are degenerative superior labral fraying, with a normal biceps tendon. Type 2 is superior labral and biceps tendon avulsion. Type 3 is a superior labral bucket handle tear, with a normal biceps tendon attached to the torn labrum. Type 4 is a labral bucket handle tear that extends into the biceps tendon. A SLAP tear can extend beyond the superior labrum and adjacent biceps into the anterior labrum, posterior labrum, or the GHLs (Fig. 5-28). There are evolving, competing arthroscopic classification systems of these more extensive tears.

Key Concepts	SLAP Tear

Superior labral anterior and posterior
Usually oriented from superior-lateral to inferior-medial
Pitfalls: Sublabral recess—follows contour of articular
  cartilage, oriented from superior-medial to inferior-lateral

tears occur after a forced extension injury or during rapid arm abduction during a fall. SLAP tears also occur or during the deceleration phase of throwing, and are an occupational hazard of throwing athletes such as baseball pitchers. The

Type 1 tears have amorphously increased signal in the superior labrum on oblique coronal MR images. This can be normal finding in older patients, especially those with a

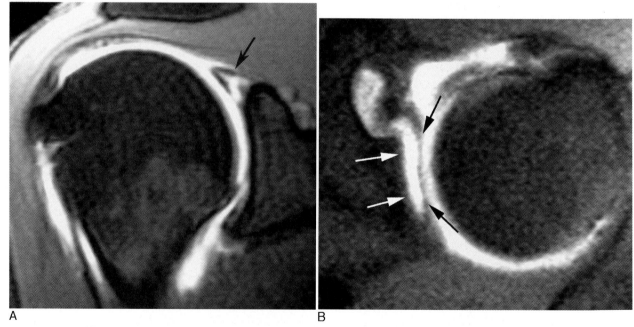

A   B

Figure 5-27 Superior labral anterior and posterior (SLAP) tears in different patients. **A,** Oblique coronal fat-suppressed T1-weighted MR arthrogram shows high signal intensity within the superior labrum oriented toward the acromion *(arrow)*. Other images (not shown) demonstrated that this pattern extended into the posterior superior labrum, consistent with a SLAP tear. **B,** Axial T2-weighted saline arthrogram image obtained at the level of the inferior margin of the superior labrum in a different patient shows fluid tracking between the labrum *(black arrows)* and the glenoid *(white arrows)*. The separation of the labrum and the glenoid extends posteriorly to the 10 o'clock position and therefore is likely to represent a SLAP tear rather than a sublabral sulcus.

(Continued)

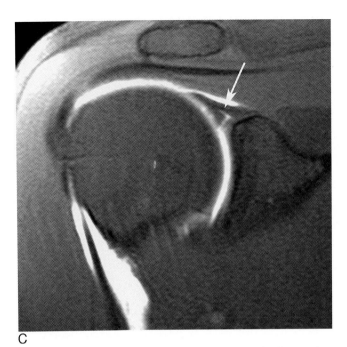

C

Figure 5-27—(Cont'd)   C, Oblique coronal T1-weighted MR arthrogram shows a subtle SLAP tear *(arrow)* dissecting between the labrum and the biceps undersurface. See also Fig. 5-8A: Can you see the SLAP tear?

chronically high-riding shoulder, such as those occurring with chronic rotator cuff tear. All other SLAP tears show a discrete defect in the superior labrum that extends from anterior to posterior, which must be distinguished from the normal variant, sublabral sulcus, discussed previously (Fig. 4-20). The radio-

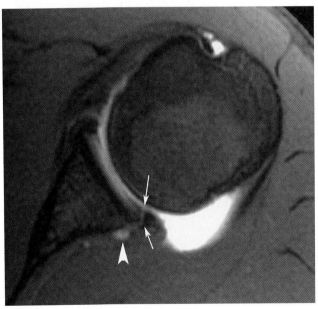

Figure 5-28   Posterior labral tear. Axial fat-suppressed T1-weighted MR arthrogram shows a subtle tear *(arrows)*, confirmed by finding of contrast medium in an adjacent paralabral cyst *(arrowhead)*.

logist's main role is to decide if any SLAP tear is present. On oblique coronal MR images, the normal variant sulcus is typically oriented in a superomedial to inferior lateral direction (toward the patient's head). In contrast, many (but not all) SLAP tears are oriented in a superior-lateral to inferior-medial direction (toward the acromion). Also, the normal variant sublabral sulcus should not extend posterior to the biceps anchor, usually not posterior to the 11 o'clock position. A third useful finding concerns the width: a defect wider than 2 to 3 mm usually indicates a SLAP tear rather than a sulcus.

Magnetic resonance arthrography is much more sensitive than plain MRI in detection of SLAP tears. Sensitivity is improved by scanning with the arm in external rotation or under caudally oriented traction. These techniques apply traction to the superior labrum transmitted through the biceps long head tendon. Even with a cooperative patient and the best scanning technique, not all SLAP tears are visible on MRI or MR or CT arthrography.

POSTOPERATIVE SHOULDER

Imaging of the previously operated shoulder presents special challenges. Normal tissue planes are disrupted, and artifact from suture anchors, hardware, and micrometal debris can be extensive. Such artifacts can be minimized with use of fast spin-echo sequences without chemical fat suppression. Conventional and CT arthrography are not affected by micrometal artifact. Suture anchors can incite a granulomatous reaction or displace into the joint or adjacent soft tissues (Fig. 5-29). Detection of rotator cuff and labral retear is enhanced with MR or CT arthrography (Figs. 5-30, 5-31).

MISCELLANEOUS SHOULDER CONDITIONS

Osteochondral injuries of the shoulder include bony Bankart and reverse Bankart injuries, already discussed, and the glenolabral articular disruption (see Fig. 5-21F). Although the shoulder is not a weight-bearing joint, considerable loads are placed across the shoulder joint during abduction, and osteochondritis dissecans or articular cartilage injuries may result. Most articular cartilage defects of the glenohumeral joint occur in the setting of osteoarthritis. The subscapularis muscle occasionally avulses the lesser tuberosity.

Shoulder arthroplasty is performed for painful arthritis or severe humeral head fractures. A humeral hemiarthroplasty is often used, although a glenoid component may also be placed (see Fig. 24-16).

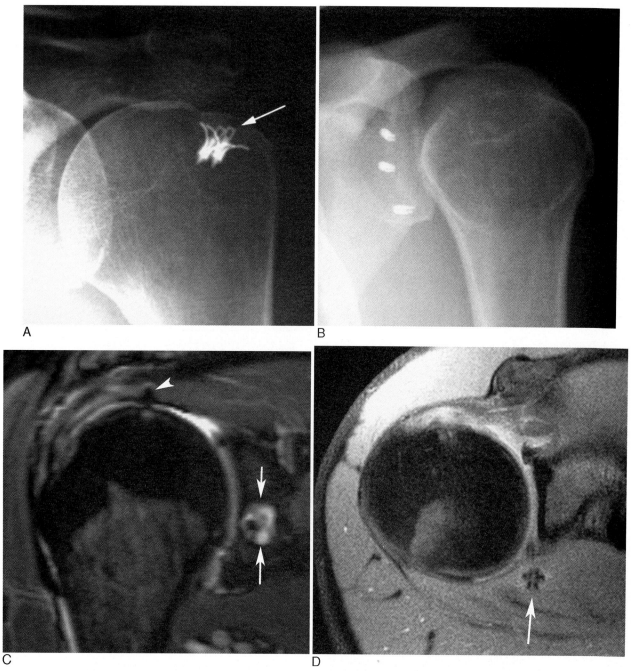

Figure 5-29 Suture anchors and tacks. **A,** Rotator cuff repair with metallic suture anchors in the greater tuberosity *(arrow)*. The suture anchors provide a site to reattach the torn supraspinatus tendon. **B,** Anterior capsular repair. The suture anchors were placed in the anterior glenoid, to allow reattachment of a stripped anterior capsule and labrum. **C,** Suture anchor complications after anterior capsule repair. Sagittal fat-suppressed T2-weighted MR image shows fluid signal surrounding low signal of a suture anchor *(arrows)*, representing a granulomatous reaction. Metallic anchors have been supplanted by various radiolucent bioabsorbable polymers, some prone to granulomatous reaction. Also note a displaced suture anchor above the humeral head, partially within the rotator cuff *(arrowhead)*. **D,** Axial fat-suppressed T2-weighted MR image in a different patient shows a bioabsorbable tack that has dissected into the infraspinatus *(arrow)*.

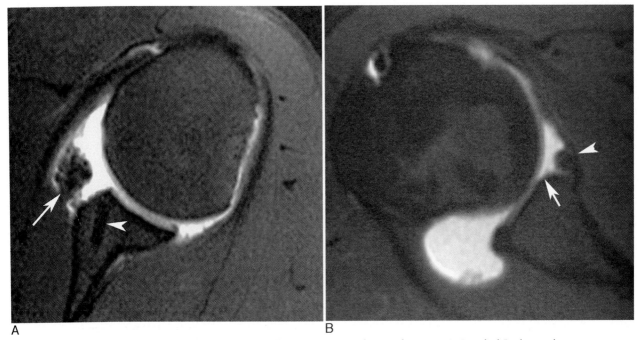

A   B

Figure 5-30 Failed Bankart repairs in different patients. Axial MR arthrograms. **A,** Detached Bankart and labral fragment. Note suture anchor seen as subtle linear low signal in the glenoid *(arrowhead).* **B,** ALPSA (anterior labral periosteal sleeve avulsion)-like recurrent Bankart lesion *(arrowhead),* with avulsion of anterior glenoid cartilage *(arrow).* Note anterior subluxation of the humeral head. Recall that ALPSA lesions are usually associated with anterior instability.

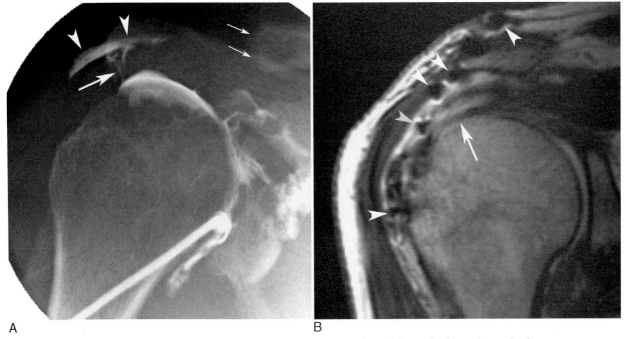

A   B

Figure 5-31 Rotator cuff retears after repair. **A,** Spot image obtained during shoulder arthrography shows contrast medium passing through a small rotator cuff perforation *(arrow)* into the subacromial subdeltoid bursa *(arrowheads).* Also note the prior distal clavicle resection *(small arrows)* and small acromion. **B,** Coronal T1-weighted MR arthrogram shows tear with retraction *(arrow).* Note low signal artifacts *(arrowheads)* caused by sutures or minute metal fragments.

CHAPTER 6

Elbow

IMAGING TECHNIQUES
ELBOW ANATOMY
ELBOW FRACTURES IN CHILDREN
ELBOW FRACTURES IN ADULTS
ELBOW LIGAMENTS AND TENDONS
MISCELLANEOUS ELBOW INJURIES
FOREARM

IMAGING TECHNIQUES

Radiographic evaluation of the traumatized elbow should include at least anteroposterior (AP) and lateral views, the latter obtained with the elbow flexed 90 degrees to assess for a joint effusion. Anteroposterior oblique views can increase detection of subtle fractures. An oblique radial head view is useful if a radial head fracture is suspected. Ultrasonography (US) can depict joint effusion and many fractures of unossified cartilage in children. Arthrography, although now rarely used, demonstrates full-thickness collateral ligament tears and some articular surface partial-thickness collateral ligament tears, as well as some chondral defects. Arthrography also can characterize chondral fractures in children and assist in characterizing osteochondritis dissecans lesions for fragment stability. Computed tomography (CT) is useful for characterizing complex articular fractures and post-traumatic complications in adults, such as intra-articular bodies, osteophytes, and fracture fragment malalignment. Computed tomographic arthrography combines the advantages of conventional arthrography and CT and offers superior assessment of intra-articular bodies and chondral defects.

Magnetic resonance imaging (MRI) of the elbow usually is performed with the elbow extended. Use of a surface coil that allows the elbow to be scanned at the patient's side enhances patient comfort but places the elbow away from the "sweet spot" of the magnet isocenter. Positioning the elbow in the center of the magnet with the arm fully abducted (elbow above the patient's head) is an alternative if off-axis imaging is unsuc-

cessful. A high-resolution coronal sequence can help in assessing the collateral ligaments. Magnetic resonance arthrography is the preferred technique for assessment of collateral ligament injury in athletes. Chondral and osteochondral lesions can be evaluated with CT arthrography or MR arthrography.

ELBOW ANATOMY

The elbow joint is enclosed by a single synovial compartment that includes the articulations of the radial head with the humeral capitellum, the proximal ulna with the humeral trochlea, the proximal radioulnar joint, and related muscles and connective tissues. The ulnar nerve is located posterior to the medial humeral epicondyle in a small groove medial to the olecranon, a superficial location that exposes this nerve to trauma. The radial and median nerves are anterior to the joint.

Key Concepts	Normal Elbow Radiographic Anatomy

AP view checklist:
   Radial head aligned with capitellum
   Ulna aligned with trochlea
   Radial head articulates with ulna
   Normal valgus ("carrying angle") approximately 165
     degrees
   Children: Ossification centers normally positioned
Lateral view checklist:
   Fat pad sign (effusion)
   Radial head aligned with capitellum
   Anterior humeral line intersects middle third of capitellum
   Ulna congruent with trochlea

The normal radiographic anatomy of the elbow is illustrated in Figure 6-1. The distal humeral shaft widens medially and laterally to form the epicondyles. The lateral epicondyle is the

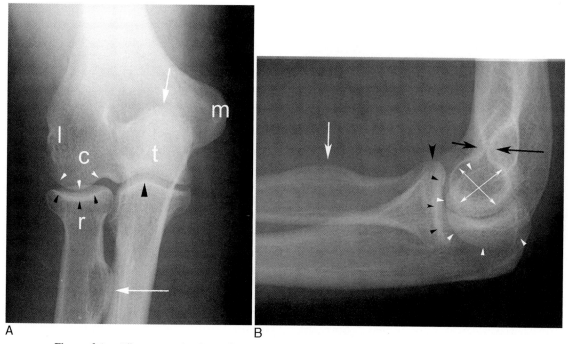

Figure 6-1   Elbow: normal radiographic anatomy. **A,** AP view. **B,** Lateral view. Small black arrowheads, radial head proximal articular surface; small white arrowheads, capitellum articular surface; large black arrowhead, coronoid process of the ulna; short white arrow, olecranon process of the ulna; long white arrow, radial tuberosity (insertion site of biceps); short black arrow (part B only), coronoid fossa; long black arrow (part B only), olecranon fossa; white double arrows (part B only), trochlea. c, capitellum; l, lateral epicondyle; r, radial neck; m, medial epicondyle; t, trochlea (superimposed over the olecranon).

common origin of the wrist extensor (dorsiflexor) muscles, and the medial epicondyle is the common origin of the wrist flexor muscles. The humeral condyles are the rounded capitellum laterally and the V-shaped trochlea medially. The condyles are anteriorly positioned relative to the epicondyles. As seen on a lateral radiograph, a line drawn along the anterior humeral shaft cortex, the *anterior humeral line,* normally passes through the middle third of the capitellum (Fig. 6-2). Variation from this arrangement is evidence for a fracture. The distal humerus has concavities on both its anterior and posterior surfaces. The shallow coronoid fossa anteriorly accommodates the ulnar coronoid process during elbow flexion. The deeper olecranon fossa posteriorly accommodates the ulnar olecranon process during elbow extension. A normal variant foramen may connect the coronoid and olecranon fossae.

The cylindrical radial head articulates with the rounded capitellum and the concave lateral margin of the proximal ulna. A line drawn through the center of the radial shaft should bisect the capitellum on any view (see Fig. 6-2). This line is called the *radiocapitellar line.* If this line does not bisect the capitellum, then a radial dislocation is present. The radial tuberosity on the proximal medial radial shaft is the insertion site of the biceps tendon. This medial insertion allows the biceps to function as a wrist supinator (turns palm forward) as well as an elbow flexor. When viewed *en face,* the radial tuberosity may simulate an aggressive lytic lesion (Fig. 6-3). The characteristic location of this finding and the exophytic contour on an orthogonal view reveal the normal nature of this finding.

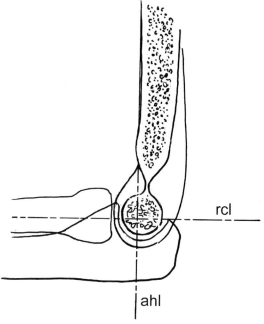

Figure 6-2   Radiocapitellar and anterior humeral lines. The anterior humeral line is drawn along the anterior cortex of the humeral shaft cortex. If this line does not pass through the middle of the capitellum, then a fracture is likely. The radiocapitellar line is drawn along the center radial shaft. If this line does not bisect the capitellum, then a radial head dislocation or subluxation is present. This diagram also illustrates the normal relationship of the trochlea (seen in cross-section) and the ulna. Note that the capitellum articular surface projects slightly anterior to the trochlea. ahl, anterior humeral line; rcl, radiocapitellar line.

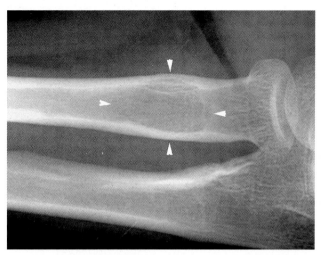

Figure 6-3   Pseudolesion of the proximal radius *(arrowheads)* caused by the normal appearance of the radial tuberosity when seen *en face*.

The proximal ulna includes the olecranon process posteriorly and the coronoid process anteriorly, and broad articular contact with the humeral trochlea. A small notch-like defect or groove may be seen on the ulnar articular surface, usually appreciated only on MR images, at the base of the coronoid process (Fig. 6-4). A similar pseudodefect may be noted on the dorsal capitellum (Fig. 6-5). The triceps tendon inserts on the posterior olecranon (see Fig. 6-4B). Distal triceps injury and avulsion of the triceps tendon insertion are often clinically apparent, but MRI can assist in determining the extent of injury.

The "carrying angle" is the angle formed by the humerus and the ulna in the coronal plane when the elbow is extended. The normal fully extended elbow joint is in about 165 degrees of valgus alignment, slightly greater in women and less in men. (Think of this as allowing the upper extremity to match the contour of the waist and hips with the arms at one's side.) A related angle in children is *Baumann's angle,* formed by the humeral shaft and the capitellar physis (Fig. 6-6). *Cubitus varus* is an abnormally increased carrying angle (i.e., loss of valgus), and *cubitus valgus* is an abnormally decreased carrying angle (i.e., too much valgus).

The subcutaneous olecranon bursa overlies the olecranon process and is the most common site of bursitis in the body. Olecranon bursitis, whether due to direct trauma, hemorrhage, or inflammatory process (e.g., rheumatoid arthritis or acute gout), causes pain and swelling over the olecranon process (Fig. 6-7). The extensor surface of the elbow and proximal forearm is one of the more common sites of rheumatoid nodules.

A fat pad normally resides within the olecranon fossa when the elbow is flexed. This fat pad is normally not visible on lateral radiographs obtained with 90-degree elbow flexion because it is superimposed on the dense bone of the distal ulna. However, a hemarthrosis or any other process that distends the joint capsule (joint effusion, pus, pannus, pigmented villonodular synovitis) can displace this fat pad

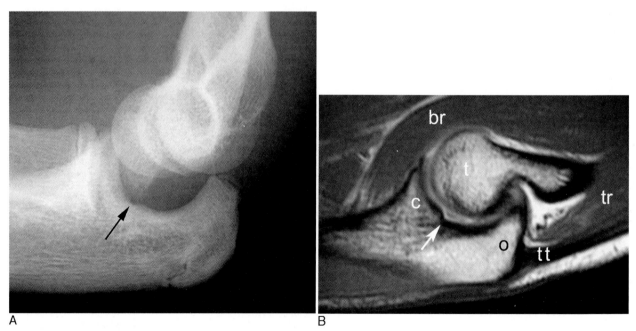

A   B

Figure 6-4   Normal variant "pseudodefect" of the ulna at the base of the olecranon process. **A,** Lateral radiograph in a patient with an elbow dislocation shows a small notch-like defect in the subchondral bone at the base of the coronoid process *(arrow)*. **B,** Sagittal T1-weighted MR arthrogram also demonstrates the normal variant pseudodefect *(arrow)*. This image also illustrates normal anatomy. br, brachialis muscle; c, coronoid process; o, olecranon; t, trochlea; tr, triceps muscle; tt, triceps tendon.

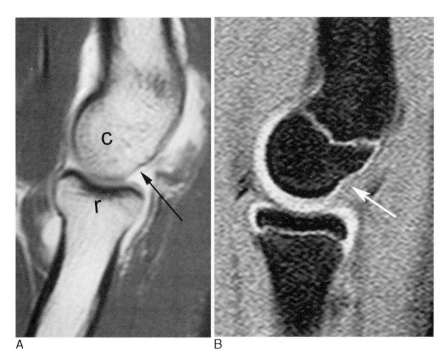

A   B

Figure 6-5 Normal "pseudodefect" of the capitellum. **A,** Sagittal T1-weighted MR arthrogram from the same study as shown in Fig. 6-4A shows a shallow concave "defect" in the dorsal capitellum *(arrow).* **B,** Sagittal fat-suppressed spoiled gradient echo sequence in a child shows the same finding *(arrow).* This normal variant should not be confused with an osteochondral defect. C, capitellum; r, radial head.

superiorly and posteriorly out of the olecranon fossa, producing the *posterior fat pad sign* on a lateral radiograph (Figs. 6-8, 6-9). A separate fat pad *anterior* to the distal humerus is a normal finding on lateral radiographs. The anterior fat pad normally has a straight anterior contour. A joint effusion can cause this fat pad to bulge anteriorly, creating the "spinnaker sail sign" or "anterior fat pad sign." The anterior fat pad sign is more sensitive, but less specific for the presence of elbow joint distention than the posterior fat pad sign. In the setting of acute trauma, a posterior fat pad sign in an adult nearly always indicates that a fracture is present. This finding is less specific in children because soft tissue injuries may cause an effusion. The absence of a fat pad sign does not exclude a significant injury, as a distal humeral fracture may be extra-articular, and a severe injury can lacerate the joint capsule and

Figure 6-6 Measurement of Baumann's angle in children. Two lines are drawn, one along the shaft of the ulna, and one parallel to the distal humeral physis along the proximal capitellum. The angle formed is measured as shown in the diagram. Both sides are compared. A difference greater than 5 degrees is considered significant and may alter therapy. An increase in Baumann's angle indicates varus alignment, and a decrease indicates valgus alignment. c, capitellum; r, radius; u, ulna.

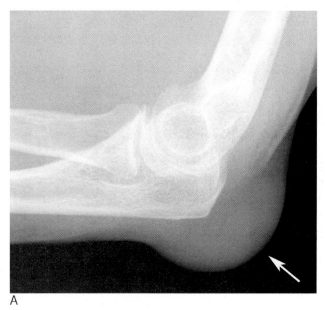

A

Figure 6-7 Olecranon bursitis. **A,** Lateral radiograph shows soft tissue swelling centered over the olecranon process *(arrow).* This case was due to hemorrhage into the bursa caused by direct trauma.

(Continued)

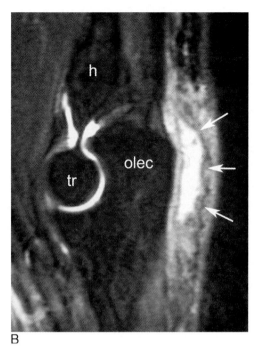

B

Figure 6-7—(Cont'd)   B, Sagittal fat-suppressed T2-weighted MR image in a different patient shows fluid-filled bursa *(arrows)* due to infection. h, distal humeral shaft; olec, olecranon; tr, trochlea.

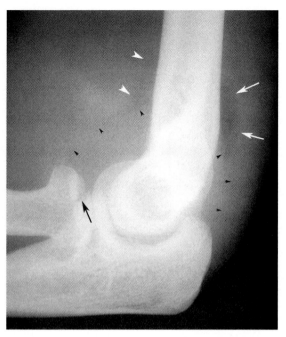

Figure 6-9   Fat pad sign in an adult with a radial head fracture *(black arrow)*. Lateral radiograph shows posterior *(white arrows)* and anterior *(white arrowheads)* fat pad signs due to hemarthrosis. Black arrowheads mark the distended joint capsule.

allow a hemarthrosis to decompress into the extra-articular soft tissues.

The *os supratrochleare dorsale* is a small ossicle that resides in the olecranon fossa. Although generally considered to be a normal variant, the os supratrochleare dorsale can cause impingement and pain during elbow extension. An intra-articular osseous body can have an identical appearance and also may cause impingement (see Fig. 2-3B). The distinction is not

important because a symptomatic ossicle will be removed and an asymptomatic ossicle generally will not.

A *supracondylar process,* or avian spur, is a rare (about 1 in 200 people) developmental variant, seen as a bony excrescence on the anterior-medial distal humeral shaft (Fig. 6-10). An

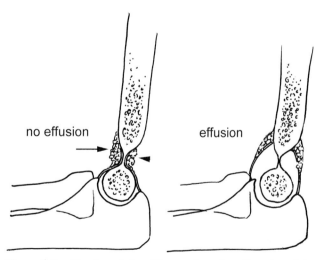

Figure 6-8   The fat pad sign. Diagram shows how distention of the elbow joint capsule displaces the posterior fat pad *(arrowhead)* out of the olecranon fossa, making it visible on a lateral view, and distorts the anterior fat pad *(arrow)*, potentially causing it to have a convex margin anteriorly, known as the "spinnaker sail sign."

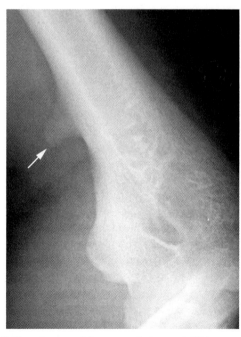

Figure 6-10   Supracondylar process (avian spur). This normal variant bony excrescence *(arrow)* projects anteriorly and slightly medially from the distal humeral shaft.

associated ligament of Struthers can connect the supracondylar process to the medial humeral epicondyle, where it may entrap the median nerve.

ELBOW FRACTURES IN CHILDREN

Most elbow fractures in children are the result of a fall on an outstretched hand. Compression injuries are unusual, but the axial load can result in forced hyperextension or valgus. Hyperextension can cause the ulna to lever against the distal humerus like a bottle opener removing a bottle cap (Fig. 6-11). This mechanism causes the most common elbow fracture of children, the *supracondylar fracture,* which is a transverse fracture of the distal humerus proximal to the humeral condyles (Fig. 6-12). Supracondylar fractures can range from obvious to subtle on radiographs, but two cardinal signs are often present: a posterior fat pad sign and posterior displacement of the capitellum relative to the anterior humeral line (Fig. 6-12B). Alignment on the AP radiograph should also be assessed for evidence of abnormal cubitus valgus or varus because either of these findings may alter therapy. Comparison with the contralateral elbow may be required. A quantitative approach is to measure the Baumann's angle formed by the humeral shaft and the capitellar physis (see Fig. 6-6). The injured and uninjured sides are measured. A difference of 5 degrees or more is considered significant.

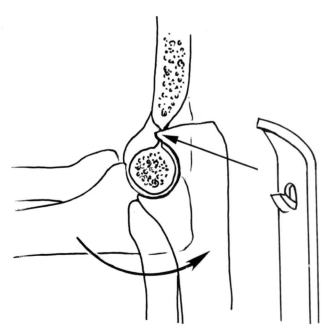

Figure 6-11 Mechanism of the pediatric supracondylar fracture. A fall on an outstretched hand can result in elbow hyperextension, especially in children since they have lax ligaments and more flexible joints. Hyperextension concentrates tension and shearing force across the relatively weak supracondylar distal humerus, analogous to the leverage applied to a bottle cap by a bottle opener, resulting in fracture with apex anterior angulation.

Key Concepts	Elbow Fractures in Children

Fat pad sign is usually present, but is less sensitive and specific for fracture than in adults
Supracondylar (65%):
    Fall on an outstretched hand causes elbow hyperextension
    Abnormal anterior humeral line
Medial epicondylar avulsion (10%):
    Fall on an outstretched hand causes valgus stress
    Possible entrapment—don't miss it!
    Little leaguer's elbow is chronic avulsive injury to medial epicondyle physis
Lateral condylar (15%):
    Lateral fall with arm at side causes varus stress across elbow
    May be incomplete, involving only part of the physis
    Most involve lateral metaphysis (at least Salter-Harris II fracture)
    Often occurs in younger children with unossified epiphyseal cartilage; rare Salter-Harris IV variant may therefore be underestimated on radiographs; US or MRI can show fractures through unossified cartilage and assist in determining whether fracture extends to the articular surface
Separation of the condyles from the metaphysis
    Usually Salter-Harris I fracture, may be Salter-Harris II fracture
    Infants: Birth injury, child abuse
    Toddlers: Child abuse, twisting injuries
Radial head dislocation:
    Congenital
    Jerked (nursemaid's) elbow

Fractures of the lateral humeral condyle are the second most common type of elbow fracture in children. Lateral condyle fractures are caused by varus stress. Varus stress across the elbow may be produced when there is a lateral blow to the forearm or when a child falls laterally with the arm at the child's side. Varus stress causes distraction force across the lateral side of the elbow that can result in an avulsion-like fracture that may be complete or incomplete. Typically, these fractures extend along or across the lateral distal humeral physis, usually with a small metaphyseal fragment (Fig. 6-13). The distal extent of the fracture is more variable. If incomplete, the fracture may not extend beyond the physis, or the fracture may extend distally into the lateral condyle, either through the ossified portion of the capitellum (true Salter-Harris IV fracture) or, far more frequently, medial to the capitellum through unossified cartilage (Fig. 6-14). Incomplete lateral condyle fractures generally are stable and are treated with casting. However, if the fracture line continues distally to the articular surface, the fracture is complete. Complete lateral condyle fractures generally are unstable and require operative fixation. Distinguishing a complete fracture from an incomplete fracture can be difficult because most of the

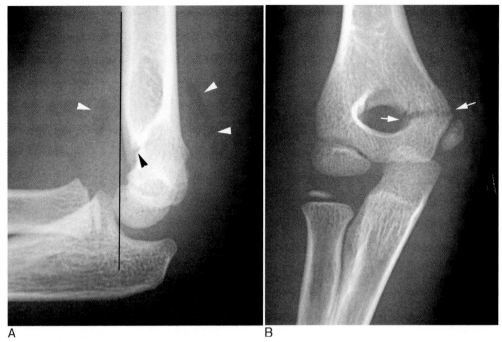

Figure 6-12   Displaced supracondylar fracture. **A,** Lateral radiographic view shows displaced anterior and posterior fat pads *(white arrowheads)* and posterior displacement of the capitellar growth center relative to the anterior humeral line. A portion of the fracture line is faintly seen *(black arrowhead)*. **B,** AP view shows the lateral aspect of the fracture line. The AP view of a supracondylar fracture often does not show the fracture. Careful attention to the appearance of the fat pads and alignment on the lateral view is necessary to make the diagnosis.

fracture extends through unossified cartilage and is therefore not visible on radiographs. Additional imaging with US, MRI, or intraoperative assessment with arthrography is often needed.

Valgus stress can result in *avulsion of the medial epicondyle ossification center* (Figs. 6-15–6-17). This injury can occur as an acute avulsion with obvious displacement, or as a chronic stress injury due to repetitive traction known as *little leaguer's elbow,* which is discussed later in this chapter. Valgus stress causes traction on the medial epicondyle by the strong medial collateral ligament and the wrist flexor-pronator muscle group. The medial epicondyle physis is the weakest link of the elbow medial stabilizers, so it yields before the other structures are injured. The avulsed medial epicondyle is displaced distally by the pull of the medial collateral ligament and the flexor-pronator muscles. Radiographs reveal displacement of the medial epicondyle ossification center, which may be subtle and require comparison with the uninjured side for confident diagnosis, or may be obvious and require no further imaging. A hemarthrosis may not be present because the injury can be entirely extra-articular. Either US or MRI can be helpful in diagnosing avulsion of an unossified medial epicondyle in a younger child. Prompt healing with normal function is achieved simply by placing the arm in a sling, although radiographs often reveal persistent widening and irregularity of the injured physis. Surgical repair is generally reserved for high-level athletes or elbow instability. Displacement of the medial epicondyle by greater than 5 mm is more likely to require fixation.

An important variant of medial epicondyle ossification center avulsion is *medial epicondyle entrapment.* The elbow may transiently dislocate posterolaterally during a medial epicondylar avulsion. The medial aspect of the elbow joint may open transiently, allowing the avulsed medial epicondyle fragment to slip between the trochlea and ulna, where it becomes

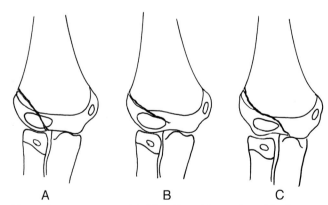

Figure 6-13   Diagram of childhood lateral humeral condylar fractures. **A,** True Salter-Harris IV fracture with osseous fracture of the capitellar growth center. **B,** Incomplete fracture with extension into the condylar cartilage. The fracture line might also terminate within the physis without extension into the condylar cartilage. **C,** Complete fracture through the condylar cartilage. This fracture can be difficult to diagnose with radiographs. This pattern is more common than seen in part A and is also potentially unstable.

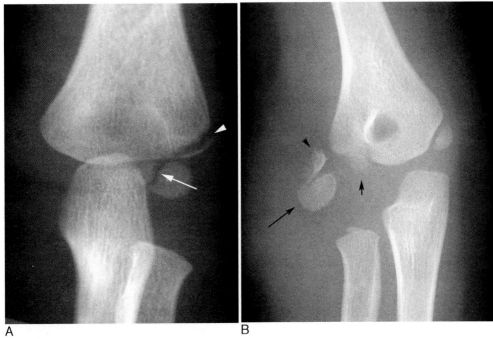

Figure 6-14   Lateral condylar fractures. **A,** Salter-Harris IV fracture. AP radiograph shows the fracture extending through the distal lateral metaphysis *(arrowhead)* and the capitellar growth center *(arrow)*, similar to Figure 6-13A. **B,** Complete fracture. The fragment is displaced laterally and rotated. Note the small metaphyseal fragment *(arrowhead)* and the capitellar growth center *(long arrow)*. Although the capitellar growth center appears to be intact on this view, there is a small nondisplaced capitellar fragment *(short arrow)*. Also note the extensive lateral soft tissue swelling. (Part B courtesy of L. Das Narla, MD.)

entrapped after the humerus and ulna attempt to return to their normal positions (see Figs. 6-15, 6-17). Rapid identification of this condition is essential because an entrapped medial epicondyle will fuse to the ulna within a few weeks, resulting in permanent disability. Radiographs of medial epicondylar entrapment may be deceptive: A fat pad sign may not be present, and the entrapped medial epicondylar ossification center may simulate a normal trochlear ossification center if the trochlea is unossified. Knowledge of the normal maturation of the elbow ossification centers is necessary to avoid this pitfall. The order of appearance on radiographs of the six ossification centers of the elbow may be recalled with the mnemonic CRITOE (Fig. 6-18). The *C*apitellum begins to ossify at about age 1 year, followed by the *R*adial head after

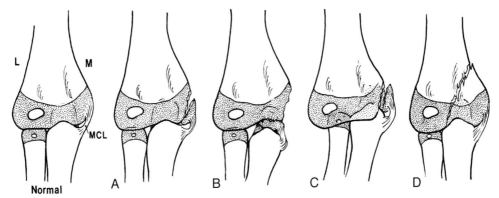

Figure 6-15   Diagram shows types of fractures involving medial epicondyle in children. Right elbow is illustrated. **A,** Simple avulsion of medial epicondyle. **B,** Avulsion with entrapment of medial epicondyle between ulna and trochlea. **C,** Avulsion in association with elbow dislocation. **D,** Salter-Harris IV fracture of medial humeral condyle. M, medial; L, lateral; MCL, medial collateral ligament. (Reprinted with permission from May DA, Disler DG, Jones EA, Pearce DA: Using sonography to diagnose an unossified medial epicondyle avulsion in a child. AJR 174:1115–1117, 2000. Modified with permission from Rogers LF: Radiology of Skeletal Trauma. New York, Churchill Livingstone, 1992, pp 772–779).

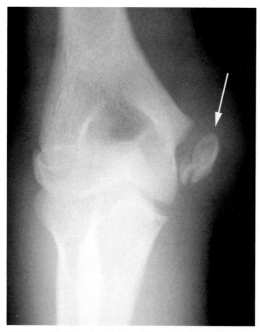

Figure 6-16   Medial epicondyle avulsion AP radiograph shows medial and slight distal displacement of the medial epicondyle ossification center *(arrow)*. There is surrounding soft tissue swelling.

age 3 years, followed by the medial ("*I*nternal") epicondyle at about age 4 to 5 years, followed, sometimes closely, by the *T*rochlea at about age 7 to 8 years, followed by the *O*lecranon at age 8 to 10 years, followed by the lateral ("*E*xternal") epicondyle at age 9 to 13 years. Ossification of each center tends to begin a year or two earlier in girls than boys. The exact ages actually are fairly variable and aren't terribly important to memorize. Rather, it is the *order of appearance* of the ossification centers that is important to know. If what appears to be a normal trochlear ossification center is seen without a normally positioned, partially ossified medial epicondylar center, the diagnosis of medial epicondylar entrapment is likely. If this diagnosis is suspected in a younger child, in whom neither the medial epicondyle nor the trochlea has begun to ossify, then US, MRI, or surgical evaluation (which is sometimes combined with intraoperative arthrography) can be used to locate the medial epicondyle.

The term *little leaguer's elbow* is often used generically to describe any traumatic abnormality of the medial epicondyle in a child. A more specific use of this term refers to a chronic repetitive traction injury seen in young baseball pitchers, other throwing athletes, and hockey players. Radiographs reveal displacement, fragmentation, or sclerosis of the medial epicondyle. Because the medial epicondyle is the last elbow secondary ossification center to fuse, little leaguer's elbow can occur late into adolescence (Fig. 6-19).

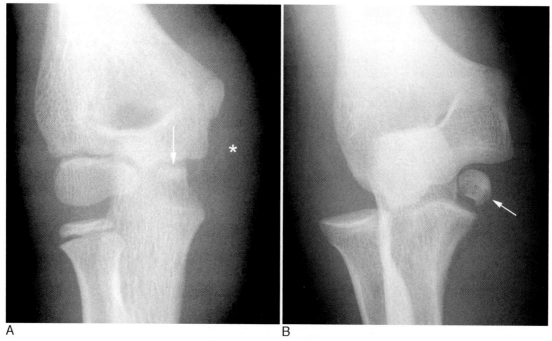

A   B

Figure 6-17   Medial epicondyle entrapment after transient elbow dislocation. **A,** The entrapped medial epicondyle simulates a normal trochlear ossification center *(arrow)*. The medial soft tissue swelling is a clue to the diagnosis, but the important finding is that a normal medial epicondyle growth center is not seen *(asterisk)*. **B,** Entrapped medial epicondyle in an older child after spontaneous partial reduction of an elbow dislocation. Diagnosis in this case is easier than for case shown in part A. Note that all the other ossification centers have fused. The medial epicondyle is the last elbow ossification center to fuse.

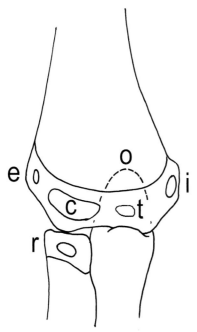

Figure 6-18 Diagram of the order of radiographic appearance of ossification centers around the elbow (CRITOE): c, capitellum; r, radial head; i, medial ("internal") epicondyle; t, trochlea; o, olecranon; e, lateral ("external") epicondyle.

Fracture-separation of the entire distal humeral physis, also termed *separation of the humeral condyles,* is a displaced Salter-Harris I (or rarely Salter-Harris II) fracture of the distal humerus. Displacement is usually medial or posteromedial, in contrast with the posterolateral displacement usually seen in

adult elbow dislocation. Significant force is required, often with a twisting component. This injury can occur during a difficult delivery, and is associated with child abuse in infants and toddlers. Clinical and radiographic diagnosis can be difficult, especially in infants, because the displaced bones are unossified, and the condition is difficult to distinguish from elbow dislocation. Arthrography, US, or MRI can reveal the diagnosis in infants and toddlers. Radiographic diagnosis is easier after the capitellum ossifies because the displacement of the capitellum relative to the humerus and the preserved radiocapitellar alignment can be appreciated.

The elbow is the most frequently traumatically dislocated joint in children younger than age 10 years. Complete dislocation of both the ulna and radius occurs after a fall with the elbow slightly flexed. The radius and ulna usually dislocate posteriorly, although displacement in almost any direction may occur. If only the radial head is dislocated, then a proximal ulnar fracture (Monteggia's fracture) must be excluded (Fig. 6-20). Childhood elbow dislocation can also occur on a congenital basis, either as a sporadic finding (Figs. 6-21, 6-22) or in association with onycho-osteodysplasia (discussed in Chapter 47). In chronic congenital radial head dislocation, the radial head becomes overgrown and dysplastic, allowing easy distinction from a postnatal traumatic dislocation.

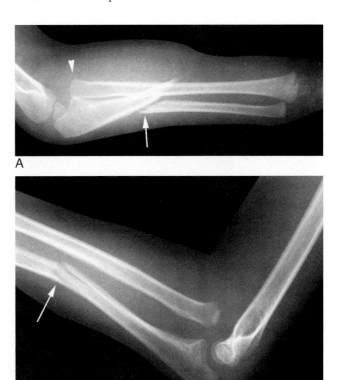

Figure 6-20 Monteggia's fracture dislocation. **A,** Lateral radiographic view of the forearm shows anterior dislocation of the radial head *(arrowhead)* and a fracture of the proximal ulna *(arrow).* **B,** In this case the ulna fracture is a greenstick fracture *(arrow).* (Part B courtesy of L. Das Narla, MD.)

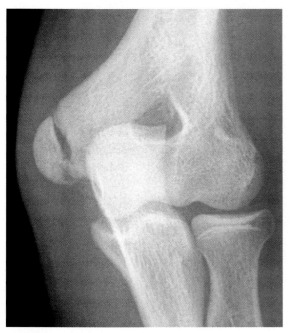

Figure 6-19 Little leaguer's elbow. AP radiograph shows wide physis of the medial epicondyle. This was a chronic, painful finding in a 17-year-old pitcher.

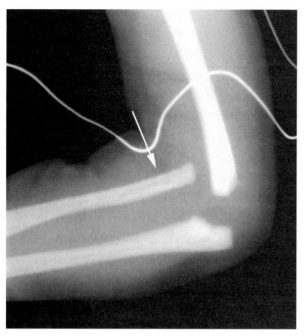

Figure 6-21 Congenital radial head dislocation: neonatal findings. Lateral radiograph in a newborn shows volar displacement of the proximal radius *(arrow)*. The humerus and ulna are normally aligned.

Subluxation of the radial head, also termed *jerked elbow, pulled elbow,* or *nursemaid's elbow,* is anterior subluxation or dislocation of the radial head in a young child with no or only partial disruption of the annular ligament. A distracting force applied to the forearm or hand with the arm extended can allow the radial head to slip out of the collar formed by the annular ligament. Excessive force is not required. The typical child with this condition is between 2 and 3 years of age, although it may occur in older children up to 6 or 7 years of age. Careful scrutiny of radiographs may reveal subtle subluxation of the radial head, but radiographs are frequently normal and, specifically, a fat pad sign is usually absent. Pulled elbow is painful. The child holds the injured elbow in flexion and pronation, and refuses to allow extension. Fortunately, the condition is usually self-limited, with eventual spontaneous reduction of the radial head to its normal position within the annular ligament. Closed reduction by elbow flexion and supination is usually elected for patient comfort. Such reduction may be unintentionally achieved by a radiographer who coaxes the child to flex and supinate her elbow for radiographs.

ELBOW FRACTURES IN ADULTS

A fall on an outstretched hand is the most common cause of radial head and neck fractures in adults. The axial load associated with a fall causes impaction of the capitellum against the radial head. Two patterns are most frequently seen. The first is a single longitudinal fracture line occurring through the proximal articular surface of the radial head, often with distal impaction of a portion of the head (see Fig. 6-9). These fractures can be subtle, but a fat pad sign is almost always present and the area over the radial head is tender. Additional views obtained at different oblique angles may be needed to reveal

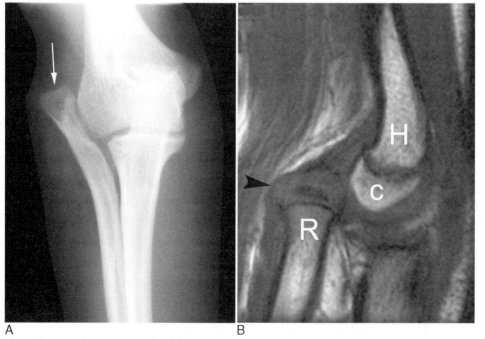

A   B

Figure 6-22 Chronic congenital radial head dislocation. **A,** Radiograph in an older child with congenital radial head dislocation shows lateral dislocation and overgrowth in the form of elongation of the proximal radius. **B,** Sagittal T1-weighted MR image in a different child shows anterior radial head dislocation with mild overgrowth of length and AP size *(arrowhead)*. Note the dysplastic capitellum, with angular contours rather than the normal semi-circular cross section. c, capitellum; H, humerus; R, radial shaft.

the fracture. Treatment is by immobilization with a sling. However, fracture displacement resulting in an articular surface stepoff of 2 mm or greater is associated with development of secondary osteoarthritis, especially if a large portion of the radial head is displaced, so open reduction with internal fixation is sometimes used. The second common fracture pattern is impaction of an intact radial head into the radial neck. The radial head is normal, but it may be angulated relative to the neck (Fig. 6-23). Some radial head fractures are quite subtle radiographically and may be detected on an MRI study performed for elbow pain (Fig. 6-24).

Key Concepts	Elbow Fractures in Adults

Fat pad sign: Sensitive and specific for fracture in the setting of trauma

Radial head and neck (50%):
    May be subtle—get additional views
    Tenderness over radial head
    Associations:
        Fractures: Capitellum, Essex-Lopresti, Monteggia's
        Dislocations

Ulna: Olecranon fracture: may be distracted by triceps pull

Distal humerus:
    Intercondylar T or Y fracture: Comminuted with
        extension into joint through trochlear ridge
    Transcondylar fracture: Older patients with osteoporosis

A comminuted radial head and neck fracture is caused by high-force trauma such as a high-speed motor vehicle crash. This fracture is associated with additional elbow and forearm injuries such as capitellar and coronoid process fractures, elbow dislocation (usually posterior), and the *Essex-Lopresti fracture*. This fracture is an acute tear of the interosseous liga-

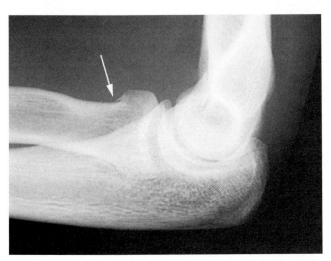

Figure 6-23   Adult impacted radial head fracture with intact articular surface. The fracture is often nondisplaced and therefore subtle *(arrow)*. (See also Fig. 6-9.)

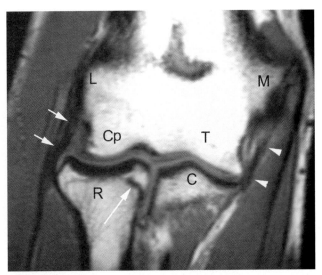

Figure 6-24   Radiographically occult radial head fracture: diagnosis with MRI. Coronal T1-weighted MR image shows an incomplete radial head fracture seen as a low signal line *(long arrow)*. It is not terribly important to diagnose such fractures, so MRI is rarely used. This image also demonstrates normal elbow anatomy. Short arrows, radial collateral ligament; arrowheads, ulnar collateral ligament; C, coronoid process of the ulna; Cp, capitellum (note its normal rounded contour); L, lateral epicondyle; M, medial epicondyle; R, radial head; T, trochlea (note its normal V-shaped contour).

ment of the forearm, comminuted fracture of the radial head and neck, and dislocation of the distal radioulnar joint (Fig. 6-25). It is important to identify this unstable fracture because resection of the radial head and neck fragments, a frequent treatment for comminuted proximal radius fractures, will allow the radial shaft to migrate proximally, resulting in abnormal alignment at the wrist.

Elbow dislocation is less frequent in adults than in children. As in children, the radius and ulna usually dislocate posteriorly, although dislocation in almost any direction may occur. Associated fractures are frequent, and there often is significant associated ligamentous, neurovascular, and muscular injury. Myositis ossificans in the muscles that surround the elbow, notably in the brachialis muscle, is a frequent sequela of elbow dislocation (Fig. 6-26). Prompt reduction of the elbow dislocation reduces the risk of post-traumatic ossification and associated reduced range of motion.

Intra-articular fracture of the olecranon can occur as a result of avulsion of the olecranon process by the triceps tendon (Fig. 6-27). Traction by the triceps displaces the proximal fragment proximally, potentially resulting in wide diastasis. This fracture is treated with internal fixation with an olecranon screw, or wires and a figure-of-eight tension band (see Fig. 6-27B).

Distal humerus fractures in older, osteoporotic patients are often simple transverse fractures. Fractures in younger adults usually also include a longitudinal component in a Y or T configuration. The intra-articular fracture line usually extends through the trochlea. Surgical fixation is required, usually

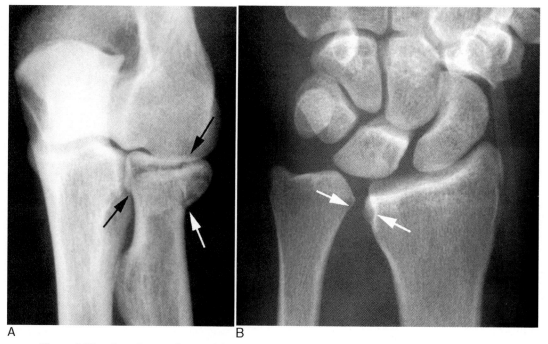

Figure 6-25 Essex-Lopresti fracture dislocation. The elbow (A) shows a comminuted radial head fracture *(arrows)*. The wrist (B) shows distal radioulnar joint dislocation seen as joint widening and distal displacement of the ulna *(arrows)*. The primary injury is an acute tear of the interosseous ligament of the forearm. This is an unstable fracture that requires specialized orthopedic management.

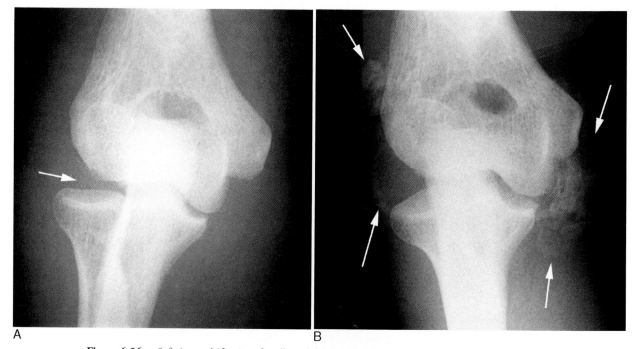

Figure 6-26 Soft tissue calcification after elbow dislocation. **A,** Initial AP radiographic view after reduction of an elbow fracture. Note that the radiocapitellar articulation is wide *(arrow)*, indicating that reduction was not complete. Because this patient sustained a severe neurologic injury, the treating physicians elected not to complete the reduction. **B,** Three weeks later, calcification can be seen around the elbow *(arrows)*. The calcification is due to myositis ossificans and calcification in other soft tissues. The patient's neurologic injury, with associated absence of motion of this joint, probably contributed to the rapidity and severity of the soft tissue calcification.

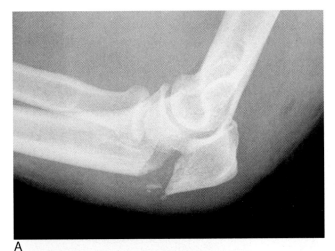

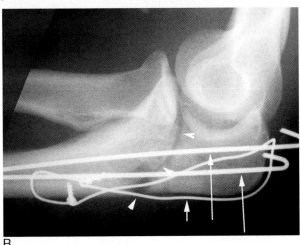

Figure 6-27 Olecranon avulsion. **A,** Transverse fracture due to avulsion by the triceps muscle. **B,** Postoperative appearance in a different patient. Fixation can be accomplished with a longitudinal screw or, as in this case, wires *(long arrows)* with a figure-of-eight tensioning band *(short arrows).* Note the fracture *(arrowheads).*

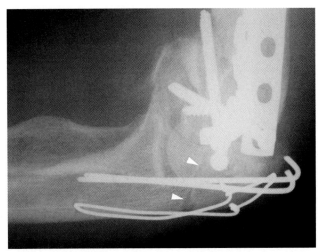

Figure 6-28 Olecranon osteotomy. This patient sustained a comminuted intra-articular distal humerus fracture that required open reduction with internal fixation. An olecranon osteotomy was performed to provide access to the articular surface of the humerus during reduction. The method of fixation of the osteotomy is similar to that used for the olecranon fracture in Fig. 6-27, but note the straight margins of the osteotomy *(arrowheads).* The presence of extensive fixation hardware in the distal humerus provides another clue that the ulna was not fractured.

accomplished with transcondylar screws and medial and lateral plates. An intra-articular approach through an olecranon osteotomy is often used during this repair. The repaired osteotomy is similar in appearance to an internally fixed olecranon fracture, except that an osteotomy has straight, smooth margins (Fig. 6-28).

ELBOW LIGAMENTS AND TENDONS

The major ligaments of the elbow are the *medial or ulnar collateral ligament (MCL) complex,* and the *radial or lateral collateral ligament (LCL) complex* that blends into the *annular ligament* that surrounds the radial head (see Figs. 6-24, 6-29–6-32).

The most important and, fortunately, easiest to image component of the MCL complex is the cord-like *anterior bundle or band* that attaches the medial epicondyle to the anterior medial ulna on the coronoid process (see Figs. 6-24, 6-29). The anterior bundle is sometimes called simply the MCL. The anterior bundle is vulnerable to injury with acute or chronic valgus stress. This ligament is best seen on coronal MR images obtained with the elbow in extension. A normal anterior bundle has sharp margins and low signal intensity on all sequences (see Fig. 6-24). Partial tears or sprains of the anterior bundle are seen on T2-weighted images as increased signal intensity within the ligament. Intra-articular contrast may enter but not pass completely through a partial-thickness tear. Complete tears reveal interruption and possibly laxity of ligament fibers, with escape of joint fluid or injected contrast into the surrounding extra-articular soft tissues (Fig. 6-33).

The other components of the MCL complex are the *posterior bundle* and the *oblique band or transverse ligament* (see Figs. 6-29, 6-32A). The oblique band connects the medial proximal olecranon to the coronoid process just posterior to the anterior bundle insertion. The posterior bundle originates at the medial epicondyle and spreads fan-like to the proximal ulna. The posterior bundle and the oblique band form the floor of the cubital tunnel and thus are adjacent to the ulnar nerve (see Fig. 6-32A). These ligaments are thin and closely apposed to the trochlea and ulna, making them difficult to distinguish as distinct structures even with high-resolution US or MRI. However, tears of these ligaments can be inferred if joint fluid or intra-articular contrast medium escapes from the medial aspect of the elbow with a normal-appearing anterior band.

The LCL extends from the lateral epicondyle in a fan-like configuration to the annular ligament (see Figs. 6-24, 6-30, 6-33). The *lateral ulnar collateral ligament* extends from the posterior aspect of the LCL origin on the lateral epicondyle

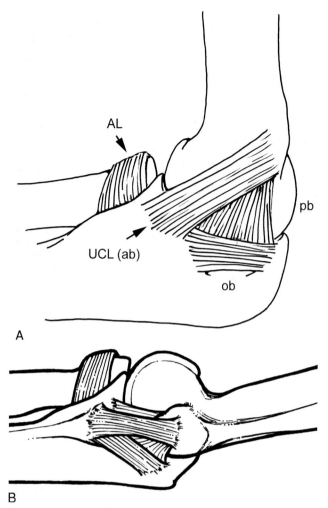

A

B

Figure 6-29 Diagram of medial ligaments of the elbow. **A**, Elbow flexed. **B**, Elbow extended. AL, annular ligament; UCL (ab), ulnar (medial) collateral ligament anterior bundle or band (the strongest and most important component of the UCL); ob, oblique (transverse) band of the UCL; pb, posterior bundle of the UCL.

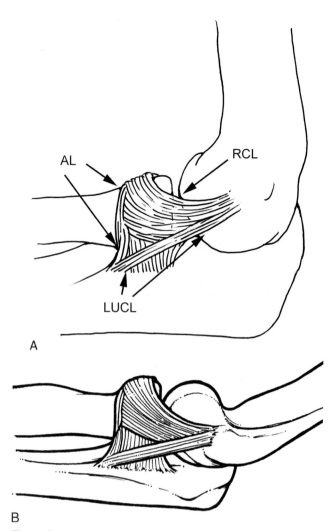

A

B

Figure 6-30 Diagram of lateral ligaments of the elbow. **A**, Elbow flexed. **B**, Elbow extended. AL, annular ligament; LUCL, lateral ulnar collateral ligament; RCL, radial (lateral) collateral ligament (note that the RCL blends into the annular ligament).

around the posterior aspect of the radial head and neck to the posterolateral ulna. This ligament is an important posterolateral elbow stabilizer. Lateral ligament injuries have an appearance on MR images similar to that of medial ligament injuries but are less common.

The *annular (orbicular) ligament* of the radius is attached to the ulna and wraps around the radial head in the transverse plane, forming a collar that prevents radial head dislocation (see Figs. 6-29, 6-30, 6-32). The annular ligament is disrupted by radial head dislocation in adults.

Lateral epicondylitis ("tennis elbow") is tendinitis of the common origin of the wrist dorsiflexors and supinators at the lateral epicondyle. Lateral epicondylitis is caused by repetitive motion and is an affliction of carpenters, golfers, and many other active individuals in addition to tennis players. Most cases recover with conservative therapy. In refractory cases, MRI can be useful in assessing the extent of injury since surgi-

cal debridement can be helpful in some cases. Tendinitis is seen as increased signal intensity on T2-weighted images or tendon thickening, in many cases with adjacent marrow edema (Fig. 6-34A). A recent therapeutic injection may produce similar soft tissue findings on MRI or US. Radiography or US of lateral epicondylitis may reveal calcification (see Fig. 6-34B). A tear is seen as a focus of very high signal intensity on T2-weighted images filling a defect within the tendon (Fig. 6-35). The high signal intensity may represent fluid or blood within a tendon defect, granulation tissue, or a combination. Ultrasonography shows low signal and interruption of the normal tendon fiber pattern (Fig. 6-36).

Medial epicondylitis is tendinitis of the common origin of the wrist flexors and pronators at the medial epicondyle. The MRI features are identical to those of lateral epicondylitis. Medial epicondylitis occurs in professional baseball pitchers and tennis players. An associated traction spur at the coronoid

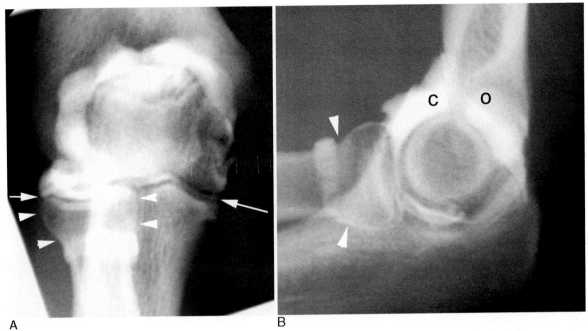

Figure 6-31   Normal arthrographic anatomy of the elbow. **A,** AP radiographic view. **B,** Lateral radiographic view. Arrowheads, impression from annular ligament around radial head; short arrow, position of radial collateral ligament (RCL) (an RCL tear would allow contrast to flow laterally); long arrow, position of ulnar collateral ligament (UCL) (a UCL tear would allow contrast medium to flow medially). C, coronoid fossa; O, olecranon fossa.

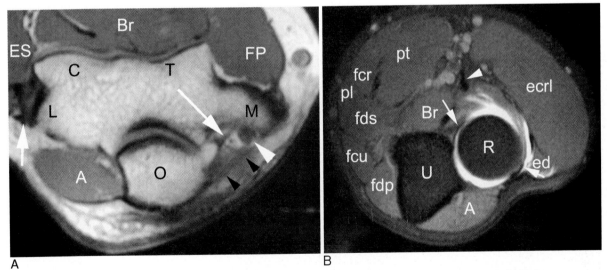

Figure 6-32   Normal MR anatomy of the elbow: axial images. **A,** Axial T1-weighted MR image obtained through the distal aspect of the humeral epicondyles. White arrowhead, ulnar nerve; black arrowheads, cubital tunnel retinaculum; short white arrow, common extensor tendon; long arrow, floor of the cubital tunnel formed by the transverse and posterior bands of the ulnar collateral ligament. **B,** Fat suppressed T1-weighted MR arthrogram more distal than in part A, through the radial head. Arrowhead, biceps tendon; short arrows, annular ligament. *Muscles:* A, anconeus; Br, brachialis; ecrl, extensor carpi radialis longus; ed, extensor digitorum; ES, extensor-supinator group; fcr, flexor carpi radialis; fcu, flexor carpi ulnaris; fdp, flexor digitorum profundus; fds, flexor digitorum superficialis; FP, flexor pronator group; pl, palmaris longus; pt, pronator teres. *Bones:* C, capitellum; L, lateral epicondyle; M, medial epicondyle; o, olecranon; R, radial head; T, trochlea; u, ulna.

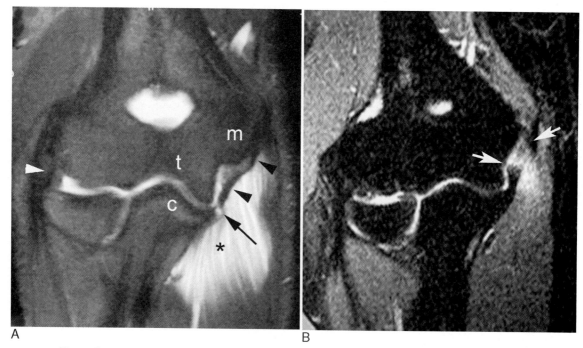

Figure 6-33   Ulnar collateral ligament tear. **A,** Coronal fat-suppressed T2-weighted MR arthrogram obtained in a professional baseball pitcher who developed medial elbow pain while pitching. Note the focal tear (black arrow) in the distal ulnar collateral ligament (UCL) with extension of contrast medium into the medial musculature. *Also note the normal low signal intensity of the remainder of the UCL *(black arrowheads)* and the normal radial collateral ligament *(white arrowhead).* **B,** Coronal inversion recovery MR image obtained in a different patient shows proximal UCL interruption *(arrows).* This is the most frequent location for UCL tears. C, coronoid process; m, medial epicondyle; t, trochlea.

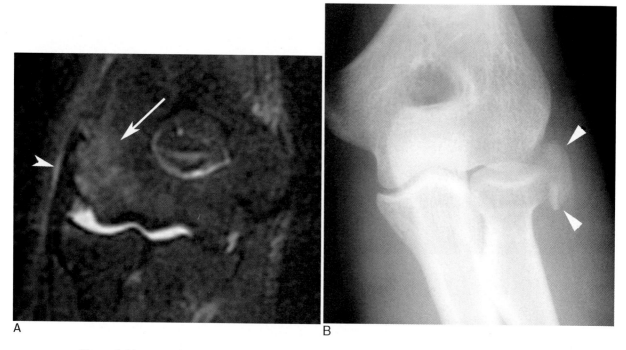

Figure 6-34   Lateral epicondylitis and "tennis elbow." **A,** Coronal inversion recovery MR images shows marrow edema in the lateral epicondyle *(arrow)* and subtle edema adjacent to the mildly thickened common extensor tendon *(arrowhead).* **B,** Calcific tendinitis of the common extensor tendon *(arrowheads).*

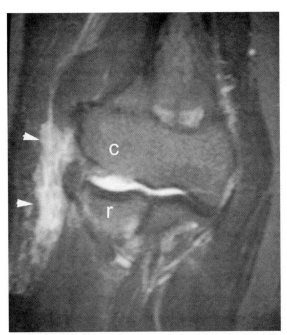

Figure 6-35   Tear of the common extensor tendon. Coronal inversion recovery MR image shows high signal intensity in and adjacent to the tendon *(arrowheads)*. C, capitellum; r, radial head.

owing to retraction of the muscle belly, but some cases are difficult to diagnose clinically. Most disruptions occur at the tendon insertion onto the radial tuberosity, but more proximal tears may occur. Magnetic resonance images of a degenerated or partially torn tendon reveal increased signal intensity on all sequences, tendon thickening, and surrounding edema. A partially or completely torn distal biceps is often surrounded by fluid. A tendon rupture is seen on MR images as interruption of tendon fibers. The normal biceps courses anterior to the brachialis muscle before curving posteriorly to the radial tuberosity. Sagittal images may allow demonstration of the torn and retracted tendon on a single image (Fig. 6-37), but serial T2-weighted axial images extending from the musculotendinous junction to the radial tuberosity are more reliable in detection or exclusion of a biceps tendon tear. Therefore, it is essential that an axial sequence extends distally to the radial tuberosity (see Figs. 6-32, 6-37).

Several clinical and imaging pitfalls are associated with biceps tendon tears. An associated hematoma may lead to clinical suspicion of an underlying sarcoma. Magnetic resonance images will reveal a mass with bizarre signal characteristics related to the hemorrhage, potentially misleading the radiologist as well. Some of the proximal medial biceps tendon fibers form the flat, broad *biceps aponeurosis (lacertus fibrosis)* that inserts into the medial fascia of the forearm. A distal tendon rupture can be clinically masked if the biceps aponeurosis remains intact, because the intact aponeurosis limits tendon retraction and allows for limited biceps function. Chronic inflammation of the small *cubital bursa* may be both a cause and an effect of biceps tendon rupture. This bursa is located between the distal tendon and the medial radius (see Fig. 6-37A). Magnetic resonance images reveal fluid distention of the bursa. Radiographs may reveal reactive changes in the adjacent radius, suggesting an aggressive process such as a neo-

insertion of the anterior bundle of the MCL may be seen. Little leaguer's elbow in skeletally immature throwing athletes may also occur in association with medial epicondylitis.

The *distal biceps tendon* can undergo degeneration and tear. Most biceps tendon tears occur in men and are due to repetitive stress. Rheumatoid arthritis, previous local steroid injection, and use of anabolic steroids increase the risk of biceps tendon tear. A chronically degenerated tendon may completely tear spontaneously or after a seemingly trivial injury. Complete rupture of the distal biceps tendon is usually clinically evident

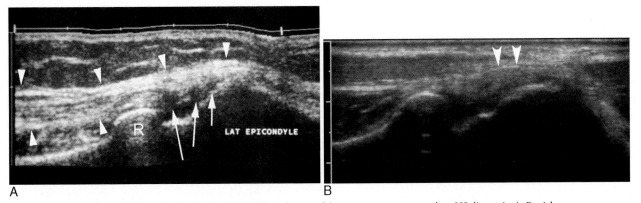

Figure 6-36   Partial-thickness tear and tendinosis of the common extensor tendon: US diagnosis. **A,** Partial tear. Coronal image (distal at the left of the image) reveals hypoechoic defects in the deep portion of the proximal tendon *(arrows)*. Note the normal US appearance of the remainder of the tendon *(arrowheads)*. **B,** Chronic tendinosis. Note thickened common extensor origin *(arrowheads)*, but no tear is seen. R, radial head. (Part A courtesy of Doohi Lee, MD.)

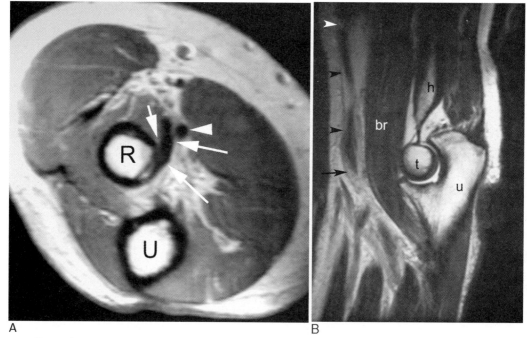

Figure 6-37   Biceps tendon insertion and tear. **A,** Normal distal biceps tendon. Axial T2-weighted MR image shows the distal tendon *(long arrows)* inserting onto the radius. Most biceps tendon tears occur at the insertion. The short arrow marks the location of the cubital bursa, which is normal in this case and therefore is not seen. Inflammation of this bursa causes local fluid accumulation and can clinically simulate a distal biceps tear or tendinitis. The arrowhead marks the ulnar artery. **B,** Biceps tendon tear. Sagittal T2-weighted MR image shows retracted biceps musculotendinous junction *(white arrowhead),* lax wavy tendon *(black arrowheads),* and frayed torn margin of the biceps tendon *(black arrow).* Note that review of serial axial T2-weighted images is the best method for detection of distal biceps tears on MR imaging. br, brachialis muscle; h, distal humeral shaft; R, radius; t, trochlea; u, proximal ulna.

plasm. All these potential pitfalls may be avoided with careful scrutiny of the biceps tendon.

Triceps tendon injuries are unusual. Complete tears are usually diagnosed by physical examination and radiographs. Both MRI and US can be helpful in problem cases (Fig. 6-38). More frequently, the olecranon fractures and is displaced proximally, as discussed previously (see Fig. 6-27). Either MRI or US can be used to characterize a partial tendon tear or degeneration.

MISCELLANEOUS ELBOW INJURIES

Cubital tunnel syndrome is ulnar neuropathy caused by trauma in the cubital tunnel located posterior to the medial epicondyle. The cubital tunnel is formed by the medial epicondyle, proximal ulna, and overlying retinaculum. Causes of cubital tunnel syndrome include ulnar nerve subluxation, nerve traction, ulnar bone spurs, a ganglion or other mass lesion, fibrosis, fracture, inflammatory process, or anatomic derangements. Clinical features include weakness of the flexor carpi ulnaris muscle and the intrinsic muscles of the hand. MRI may reveal a causative lesion, or simply signal alteration in the fat that normally surrounds the ulnar nerve within the tunnel. T2-weighted and inversion recovery MR images may reveal

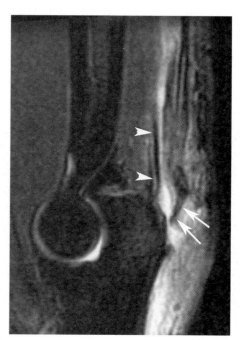

Figure 6-38   Triceps tendon tear in 30-year-old man with posterior elbow pain and limited elbow extension. Sagittal fat-suppressed T2-weighted MR image shows large tear *(arrows),* but the deepest portion of the tendon is intact *(arrowheads);* this explains why limited elbow extension was possible.

nerve or perineural edema (Fig. 6-39). Treatment depends on the cause. Offending masses are resected. The retinaculum may be released (Fig. 6-40). Sometimes, the nerve is transferred out of the cubital tunnel into medial subcutaneous fat.

The radial nerve is vulnerable to a compressive neuropathy just distal to the elbow where the deep branch passes into the supinator muscle. Clinical features include weakness of finger extensor muscles and pain and tenderness adjacent to the lateral epicondyle. The latter symptoms may simulate lateral epicondylitis. Potential causes include previous elbow dislocation or fracture, a mass lesion, or fibrosis. Magnetic resonance images may reveal a mass-like lesion such as a hematoma or neoplasm, but usually are unrevealing.

The median nerve is vulnerable to entrapment neuropathy as it courses between the two heads of the pronator teres muscle anterior and slightly distal to the elbow. Clinical features include weakness of the first three fingers and pain with writing, weightlifting, and other activities that use the pronator teres muscle. As with radial nerve entrapment, MR images are usually unrevealing unless a mass lesion is present. The median nerve may be entrapped proximal to the elbow by a ligament of Struthers, as noted previously. The median nerve is also vulnerable to compressive neuropathy just distal to the elbow as it passes through the flexor carpi ulnaris muscle. Imaging findings are usually absent, although a mass may be seen.

Osteochondritis dissecans of the capitellum (OCD, Panner's disease, Figs. 6-41, 3-9B) can be considered a variant type of traumatic elbow injury. The distal and posterior portions of the capitellum are vulnerable to direct impaction when the elbow is flexed. This mechanism is a likely cause of capitellar OCD. The capitellum is also vulnerable to post-traumatic avascular necrosis (Fig. 22-5D).

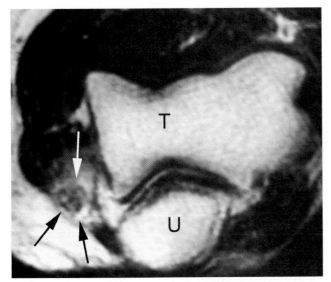

Figure 6-39   Ulnar nerve injury. Axial T2-weighted MR image distal to the medial epicondyle shows thickening and heterogeneously increased signal intensity in the ulnar nerve *(black and white arrows)*. The cause of the injury in this case was trauma due to repetitive overstretching of the nerve. The ulnar nerve must normally stretch to accommodate elbow flexion. In this case, a portion of the nerve was fixed by fibrosis in the cubital tunnel, which focused the stretching forces on a short segment of the nerve. T, trochlea; U, proximal ulna.

FOREARM

Isolated fracture of the ulnar shaft *(nightstick fracture)* is caused by a direct blow. A classic nightstick fracture occurs when the forearm is raised to protect the head from a blow from a blunt object such as a policeman's nightstick.

Most forearm shaft fractures usually include both bones, either with fracture of both (Fig. 6-42) or fracture of one and dislocation of the other. *Both bones fractures* are of the ulna and radius and are treated with casting in children. These fractures heal rapidly and can remodel after the fracture has healed. Both bones fractures in adults are usually treated by internal fixation of each bone (Fig. 1-21C). *Post-traumatic radioulnar synostosis* (i.e., osseous union of the ulna to the radius) is an unusual complication of a both bones fracture. Treatment is by resection of the synostosis.

Galeazzi's fracture is a fracture of the radial shaft and dislocation of the distal ulna (Fig. 6-43). The distal radioulnar joint is injured and may develop chronic instability. *Monteggia's fracture* is dislocation of the radial head and fracture of the proximal ulnar shaft (see Fig. 6-20). The rare Essex-Lopresti fracture (see Fig. 6-25) was discussed earlier.

As noted in Chapter 2, the volar forearm musculature is vulnerable to *compartment syndrome. Volkmann's contracture* is a devastating result of volar forearm compartment syndrome. The fingers and wrist develop progressive fixed flexion defor-

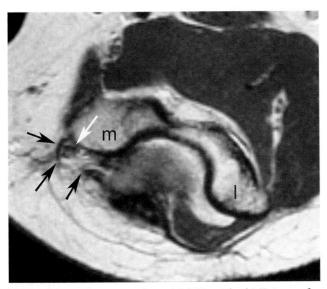

Figure 6-40   Ulnar nerve release. Axial T2-weighted MR image after release of the cubital tunnel retinaculum. Note surgically divided retinaculum *(black arrows)* and ulnar nerve, which is displaced medially *(white arrow)*. l, lateral epicondyle; m, medial epicondyle.

mity due to fibrosis of the necrosed forearm muscles. Early detection is imperative to avoid this devastating outcome. When acute compartment syndrome is suspected, direct measurement of intracompartmental pressure is the appropriate test. This should not be delayed in order to perform MRI or other imaging study. Treatment of acute compartment syndrome is by decompression of the affected compartment by fasciotomy.

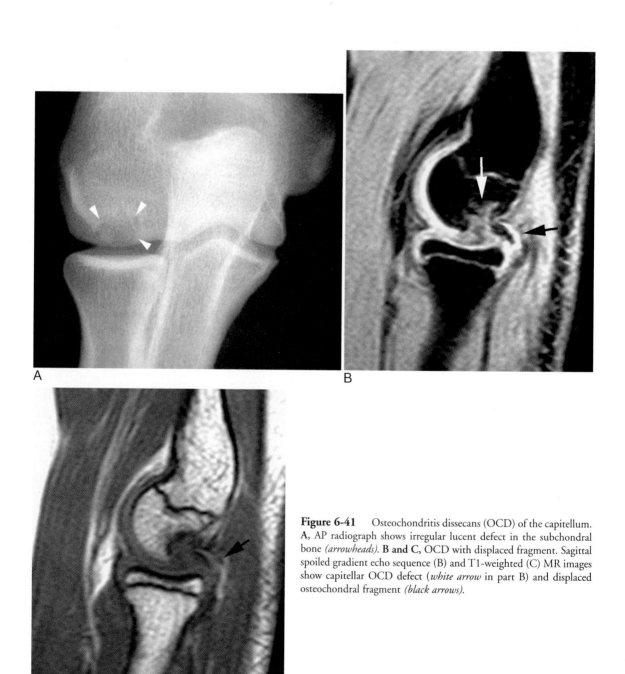

Figure 6-41   Osteochondritis dissecans (OCD) of the capitellum. **A,** AP radiograph shows irregular lucent defect in the subchondral bone *(arrowheads).* **B and C,** OCD with displaced fragment. Sagittal spoiled gradient echo sequence (B) and T1-weighted (C) MR images show capitellar OCD defect *(white arrow* in part B) and displaced osteochondral fragment *(black arrows).*

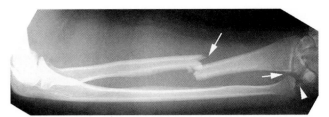

Figure 6-43   Galeazzi's fracture. Note the radial shaft fracture *(long arrow)* and distal ulnar dislocation *(short arrow)*. This patient also has an ulnar styloid fracture *(arrowhead)*.

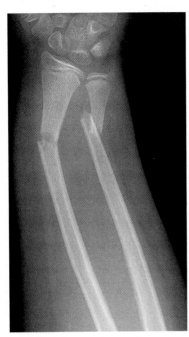

Figure 6-42   Both bones forearm fracture in a child.

CHAPTER 7

Wrist

IMAGING TECHNIQUES
DISTAL FOREARM AND DISTAL RADIOULNAR JOINT
DISTAL FOREARM FRACTURES
TRIANGULAR FIBROCARTILAGE COMPLEX
RADIOCARPAL JOINT
CARPAL BONES
CARPAL BONE FRACTURES AND DISLOCATIONS
CARPAL INSTABILITY
MISCELLANEOUS CARPAL CONDITIONS

The wrist includes the tissues between the proximal aspect of the distal radioulnar joint and the base of the metacarpals, and therefore includes the distal ulna and radius; the eight carpal bones; the proximal metacarpals; the triangular fibrocartilage; and numerous related ligaments, tendons, and synovial compartments. The wrist is a marvelously, maddeningly complex joint, made all the more challenging for the radiologist by the comparatively small size of many important soft tissue structures that test the limits of both our scanners and our diagnostic skills.

Key Concepts	Normal Wrist Alignment

Distal radius articular surface: palmar tilt, ulnar inclination
Distal ulna: May be a few millimeters shorter than distal radius, not longer
Carpal bone alignment (wrist in neutral position):
PA view:
Proximal and distal rows form smooth arcs
Lateral view:
Scaphoid tilted palmar, scapholunate angle 30 to 60 degrees
Lunate aligned within 10 degrees of capitate
Carpometacarpal joints: Normal zig-zag pattern on PA radiograph

IMAGING TECHNIQUES

Radiographic evaluation of the traumatized or painful wrist should include, at a minimum, posteroanterior (PA) and lateral radiographs, the latter obtained with wrist in neutral position to properly assess carpal alignment. Dedicated views of the scaphoid are required if the patient has snuff box tenderness or any other evidence of a scaphoid fracture. A variety of other specialized radiographic projections of the wrist have been described. Ultrasonography (US) is useful for assessing for a joint or tendon sheath effusion, tendon pathology, or for a mass lesion in the carpal tunnel. Fluoroscopy can provide extensive evidence about the functional status of ligaments and tendons, based on the alignment and motion of the carpal bones. Arthrography can reveal tears of the lunotriquetral and scapholunate interosseous ligaments and the triangular fibrocartilage. Computed tomography (CT) is useful for characterizing complex fractures and post-traumatic complications such as malunion or nonunion of the scaphoid.

Magnetic resonance imaging (MRI) of the wrist is extremely sensitive in the detection of fractures, avascular necrosis, tenosynovitis, and mass lesions. These abnormalities may be detected in a cooperative patient with almost any scanner. However, assessment of carpal ligaments and the triangular fibrocartilage complex requires extremely high-quality imaging with a dedicated coil and a high-field magnet, and is improved with MR arthrography. Imaging sequences are a matter of personal preference but generally include coronal high-resolution T2-weighted or gradient echo images to assess the interosseous ligaments and the triangular fibrocartilage complex, and T1-weighted and fluid-sensitive (fat-suppressed T2 or inversion recovery) images to assess the bone marrow for edema or fracture. Axial images are needed to assess the nerves and tendons, notably those in the carpal tunnel. These structures also can be studied with US.

Normal wrist anatomy is reviewed in Figures 7-1 and 7-2.

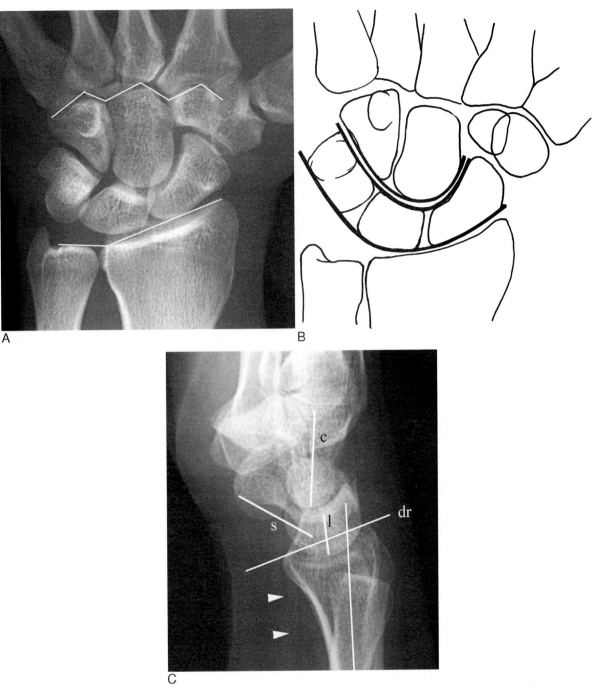

Figure 7-1   Normal radiographic anatomy of the wrist. **A,** PA view. Note the normal ulnar inclination of the distal radius *(long white line)*. Also note the approximately equal length of the distal ulna and radius *(short transverse line)* and the "zig-zag" contour formed by the carpometacarpal joints. **B,** Diagram of the normal smooth carpal arcs. Interruption of one of these arcs is evidence of a ligamentous injury or carpal dislocation. **C,** Lateral view. The long axes of the radius, capitate, scaphoid, and lunate are marked with lines (r, c, s, and l, respectively). Note how the long axis of the scaphoid is estimated by connecting the two most volar projections, which are relatively easy to identify. The radius, capitate, and lunate are approximately colinear. The scaphoid is angled approximately 45 degrees palmar compared to the lunate. Note the palmar tilt of the distal radial articular surface. Also note the normal fat pad volar to the pronator quadratus muscle *(arrowheads)*. dr, distal radial articular surface.

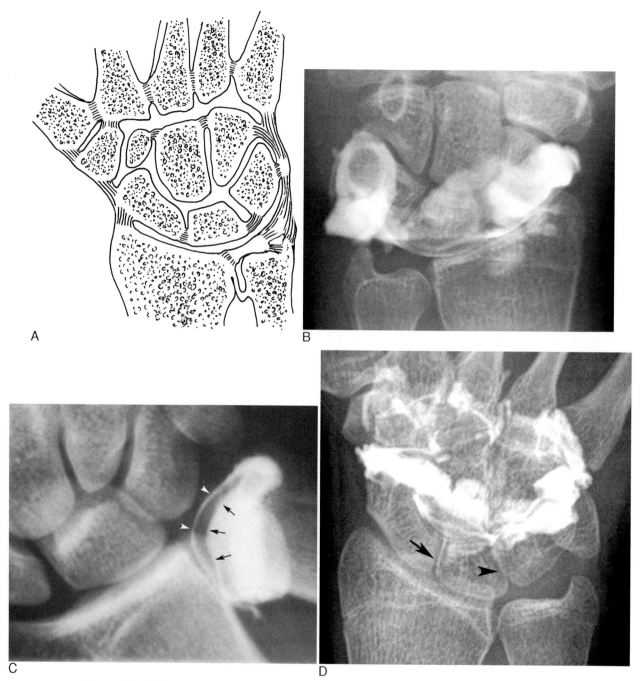

Figure 7-2   Wrist compartmental anatomy. **A,** Diagram shows the synovial compartments of the wrist. Note the structures that separate the compartments: the scapholunate and lunotriquetral interosseous ligaments separate the radiocarpal and midcarpal compartments. The triangular fibrocartilage complex separates the radiocarpal joint from the distal radioulnar joint. Note the ligamentous fixation of the triangular fibrocartilage to the radius, ulna, and medial joint capsule. **B,** Normal radiocarpal arthrogram. Note that contrast medium does *not* flow through the interosseous ligaments of the proximal carpal row into the midcarpal joint or through the triangular fibrocartilage into the distal radioulnar joint. **C,** Normal distal radioulnar joint arthrogram. Note the radiolucent articular cartilage of the distal ulna *(arrows)*. *Arrowheads* mark the proximal margin of the triangular fibrocartilage. **D,** Midcarpal joint arthrogram. Contrast medium extends between the scaphoid and lunate *(arrow)* and lunate and triquetrum *(arrowhead)*, but is contained by the scapholunate and lunotriquetral interosseous ligaments. DRUJ, distal radioulnar joint; lt, lunotriquetral; MC, midcarpal joint; RC, radiocarpal joint; sc, scapholunate; tfc, triangular fibrocartilage complex.

DISTAL FOREARM AND DISTAL RADIOULNAR JOINT

The articular surface of the distal radius is normally tilted toward the ulna by approximately 20 to 25 degrees and toward the palm by approximately 11 degrees (see Fig. 7-1). Deviation from this pattern is most frequently due to an old fracture that healed with deformity, although developmental conditions such as Madelung deformity also should be considered. The articular surface of the radius frequently contains two shallow depressions that correspond to the scaphoid and lunate bones, respectively termed the *scaphoid fossa* (or facet) and the *lunate fossa* (or facet). These are useful landmarks for localizing an intra-articular fracture of the distal radius.

The distal ulna is normally no longer than the adjacent radius, and may be a few millimeters shorter. The term *ulna* (or *ulnar*) *positive* (or *plus*) *variance* indicates that the distal ulna is longer or extends more distally than the radius. A long ulna can impact against the triangular fibrocartilage and the medial lunate. *Ulnar negative* (or *ulnar minus*) *variance* indicates that the distal ulna is more than a few millimeters shorter than the distal radius, which results in ulnar impaction syndrome. Ulna minus is associated with an increased risk of *Kienböck's disease,* also termed lunatomalacia or avascular necrosis of the lunate (see also Fig. 22-8). Accurate identification of ulnar variance requires a properly positioned PA radiograph with the wrist and forearm in neutral alignment (see Fig. 7-1A). If the PA radiograph is obtained with the wrist dorsiflexed and the hand flat on the film cassette, the dorsal ulna will project distally on the image, simulating ulna posi-

tive variance (Fig. 7-3). Wrist supination "shortens" the ulna and wrist pronation "lengthens" the ulna relative to the distal radius (see Fig. 7-3).

Key Concepts	Wrist Compartments

Distal radioulnar joint (DRUJ) allows supination/pronation. Arthrogram capacity, 1 mL
Radiocarpal joint: Arthrogram capacity, 3–5 mL
Intercarpal (midcarpal) joint: can communicate distally with the carpometacarpal joints; Arthrogram capacity, 3–5 mL
Pisotriquetral joint: Usually communicates with radiocarpal joint as a normal variant; when a separate compartment, arthrogram capacity, approximately 1 mL; not routinely injected during arthrography

The distal radioulnar joint (DRUJ) is anatomically and functionally distinct from the more distal synovial compartments around the carpal bones. The DRUJ, paired with the proximal radioulnar joint at the elbow, allows wrist pronation and supination. The distal ulna has a cylindrical cross-section contour that articulates with a concave depression in the distal radius, the sigmoid notch; this is exactly the reverse of the arrangement at the elbow between the smaller, cylindrical radial head and the concave articular surface of the proximal ulna.

The DRUJ has a relatively small volume and is well distended at arthrography by injection of just 1 mL of contrast medium (see

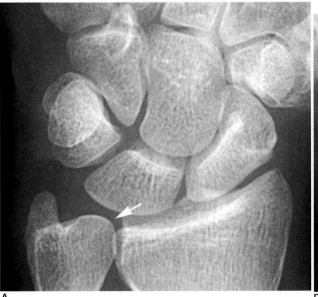
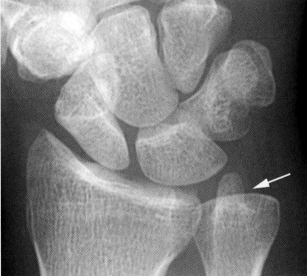

A   B

Figure 7-3 Effect of wrist position on apparent ulnar variance. All images are of the same patient. A properly positioned PA radiograph is obtained with the wrist in neutral position (see Fig. 7-1A). Pronation (A) causes apparent lengthening of the ulna *(arrow).* Supination (B) causes apparent shortening of the ulna *(arrow).*

(Continued)

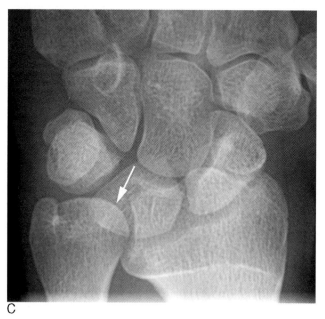

C

Figure 7-3—(Cont'd)   Wrist dorsiflexion (C), as can occur with the hand flat on the x-ray cassette but with the elbow elevated, causes apparent lengthening of the ulna *(arrow)*.

Fig. 7-2). The DRUJ is bounded distally and separated from the radiocarpal joint by the triangular fibrocartilage complex (TFCC). Communication between the DRUJ and the radiocarpal compartment at arthrography indicates a perforation in the TFCC. Communication between the DRUJ and the extensor carpi ulnaris tendon sheath can occur following wrist trauma with capsular injury or in rheumatoid arthritis.

Subluxation and instability of the DRUJ can occur as an isolated injury or as a component of a more complex injury such as a Colles fracture or Galeazzi's or Essex-Lopresti fracture-dislocation. The distal ulna is normally slightly posterior relative to the radius. In most instances of DRUJ subluxation, the distal ulna subluxes further dorsally. Diagnosis is suggested by physical examination, and axial CT or MRI can be used for confirmation. A suggested protocol is to obtain limited axial images through the DRUJ with the wrist in neutral, extreme pronation and extreme supination. The convex articular surface of the lateral distal ulna should be congruent with the sigmoid notch of the medial distal radius, regardless of wrist position. Wrist pronation (thumbs point medially and posteriorly) tends to accentuate any subluxation. Imaging the uninjured side for comparison purposes is helpful, as there may be some normal variation in joint laxity.

DISTAL FOREARM FRACTURES

Distal forearm fractures are among the most common musculoskeletal injuries. Most are the result of a fall on an outstretched hand. The age of the patient is an excellent predictor of the fracture pattern. Younger children usually sustain a transverse fracture of the metaphysis of the distal radius, and

often a fracture of the distal ulna as well. These fractures are frequently buckle or torus fractures, and are proximal to the physis (see Fig. 1-10). Adolescents have stronger bones, so the fracture almost always extends partially through the comparatively weak physis, usually in a Salter-Harris II pattern. Also seen in preteens and adolescent gymnasts is a Salter-Harris I variant stress injury of the distal radius. Radiographs in these children reveal widening of the physis with irregular, sclerotic margins (see Fig. 3-7). After closure of the physes in young adults, most wrist fractures involve the scaphoid. As middle-age approaches, the distal radius again becomes the most common site of fracture. The fractures seen in children and adolescents may be subtle but are usually straightforward to describe and treat. Fractures in adults are more variable in terms of comminution, alignment, intra-articular extension, and treatment.

Key Concepts	Common Wrist and Distal Forearm Fracture Patterns by Age
4–10 years: Distal radius and ulna transverse metaphyseal; often incomplete (buckle or torus)	
11–16 years: Distal radius, usually Salter-Harris II fracture; dorsal displacement—best seen on lateral view	
17–40 years: Scaphoid, occasionally triquetrum or both; may be occult on radiographs	
≥40 years: Colles fracture; more frequent in women; associated with osteoporosis	

Several "named" distal radius fracture patterns are so deeply ingrained in the orthopedic and radiology lexicon that radiologists should be familiar with these named injuries. A *Colles fracture* of the distal radius, with apex volar angulation and dorsal impaction, is by far the most frequent wrist fracture in middle-aged and older adults (Fig. 7-4A, B). The clinical deformity that accompanies a Colles fracture is sometimes likened to an upside-down fork, with the forearm representing the handle and the wrist and hand representing the tines. Colles fracture is more common in women because of their relatively weaker bones, and is associated with hip and proximal humerus fractures in elderly patients. The dorsal impaction often worsens after casting, owing to compressive forces across the wrist from the dorsal and palmar tendons. Even with external fixation, anatomic alignment may be difficult to maintain. Thus, Colles fractures often heal with loss of normal palmar tilt and ulnar inclination, and frequently heal with dorsal tilt, as well as loss of radial length. This alteration in radial articular surface alignment, combined with frequently coexisting ligamentous injuries, results in alteration of wrist mechanics with potential for development of chronic pain and post-traumatic osteoarthritis. Reflex sympathetic dystrophy and acquired ulna positive variance with ulnar impaction syndrome also may occur after a Colles or any other distal radius fracture. Intra-articular extension increases the risk for these complications. A *Smith's fracture* is a reverse Colles fracture, with apex dorsal angular deformity resulting in volar tilt of the distal radius articular surface. A *Barton's fracture* is an unstable intra-articular fracture of the dorsal lip of the radius, with dorsal subluxation of the carpus along with the dorsal radius fragment. Surgical reduction and fixation are required. A *reverse Barton's fracture* is a similar injury with volar displacement (see Fig. 7-4C). A *Hutchinson's fracture (chauffeur's fracture)* is an intra-articular fracture of the radial styloid (see Fig. 7-4D). Hutchinson's fractures are caused by

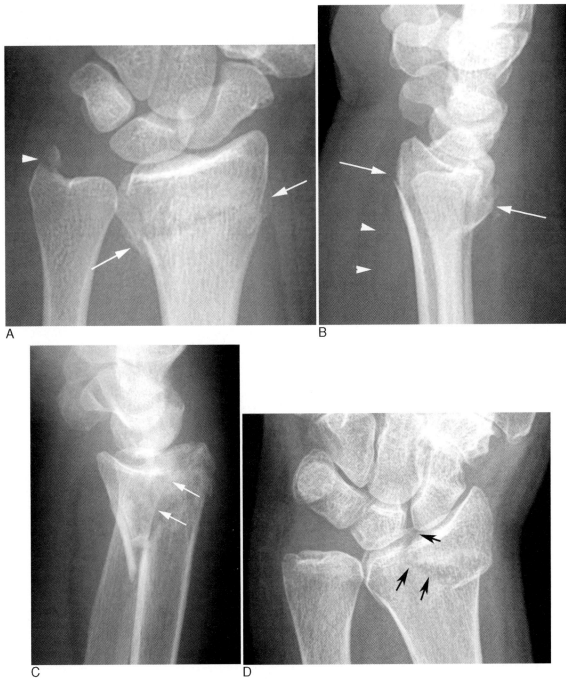

Figure 7-4   Distal radius fractures. **A and B,** Colles fracture: PA (A) and lateral (B) views show a dorsal impaction fracture of the distal radius *(arrows)* that results in dorsal, rather than the normal palmar, tilt of the articular surface of the distal radius. Also note the ulnar styloid fracture *(arrowhead in* part A). On the lateral view (B), the normal pronator fat pad is absent *(arrowheads* mark normal position of this fat pad). **C,** Reverse Barton's fracture of the volar lip of the radius *(arrows),* with volar subluxation of the carpus along with the radius fragment. This is an unstable fracture. **D,** Hutchinson's (chauffeur's) intra-articular fracture of the radial styloid *(arrows).*

avulsion by the radial collateral ligament, or a direct blow. The latter often is associated with a fracture dislocation. Hutchinson's fractures are associated with scapholunate interosseous ligament tears. This fracture is also known as a chauffeur's fracture because it was an affliction of chauffeurs before the introduction of electric starters. The chauffeur was required to start the car with a crank inserted through the front grill into the engine. If the engine suddenly misfired or started during cranking, the crank would violently accelerate in the hands of the chauffeur, placing an enormous load across the radial styloid. A fall on an outstretched hand is now the most frequent cause of this fracture.

Numerous classification systems of distal radius fractures have been described, each having advantages and disadvantages. It may be worth learning a system used by your local orthopedic surgeons in order to enhance communication of abnormal findings. Otherwise, it is suggested that you limit your report to a clear description of the findings, with specific reference to the presence or absence of articular extension into the DRUJ or into the radiocarpal joint. The presence or absence of an ulnar styloid fracture also should be noted. If intra-articular extension is present, articular step-off or diastasis should be measured, as defects of 2 mm or greater are associated with development of post-traumatic osteoarthritis and thus serve as an indication for operative reduction.

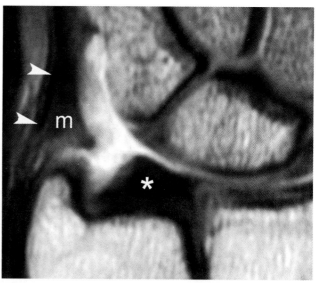

Figure 7-5   The triangular fibrocartilage complex. Coronal T1-weighted MR arthrogram shows normal appearance of the triangular fibrocartilage *(asterisk),* with low signal intensity and smooth margins. This patient has a normal variant "meniscal homologue" attached to the ulnar collateral ligament *(arrowheads).* The meniscal homologue is partially composed of fibrocartilage and is triangular in shape, hence its name. M, meniscal homologue. (Courtesy of Charles Pappas, MD.)

TRIANGULAR FIBROCARTILAGE COMPLEX

The TFCC is located between the distal ulna and the proximal carpal row (Figs. 7-2, 7-5). The TFCC is the primary stabilizer of the DRUJ and also allows wider distribution of forces across the radiocarpal joint. The TFCC consists of several components that are not discrete structures but rather blend continuously from one structure to the next. The TFCC includes a central disk-shaped fibrocartilaginous portion, termed the *triangular fibrocartilage* (TFC), and sometimes the triangular fibrocartilage disk. The TFC blends into the thick, strong dorsal and volar *radioulnar ligaments* that fix the TFC to the radius laterally and to the ulnar head and styloid process medially. The extensor carpi ulnaris tendon sheath and the volar medial portions of the wrist capsular ligaments, the ulnotriquetral and ulnolunate ligaments, also are components of the TFCC. Finally, the *meniscal homologue,* a wedge-shaped fibrofatty thickening of the medial joint capsule distal to the TFC occasionally identified at wrist arthrography, is considered by some authors to be a component of the TFCC. Many TFCC injuries occur during a wrist fracture and are not immediately apparent. Tears of the TFCC cause ulnar sided wrist pain and weakness. A click or pop with wrist motion may be present. Arthrography or MRI may reveal a defect in the TFC or communication between the radiocarpal joint and the DRUJ (Fig. 7-6). Patterns of TFCC tears are complex, but generally occur as a perforation of the TFC or a tear of the TFC fixation to the radius, ulna, or dorsal or volar joint capsule. Occasionally, similar, asymptomatic defects may be observed in older individuals, thought to represent a consequence of "normal" age-related degeneration. This potential pitfall of false-positive diagnosis is similar to age-related partial separations of the glenoid labrum of the shoulder, small perforations in the lunotriquetral and scapholunate interosseous ligaments of the wrist, and "degenerative" signal alterations in the menisci of the knee.

Key Concepts	Triangular Fibrocartilage Complex (TFCC)

TFCC = fibrocartilage disc (the TFC), ligamentous fixation of the disc to the joint capsule and the ulnar styloid. Many authors also include adjacent wrist ligaments, tendon sheath of extensor carpi ulnaris, and meniscal homologue

Separates distal radioulnar joint (DRUJ) from radiocarpal joint

Extends joint surface of distal radius medially

Ulnar impaction (or abutment) syndrome is impingement of the distal lateral ulna against the TFCC and the proximal carpal row, in particular the proximal medial lunate (Figs. 7-7). Chronic impingement causes degeneration of the TFC and

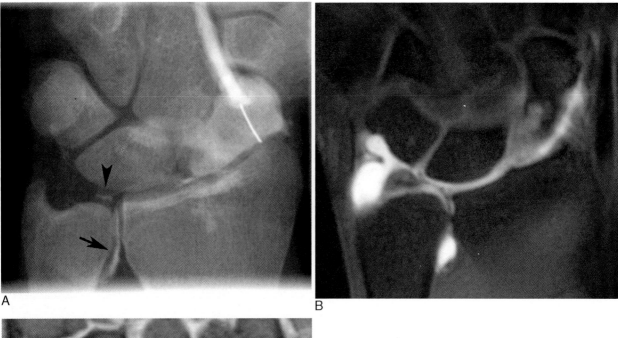

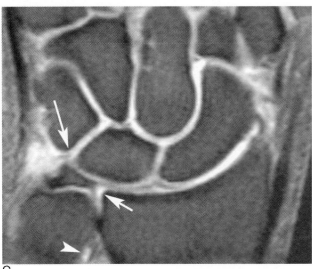

Figure 7-6   Triangular fibrocartilage tear. **A,** Spot image during radiocarpal joint injection shows contrast medium in the distal radioulnar joint *(arrow),* indicating triangular fibrocartilage complex (TFCC) tear. The tear is visible as contrast medium in the expected position of the triangular fibrocartilage *(arrowhead).* **B,** Coronal fat-suppressed T1-weighted MR arthrogram obtained after radiocarpal injection in a different patient shows a TFC tear. **C,** MR arthrogram in another patient shows TFC avulsion from its radial attachment *(short white arrow).* Contrast medium has entered the distal radioulnar joint through this defect *(white arrowhead).* Also note the high signal intensity within the midcarpal joint due to contrast medium passing through a lunotriquetral ligament tear *(long white arrow).*

lunate cartilage. Clinical features are similar to a those of a TFCC tear. Radiographs may reveal ulna positive variance and subchondral cysts, sclerosis or osteophytes in the proximal medial lunate, proximal radial triquetrum, or distal ulna. An old radial fracture as the cause of the ulnar positive variance may be evident. Associated TFCC tears or degeneration may be documented by arthrography or MRI. Treatment is by surgical shortening of the ulna, with resection of a short segment of the distal shaft.

Ulnar impingement syndrome is impaction, often with pseudarthrosis, of a markedly shortened ulna against the distal metaphysis of the radius. Clinical features may mimic those of ulnar impaction but are often more severe. Ulnar impingement is a potential complication of ulnar growth arrest, surgical ulnar shortening, or any traumatic or growth abnormality that reduces the length of the ulna.

RADIOCARPAL JOINT

The radiocarpal joint is a synovial compartment that is bounded by the proximal carpal row distally and the radius and the TFCC proximally (see Fig. 7-2). The capacity of the radiocarpal joint at arthrography is approximately 3 to 5 mL. Communication between the radiocarpal and midcarpal joints indicates a tear of the scapholunate or the lunotriquetral interosseous ligament. Such tears usually are significant in younger individuals but also can occur in the form of asymptomatic perforations in older individuals (see discussion later in this chapter). Communication between the radiocarpal joint and the DRUJ indicates a perforation of the TFCC, which is less frequently seen as an incidental, age-related finding. As with the DRUJ, wrist trauma or rheumatoid arthritis

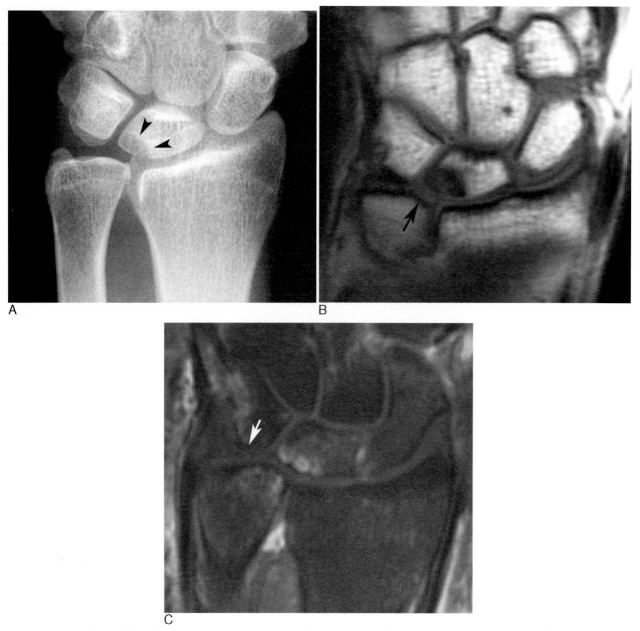

Figure 7-7   Ulnar impaction syndrome. **A,** PA radiograph shows mild ulna positive variance. Note the small cyst-like lucencies in the proximal medial lunate *(arrowheads)* that are due to impaction against the ulna. **B and C,** Coronal T1-weighted (B) and inversion recovery (C) images in a different patient show ulna positive and cyst-like lesions in the lunate and adjacent ulna with adjacent marrow edema. The triangular fibrocartilage disc in torn *(arrow* in B), with only a small residual, degenerated medial portion *(arrow* in C).

can cause communication between the radiocarpal joint and the extensor carpi ulnaris tendon sheath.

CARPAL BONES

A useful approach to understanding the anatomy of the carpus (the carpal bones as a unit) begins with the concept of carpal rows. The carpal bones are arranged in two rows. The proximal carpal row consists of the triquetrum, lunate, and scaphoid. The distal carpal row consists of the hamate, capitate, trapezoid, and trapezium. (The pisiform is positioned palmar to the triquetrum.) A PA radiograph of a normal wrist reveals the margins of the carpal rows to form smooth arcs, termed *carpal arcs* or *Gilula's arcs* in honor of the radiologist, Louis Gilula, MD, who described them (see Fig. 7-1). The lateral view of the wrist superimposes most of the carpal bones. However, a well-positioned lateral wrist radiograph will allow identification of the radius, lunate, capitate, and third metacarpal. These bones should be roughly colinear when the wrist is in neutral alignment (*not* dorsiflexed, see Fig. 7-1C).

The long axis of the scaphoid is normally in approximately 45 degrees palmar flexion relative to the lunate at neutral wrist positioning.

Carpal motion is complex but may be simplified by considering the concept of carpal rows. A useful simplification is that each carpal row functions as a unit, with carpal motion occurring at the radiocarpal joint and the *midcarpal joint* between the carpal rows. Approximately 50% of wrist flexion and extension occurs at the radiocarpal joint and 50% at the midcarpal joint. Thus, a lateral radiograph of the wrist in palmar flexion should show the lunate palmar flexed relative to the radius and the capitate palmar flexed relative to the lunate. Motion in the coronal plane, that is, ulnar and radial deviation, is more complex (Fig. 7-8) because the carpus pivots around a center of rotation in the proximal capitate. When the wrist is in neutral position, the lunate straddles the junction of the radius and the TFC. Ulnar deviation slides the proximal carpal row *radially* (laterally) as the fingers angle medially. In addition, the scaphoid and lunate tilt dorsally during ulnar deviation. The lunate articulates exclusively with the radius when the wrist is in ulnar deviation.

Radial deviation slides the proximal carpal row *medially* as the hand angles laterally. In addition, the scaphoid and lunate tilt palmarly during radial deviation. Only about 30% to 50% of the lunate articulates with the radius when the wrist is in radial deviation. Variation from these normal carpal alignment and motion patterns may be the only telltale sign of a significant ligamentous injury or carpal instability, further discussed later in this chapter.

CARPAL BONE FRACTURES AND DISLOCATIONS

The most frequently fractured carpal bone is the scaphoid (Figs. 7-9, 7-10, 1-7, 1-30). Most scaphoid fractures occur through the waist (midportion) and are nondisplaced. Like other bones that are largely covered with articular cartilage, such as the femoral head and the talar dome, the proximal pole of the scaphoid has a tenuous blood supply and is vulnerable to avascular necrosis, delayed union, or nonunion if the blood supply is interrupted by trauma (see Figs. 1-30, 7-10). The distal pole has an excellent blood supply and heals promptly. In an unfortunate anatomic arrangement, the blood supply to the proximal pole enters the scaphoid at the waist and courses proximally within the bone. Therefore, a scaphoid waist or proximal pole fracture has a high likelihood of injuring the only available blood supply to the proximal pole. A delay in immobilization increases the risk that this blood supply will be

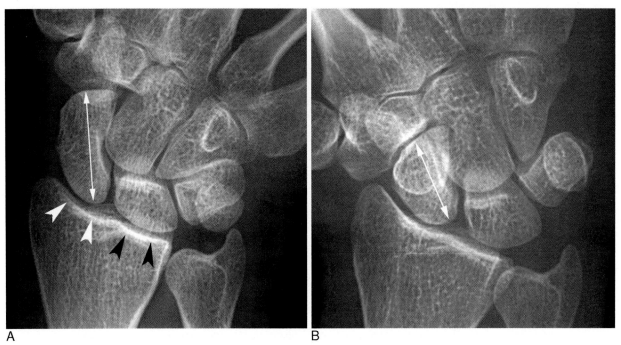

A   B

Figure 7-8   Normal carpal motion in ulnar (A) and radial (B) deviation. Note that the proximal carpal row slides along the radius. Also note that the scaphoid appears to shorten with radial deviation (B) as it tilts more volarly, and appears to elongate with ulnar deviation, as it tilts toward the coronal plane. The spaces between the scaphoid, lunate, and triquetrum change only slightly between the two images. Also note the concavities in the articular surface of the distal radius, which are the normal scaphoid and lunate fossae, marked with white and black arrowheads, respectively in part A. These fossae may be well developed, as in this patient, or nearly absent. Slight angulation of the x-ray beam also can make these fossae more or less apparent.

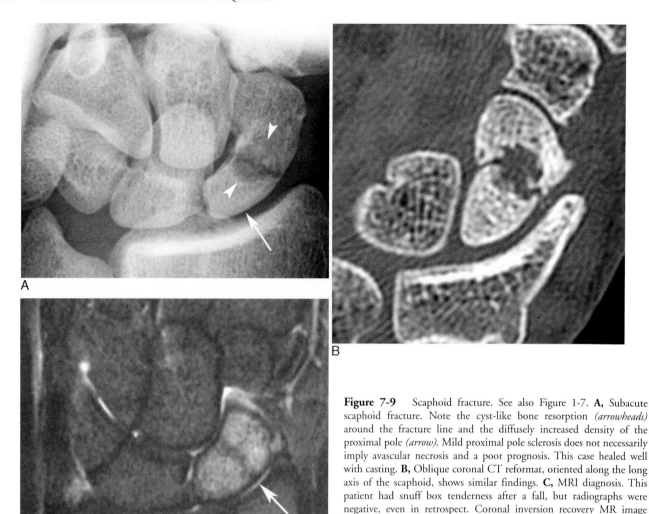

Figure 7-9   Scaphoid fracture. See also Figure 1-7. **A,** Subacute scaphoid fracture. Note the cyst-like bone resorption *(arrowheads)* around the fracture line and the diffusely increased density of the proximal pole *(arrow)*. Mild proximal pole sclerosis does not necessarily imply avascular necrosis and a poor prognosis. This case healed well with casting. **B,** Oblique coronal CT reformat, oriented along the long axis of the scaphoid, shows similar findings. **C,** MRI diagnosis. This patient had snuff box tenderness after a fall, but radiographs were negative, even in retrospect. Coronal inversion recovery MR image shows diffuse scaphoid marrow edema. The fracture line is seen as a low-signal-intensity band traversing the scaphoid waist *(arrow)*.

interrupted. Thus, prompt diagnosis and treatment are essential. Some scaphoid fractures are simply not visible on initial radiographs, even with dedicated views. Negative radiographs in the presence of snuff box tenderness and a history of wrist trauma necessitate immobilization or further imaging with CT or MRI (see Fig. 7-9C). If immobilization is selected (it usually is), repeat radiographs obtained after 7 to 10 days usually reveal bone resorption or faint sclerosis around a fracture. Some fractures remain radiographically occult. Scaphoid waist and proximal pole fractures may take up to 2 years to heal. Cystic changes and fragmentation along the fracture margins can occur in slowly healing fractures and in cases of nonunion (see Fig. 7-9). Screw fixation and bone grafting are occasionally required (see Fig. 7-10). In addition to the complications of delayed union, nonunion, and avascular necrosis, a scaphoid fracture may heal with apex dorsal angular deformity, termed

the *humpback deformity* (see Fig. 7-10). Thin-section CT sections obtained parallel to the long axis of the scaphoid exquisitely demonstrate complications such as the humpback deformity, and allow detailed assessment of presence or absence of fracture healing (see Figs. 1-28, 7-10).

The second most frequent carpal bone fracture is an avulsion fracture of the joint capsule from the dorsal triquetrum. This fracture is usually visible only on a lateral or slightly off-lateral radiograph, where it is seen as a small cortical chip displaced a few millimeters from the triquetrum (Fig. 7-11). Point tenderness over the fracture is an important clue to this diagnosis. Transverse fractures across the capitate and proximal hamate can be seen as part of complex fracture-dislocations. The hook of the hamate (hamulus) can fracture with a direct blow to the palm or as a stress fracture in carpenters or golfers. The hook is seen "on end" on PA radiographs as a dense C

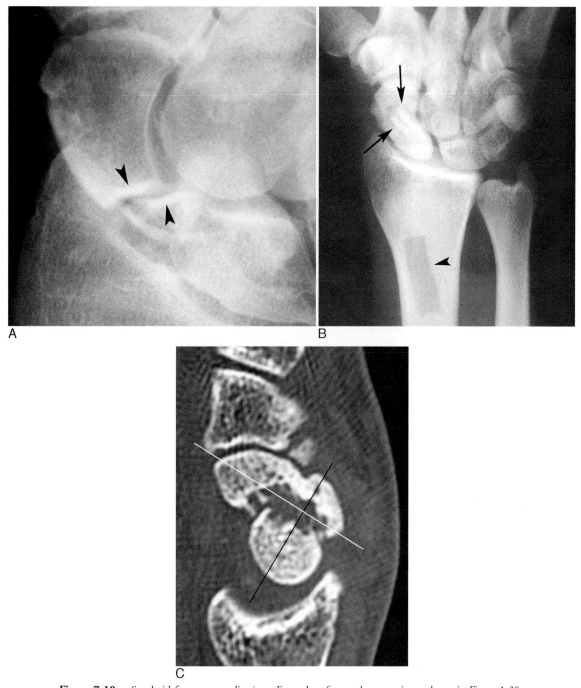

Figure 7-10   Scaphoid fracture complications. Examples of avascular necrosis are shown in Figure 1-30. **A,** Nonunion. Note the sclerosis and smooth margins of the old fracture *(arrowheads),* indicating that this is a chronic finding. **B,** Delayed union, successfully treated with bone grafting. Note the graft fragments *(arrows)* and the graft donor site in the distal radius *(arrowhead).* **C,** Humpback deformity. Oblique coronal CT image aligned with the scaphoid shows dorsal tilt of the proximal fragment *(black line)* and palmar tilt of the distal fragment *(white line),* resulting in the "humpback" deformity. Other images (not shown) showed that the fracture had healed in this position.

projecting over the mid-distal hamate. If the hook is displaced, this C may not be seen. A carpal tunnel view or other dedicated views may reveal this fracture (Fig. 7-12). Computed tomography or MRI usually is definitive. Lunate fractures are rare. However, the lunate is vulnerable to avascular necrosis (Kienböck's disease, see Fig. 22-8), especially in the presence of negative ulna variance, which can progress to lunate fragmentation and collapse.

Carpal trauma concentrates disruptive forces along arcs that run perpendicular to Gilula's arcs (Fig. 7-13). This results in

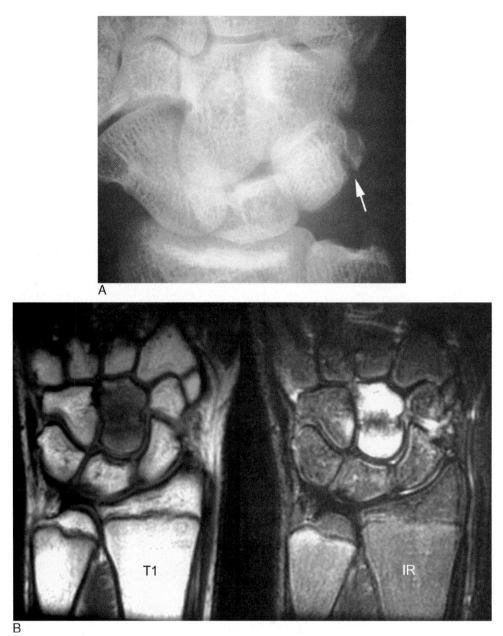

Figure 7-11   Subtle carpal fractures. **A,** Triquetral dorsal avulsion fracture *(arrow)*. These fractures may only be seen on an oblique view as in this example. **B,** Radiographically occult transverse capitate fracture easily detected with MRI.

injury patterns known as greater and lesser arc injuries. *Greater arc* injuries extend through the radial styloid and scaphoid, and across the proximal capitate, hamate, triquetrum, and ulnar styloid, or through the ligaments adjacent to these bones. This accounts for the relative frequency of scaphoid and radial and ulnar styloid fractures, as well as the ligamentous injuries that can accompany these fractures. A relatively common greater arc injury is the *trans-scaphoid perilunate fracture-dislocation,* in which the arc of injury passes through the scaphoid waist, across the ligaments fixing the distal carpal row and the triquetrum to the lunate, and the ulnar styloid. Other

greater arc injuries include the trans-scaphoid, transcapitate, perilunate fracture-dislocation (Fig. 7-14) and the rare and severe trans-scaphoid, transcapitate, transhamate, transtriquetral fracture-dislocation. Restoration of normal function is difficult with any of these injuries. The bones can be restored to their proper positions, and the fractures can heal, but the extensive associated ligamentous damage often results in abnormal carpal motion with pain and loss of function.

Lesser arc injuries, also termed *rotary subluxation of the lunate,* are confined to the ligaments surrounding the lunate. Lesser arc injuries result from forced hyperextension

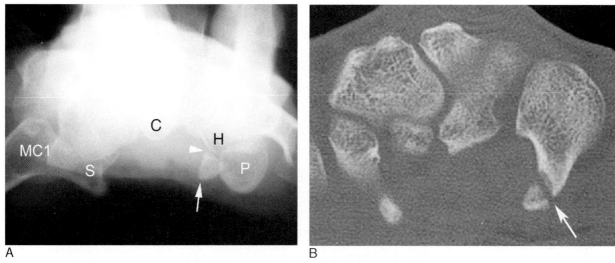

Figure 7-12   Carpal tunnel view and hamate hook (hamulus) fracture. **A,** Carpal tunnel view radiograph is obtained with the wrist dorsiflexed and the x-ray beam tangential to the wrist. Arrow, hook of hamate. This patient has an unfused hook of the hamate *(arrowhead)*. Note the straight, smooth, sclerotic margins, suggesting that this finding may be due to a developmental variant or a chronic ununited fracture. **B,** CT image in a different patient shows an acute hamate hook fracture *(arrow)*. C, capitate; H, hamate; MC1, thumb metacarpal; P, pisiform; S, scaphoid and trapezium.

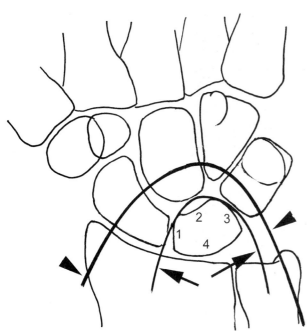

Figure 7-13   Carpal trauma tends to concentrate disruptive forces along or close to these greater *(arrowheads)* or lesser *(arrows)* arcs. The greater arc *(arrowheads)* passes across the scaphoid waist; thus, greater arc injuries are usually fracture dislocations that include a scaphoid waist fracture. The lesser arc *(arrows)* surrounds the lunate. Lesser arc injuries cause a spectrum of ligamentous injuries and dislocations that involve the lunate in a predictable pattern of increasing severity. The mildest form (stage 1) disrupts only the scapholunate ligaments, causing scapholunate dissociation (see Fig. 7-22). Stage 2 is more severe, as it also disrupts the ligamentous fixation of the lunate to the capitate. Further ligamentous disruption continues around the lunate to stage 4, resulting in lunate dislocation (see Fig. 7-16).

(dorsiflexion) force applied to the thenar eminence. Ligamentous injury around the lunate occurs in a predictable pattern with increasing force (Figs. 7-15, 7-16). This is an advanced concept for an introductory text, but is included for completeness. The stage 1 injury is interruption of the scapholunate ligaments and results in scapholunate dissociation (discussed later in this chapter). Stage 2 injury releases the fixation between the lunate and capitate (see Fig. 7-15). Capitolunate instability or a perilunate dislocation are classic presentations of stage 2 rotary subluxation. Stage 3 injury continues around the circumference of the lunate with interruption of ligamentous fixation of the lunate and triquetrum. A stage 3 injury may present as a *midcarpal dislocation,* in which the lunate is tilted palmarly and the other carpal bones dislocated dorsally relative to the lunate and the radius. In stage 4 injury, there is complete disruption of the ligamentous fixation of the lunate to the radius, resulting in palmar lunate dislocation (see Fig. 7-16). The radiographic appearance of perilunate and midcarpal dislocations can overlap, blurring the distinction between some stage 2 and stage 3 injuries. Similarly, there can be overlap of the radiographic appearance of midcarpal and lunate dislocation, blurring the distinction between some stage 3 and stage 4 injuries. Usually the distinction is not terribly important.

CARPAL INSTABILITY

Carpal instability can be a confusing and intimidating subject for the radiologist. This discussion will attempt to simplify this topic by beginning with a review of necessary terminology,

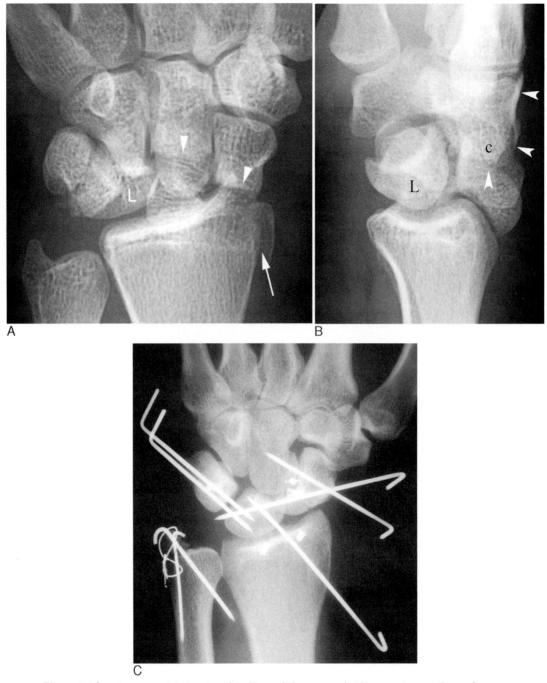

Figure 7-14   Greater arc injuries. **A and B,** Transradial, trans-scaphoid transcapitate perilunate fracture-dislocation. The PA view (A) shows fractures of the radial styloid *(arrow),* and the scaphoid waist and proximal capitate *(arrowheads),* with ligamentous disruption medially completing the greater arc. The lateral view (B) shows the lunate has normal relation with the radius, but the capitate is dislocated dorsally (*arrowheads* mark the proximal capitate in B). This pattern is termed perilunate dislocation. **C,** Surgical reconstruction of the wrist after a trans-scaphoid perilunate fracture-dislocation in a different patient. The extensive fixation illustrates the severity of the ligamentous injuries associated with greater arc injuries. c, capitate; L, lunate.

followed by a simplified anatomic overview and a brief discussion of the important instability patterns.

Normal osseous carpal anatomy and motion have been discussed previously. *Translocation* describes a shift of the entire carpus from its normal position relative to the radius (e.g.,

ulnar translocation). *Dissociation* usually implies abnormal motion between bones within the same carpal row, often in association with interruption of the corresponding interosseous ligament, such as *scapholunate dissociation.* Because the proximal carpal row has no tendinous attachments, its position is

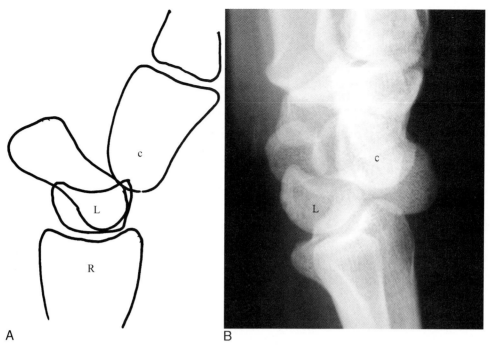

Figure 7-15   Stage 2 lesser arc injury: perilunate dislocation. **A,** Diagram shows alignment findings in perilunate dislocation. The lunate is not displaced volarly, although it is often tilted volarly. The capitate is displaced dorsally relative to the lunate and radius. Stage 3 lesser arc injury results in midcarpal dislocation (not shown), in which the lunate is volarly subluxed but not dislocated relative to the radius and the capitate is dorsally *dislocated* relative to the lunate. **B,** Lateral radiograph shows perilunate dislocation, with alignment similar to that seen in part A. c, capitate; L, lunate; R, radius.

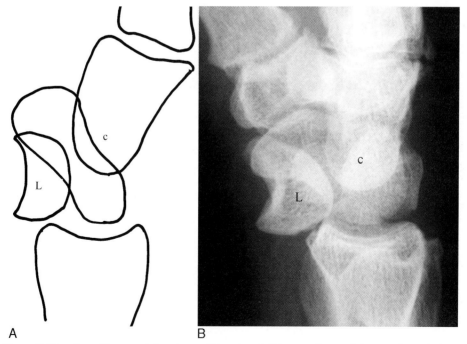

Figure 7-16   Stage 4 lesser arc injury: lunate dislocation. **A,** Diagram of lunate dislocation shows the lunate to be tilted and dislocated volarly. The capitate is collinear with the radius. **B,** Lateral radiographic view shows the palmar lunate dislocation, with alignment similar to that shown in part A. In this dislocation pattern, there is true dislocation both at the radiolunate and lunocapitate articulations.

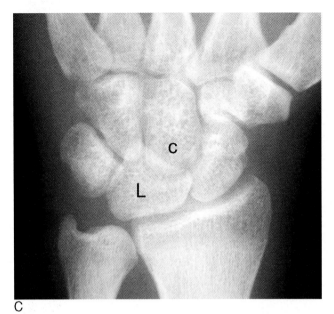

C

Figure 7-16—(Cont'd)   **C,** PA radiographic view shows disruption of the carpal arcs and abnormal contour of the lunate due to the dislocation. C, capitate; L, lunate; R, radius.

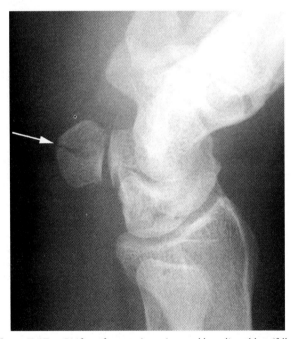

Figure 7-17   Pisiform fracture *(arrow),* caused by a direct blow (fell on palm of hand onto a hard surface).

determined by the position of the radius and the distal carpal row. In the language of mechanical engineering, this makes the proximal carpal row an *intercalated segment.* Intercalated segment instability patterns represent instability *between carpal rows.* Thus, the terms "dorsal intercalated segment instability

(DISI)" and "volar intercalated segment instability (VISI)" refer to abnormal alignment between the carpal rows, with particular focus on alignment of the lunate and capitate. *Carpal columns* run perpendicular to the carpal rows. There are three carpal columns: central (radius-lunate-capitate), ulnar (ulna-triquetrum-hamate), and radial (radius-scaphoid-trapezoid and trapezium). The carpal columns transmit force from the hand to the forearm, primarily through the central column. Instability can be confined to one of the carpal columns. *Static carpal instability* produces abnormal carpal alignment on standard radiographs obtained with the wrist in neutral alignment. In contrast, *dynamic* carpal instability requires wrist fluoroscopy or special radiographs such as a clenched fist view or for detection. For example, fluoroscopy may reveal abnormal carpal motion in a patient with a painful wrist click or clunk.

WHAT THE CLINICIAN WANTS TO KNOW: CARPAL INSTABILITY

Carpal alignment

Dynamic instability as shown by fluoroscopy/stress maneuvers

Arthrography or MRI: ligament or triangular fibrocartilage complex tears

Complications: Osteoarthritis, SLAC wrist (scapholunate dissociation with advanced collapse)

Associated conditions: Old fractures, inflammatory arthritis, calcium pyrophosphate deposition (CPPD) arthropathy

---

Instability results from ligament injury. Wrist ligaments are most frequently injured by trauma, but inflammatory arthritis, usually rheumatoid arthritis, also may cause significant ligament damage. Ligamentous anatomy of the wrist is complex. The most important *intrinsic ligaments* are the *scapholunate* (SL) and the *lunotriquetral* (LT) interosseous ligaments located along the proximal margins of these bones (Figs. 7-2A, 7-18–7-20). The SL and LT ligaments can be directly studied with arthrography and high-quality MRI and CT and MR arthrography. Both of these ligaments have thicker, stronger dorsal and palmar components that blend into the extrinsic ligaments of the joint capsule, and thinner central portions. The dorsal portion of the SL and palmar portion of the LT probably are the most important parts of these ligaments. Perforation of the thin central portion can occur as an incidental finding, especially in older patients. Such perforations do not indicate ligament failure and therefore are an important pitfall in arthrography in older patients. Thin-section MRI often reveals portions of the interosseous ligaments to be triangular in cross-section. The ligaments may appear to attach onto the articular cartilage, or through the cartilage into bone. Both the LT and SL ligaments can stretch by approximately 50% to 100% of their length before tearing. Another set of interosseous ligaments unite the bones of the distal carpal row. These ligaments are rarely interrupted and are not discussed further.

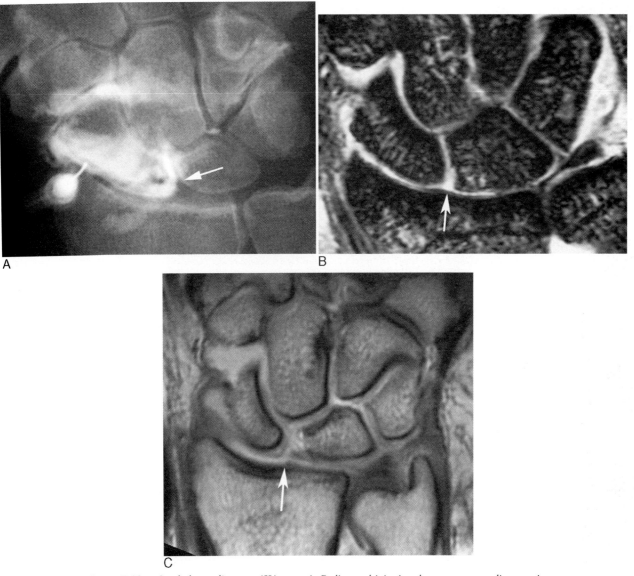

Figure 7-18   Scapholunate ligament (SL) tears. **A,** Radiocarpal injection shows contrast medium passing through a scapholunate tear *(arrow)* into the midcarpal joint. **B,** Coronal gradient echo MR image shows high signal intensity similar to joint fluid in the normal location of the SL ligament. **C,** Coronal T1-weighted MR arthrogram obtained after radiocarpal injection shows SL ligament tear *(arrow)* with wide scapholunate interval.

Key Concepts	Carpal ligaments

Intrinsic ligaments:
  Scapholunate (SL) and lunotriquetral
    (LT) interosseous ligaments
  Separate radiocarpal from midcarpal joints
  Dorsal portion of SL probably most important for carpal
    stability
  Small perforations may not be significant
Capsular (extrinsic ligaments):
  Complex arrangement of dorsal and palmar capsular
    thickening
  Necessary for carpal stability

The *extrinsic wrist ligaments,* also termed the *capsular ligaments,* are a complex set of organized thickenings of the palmar and dorsal joint capsule (see Fig. 7-20). These ligaments are very important functionally but are difficult to image directly. The palmar (volar) capsular ligaments are thought to be stronger and more important in maintaining wrist stability than the dorsal ligaments. Many of the capsular ligaments are named by the bones they connect. A limited enumeration of the most important capsular ligaments is included here. The main palmar ligaments include the radioscaphocapite, radiolunotriquetral, and the ulnotriquetral and ulnar collateral ligaments. The main dorsal ligaments include the radioscaphoid, dorsal radiolunotriquetral, and a variable transverse ligament or ligaments that extend from the triquetrum laterally across

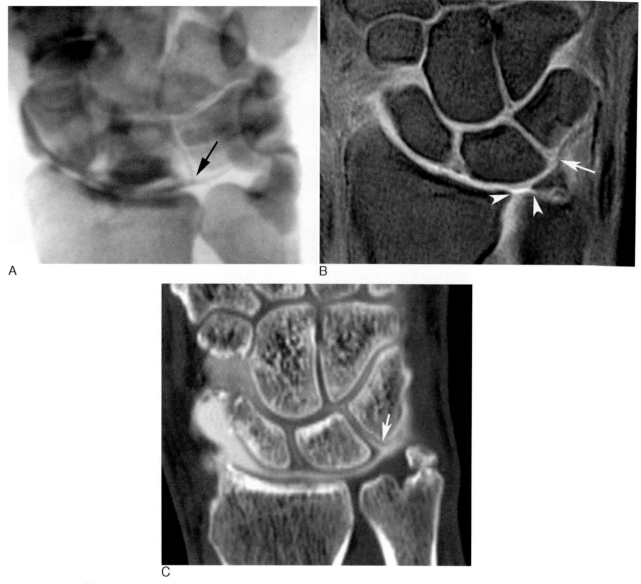

Figure 7-19   Lunotriquetral ligament (LT) tears. **A,** Ulnar deviation view obtained after radiocarpal injection shows a lunotriquetral tear *(arrows)* with contrast medium filling the midcarpal compartment. **B,** Coronal T1-weighted MR arthrogram image after radiocarpal injection shows LT ligament tear *(arrow)* and wide triangular fibrocartilage (TFC) tear *(arrowheads)*. **C,** CT arthrogram reformat in a different patient with LT tear *(arrow)*. Note the intact SL ligament and TFC.

the capitate to the scaphoid and trapezoid. Limited demonstration of these extrinsic ligaments is possible with thin-section MRI. Much can be inferred about their functional status by assessment of carpal alignment and motion on radiographs and fluoroscopy (Figs. 7-21–7-23).

Scapholunate dissociation (rotary or rotatory subluxation of the scaphoid) is caused by disruption of the SL interosseous ligament *and* the extrinsic ligaments that stabilize this articulation (see Figs. 7-21, 7-22). This is the most common carpal instability pattern. A normal lateral radiograph obtained with the wrist in neutral alignment shows the scaphoid in approximately 45 degrees of palmar angulation (normal range, 30 to

60 degrees) and the lunate in neutral alignment. Compressive forces across the wrist due to dorsal and palmar muscle contraction tend to force the scaphoid into further palmar flexion. However, the normal ligamentous fixation of the scaphoid to the lunate prevents the scaphoid from further palmar angulation. In scapholunate dissociation, the scaphoid is released from the lunate and can rotate into greater palmar flexion. Thus, the key finding on the lateral radiograph is that the scapholunate angle will exceed 60 degrees. Additionally, the lunate may roll dorsally from its normal neutral alignment, although this is not always present. When present, dorsal rotation of the lunate alters its appearance on a PA radiograph

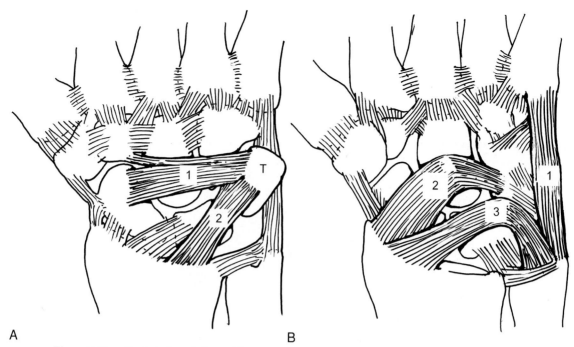

Figure 7-20 Extrinsic (capsular) carpal ligament anatomy. **A,** Diagram of the dorsal carpal ligaments. The most important are labeled: 1, dorsal intercarpal (transverse) ligament; 2, dorsal radiocarpal (radiolunotrique-tral) ligament. Note that both insert onto the triquetrum. **B,** Diagram of the palmar carpal ligaments. The most important are labeled: 1, ulnar carpal complex (includes the ulnar collateral ligament); 2, distal arc (radioscaphocapitate and capitotriquetral, blends into 1); 3, proximal arc (radiolunotriquetral, also termed long radiolunate, and ulnotriquetral). T, triquetrum.

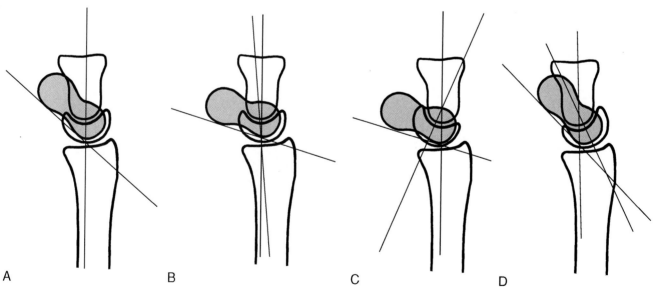

Figure 7-21 Diagram of carpal instability patterns as seen on a lateral radiograph. All measurements require a well-positioned lateral view with the wrist in neutral alignment, not dorsiflexed. **A,** Normal. Scapholunate angle is between 30 and 60 degrees and capitate and lunate are aligned. **B,** Scapholunate dissociation. Scapholunate angle is greater than 60 degrees, but capitate and lunate are approximately aligned. **C,** Dorsal intercalated segment instability (DISI). Scapholunate angle is greater than 60 degrees and lunate is tilted dorsally with capitolunate angle greater than 10 to 20 degrees. **D,** Volar intercalated segment instability (VISI). Scapholunate angle is less than 30 degrees and lunate is tilted palmar with capitolunate angle greater than 10 to 20 degrees.

from the normal trapezoidal configuration into a triangular shape (see Fig. 7-22A). A PA radiograph may also reveal widening of the scapholunate interval above its normal value of 2 mm; 4 mm is considered to be pathognomonic (see Figs. 7-18C, 7-22). A gap between the scaphoid and lunate has been called the "Terry Thomas sign" in reference to the late, gap-toothed British comedian. A more current popular reference might be the "David Letterman sign." A PA view obtained with a clenched fist or a PA view in ulnar deviation may elicit or increase this finding. Fluoroscopy reveals the scaphoid and

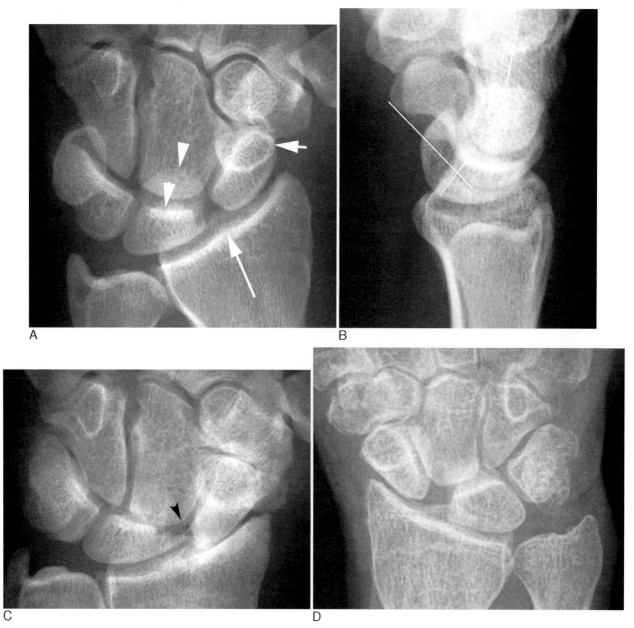

Figure 7-22   Scapholunate dissociation and dorsal intercalated segment instability (DISI). **A,** PA radiographic view shows a widened scapholunate interval *(long arrow)*. The arrowheads mark the dorsal and volar margins of the distal lunate, which should be superimposed on a PA view. They do not overlap because the lunate is rotated dorsally. The scaphoid is rotated volarly, causing it to appear shortened on this PA view *(short arrow)*. These findings suggest scapholunate dissociation. **B,** Lateral view with the wrist in neutral alignment. Note lines drawn through the long axes of the lunate, scaphoid, and capitate show the scapholunate angle to be greater than 60 degrees, indicating scapholunate dissociation. Additionally, the capitolunate angle is greater than 20 degrees, indicating DISI also is present. **C,** Follow-up PA radiograph obtained 3 years later shows progression to scapholunate advanced collapse (SLAC) wrist, with collapse of the capitate into the lateral lunate and medial scaphoid *(arrowhead)* and secondary osteoarthritis. **D,** Clenched fist view in a different patient with scapholunate dissociation accentuates the wide scapholunate interval *(arrow)*.

(Continued)

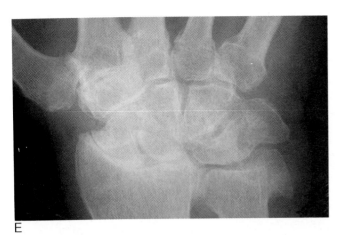

Figure 7-22—(Cont'd)   **E,** SLAC wrist, more advanced case.

lunate to move independently of one another. In some cases of scapholunate dissociation, PA and lateral radiographs are normal, and the abnormality becomes evident only with fluoroscopy or a stress series of radiographs that reproduces the range of motion examined with fluoroscopy. Provocative maneuvers may be required. A popular example is the Watson's test (scaphoid shift test). The patient's wrist is held in neutral alignment with the examiner's thumb pressed against the palmar distal pole of the scaphoid. The wrist is then moved into radial deviation while maintaining this pressure. The scaphoid will rotate further palmar in a normal wrist, but will not if scapholunate dissociation is present. This test is clinically pos-

itive if painful, but may also be performed during fluoroscopy to document the absence of scaphoid palmar flexion during radial deviation.

Abnormal motion and distribution of forces associated with scapholunate dissociation can result in degeneration and collapse of the medial scaphoid and lateral lunate bones and radiocarpal joint, termed *scapholunate advanced collapse* (SLAC wrist, Fig. 7-22).

Dorsal intercalated segment instability (DISI, dorsiflexion instability) is usually but not necessarily associated with scapholunate dissociation. Like scapholunate dissociation, DISI is a derangement of the radial side of the wrist and is often associated with radial-sided symptoms. The lunate tilts *dorsally,* increasing the lunocapitate angle above 20 degrees. Note that some authors use 30 degrees to reduce false-positive diagnoses of DISI. Scapholunate dissociation usually is present, with the scapholunate angle greater than 60 degrees (see Fig. 7-22). Lateral fluoroscopy of the wrist in flexion in DISI shows that the lunate fails to flex relative to the radius, or that the capitate fails to flex relative to the lunate. It should be noted that static radiographic configuration of DISI can occasionally be seen as a normal variant, with normal motion seen at fluoroscopy.

Volar intercalated segment instability (VISI, volar flexion instability) is a consequence of ulnar-sided ligament derangement. The lunate is turned volarly and the capitolunate angle is greater than 20 degrees (Fig. 7-23). As with DISI, some authors use 30 degrees to reduce false-positive diagnoses. Comparing the alignment of the lunate and radius also can

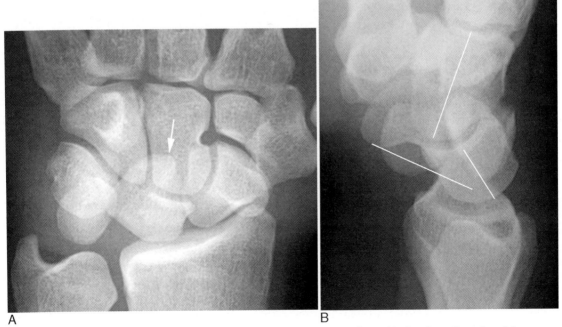

Figure 7-23   Volar intercalated segment instability (VISI). **A,** PA radiographic view shows disruption of the carpal arcs. Note the triangular or wedge shape of the lunate *(arrow),* indicating that it is rotated. **B,** Lateral view with lines drawn through the long axes of the lunate, scaphoid, and capitate shows VISI alignment, with the scapholunate angle less than 30 degrees and the capitolunate angle greater than 20 degrees.

reduce false-positive diagnoses because the lunate is usually palmar-flexed by at least 10 degrees relative to the radius. Lunotriquetral dissociation is usually also present, so the scapholunate angle is decreased below 30 degrees. Fluoroscopy of palmar and dorsiflexion in VISI does not show symmetric motion at the radiolunate and lunocapitate joints. Both lunotriquetral dissociation and VISI are associated with ulnar-sided pain. VISI is much less common than DISI. The former may result from a fall onto the hypothenar eminence but is also the most frequent carpal instability pattern encountered in patients with rheumatoid arthritis.

Lunotriquetral dissociation or instability results from disruption of the ligamentous fixation of the lunate and triquetrum. The condition is conceptually similar to scapholunate dissociation, but lunotriquetral instability does not typically result in LT widening. Subtle interruption of the carpal arcs may be seen, and the scapholunate angle may decrease to less than 30 degrees. A clenched fist maneuver will roll the scaphoid and lunate into palmar flexion. Lunotriquetral instability usually occurs in association with VISI.

Capitolunate instability (*c*apitolunate *i*nstability *p*attern, CLIP wrist) is a dynamic instability pattern of the central column centered at the lunocapitate joint. Manipulation of the capitate and lunate during fluoroscopy with the "CLIP maneuver," described in Chapter 48, may be needed to detect this condition.

Triquetrohamate instability is a dynamic instability of the medial column. Patients have ulnar-sided pain and a reproducible click. Fluoroscopy reveals the click to correspond to the abnormal motion between the hamate and triquetrum. Normally, the proximal carpal row smoothly swings into dorsiflexion as the wrist goes into ulnar deviation. In triquetrohamate instability, the dorsiflexion is delayed until the wrist is fairly far into ulnar deviation, when the proximal carpal row abruptly flips into dorsiflexion with a painful clunk. Triquetrohamate instability is caused by forced pronation and radial deviation.

Carpal translocation can occur in any direction. Ulnar translocation of the entire carpus is associated with rheumatoid arthritis. Radial and dorsal carpal translocation is associated with a prior Colles fracture. Palmar carpal translocation is associated with a prior reverse Barton's fracture.

MISCELLANEOUS CARPAL CONDITIONS

The tendons of the wrist are grouped in anatomic compartments (Fig. 7-24). The tendons of the wrist can be studied with MRI, US, and injection of contrast medium into a tendon sheath under fluoroscopic guidance (tenography). Tendons of the wrist are vulnerable to overuse and traumatic injury, similar to tendons elsewhere in the body (Fig. 7-25). Rheumatoid arthritis causes pannus formation as well as fluid accumulation within the tendon sheaths. *De Quervain's disease*

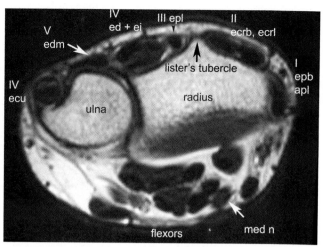

Figure 7-24 Wrist tendon compartments. Axial T1-weighted MR image shows the flexor and six extensor tendon compartments. Clockwise, from the left (medial) side of the image: ecu, extensor carpi ulnaris (note the thickened tendon indicating tendinosis); edm, extensor digiti minimi; ed, extensor digitorum; ei, extensor indicis; epl, extensor pollicis longus; ecrb, extensor carpi radialis brevis; ecrl, extensor carpi radialis longus; epl, extensor pollicis brevis; apl, abductor pollicis longus; med n, median nerve.

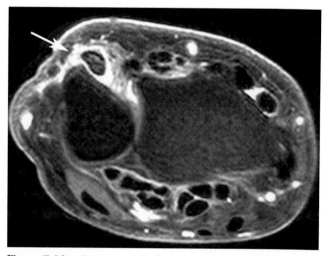

Figure 7-25 Extensor carpi ulnaris partial tear and tenosynovitis. Axial fat-suppressed T2-weighted MR image shows thickened, edematous extensor carpi ulnaris tendon with tendon sheath fluid *(arrow)*. Patients with ECU tendinitis present with medial wrist pain that can mimic a triangular fibrocartilage (TFC) or lunotriquetral (LT) ligament tear or lunate avascular necrosis.

is stenosing tenosynovitis of the extensor pollicis brevis and abductor pollicis longus tendons. *Palmar fibromatosis*, also know as *Dupuytren's contracture*, is fibromatosis of the palmar hand. Fibrotic bands tether the hand flexor tendons, causing flexion contractures, most frequently of the medial fingers (see Fig. 33-8). This is a common condition in the elderly. The extensor carpi ulnaris tendon can dislocate from its groove in the distal ulna.

Key Concepts	**Frequently Missed Wrist Injuries**
Scaphoid waist fracture	
Triquetrum fracture	
Carpometacarpal (CMC) dislocation	
Hamate hook fracture	

Ganglion cysts are common around the wrist, and most discovered on MRI or US are incidental. However, these may be associated with wrist pain, and correlation of the imaging findings with clinical symptoms is necessary. Ganglion cysts contain free water and are seen on US as well-circumscribed uniloculate or multiloculate cysts. Magnetic resonance imaging shows uniform high T2 signal intensity and intermediate T1 signal intensity. Magnetic resonance images with gadolinium may show only peripheral enhancement. These lesions often develop at areas of relative weakness in the joint capsule, but some originate from tendon sheaths. Contrast enhancement may better outline the ganglion neck (i.e., the frequently narrow attachment of the ganglion to the joint capsule). Resected ganglia tend to recur if the neck is not also removed, so identification of the source of the ganglion relative to the joint capsule is important information for the surgeon.

Carpal tunnel syndrome is median nerve dysfunction caused by increased pressure within the carpal tunnel. The many potential causes of carpal tunnel syndrome include fracture, tenosynovitis, rheumatoid arthritis, gout, amyloid, tuberculosis, tumors, pregnancy, diabetes, anomalous muscles, and repetitive stress. Many cases are idiopathic. Some authors believe that MRI and US can make or exclude the diagnosis of carpal tunnel syndrome, but most believe that the syndrome is a clinical or electromyographic diagnosis. Both MRI and US can be useful in identifying or excluding a surgically correctable cause, such as a mass lesion within the carpal tunnel (Figs. 7-26, 7-27).

Guyon's canal on the palmar medial wrist between the pisiform and the hook of the hamate contains the ulnar nerve

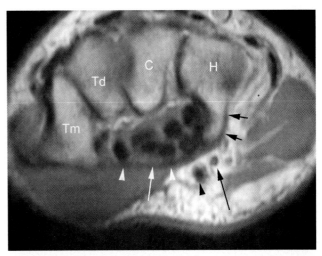

Figure 7-26   Carpal tunnel and Guyon's canal. Axial proton density MR image shows normal anatomy of the carpal tunnel and Guyon's canal. The carpal tunnel is bounded by the trapezium, trapezoid, capitate, hamate (with the hook marked by *short black arrows*), and retinaculum *(white arrowheads)*. The median nerve *(white arrow)* has intermediate signal intensity on this sequence because it contains myelin, which has signal characteristics similar to those of fat. A normal median nerve is difficult to identify on a fat-suppressed sequence unless it is edematous. Guyon's canal is a triangular shaped space located palmar to the hook of the hamate. It contains the ulnar nerve *(long black arrow)* and the ulnar artery *(black arrowhead)*. Can you identify the same structures in Figure 2-32? C, capitate; H, hamate; Td, trapezoid; Tm, trapezium.

and artery (see Fig. 7-27). The same list of conditions that can cause median nerve impingement within the carpal tunnel can similarly afflict the ulnar nerve within Guyon's canal.

The wrist is prone to cartilage degeneration just as any other joint. Two sites deserve special mention. Ulna abutment syndrome, discussed previously, causes cartilage loss at the proximal lunate. In about 50% of individuals, the proximal pole of the hamate articulates with the lunate, termed a type II hamate. (Type I hamate does not articulate with the lunate.) This normal variant carries a risk of symptomatic chondromalacia and subchondral marrow edema at the hamate proximal pole, or occasionally the adjacent lunate, which are often extremely subtle on MRI (Fig. 7-28).

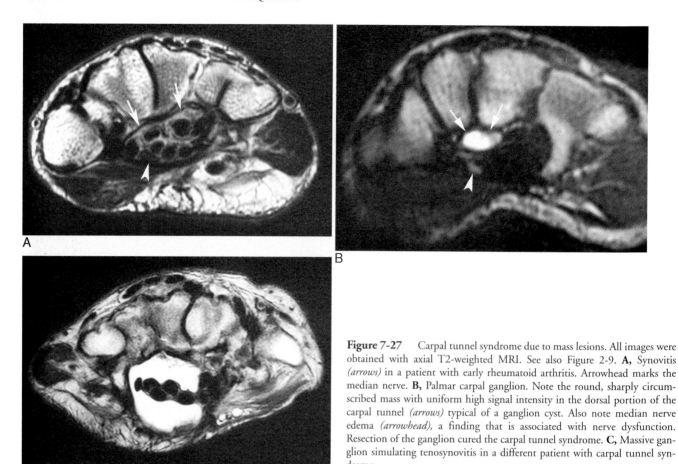

Figure 7-27   Carpal tunnel syndrome due to mass lesions. All images were obtained with axial T2-weighted MRI. See also Figure 2-9. **A,** Synovitis *(arrows)* in a patient with early rheumatoid arthritis. Arrowhead marks the median nerve. **B,** Palmar carpal ganglion. Note the round, sharply circumscribed mass with uniform high signal intensity in the dorsal portion of the carpal tunnel *(arrows)* typical of a ganglion cyst. Also note median nerve edema *(arrowhead),* a finding that is associated with nerve dysfunction. Resection of the ganglion cured the carpal tunnel syndrome. **C,** Massive ganglion simulating tenosynovitis in a different patient with carpal tunnel syndrome.

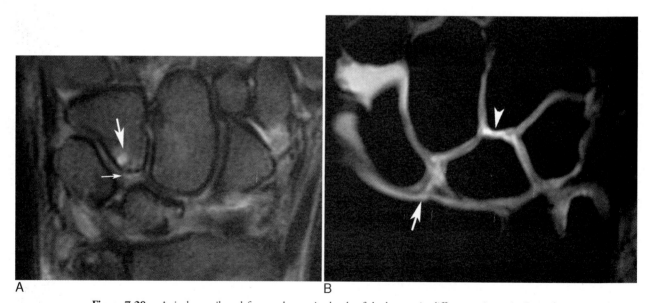

Figure 7-28   Articular cartilage defects at the proximal pole of the hamate in different patients. **A,** Coronal inversion recovery MR image shows subchondral edema and cysts in the hamate *(large arrow)* and high signal intensity in proximal pole cartilage *(small arrow).* **B,** Coronal fat-suppressed T1-weighted MR arthrogram. The image is adjusted to display articular cartilage gray. Note high-signal-intensity contrast medium *(arrowhead)* abutting the hamate. Also note scapholunate ligament tear *(arrow).*

The thumb metacarpal (MC) articulates with the trapezium, constituting the first carpometacarpal (CMC) joint (CMC I joint). The second MC articulates with the trapezoid, the third MC articulates with the capitate, and the fourth and fifth MCs articulate with the hamate. The proximal second through fifth MCs also articulate with adjacent MCs. The articulation of the second through fifth metacarpals and the distal carpal row form a single synovial compartment, the CMC II-V joint. This compartment frequently communicates with the midcarpal joint as a normal variant. The articulations of the CMC II-V joint normally have a "zig-zag" pattern on a true posteroanterior (PA) radiograph obtained with the palm and fingers flat against the cassette (see Fig. 7-1A). Disruption of this pattern suggests a dislocation (Fig. 8-1). Carpometacarpal II-V dislocations are usually dorsal, may be multiple, and are often associated with small fractures. Conversely, the presence of a small fracture fragment at or adjacent to a CMC joint suggests that a dislocation is or was present.

Thumb injuries require dedicated radiographs because routine hand radiographs do not profile the thumb in true PA and lateral projections. Extra-articular fractures of the first metacarpal tend to maintain anatomic alignment because the muscle attachments along the shaft resist displacement. However, intra-articular fractures at the base of the thumb can displace and are frequently unstable. A *Bennett's fracture* is an intra-articular fracture-dislocation of the proximal first MC. The mechanism of injury is axial loading of a partially flexed first metacarpal, often sustained during a fistfight. The volar ligamentous fixation of the first MC is very strong, so a small volar bone fragment is avulsed from the first MC and retains a normal position while the larger fragment subluxes or dislocates dorsally. A Bennett's fracture is unstable and is treated by open reduction and internal fixation (ORIF). The unusual *Rolando's fracture* is a comminuted Bennett's fracture (Fig. 8-2). Restoration of anatomic alignment is often impossible because of the comminution, so Rolando's fractures are frequently treated with casting or traction rather than ORIF.

A *boxer's fracture* is a metacarpal fracture caused by abrupt axial loading, usually during delivery of a punch (Fig. 8-3). The neck of the fifth MC is the most frequent location, with the fourth MC similarly fractured in many cases. Apex dorsal angulation with volar comminution is common, and healing with this angular deformity is frequent. A boxer's fracture may be complicated by an infection due to contamination by the teeth of the recipient of the punch.

Extra-articular fractures of the phalanges, particularly of the tufts, are often the result of blunt or sharp trauma (e.g., with a hammer, car door, or table saw). Accurate assessment of fracture angulation requires a true lateral radiograph. Rotational deformity is also important but may be assessed clinically.

Key Concepts	Frequently Missed Hand Injuries
Carpometacarpal (CMC) joint dislocation Palmar and dorsal avulsion fractures of the bases of the middle and distal phalanges Thumb metacarpal (MC) base fracture (e.g., Bennett's fracture)	

The metacarpophalangeal (MCP) and interphalangeal joints are stabilized against valgus and varus stress by ulnar (medial) and radial (lateral) collateral ligaments, respectively. Collateral ligament injuries can occur at any of these joints. The injured ligament may stretch, partially or completely tear, or avulse a small chip fragment. Posteroanterior views with valgus or varus stress may be required for diagnosis of a collateral ligament injury. Comparison with the uninjured side can be helpful, as some laxity of the collateral ligaments is normal.

The most frequently injured collateral ligament in the hand is the ulnar collateral ligament (UCL) of the thumb MCP joint. This injury, better known as *gamekeeper's thumb* or *skier's thumb*, is caused by valgus stress across the thumb, often

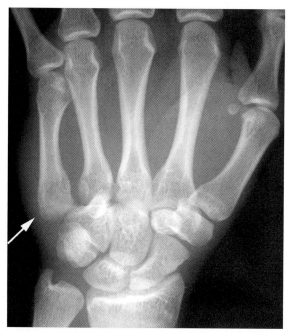

Figure 8-1   Dislocation of the base of the fifth metacarpal. Note the lateral position of the base of the fifth metacarpal as well as the abnormal finding of a gap between the bases of the fourth and fifth metacarpals.

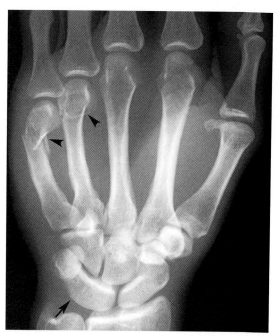

Figure 8-3   Boxer's fractures. The fourth and fifth metacarpals show typical neck fractures with apex dorsolateral angulation *(arrowheads)*. Also note the incidentally detected normal variant lunotriquetral coalition *(arrow)*.

combined with hyperextension (Fig. 8-4). Gamekeeper's thumb was first recognized as an occupational hazard of British gamekeepers, whose method of killing wounded rabbits placed valgus stress across the thumb. After several years of this overuse, the gamekeeper's UCL became stretched or torn, and the consequent instability resulted in pain and disability.

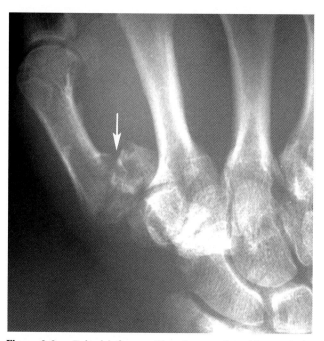

Figure 8-2   Rolando's fracture. Note the comminuted intra-articular fracture at the base of the thumb *(arrow)*.

Today, an injury to the thumb MCP UCL is often acute, sustained while falling on an outstretched hand while holding a ski pole. The tip of the thumb extends beyond the ski pole handle into the snow as the skier's forward momentum drives the hand forward along the snow surface, resulting in thumb valgus and hyperextension. A faulty pole plant has also been suggested as a cause of a UCL injury in skiers. Most UCL sprains and partial tears, as well as some minimally displaced complete tears or avulsions, are managed by immobilization. However, complete tears often require surgical exploration to locate and reattach the free edges of the torn UCL. In particular, the thumb adductor tendon aponeurosis can become interposed between the torn edges of the UCL, a situation termed the *Stener lesion*. High-resolution magnetic resonance imaging (MRI) can help identify the position of the ligament (Fig. 8-4C). Because a displaced ligament will not heal appropriately, Stener lesions are surgically corrected with anatomic reattachment of the displaced ligament.

Dislocations of the finger joints are associated with collateral ligament injuries and often with small avulsion fragments. The proximal interphalangeal (PIP) joints are the most frequently dislocated, usually dorsally or laterally (Fig. 8-5). These dislocations often reduce spontaneously or are reduced by the patient or nonmedical personnel before medical attention is reached. Residual soft tissue swelling, mild subluxation, or small avulsion fragments may be the only radiographic evidence of the prior dislocation. However, more severe associated fractures can occur (Fig. 8-5B).

Intra-articular fractures of the phalanges can occur on the medial, lateral, volar, or dorsal surfaces. Medial and lateral

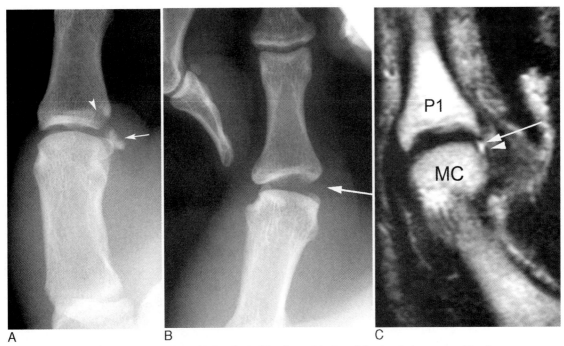

A   B   C

Figure 8-4   Skier's (gamekeeper's) thumb. **A,** AP radiographic view of the thumb shows an avulsion fracture at the distal insertion of the ulnar collateral ligament (UCL). Note the small avulsion fragment *(arrow)* and the donor site on the proximal phalanx *(arrowhead).* **B,** UCL injury without avulsion fracture in a different patient. The MCP joint has widened medially with stress *(arrow),* indicating laxity or disruption of the UCL. **C,** MR diagnosis. Coronal T2-weighted image shows high signal intensity of joint fluid passing through the interruption of the UCL *(arrow).* The arrowhead marks the intact, proximal portion of the UCL. MC, thumb metacarpal; P1, proximal phalanx.

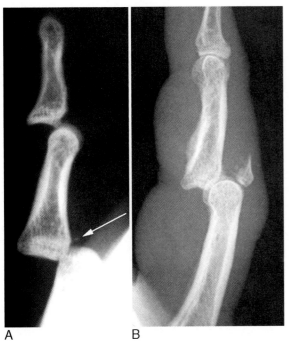

A   B

Figure 8-5   Finger dislocations. **A,** Dorsal dislocation of the thumb MCP *(arrow)* and interphalangeal joints. A tiny chip fragment at the MCP joint is faintly visible at the tip of the *arrow.* **B,** Second (index) finger PIP fracture dislocation. This injury required surgical reduction and fixation.

fractures are associated with collateral ligament avulsions, as noted previously. An avulsion fractures of the proximal volar aspect of the middle phalanx is termed a *volar plate fracture.* The volar plates are fibrocartilaginous structures that span the volar aspect of the PIP and MCP joints. Hyperextension can avulse the distal attachment of the volar plate at the PIP joint. A lateral radiograph reveals a small avulsion fragment displaced proximally from the donor site at the base of the middle phalanx (Fig. 8-6). A radiographically similar injury known as a

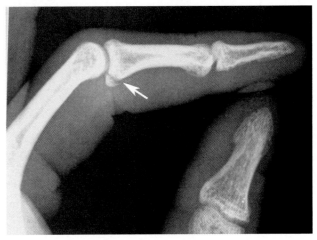

Figure 8-6   Volar plate fracture *(arrow).*

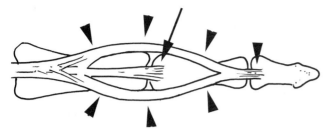

Figure 8-7   Diagram of the extensor tendon anatomy of the fingers. This dorsal view shows the middle slip *(arrow)* inserting onto the middle phalanx and the lateral slips *(arrowheads)* that unite distally before inserting onto the distal phalanx. (Modified with permission from Manaster BJ: Handbook of Skeletal Radiology, ed 2. St. Louis, Mosby, 1997.)

"Jersey finger" occurs at the distal interphalangeal (DIP) joint, due to avulsion of the flexor digitorum profundus tendon from its insertion onto the volar base of the distal phalanx. This injury is caused by forced extension while in flexion, such as when grabbing the jersey of an escaping football player. Physical examination reveals that the DIP joint cannot be flexed. Both volar plate and Jersey finger injuries can result in loss of function if not treated appropriately.

Similar injuries, with similar potential for disability if undiagnosed or improperly treated, occur on the *dorsal* margins of the middle and distal phalanges. The extensor mechanism of the fingers consists of a middle tendon slip that inserts at the base of the middle phalanx, and two lateral

tendon slips that course around the middle phalanx and unite as the common extensor tendon to insert at the base of the distal phalanx (Fig. 8-7). A fracture of the dorsal base of the distal phalanx is caused by avulsion of the common extensor tendon and is termed a *baseball finger* or a *mallet finger*. This injury occurs when an extended DIP joint is forcibly flexed, as may occur when the finger is "jammed" by a baseball striking the tip of the finger. Most baseball finger injuries are confined to the extensor tendon and radiographs reveal no fracture, but do reveal the DIP joint to be flexed (Fig. 8-8). In fact, the combination of DIP flexion and PIP extension should suggest this diagnosis. In addition, baseball finger injuries are associated with volar plate fractures; if you see one, look for the other.

A tear or avulsion of the middle slip with preservation of the remainder of the extensor mechanism can result in the *boutonnière (buttonhole) deformity* (Figs. 8-9, 8-10). The *boutonnière* deformity is flexion of the PIP joint with hyperextension of the DIP joint. Middle slip interruption allows the PIP joint to flex while the DIP is extended. With time, the PIP can pass between the lateral tendon slips like a button through a buttonhole, and become fixed in this position.

The flexor tendons of the fingers are held close to the volar surfaces of the proximal and middle phalanges by fibrous bands termed *flexor annular pulleys* (Fig. 8-11A). Repetitive flexion of the fingers while under extreme load (e.g., by rock climbers supporting their entire body weight

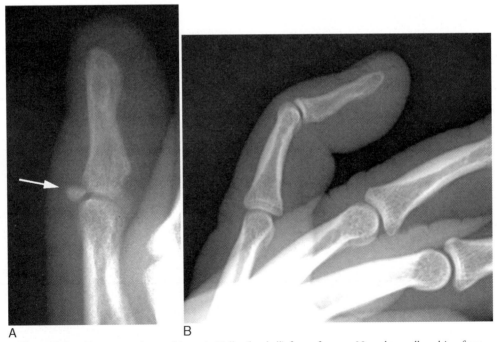

Figure 8-8   Extensor tendon avulsions. **A,** Mallet (baseball) finger fracture. Note the small avulsion from the dorsal base of the distal phalanx *(arrow)*. **B,** Tendon injury without fracture. The patient was unable to extend his distal phalanx. Note that the PIP joint is extended. This is not a natural position, and indicates a soft tissue mallet finger injury. Surgical repair of the extensor tendon was required.

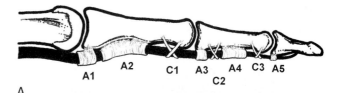

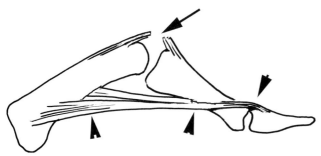

Figure 8-9   Diagram of boutonnière (buttonhole) deformity. Lateral diagram demonstrates how interruption of the middle slip of the extensor tendon *(arrow)* allows the PIP joint to flex while the dorsal interphalangeal (DIP) joint is extended. The PIP joint has herniated between the lateral slips *(arrowheads)* (like a button through a buttonhole) and become fixed in this position. (Modified with permission from Manaster BJ: Handbook of Skeletal Radiology, ed 2, St. Louis, Mosby, 1997.)

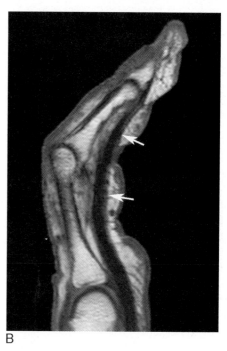

Figure 8-11   Pulley injury. **A,** Diagram of the flexor pulleys of the finger, which hold the flexor tendons close to the palmar surface of the phalanges. The annular pulleys (A1, A2, etc.) are usually of greater interest to surgeons than the cruciate pulleys (C1, etc.). **B,** Pulley failure. Sagittal T1-weighted MR image shows abnormal volar displacement of the long flexor tendon *(arrows)* due to failure of the distal A2, A3, and A4 pulleys.

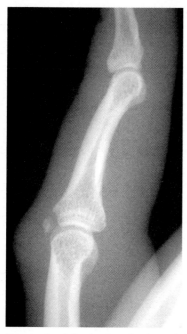

Figure 8-10   Boutonnière deformity. Lateral radiograph shows the dorsal avulsion fragment arising from the base of the middle phalanx. The PIP joint is fixed in flexion while the dorsal interphalangeal (DIP) joint is fixed in extension, causing the boutonnière deformity.

by the flexed fingertips of one hand) can cause a pulley to tear. Such injuries cause the flexor tendon to move away from the palmar surface of the phalanges during flexion like a bowstring of a violin, which can be seen on MRI or ultrasonography as abnormal palmar position of an affected flexor tendon (Fig. 8-11B).

SPINE TRAUMA BASICS
CERVICAL SPINE
CERVICAL SPINE NORMAL VARIANTS
CERVICAL SPINE FRACTURES
THORACIC AND LUMBAR SPINE
THORACIC AND LUMBAR FRACTURES

This chapter reviews imaging in acute spine trauma. Spine infection is discussed in Chapter 40, and pediatric spine conditions are reviewed in Chapter 43.

Key Concepts	Spine Trauma

First-line test: High-quality radiography or CT
Patterns of injury, some of which can be very subtle on radiographs
CT or MRI sometimes needed to detect or fully characterize a spine injury
Three-column model helps predict whether a spine injury is stable or unstable

SPINE TRAUMA BASICS

A useful concept in spine trauma is the *three-column model* of spine stability. The *anterior column* consists of the anterior longitudinal ligament and the anterior half of the vertebral bodies, intervertebral discs, and supporting soft tissues. The *middle column* consists of the posterior longitudinal ligament and the posterior half of the vertebral bodies, intervertebral discs, and supporting soft tissues. The *posterior column* consists of the posterior elements, the facet joints, and the numerous associated ligaments. Disruption of only one column generally does not result in spine instability, whereas disruption of two or three columns does. Because a column disruption may involve only the soft tissues, spine instability may be present even in the absence of a fracture. Lateral flexion-extension films can be valuable to exclude ligamentous instability. If there is concern on the radiographic series relating to fracture, computed tomography (CT) with sagittal and coronal reformation can further define osseous injury. Finally, additional critical soft tissue injuries may accompany spine trauma, such as epidural hematoma or injury to the spinal cord, vertebral arteries, conus medullaris, or nerve roots. Magnetic resonance imaging (MRI) may be needed to detect these lesions.

The same basic forces that cause fractures in the appendicular skeleton cause spine fractures: compression, tension, and shear. Rotational forces, which combine the basic forces, are a frequent factor in spine trauma.

CERVICAL SPINE

Cervical spine injuries can be extremely subtle radiographically, yet clinically devastating. Radiographic assessment of the traumatized cervical spine must include high-quality anteroposterior (AP), lateral, and open-mouth odontoid views. Many trauma centers also include oblique views in adults. An alternative approach that can be useful in large or polytrauma patients is combining lateral radiographs with CT of the entire spine. The following discussion pertains to radiographs.

Familiarity with normal anatomy and subtle signs of injury is essential. Most of the relevant information can be found on the lateral radiograph. The lateral radiograph must show the anatomy from the clivus to the top of the T1 vertebral body. A swimmer's view is often necessary to demonstrate the lower cervical spine. The following items must be evaluated:

1. The prevertebral soft tissues should be normal in width. In adults, the normal measurement is less than 5 mm at the level of C3 and C4, increasing to less than 22 mm at C6. In children, the prevertebral soft tissues should measure no more than two thirds the width of the C2 body at the level of C3 and C4 and no more than 14 mm at C6.

2. Normal cervical alignment is lordosis. However, it should be remembered that loss of lordosis is expected in patients on a backboard or in a cervical collar. Loss of lordosis may also represent muscle spasm or can even be attributed to patient positioning, as lordosis of the cervical spine is absent in 70% of uninjured persons if the chin is depressed by 1 inch.

3. Four continuous curves (Fig. 9-1) describe the normal position of the bony elements, including the anterior vertebral body line, posterior vertebral body line, spinal laminar line, and the posterior spinous process line. The spinal laminar line should form a continuous line, regardless of the degree of flexion or extension. The exception of the continuous alignment of the three other curves is found in children, where there is often a physiologic offset of 2 to 3 mm at the C2–C3 and C3–C4 levels with flexion and extension.

4. In the absence of degenerative disk disease, the distance between adjacent posterior vertebral bodies is uniform at all levels. A gap at one level suggests posterior ligamentous injury, a finding that can be supported by distraction of the associated spinous processes. Note that the normal "fanning" of the spinous processes is normally not uniform because it is greater for the proximal and distal cervical elements than for the middle elements.

5. On a perfectly positioned lateral view, the right and left facet joints are superimposed. A slightly off-lateral radiograph will show partial overlap of the right and left facet joints. In the absence of rotation, the degree of overlap should be uniform at all levels in the cervical spine. An abrupt change in the amount of overlap in adjacent levels indicates abnormal rotation along the longitudinal axis of the spine. Therefore, the degree of overlap at each level must be evaluated. Furthermore, the articular surfaces of each facet must be congruent. Absence of such congruence indicates a subluxed, perched, or dislocated facet.

6. The odontoid process normally is tilted posteriorly on the body of C2. If this posterior tilt is not seen, consider that there may be a fracture of the odontoid at its waist, with anterior subluxation of the odontoid process. This can be confirmed by spinal laminar line disruption.

7. The atlantoaxial distance is measured at the base of the dens between the anterior cortex of the dens and the posterior cortex of the atlas's anterior arch. In adults, this distance is not more than 2.5 mm and does not change with flexion. In children, the distance may be as great as 5 mm and may change by 1 to 2 mm with flexion.

8. Radiographic signs of instability include abnormal spinous process fanning, widening of the intervertebral disk space, horizontal displacement of one body on another more than 3.5 mm, angulation greater than 11 degrees, disruption of facets, or severe injury, such as multiple fractures at one segment (Fig. 9-2).

9. On an AP radiograph, the spinous processes should form a fairly continuous, although often slightly irregular, line. A fractured spinous process may be obviously displaced from this line, or what appears to be two spinous processes may be seen, one representing the nondisplaced base of the fractured process and the other representing the displaced fragment.

10. The open-mouth odontoid view is used to detect odontoid process fractures and the integrity of the ring of C1. In neutral position, there is alignment of the lateral margins of the lateral masses of C1 and C2. With rotation, the atlas normally moves as a unit with lateral facet offset on one side and medial offset on the contralateral side. Bilateral-lateral offset of the lateral margins of the lateral masses of C1 indicates a C1 ring fracture in adults. In children, bilateral offset is a normal variant due to discrepant growth of C1 and C2.

11. Oblique radiographs may be used to evaluate the posterior elements for fracture and to confirm the normal alignment of the facets. On the oblique view, facets line up like roof shingles, with each more superior facet placed posterior to the facet below.

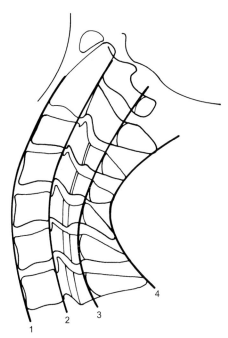

Figure 9-1 Diagram of the lateral cervical spine, with the four lines that should be evaluated for following a continuous curve. 1, anterior vertebral line; 2, posterior vertebral line; 3, spinal laminar line; 4, posterior spinous line. (Reproduced with permission from Manaster BJ: Handbook of Skeletal Radiology, ed 2. St. Louis, Mosby, 1997.)

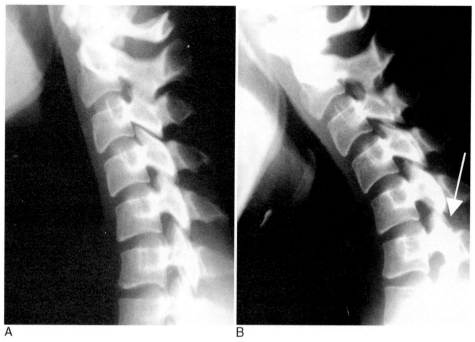

A   B

Figure 9-2   Cervical spine instability. **A,** Lateral radiographic view in the patient's neutral position. It demonstrates a mild kyphosis of the cervical spine, centered at the C5–C6 level. There is, however, no subluxation, along with only minimal uncovering of the posterior facets at C5–C6. **B,** The lateral flexion view demonstrates that this is indeed an unstable spine, with C5–C6 showing significant posterior gapping at the spinous processes, and near-complete uncoverage of the facets *(arrow)*. Even in flexion, facets should remain normally covered, as at the other levels in this spine.

CERVICAL SPINE NORMAL VARIANTS

Several developmental variants can simulate an upper cervical spine fracture. *Occipitalization of the atlas* is lack of segmentation at the atlanto-occipital junction. This presents radiographically with atlantoaxial subluxation, which can simulate a traumatic disruption (Fig. 9-3). In this situation, there is an abnormally large gap between the spinous processes of C1 and C2, with the atlas located unusually close to the occiput. The diagnosis is established by a flexion radiograph, which demonstrates fixation of the atlas to the occiput. In addition, the odontoid often has a bizarre shape. Computed tomography may also be used to establish the diagnosis.

Normal variant absence or lack of fusion of ossification centers can be especially confusing at C1 and C2. At C1, the body is occasionally bifid. The neural arches of C1 and C2 may have focal defects or absence of the normal synchondrosis between the arch and the body. In C2, there are four ossification centers: one for each neural arch, one for the body (which occasionally may be bifid), and one for the odontoid process. The body/neural arch synchondroses fuse asymmetrically between the ages of 3 and 6 years. The body/odontoid synchondrosis also fuses at this time. A lucent synchondrosis may persist into adult life, located well below the level of the apparent "base" of the odontoid, seen as a thin, straight, well-defined transverse lucency in the body of C2 below the base of the dens. This must be differentiated from an odontoid fracture, which usually occurs at the true base of the odontoid (Fig. 9-4). A transverse dens fracture may also be simulated by a Mach line from the superimposed bottom of the teeth incisors or the arch of the atlas.

The *os terminale* is an ossification center located at the superior tip of the odontoid process. Before it ossifies, the tip of the dens is V-shaped on radiographs. The os terminale normally fuses by age 12, but may persist unfused, simulating a fracture of the odontoid tip.

The *os odontoideum* is an anatomic variant, large ossicle that occupies the space normally occupied by the odontoid process. This ossicle is separated from the hypoplastic odontoid by a wide gap. It is fixed to the arch of the atlas, and moves with C1 on flexion and extension. It may appear quite bizarre and may simulate a fracture (Fig. 9-5). The cause of os odontoideum is controversial. An old ununited fracture may cause this finding, and previous trauma no doubt accounts for many of these lesions. However, many authors believe that a large os terminale may enlarge to form an os odontoideum in the setting of a hypoplastic odontoid process.

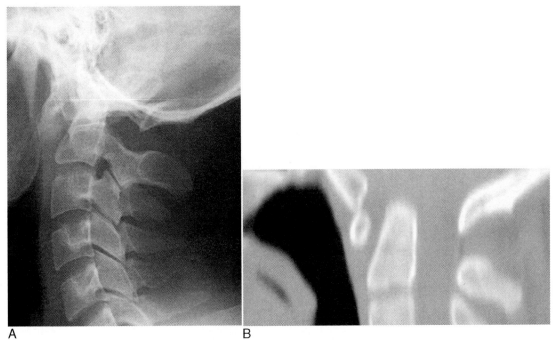

Figure 9-3 Occipitalization of the atlas. **A,** Lateral radiograph demonstrating no significant separation between the occiput and the atlas. **B,** CT demonstrates that the anterior arch as well as the hypoplastic posterior arch of the atlas are fused to the occiput. The odontoid moves independently of the occipitalized atlas, hence the abnormal atlantoaxial distance.

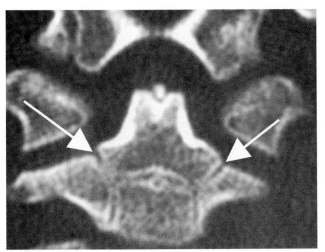

Figure 9-4 Normal synchondroses of C2. Coronal CT shows the multiple synchondroses of C2. The body of C2 is seen with the adjacent ossification centers of the posterior arches. The odontoid is a large structure that extends below the level of the apparent "base of the odontoid." This synchondrosis *(arrows)* normally fuses between the ages of 3 and 6 years, but may remain unfused throughout life, potentially simulating a type 3 dens fracture. Finally, there is a small os terminale, which is located at the superior tip of the odontoid process. Before its ossification, the tip may be seen as a V-shaped defect. The os terminale normally fuses by age 12, but may also persist unfused, simulating a tip of odontoid fracture. (Reprinted with permission from the American College of Radiology learning file.)

CERVICAL SPINE FRACTURES

Cervical spine injuries usually occur in predictable patterns based on the mechanism of injury. Knowledge of these patterns can help the radiologist to avoid missing an important injury.

Fracture of the occipital condyle is more common than was previously understood, and often requires CT for diagnosis. These fractures may involve the hypoglossal canal or jugular foramen, so clinical features of injury to cranial nerves IX to XII may be found (Fig. 9-6).

Occipital vertebral dissociation (craniocervical dissociation) can be a surprisingly easy injury to miss radiographically. The normal occipital vertebral relationship is maintained by ligaments extending from the axis to the clivus. In patients with injuries resulting in severe facial trauma, trauma to this portion of the neck may also occur. A true dislocation is often fatal and obvious on a lateral film (Fig. 9-7). Subluxation is rare and may not have a neurologic deficit or obvious radiographic findings. In such a case, a line drawn from the interior tip of the clivus (the basion) to a line drawn along the posterior body of C2 should show a distance less than 12 mm. Also, a line from the basion to the top of the odontoid process should be less than 12 mm.

Axial loading can cause bilateral vertical fractures through the neural arch of the atlas. This must be differentiated from congenital defects of the atlas. A *Jefferson fracture* is a C1 ring fracture that involves both the anterior and posterior arches. The normal angulation of the C1 facets tends to spread the C1 fragments

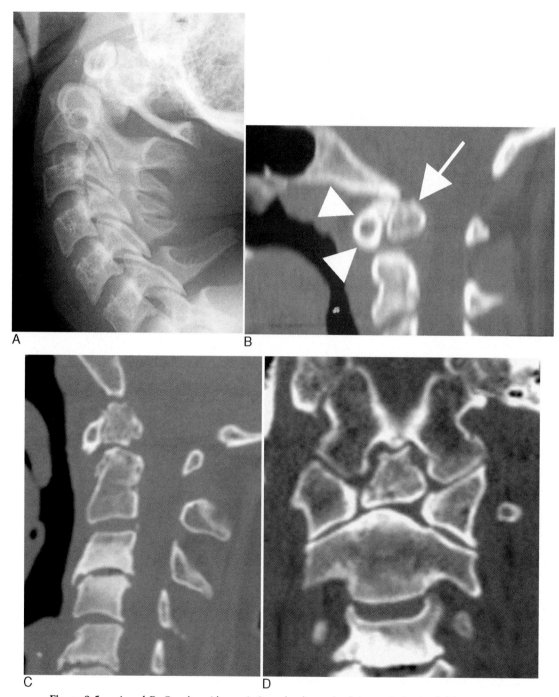

Figure 9-5 **A and B,** Os odontoideum. **A,** Lateral radiograph of the cervical spine held in extension shows that C1 is posteriorly displaced relative to C2, with the enlarged anterior arch of C1 appearing to be in the expected position of the odontoid relative to the body of C2. The odontoid is not well seen. This simulates a fracture of the odontoid and there would be abnormal motion of C1 relative to C2. This represents a variant termed os odontoideum, where the actual odontoid is hypoplastic. **B,** Sagittal reconstructed CT clearly shows the hypoplastic odontoid which is fused to the body of C2, the overgrown os terminale *(arrow),* and the overgrown anterior arch of the atlas *(arrowheads).* The os terminale moves with the atlas, and independent of C2. **C and D,** Sagittal and coronal CT reformats in a different patient with os odontoideum show anterior subluxation of the os and C1 relative to C2.

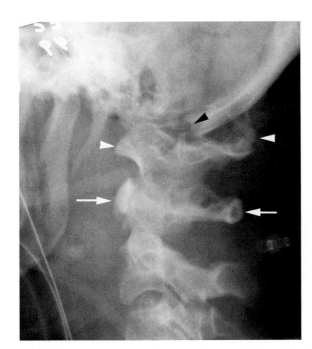

Figure 9-6 Occipital condyle fractures. Condylar fragments *(white arrowheads)* are inferiorly and posteriorly displaced. Note the fracture margin at the skull base *(black arrowhead)*. Arrows mark C1.

laterally. Surprisingly, this may be a stable fracture with minimal fragment displacement and no neurologic deficit unless there is also disruption of the transverse atlantal ligaments, which normally fixes the odontoid to the anterior arch of the atlas. Either CT or MRI can be helpful in diagnosing and characterizing this fracture and associated soft tissue injuries (Fig. 9-8).

Atlantoaxial rotatory displacement is rotation injury with locking of the facets of C1 and C2, usually seen in childhood and presenting as torticollis. Radiographs of this condition can be difficult to interpret owing to the alteration of familiar landmarks by the cervical rotation. On the open-mouth view, one lateral mass of C1 appears wider and closer to the midline with the opposite appearing narrower and laterally offset. Overlapping osseous and soft tissue structures may obscure the facets. Computed tomography with reconstruction may be extremely helpful in diagnosing this condition (Fig. 9-9).

Odontoid fractures are the most commonly missed significant cervical spine fracture. Odontoid fractures may be classified by the location of the fracture. Type 1 dens fractures involve only the tip.

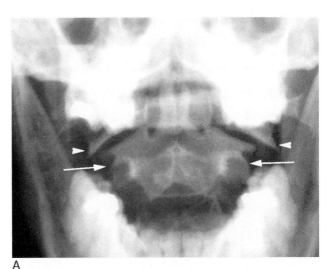

A

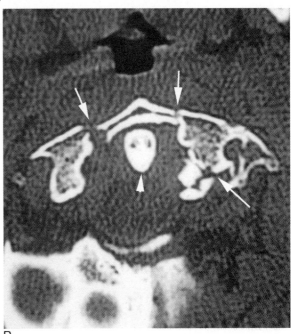

B

Figure 9-8 Burst fracture of C1. **A,** Open-mouth odontoid view shows lateral translocation of the lateral masses of C1 *(arrowheads)* relative to C2 *(arrows)*. **B,** Axial CT image shows multiple breaks in the ring of C1 *(arrows)*. Arrowhead marks the dens. (Courtesy of W. Smoker, MD.)

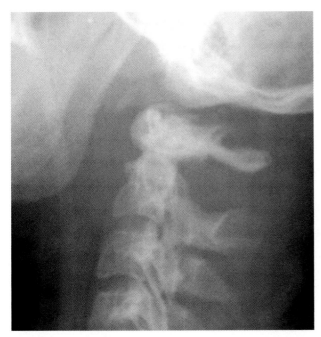

Figure 9-7 Occipital atlas dissociation. This lateral radiograph demonstrates a critical injury. Note the tremendous prevertebral soft tissue swelling and complete dissociation of the occiput from the atlas. Also note the wide interval between the posterior margin of the mandible and the cervical spine.

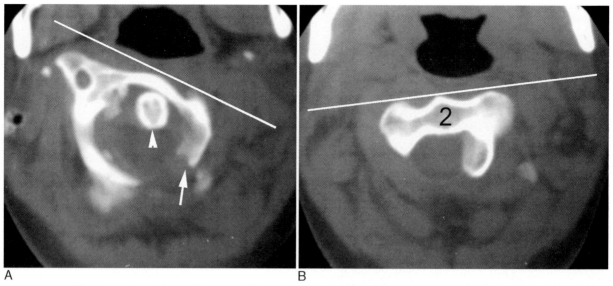

Figure 9-9   Rotatory subluxation of C1 on C2. Axial CT images obtained through the ring of C1 and the body of C2 show rotation of C1 (A) relative to C2 (B). Also note the fracture of C1 (*arrow* in part A). Arrowhead marks the dens in part A. (Courtesy of W. Smoker, MD.)

These usually but not always are stable injuries. Type 2 dens fractures are through the waist or base. This is the most common pattern, with the base of the dens the most frequent site. Type 3 dens fractures extend below the base of the dens through the body of C2. Type 2 and 3 dens fractures are unstable injuries. Transverse dens fractures can be difficult to detect with CT because the CT beam is parallel to the fracture line. Thus, attention to the odontoid view and the spinal laminar alignment on the lateral view are critical for diagnosing these fractures. However, if the fracture has an oblique extension into the vertebral body anteriorly, it may not be seen on the open-mouth view (Fig. 9-10), but thin-section CT with reformats will depict the fracture.

The *Hangman's fracture* (or, more appropriately, "hanged man") is most frequently seen at C2, but can be seen at other levels. This most frequently occurs from a hyperextension injury that results in bilateral neural arch fractures (traumatic spondylolysis).

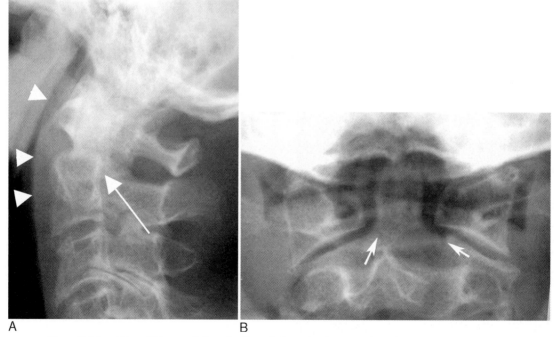

Figure 9-10   Odontoid fracture. **A,** Lateral radiograph shows that this patient has only mild prevertebral swelling, which is centered at the odontoid *(arrowheads).* The odontoid is displaced posteriorly relative to the C2 body *(arrow)* and is angled posteriorly. These findings indicate a fracture. **B,** The fracture is extremely subtle on the open-mouth odontoid radiograph *(arrows).*

(Continued)

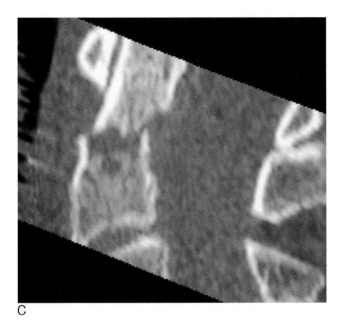

C

Figure 9-10—(Cont'd) **C,** Sagittal CT reconstruction shows the fracture.

Interruption of the spinal laminar line is the radiographic hallmark of this injury (Fig. 9-11). The odontoid and its attachments are usually intact, and cord damage is uncommon owing to the width of the cervical canal at this level. Most Hangman's fractures are type I, involving the posterior part of the body of C2 or any part of the ring without displacement or angulation and leaving the

C2–C3 disk intact. If there is greater than 3-mm displacement of C2 on C3 or a 15-degree angulation at this level, the C2–C3 disk is probably disrupted, leading to a type II or III designation and implied instability (Fig. 9-12).

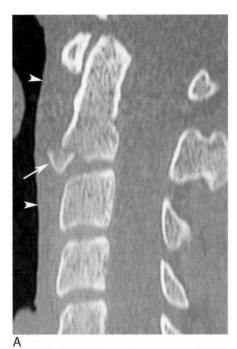

A

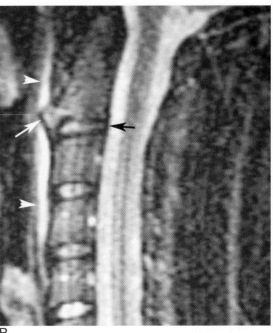

B

Figure 9-12 Hyperextension teardrop fracture of C2 with intact posterior ligaments. **A and B,** Sagittal CT reformat (A) and inversion recovery MR image (B) show anterior inferior C2 corner fracture *(arrow)* with anterior soft tissue swelling and edema *(white arrowheads)*. The posterior longitudinal ligament *(black arrowhead)* is intact, and there is no posterior element fracture or ligament injury. Because this fracture frequently occurs in conjunction with a Hangman's fracture, it is essential to evaluate the neural arch of C2 before diagnosing a hyperextension teardrop fracture of C2.

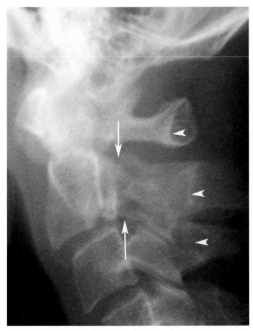

Figure 9-11 Hangman's fracture. Lateral radiograph shows the bilateral neural arch fractures at C2 that constitute a hangman's fracture *(arrows)*. The fracture extends into the posterior body of C2 and there is anterior subluxation of C2 on C3, making this a type III injury. Note the disruption of the normally straight spinal laminar line at C1–C3 *(arrowheads)*.

Flexion injuries may range from the innocuous *anterior wedge compression* to the devastating *flexion teardrop (burst)* fracture. Anterior wedge compression generally affects only the anterior column and thus is a stable injury. However, if the posterior ligamentous complex is disrupted, then there is a potentially unstable, two-column injury. Severe flexion injuries often disrupt the posterior longitudinal ligament, in which case there may be localized increased height of the intervertebral disk space, associated with fanning of spinous processes and a local kyphotic angulation. These findings are accentuated on flexion films and may allow facet subluxation or even locking. However, cervical stability may be maintained, at least temporarily, by surrounding soft tissues and muscle spasm. Delayed instability is found in 20% of these patients (Fig. 9-13). The *teardrop burst* (flexion teardrop) fracture is the most severe flexion injury compatible with life, with 80% of patients sustaining neurologic injury. The mechanism of a teardrop burst fracture is combined flexion and compression, with diving and motor vehicle accidents being most frequent. In these cases, there are coronal and sagittal comminuted vertebral body fractures with a triangular fragment found at the anterior-inferior border of the vertebral body. The posterior body is displaced into the spinal canal, with a high probability of neural damage. A classic associated neurologic injury is anterior cord syndrome of diminished motor function and loss of pain and temperature sensation, with intact vibration and proprioception, caused

by injury of the anterior spinal cord. The extent of injury is often underestimated on radiography but is well demonstrated on CT. Spinal cord and ligamentous injury and epidural hematoma are best shown by MRI (Fig. 9-14).

A *unilateral locked facet*, or, more precisely, *unilateral interfacetal dislocation,* results from flexion, distraction, and rotation. Radiographically, there is an abrupt change in the amount of facet overlap seen on the lateral image (Fig. 9-15). The most common locations for a unilateral locked facet are C4–C5 or C5–C6. Thirty-five percent of these cases are associated with fracture, most frequently of the facet. With a unilateral locked facet, there need not be significant subluxation of the vertebral body. *Bilateral locked facets (bilateral interfacetal dislocation)* are also due to flexion, but with enough distraction for the facets to become disarticulated. With a bilateral lock, the vertebral body is displaced, usually 50% of the body length as seen on the lateral radiograph (Fig. 9-16). Both lateral and oblique films show the "jumped" and locked facets. There is a high incidence of cord injury with bilateral locked facets.

Extension injuries may have extremely subtle radiographic signs. With extension injuries, there may be a tear or stretch of the anterior longitudinal ligament and disruption of the anterior annulus fibrosis. This may result in avulsion of the adjacent anterior vertebral body endplate. More severe extension injuries may also involve the middle and posterior columns and result in profound instability. Despite the serious soft tissue disruptions, these injuries

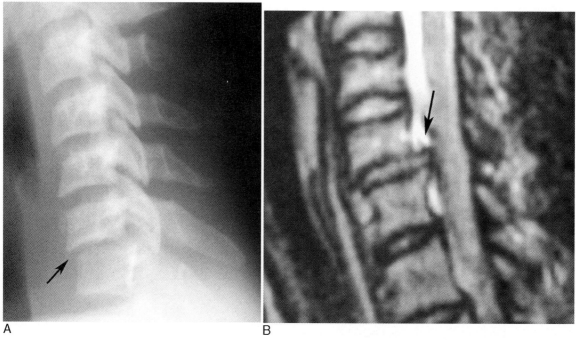

A   B

Figure 9-13   Hyperflexion injury. **A,** Lateral flexion radiograph of the cervical spine in a patient who sustained a neck injury in a motor vehicle accident. Although the neutral view (not shown) showed no abnormality, the flexion view shows anterolisthesis of C6 on C7 *(arrow)*, as well as narrowing of the disk space. This is not normal in a 14-year-old. **B,** T2-weighted sagittal MR image demonstrates the anterolisthesis of C6 on C7, along with the disk herniation and posterior longitudinal ligament disruption *(arrow)*.

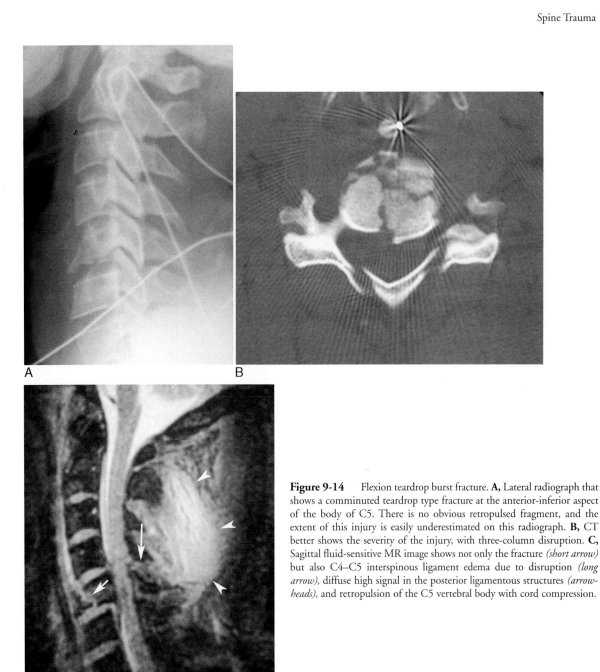

Figure 9-14   Flexion teardrop burst fracture. **A,** Lateral radiograph that shows a comminuted teardrop type fracture at the anterior-inferior aspect of the body of C5. There is no obvious retropulsed fragment, and the extent of this injury is easily underestimated on this radiograph. **B,** CT better shows the severity of the injury, with three-column disruption. **C,** Sagittal fluid-sensitive MR image shows not only the fracture *(short arrow)* but also C4–C5 interspinous ligament edema due to disruption *(long arrow),* diffuse high signal in the posterior ligamentous structures *(arrowheads),* and retropulsion of the C5 vertebral body with cord compression.

can spontaneously reduce, so radiographs may not reveal the true extent of injury. Prevertebral soft tissue swelling is an important clue. There may be posterior body displacement or a widened intervertebral disk space, especially anteriorly. A vacuum phenomenon at the annulus fibrosis is highly suggestive of an extension injury. When present, anteroinferior vertebral body avulsion, usually found at C2 or C3, may suggest the diagnosis of hyperextension injury (Figs. 9-12, 9-17). Facet compression fractures can result from hyperextension with rotation but are subtle injuries

to diagnose, even with CT. Facet compression fractures may result in nerve root compression. Hyperextension injuries can cause spinal cord injury even without fracture or dislocation. When hyperextension injury is suspected, MRI should be performed to delineate the soft tissue injury and to determine the likelihood of instability. With MRI, the spinal cord, any disk herniation, and epidural hematoma are directly visualized (Fig. 9-17B). Vertebral artery injury must be suspected in patients with facet fractures or instability.

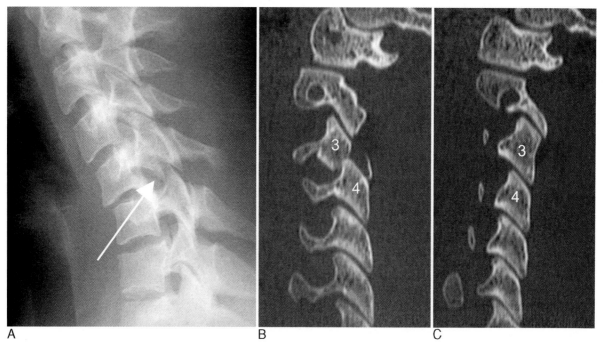

Figure 9-15   Unilateral locked facet (unilateral interfacetal dislocation, UID). **A,** Lateral radiograph shows an abrupt transition in alignment at C5–C6, where there is mild anterolisthesis of C5 on C6, splaying of the spinous processes, and a change in alignment of the facets *(arrow).* The facets at C3, C4, and C5 are in a bow-tie configuration; at C6 and C7 they are in a pure lateral configuration. There is a lock of the more anterior-inferior C5 facet on the superior facet of C6. **B and C,** Sagittal CT reformats in a different patient with UID show fracture dislocation (B) at C3–C4. Compare with normal side (C).

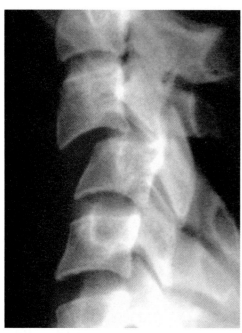

Figure 9-16   Bilateral locked facets. Lateral radiograph shows bilateral locked facet of C3–C4 with near-complete anterolisthesis of C3 on C4 and abnormal alignment of the posterior facets.

A *clay shoveler's fracture* is an isolated avulsion of the C7 or T1 spinous process. It is caused by abrupt contraction of the trapezius and other muscles that attach to these spinous processes.

THORACIC AND LUMBAR SPINE

Traumatic injury to the thoracic and lumbar spine is easier to understand than injury to the cervical spine because the anatomy is less complex. The thoracic and lumbar spine also differ from the cervical spine because of the generally larger, stronger disks, supporting ligaments, and muscles. In addition, the rib cage and the orientation of the thoracic facets above T11 help to stabilize the thoracic spine, and the exceptionally strong ligaments and muscular support help to stabilize the lower lumbar spine. As a result, forces acting on the thoracic and lumbar spine are focused at the thoracolumbar junction, with 60% of fractures occurring at the T12–L2 levels and 90% at T11–L4.

Routine radiographs of the traumatized thoracic and lumbar spine should include AP and lateral views. Suspected tho-

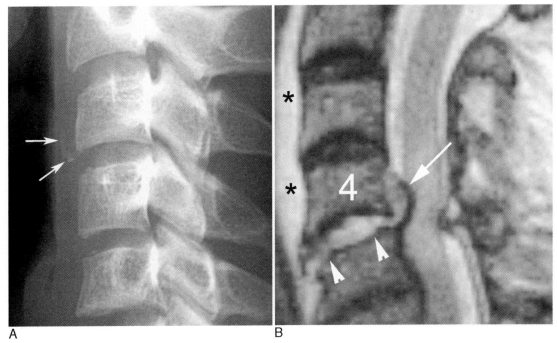

Figure 9-17   Hyperextension injury. **A,** Lateral radiograph shows no prevertebral soft tissue swelling. However, there is a subtle avulsion fracture of the anteroinferior C3 vertebral body endplate *(arrow)*. This is an indicator of a hyperextension injury, and MRI should be performed for evaluation of possible spinal cord injury. **B,** Sagittal T2-weighted MR image of a different patient with hyperextension injury shows disruption of the C4–C5 disk *(arrowheads)* and epidural *(arrow)* and prevertebral *(asterisks)* hematomas. (Courtesy of W. Smoker, MD.)

racolumbar region injuries may require dedicated views. On the AP radiograph, careful attention should be given to the interpediculate distances because widening at a single level suggests a burst fracture. Widening of the paraspinous soft tissues may be caused by a hematoma. A mid- or upper-thoracic fracture is more likely to be unstable if multiple rib fractures or a sternal fracture is present (Fig. 9-18).

The normal appearance of the lumbar spine includes a gradual widening of the interpediculate distances from L1 to L5 as seen on the AP radiograph. On the lateral view, the disk spaces gradually increase in height from the L1–L2 level to L4–L5, with L5–S1 being slightly narrower.

A *limbus vertebra* is an oblique radiolucent cleft at a superior (or occasionally inferior) corner of a vertebral body anteriorly. Limbus vertebra is thought to be an unfused ring apophysis or due to an intravertebral anterior inferior disk herniation, and is generally considered an incidental finding that could simulate a fracture (Fig. 9-19).

The presence of a calcaneus fracture after a fall from a height is associated with a significantly increased risk of a thoracic or lumbar spine fracture (and vice versa). Thus, if a calcaneus fracture is found, thoracic and lumbar radiographs should be considered.

THORACIC AND LUMBAR FRACTURES

As with the cervical spine, thoracic and lumbar injuries usually occur in predictable patterns based on the mechanism of injury.

Compression and flexion injuries tend to overlap in the thoracic and lumbar spine, as the strong posterior and middle columns can convert flexion force into vertebral body compression in a nutcracker-like mechanism. Compression and flexion account for 75% of injuries. Most are vertebral body *compression fractures* with anterior wedging or depression of the superior endplate but intact posterior elements. This is a one-column injury and hence is stable. However, 20% of lumbar injuries are fracture dislocations, involving the posterior elements as well. Most of these are *burst fractures* and require CT to evaluate for bony fragments in the spinal canal and to guide therapy and surgical approach. With burst fractures the facets may be fractured, subluxed, perched, dislocated, or locked (Fig. 9-20). The presence of a burst fracture is associated with a 40% chance that another spine fracture is present. Thus, if a burst fracture is found, the entire spine must be radiographed.

Osteoporotic compression fractures are especially common in the elderly (see Fig. 1-3) and are a common cause of disabling pain. *Vertebroplasty* (i.e., injection of methyl methacrylate into the fractured vertebral body) is an effective technique for managing these patients. *Kyphoplasty* is a similar technique that places a balloon within a compressed body, followed by inflation of the balloon and filling this space with methyl methacrylate. Compressed vertebral bodies with marrow edema are most likely to benefit from these techniques. Thus, MRI with inversion recovery imaging, which can reliably depict marrow edema, is often requested as a screening examination before vertebroplasty or kyphoplasty.

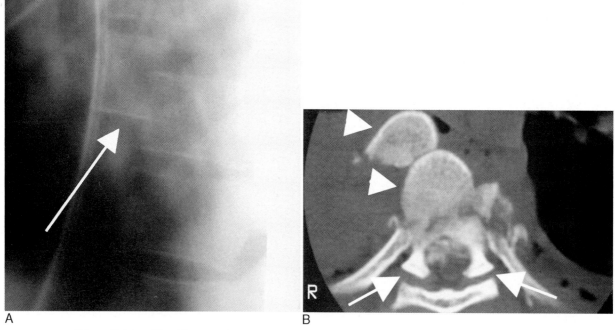

A B

Figure 9-18   Unstable upper thoracic spine injury. **A,** Lateral radiograph shows severe anterolisthesis in the midthoracic spine *(arrow)*. This degree of displacement implies sternal and probably multiple rib fractures. **B,** CT image at the level of anterolisthesis shows the two vertebral bodies as they overlap *(arrowheads)*, as well as retropulsed fragments narrowing the spinal canal, and diastasis of the facets *(arrows)*. (Reprinted with permission of the American College of Radiology learning file.)

Chance fractures (seat belt fractures) are less frequent and may be subtle because of spontaneous reduction. In this injury, fixation at the waist by a lap-type seat belt acts as a fulcrum during rapid deceleration in a motor vehicle crash, resulting in distraction of the midlumbar and lower lumbar spine. A transverse fracture extending through the posterior elements and the vertebral body or disk space with little or no vertebral body compression may be seen (Fig. 9-21). There may be an associated abdominal wall hematoma or intra-abdominal injury. The introduction of shoulder belts and, more recently, air bags has reduced the frequency of Chance fractures. These injuries are now most frequently seen after a fall from a height, with hyperflexion occurring as the victim's feet strike the ground while the victim is flexed at the waist.

The current use of a lap *and* shoulder belt concentrates forces in a motor vehicle crash at the cervicothoracic junction, often with a twisting component as only one shoulder is braced by the shoulder belt. Cervicothoracic transverse process fractures may be seen.

A *lateral compression fracture* is caused by lateral flexion. An AP radiograph reveals a vertebral body compression that is asymmetrically greater on the right or left side, often with associated scoliosis.

Hyperextension injuries of the thoracic and lumbar spine are unusual, but can disrupt the anterior longitudinal ligament and cause posterior element and facet compression injuries.

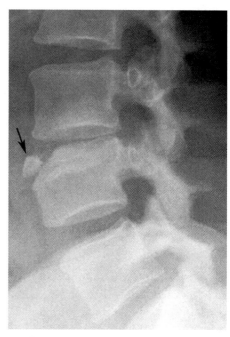

Figure 9-19   Limbus vertebra *(arrow)*.

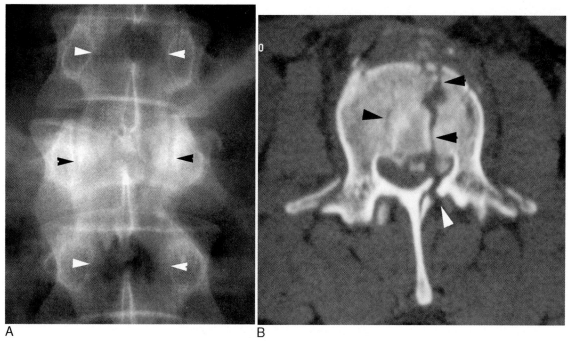

Figure 9-20   Burst fracture. **A,** AP radiograph shows widened interpediculate distance at L2 *(arrowheads)*. This indicates the "burst" nature of the fracture. **B,** CT confirms fractures through the posterior vertebral body and posterior elements *(arrowheads)*. Note the severe spinal canal narrowing.

Transverse process fractures can occur as an isolated finding or as part of a more extensive spine injury. A finding of multiple lumbar transverse process fractures on radiographs is associated with an increased risk of significant intra-abdominal injury.

Spondylolysis is interruption of the pars interarticularis. In the lumbar spine, this is generally considered a stress fracture variant rather than a consequence of an acute traumatic injury. Spondylolysis is discussed further in Chapter 43.

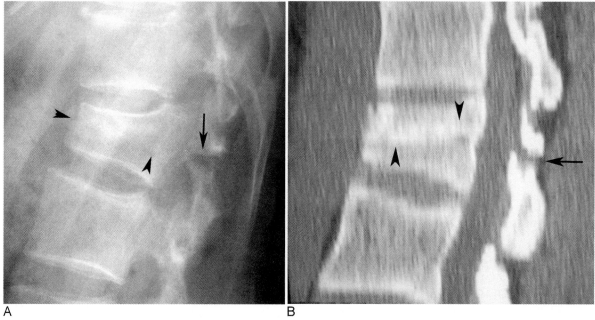

Figure 9-21   Chance fracture. **A and B,** Lateral radiograph (A) and sagittal CT reconstruction (B) show an L1 compression fracture and a transverse fracture line *(arrowheads)* that continues through the posterior elements *(arrow)*.

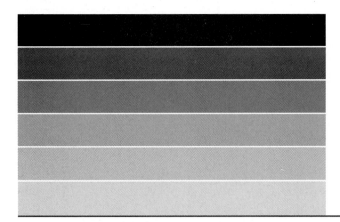

Part II Sources and Suggested Readings

Aina R, Cardinal E, Bureau N, et al: Calcific shoulder tendinitis: Treatment with modified US-guided fine-needle technique. Radiology 221:455–461, 2001.

Beltran J, Bncardino J, Mellad J, et al: MR arthrography of the shoulder: Variants and pitfalls. Radiographics 17:1403–1412, 1977.

Beltran J, Rosenberg ZS: Diagnosis of compressive and entrapment neuropathies of the upper extremity: Value of MR imaging. Am J Roentgenol 163:525–531, 1994.

Bergin D, Parker L, Zoga A, Morrison W: Abnormalities on MRI of the subscapularis tendon in the presence of a full-thickness supraspinatus tendon tear. AJR 186:454–459, 2006.

Chung C, Dwek J, Feng S, Resnick D: MR arthrography of the glenohumeral joint: A tailored approach. AJR 177:217–219, 2001.

Clavero J, Alomar X, Morrill J, et al: MR imaging of ligament and tendon injuries of the fingers. Radiographics 22:237–256, 2002.

Farmer KD, Hughes PM: MR arthrography of the shoulder: Fluoroscopically guided technique using a posterior approach. AJR 178:433–434, 2002.

Gilula LA, Yin Y: Imaging of the Wrist and Hand. Philadelphia, W.B. Saunders, 1996.

Goldfarb CA, Yin Y, Gilula LA, et al: Wrist fractures: What the clinician wants to know. Radiology 219:11–28, 2001.

Harper K, Helms C, Haystead C, Higgins L: Glenoid dysplasia: Incidence and association with posterior labral tears as evaluated by MRI. AJR 184:984–988, 2005.

Holsbeeck MV, Introscaso JH: Musculoskeletal Ultrasound, ed 2. St. Louis, Mosby-Year Book, 2001.

Kaplan PA, Helms CA, Dussault R, et al: Musculoskeletal MRI. Philadelphia, W.B. Saunders, 2001.

Kassarjain A, Torriani M, Ouellette H, Palmer W: Intramuscular rotator cuff cysts: Association with tendon tears on MRI and arthroscopy. AJR 185:160–165, 2005.

Kijowski R, DeSmet AA: MRI findings of osteochondritis dissecans of the capitellum with surgical correlation. AJR 185:1453–1459, 2005.

Kon DS, Darakjian AB, Pearl ML, Kosco AE: Glenohumeral deformity in children with internal rotation contractures secondary to brachial plexus birth palsy: Intraoperative arthrographic classification. Radiology 231:791–795, 2004.

Krief OP: MRI of the rotator interval capsule. AJR 184:1490–1494, 2005.

Levin D, Nazarian L, Miller T, et al: Lateral epicondylitis of the elbow: US findings. Radiology 237:230–234, 2005.

Manaster BJ: Handbook of Skeletal Radiology, ed 2. St. Louis, Mosby, 1997.

Massengill AD, Seeger LL, Yao L, et al: Labrocapsular ligamentous complex of the shoulder: Normal anatomy, anatomic variations, and pitfalls of MR imaging and MR arthrography. Radiographics 14:1211–1223, 1994.

Mohana-Borges AVR, Chung C, Resnick D: Superior labral anteroposterior tear: Classification and diagnosis on MRI and MR arthrography. AJR 181:1449–1462, 2003.

Mohana-Borges AVR, Chung C, Resnick D: MR imaging and MR of the postoperative shoulder: Spectrum of normal and abnormal findings. Radiographics 24:69–85, 2004.

Morag Y, Jacobson JA, Shields G, et al: MR arthrography of rotator interval, long head of the biceps brachii, and the biceps pulley of the shoulder. Radiology 235:21–30, 2005.

Moschilla G, Breidahl W: Sonography of the finger. AJR 178: 1451–1457, 2002.

Oneson SR, Scales LM, Timins ME, et al: MR imaging interpretation of the Palmer classification of triangular fibrocartilage complex lesions. Radiographics 16:97–106, 1996.

Rao S, Wasyliw C, Nunex D: Spectrum of imaging findings in hyperextension injuries of the neck. Radiographics 25:1239–1254, 2005.

Resnick D, Kang HS: Internal Derangements of Joints. Philadelphia, W.B. Saunders, 1997.

Rockwood CH, Green DP, Bucholz RW, Heckman JD, eds: Fractures in Adults, ed 4. Philadelphia, Lippincott-Raven, 1996.

Rockwood CH, Wilkins KE, Beaty JH (eds): Fractures in Children, ed 4. Philadelphia, Lippincott-Raven, 1996.

Smith DK: MR imaging of normal and injured wrist ligaments. Mag Res Imaging Clin North Am 3:229–248, 1995.

Sonin AH, Tutton SM, Fitzgerald SW, Peduto AJ: MR imaging of the adult elbow. Radiographics 16:1323–1336, 1996.

Steinbach LS, Peterfy CG (eds): Shoulder Magnetic Resonance Imaging. Philadelphia, Lippincott Williams & Wilkins, 1998.

Stoller D: Magnetic Resonance Imaging in Orthopaedics and Sports Medicine, ed 2. Philadelphia, Lippincott-Raven, 1997.

Tuite MJ, Cirillo RL, De Smet AA, Orwin JF: Superior labrum anterior-posterior (SLAP) tears: Evaluation of three MR signs on T2-weighted images. Radiology 21:841–845, 2000.

Wong SM, Griffith JF, Jui ACF, et al: Carpal tunnel syndrome: Diagnostic usefulness of sonography. Radiology 232:93–99, 2004.

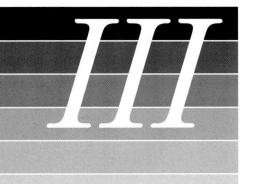

III LOWER EXTREMITY

Pelvis

ANATOMY
SACRAL FRACTURES
PELVIC FRACTURES: BIOMECHANICAL CLASSIFICATION
PELVIC FRACTURES: PELVIC RING CLASSIFICATION
    Class I and Class II Fractures
    Class III Fractures
ACETABULAR FRACTURES

ANATOMY

The pelvis is a complex anatomic region created by three bones: the two innominate bones and the sacrum. Each innominate bone is formed by synostosis of the ilium, pubis, and ischium that join at the medial wall of the acetabulum, physically recognized in childhood as the *triradiate* or *Y cartilage* of the acetabulum. In skeletally immature patients, this region may be confused with fracture. Medially, the innominate bones are adjoined at the symphysis pubis, which is a synchondrosis similar embryologically and morphologically to the disks of the spine. The sacrum and ilium are adjoined at the sacroiliac joints, which are a complex form of articulation consisting partly of synovial joint and partly of syndesmosis. The true synovial joint is in the anterior third and inferior half of the articulation, whereas the strong ligamentous attachments of the syndesmosis are present in the remaining areas. The pelvis is joined with the spine at the L5–S1 disk. The pelvis is attached at the lower extremity at the hip joints, two synovial joints that act as a ball-and-socket form of articulation.

The pelvis can be considered a ring-like structure formed by two dominant arches. The major arch is posterior and superior, formed by the iliac wings and sacrum, joined at the sacroiliac joints. The smaller arch is anterior and inferior formed by the pubic and ischial bones, joined at the symphysis pubis. There are in fact three rings in the pelvis. The largest is the ring that connects the sacrum, sacroiliac joints, iliac and pubic bones, and symphysis pubis. The pelvic inlet is the part of this ring. The other two rings are the obturator foramena of the pubic bones and ischia. As with any ring, a break in one portion of the ring is usually accompanied by a break in

another portion of the ring. Breaks may occur through a bone or an articulation. When isolated fractures of the pelvis occur, they are usually in the form of an iliac wing impaction fracture or an ischial tuberosity or iliac spine or iliac crest avulsion fracture.

The bones of the pelvis are strong and are supported by extremely strong ligaments. It therefore requires enormous force to cause a fracture of the pelvis. In addition, the pelvis is rich in vascular supply and therefore prone to life-threatening hemorrhage after trauma. Injury to the smaller nerves of the pelvis is common after pelvic trauma. As an example, erectile dysfunction is a common complication after injury in males, and results from a combination of neurologic and vascular injury. Furthermore, the sciatic nerve, although only rarely transected, often is affected by adjacent hematoma, edema, or post-traumatic fibrosis that results in a variable degree and duration of neurologic dysfunction. Urologic injury is also common after pelvic trauma with extraperitoneal and intraperitoneal bladder ruptures and, in males, urethral disruption.

Five major vertically oriented radiographic lines in the innominata bone require careful scrutiny on the anteroposterior (AP) pelvis radiograph (Fig. 10-1). The first is the *iliopectineal* (iliopubic) *line*. This line runs along the inner margin of the ilium and around the superior margin of the pubis. The second is the *ilioischial line*, which runs along the inner margin of the ilium and then inferiorly along the medial margin of the ischium. The third is the *teardrop*, which is a summation opacity related to the medial margin of the acetabulum and posterior acetabular wall. Finally, the fourth and fifth lines are the *anterior and posterior rims of the acetabulum*. These represent the lateral margins of the anterior and posterior walls of the acetabulum. Each of these lines should be smoothly contoured. Any interruption or irregularity of the line should be viewed with suspicion for the presence of fracture, and absence suggests bone destruction (Figs. 10-2, 37-19). Evaluation of the anterior and posterior acetabular rims is particularly difficult on frontal pelvis radiographs because isolated fractures are oriented in the coronal plane and thus may be obscured on the radiograph. Usually the presence of a posterior

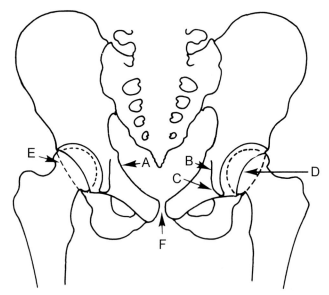

Figure 10-1 Diagram of AP pelvis demonstrating anatomic landmarks to assess in the setting of trauma. A, iliopubic line; B, ilioischial line; C, teardrop; D, anterior acetabular rim; E, posterior acetabular rim; F, symphysis pubis. (Reproduced with permission from Manaster BJ: Handbook of Skeletal Radiology, ed 2. St. Louis, Mosby, 1997.)

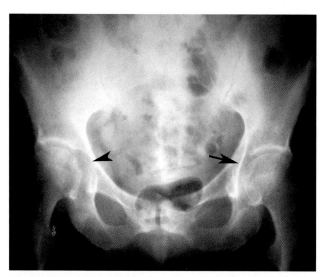

Figure 10-2 Absent ilioischial line due to metastasis. AP radiograph shows normal left line *(arrow)* but absent right line *(arrowhead)* caused by a lytic bronchogenic carcinoma metastasis.

wall fracture is inferred only by obscuration of visualization of the posterior rim.

Radiography of the pelvis is limited in its sensitivity for detection of pelvic fracture. The addition of Judet views (i.e., 45-degree bilateral oblique views) increases sensitivity and helps delineate fracture patterns in the pelvis. Note that to many radiology technologists, an "oblique pelvis view" means 30-degree oblique, so "Judet" must be specified as the desired view. This is because the 45-degree oblique view allows better

evaluation of the ischium and pubis in elongated projection. The bilateral Judet views are complementary views: one view will show the ipsilateral posterior wall and ischium, and contralateral anterior wall and pubis (Fig. 10-3). This is critical anatomy for assessment of acetabular fracture patterns. Orthopedic surgeons use these landmarks when describing Judet views. For example, the left posterior oblique Judet view (i.e., the view with the left hip rolled on to the film cassette) is termed the "left iliac oblique" view because it profiles the left iliac wing. This view is also termed the "right obturator oblique" view because it also profiles the right obturator foramen and acetabulum.

With the wider availability of spiral and multidetector computed tomography (CT) scanners, CT is now used frequently for detection and evaluation of pelvic fractures, and Judet views are requested less frequently. CT allows multiplanar and three-dimensional (3D) reformations for preoperative planning, often preferred by surgeons. The soft tissues can be evaluated for hematoma and bladder rupture. Magnetic resonance imaging (MRI) has a particularly useful role in the assessment of radiographically occult fracture, stress fracture (especially sacral stress fracture), and muscle strain. It is useful in studying patients with post-traumatic pelvic pain in the absence of radiographic or CT findings. It can also help explain patient symptoms, thus directing further therapy. Radionuclide bone scanning also can depict radiographically occult fractures,

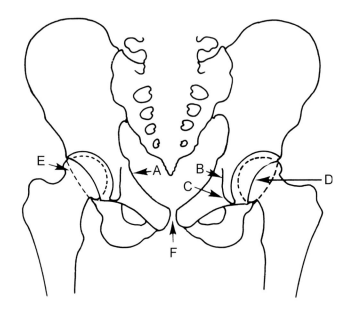

Figure 10-3 Judet (45-degree oblique) view of the pelvis. Note that the anterior (obturator) oblique view shows the anterior column and posterior acetabular rim best, whereas the posterior (iliac) oblique view shows the posterior column and anterior acetabular rim best. A, anterior column and iliopubic line; B, posterior column and ilioischial line; C, anterior acetabular rim; D, posterior acetabular rim; E, ischial spine; F, ischial tuberosity; G, obturator foramen. (Reproduced with permission from Manaster BJ: Handbook of Skeletal Radiology, ed 2. St. Louis, Mosby, 1997.)

although it less sensitive and specific than MRI. Bone scanning is not used in the acute setting in elderly patients because fractures do not accumulate radiotracer until the healing process progresses a few days after the injury.

SACRAL FRACTURES

Sacral fractures can be extraordinarily subtle in appearance on radiographs. The neuroforaminal lines of the sacrum require careful evaluation because subtle irregularity usually indicates a fracture. The presence of a transverse process fracture at L5 suggests the presence of occult sacral fracture, as forces that produce this fracture are similar to those that produce a sacral fracture. The margins of the sacroiliac joints and symphysis pubis should be parallel and smoothly contoured. Sacroiliac joints are normally no greater than 4 mm wide in adults. Any asymmetry should be viewed with suspicion for diastasis. The symphysis pubis may be up to 5 mm wide in adults and 10 mm wide in skeletally immature patients. Superoinferior offset up to 2 mm is normal when the superior pubic margins are evaluating. However, the inferior margins at the symphysis pubis should be symmetrically placed. Transverse sacral fractures may occur acutely because of direct blows. Insufficiency fractures may occur in the sacrum (see Fig. 1-19), most often in the setting of osteoporosis or after radiation therapy, and are seen as vertical areas of mixed lucency and density along the sacral wings, often with a horizontal portion through the mid-S2 or -S3 levels (like the letter "H"). More commonly, they are radiographically occult and are only detected with CT, MRI, or radionuclide bone scanning.

PELVIC FRACTURES: BIOMECHANICAL CLASSIFICATION

Pelvic ring fractures can be due to anteroposterior compression, lateral compression, or vertical shear forces. Each mechanism produces a unique fracture pattern. In *lateral compression,* the most common pattern, the essential forces result from lateral impaction injury, such as a "T-bone" motor vehicle crash in which one car strikes the door (and hence the occupant) of another at a 90-degree angle. The clue to lateral compression is the presence of *horizontal* fractures of the superior and inferior pubic rami (Fig. 10-4). Type I injury involves a direct blow to the acetabulum with fractures involving the medial acetabular wall without substantial associated innominate bone rotation. In a type II fracture the lateral compressive force is located more anteriorly, resulting in internal rotation of the ipsilateral iliac wing. This, in turn, causes not only pubic and ischial fracture but also disruption of the posterior sacroiliac joint

ligaments (or a fracture through the posterior iliac wing or sacrum). A type III lateral compression involves a greater force in which there are internal rotation of the ipsilateral innominate bone and external rotation of the contralateral innominate bone. With the exception of type III injury, incidence of substantial arterial hemorrhage is low with lateral compression.

In *anteroposterior compression,* injury results from frontal or dorsal forces, usually in a motor vehicle crash. With this injury pattern, the identifying fractures are the *vertical* fractures of the superior and inferior pubic rami (Fig. 10-5). The following grading system of anteroposterior compression fractures is often used. A type I fracture shows only vertical pubic ramus fractures, a type II fracture is an "open-book" type fracture with symphysis

Key Concepts	Pelvic Fractures: Biomechanical Classification

Lateral compression
Clue: *Horizontal* fractures of the superior and inferior pubic rami
Type 1
　Medial acetabular wall without substantial associated innominate bone rotation
Type II
　Internal rotation of ipsilateral iliac wing
　Pubic and ischial fractures
　Disruption of the posterior sacroiliac joint ligaments or a fracture through the posterior iliac wing or sacrum
Type III
　Internal rotation of the ipsilateral innominate bone
　External rotation of the contralateral innominate bone
　Only lateral compression (LC) fracture with substantial risk of arterial hemorrhage
Anteroposterior compression
Clue: *Vertical* fractures of the superior and inferior pubic rami
Type I
　Vertical pubic ramus fractures
Type II
　"Open-book" type fracture
　Symphysis pubis diastasis
　Disruption of the anterior sacroiliac ligaments
Type III
　"Sprung pelvis"
　Diastasis of the symphysis pubis and sacroiliac joints
　Disruption of the anterior and posterior sacroiliac joint ligaments
　Type II and III fractures are unstable and have a higher likelihood of associated arterial hemorrhage
Vertical shear
Clue: *Vertical displacement* of a portion of the pelvis
Malgaigne fracture
　Unstable injury most associated with arterial hemorrhage

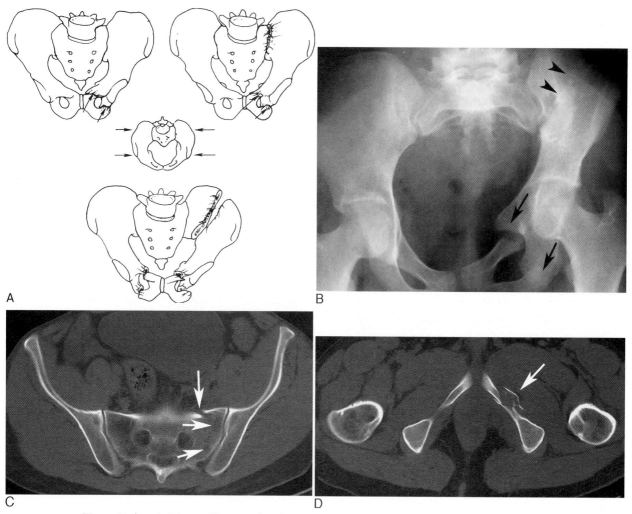

Figure 10-4   **A,** Diagram illustrating lateral compression injury. Central figure with arrow demonstrates direction of force. Note that the signature fracture pattern is horizontal fractures of the superior and inferior pubic rami *(arrows)*. Upper left part of figure is type 1 injury. Note that greater degrees of force result in internal rotation of ipsilateral iliac wing with sacroiliac joint disruption or iliac wing fracture (upper right part of figure). Greater force will result in contralateral innominate bone external rotation (lower part of figure). **B,** Radiograph demonstrating features of lateral compression with horizontal fractures of superior and inferior pubic rami *(arrows)*, iliac wing fracture *(arrowheads)*, and internal rotation of ipsilateral innominate bone. **C and D,** Axial CT in an automobile driver struck on the left side by another car. Note fractures *(arrows)* of the sacrum (C) and inferior pubic ramus/ischium (D).

pubis diastasis and disruption of the anterior sacroiliac ligaments, and a type III fracture is a "sprung pelvis" involving diastasis of the symphysis pubis and sacroiliac joints with disruption of the anterior and posterior sacroiliac joint ligaments. Type II and III fractures are unstable and have a higher likelihood of associated arterial hemorrhage. Variations in anteroposterior compression injuries do occur. In the "bucket handle" fracture, there are ipsilateral vertical fractures of the superior and inferior pubic rami associated with contralateral sacroiliac joint diastasis or adjacent vertical fracture. Impact directly to the symphysis pubis may result in bilateral superior and inferior pubic rami fractures, called a *straddle* fracture. Posterior acetabular fractures often occur with anteroposterior compression fractures.

In *vertical shear,* superior-inferior forces predominate, resulting in *vertical displacement* of a portion of the pelvis

(Fig. 10-6). The appearance of ipsilateral rami and sacroiliac disruptions is termed a *Malgaigne* fracture. The site of displacement may be at the symphysis pubis and sacroiliac joint or adjacent pubis, ilium, and sacrum. This injury is an unstable injury, with the highest association with arterial hemorrhage. A straddle fracture also may result from a superiorly oriented blow to the symphysis region. Associated urethral injury is common in males with this injury.

In the acute setting, the initial management of pelvic fractures is the control of life-threatening hemorrhage. Hemorrhage is most highly associated with type III lateral compression, types II and III anteroposterior compression, and vertical shear injuries. Initial orthopedic management is to stabilize the pelvis, most commonly with the placement of external fixation pins in the iliac wings. This is usually performed in the emergency department. Sacroiliac joint diastasis or sacral distraction can be treated with placement of percutaneous or surgically placed transverse lag screws. Symphysis pubis, pubic ramus, and iliac wing fractures are usually reduced intraoperatively with malleable plates. The adoption of percutaneous external fixation has resulted in reduced bleeding complications and has diminished the need for arteriographic embolization. Hemodynamically unstable patients, however, require immediate arteriography and embolization. Retrograde cystography and, in males, retrograde urethrography often are indicated, particularly when hematuria is present.

PELVIC FRACTURES: PELVIC RING CLASSIFICATION

Pelvic fractures can also be classified by the degree of disruption of the pelvic ring. Class I fractures (Figs. 10-7, 1-13B) are isolated fractures that do not disrupt the pelvic ring. Class II fractures disrupt the ring in one location. Because the pelvic ring is quite rigid, class II fractures are unusual unless associated with sacroiliac or symphysis pubis disruption. Class III fractures disrupt the ring in at least two locations, and class IV fractures disrupt the acetabulum.

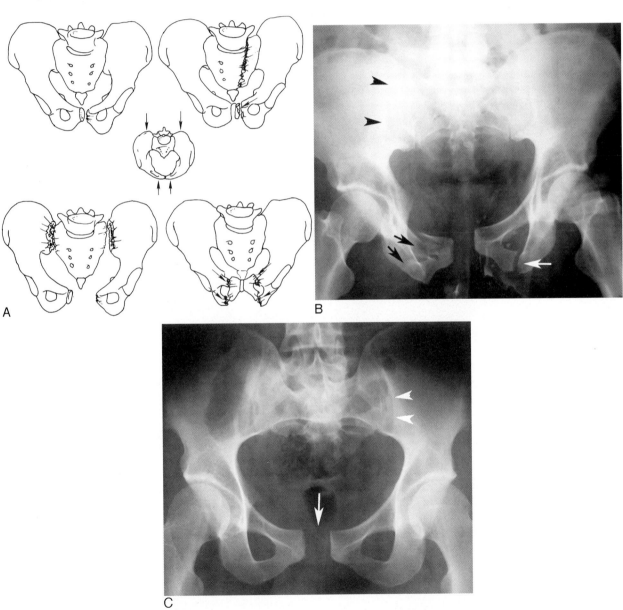

Figure 10-5   Anteroposterior compression. **A,** Diagram demonstrates features of anteroposterior compression. Central figure demonstrates direction of forces. Signature fracture pattern is vertically oriented fractures of superior and inferior pubic rami *(arrows)* or symphysis pubis diastasis. With increasing force there is variable sacroiliac diastasis or sacral fracture. **B,** Radiograph demonstrates features of anteroposterior compression with vertically oriented fractures of superior and inferior pubic rami *(arrows)*, symphysis pubis diastasis, and right sacroiliac joint diastasis *(arrowheads)*. **C,** Radiograph demonstrating features of AP force with symphysis pubis *(arrow)* and left sacroiliac joint diastasis *(arrowheads)*.

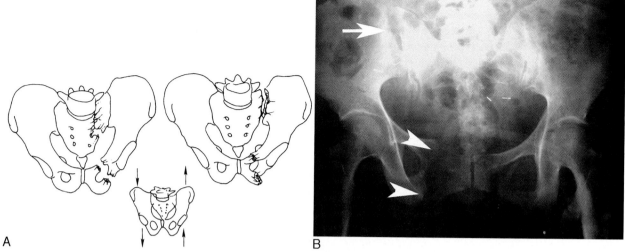

Figure 10-6   Vertical shear. **A,** Diagram demonstrating features of vertical shear. Central lower figure demonstrates direction of forces. Signature feature is that of vertical malalignment of pelvis. **B,** Malgaigne fracture. This pelvic fracture demonstrates ipsilateral fractures of the inferior and superior pubic rami *(arrowheads)* as well as the iliac wing adjacent to the sacroiliac joint *(arrow)*. Note the superior displacement of the right innominate bone relative to the sacrum and left side. This is an unstable fracture.

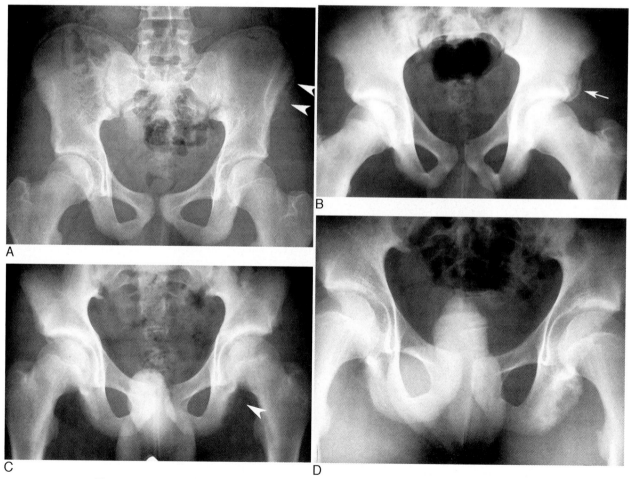

Figure 10-7   Examples of class I fracture. **A,** Frontal radiograph of pelvis demonstrates avulsion of left anterior superior iliac spine (sartorius origin, *arrowheads*). **B,** Avulsion of the anterior inferior iliac spine (rectus femoris insertion, *arrowheads*). **C and D,** Left ischial tuberosity avulsion (hamstring origin, *arrowhead* in part C). Follow-up radiograph (D) obtained 13 months later shows new bone formation in a chronic avulsion, mimicking osteosarcoma.

Class I and Class II Fractures

Apophyseal avulsion injuries are one form of class I fracture (see Figs. 10-7, 1-13). There are five pelvic apophyses that appear by puberty and fuse by the middle of the third decade: the iliac crest, the anterior-superior iliac spine (the origin of the sartorius muscle), the anterior-inferior iliac spine (the origin of the rectus femoris muscle), the inferior pubic ramus (the origin of the adductor muscles), and the ischial tuberosity (the origin of the hamstring muscles). Avulsion injuries may be confusing both clinically and radiographically. These injuries may be subtle in the skeletally immature patient because they are Salter-Harris I equivalent fractures, often with minimal or no visible displacement of an otherwise normal-appearing apophyseal ossification center. Subtle asymmetry in the width of the growth plates may be present at the time of injury. In younger children, the displaced apophysis may be unossified and therefore invisible on radiographs. However, apophyseal avulsion injuries usually become evident on subsequent radiographs when healing and heterotopic bone formation between the pelvis and the avulsed fragment becomes apparent. In early stages of healing, the healing bone is immature and may be confused with osteosarcoma. Such avulsions are particularly confusing at the ischial tuberosity and the inferior pubic ramus, with the occasional appearance of osseous enlargement and sclerosis further confusing the correct diagnosis. Clinical correlation and close radiographic follow-up should demonstrate maturation of the new bone, allowing distinction from osteosarcoma.

Key Concepts	Pelvic Fractures: Pelvic Ring Classification

Class I: Isolated fractures that do not disrupt the pelvic ring
Class II: Pelvic ring disrupted in one location
Class III: Pelvic ring disrupted in at least two locations
Class IV: Acetabular fractures

Other forms of class I and II fractures are iliac wing fractures, isolated sacral fractures, and isolated ischial or pubic rami fractures. An isolated pubic ramus fracture may also occur from a direct blow and, like the sacrum, is also prone to insufficiency fracture among osteoporotic patients and patients after radiation therapy. These fractures may assume bizarre appearances, with bone expansion and aggressive-appearing new bone formation mimicking osteosarcoma. Sacral fractures were previously discussed. The pubic bones are also common locations for pseudofractures of osteomalacia (Looser's zones). Among patients with normal bone mineralization, pubic stress fractures are most common at the junction of the pubis and ischium, especially among long-distance runners. This is also the location of the developmental ischiopubic synchondrosis, which has variable appearance in the skeletally immature patient that can simulate a healing fracture.

Class III Fractures

Class III fractures are unstable fractures and represent one third of cases of pelvic trauma. These involve pelvic disruption in two or more locations and can assume any of the patterns as described under the biomechanics section. These are unstable fractures due to the presence of extensive ligamentous injury and are associated with significant risk for visceral injury and internal hemorrhage.

ACETABULAR FRACTURES

Acetabular fractures are class IV fractures in the pelvic ring classification system. Acetabular fractures occur in the setting of forces directed to the acetabulum through the femoral head. Depending on the direction of forces and the position of the femoral head at the time of injury, a variety of fracture patterns may be found (Fig. 10-8). The most commonly used

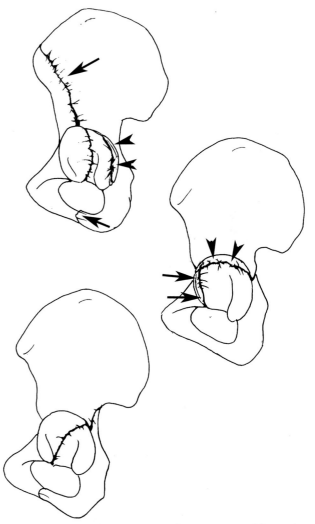

Figure 10-8   Diagram demonstrating fracture patterns of the acetabulum. Top diagram shows anterior column *(arrows)* and posterior wall *(arrowheads)* patterns. Middle diagram demonstrates anterior wall *(arrows)* and transverse *(arrowheads)* patterns. Bottom image demonstrates posterior column pattern.

classification system is that of Letournel and Judet. This classification system is based on an understanding of the anterior and posterior column anatomic description of load bearing. The *anterior column* is the anterior portion of the pelvis that allows load bearing from the spine to the lower extremity. The *posterior column* is the posterior portion of the pelvis that allows load bearing from the spine to the lower extremity. The anterior and posterior columns are not the anterior and posterior walls. Instead, they are the entire load-bearing portion of the hemipelvis anteriorly and posteriorly. Thus the posterior column consists of the sciatic notch region of the hemipelvis, the posterior acetabular wall, and the ischium. The anterior column consists of the iliopectineal line, the anterior acetabular wall, and the superior and inferior pubic rami.

There are five primary or elemental fracture patterns of the acetabulum: anterior wall, posterior wall, transverse, anterior column, and posterior column fractures. The most common primary fracture of the acetabulum is a *posterior wall* fracture, occurring in 17% of all acetabular fractures (Fig. 10-9). Wall fractures refer to fracture lines in the non–weight-bearing lips or rims of the anterior and posterior acetabulum. Column fractures refer to separation of the anterior or posterior weight-bearing portions of the pelvis from the remainder of the pelvis. For example, in the *posterior column* fracture, the fracture line extends from the sciatic notch through the medial wall of the acetabulum, the acetabular floor, and the ischiopubic junction. Thus, the ischium, posterior acetabulum, and sciatic notch region are separated from the remainder of the hemipelvis. *Anterior column* fractures appear as fracture lines extending through the iliac wing, the medial wall of the acetabulum, the acetabular floor, and the ischiopubic

junction. Thus, an anterior column fracture separates the anterior weight-bearing portion of the hemipelvis from the remainder of the hemipelvis. A transverse fracture (Fig. 10-10) separates the upper hemipelvis from the lower hemipelvis and can occur above, at, or inferior to the roof of the acetabulum. Transverse fractures occur in 10% of acetabular fractures.

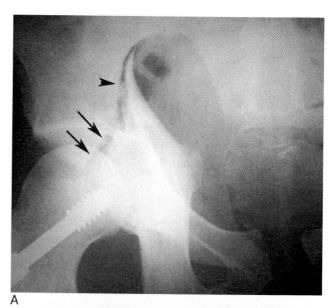

A

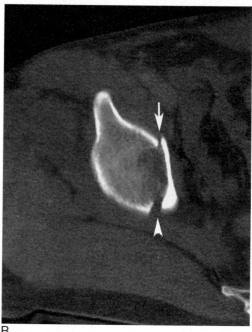

B

Figure 10-10   Transverse fracture of acetabulum. **A,** Frontal radiograph demonstrates fracture line through the superior acetabulum with extension across the ilioischial line *(arrowhead)*. Note transverse orientation of fracture line through the acetabulum *(arrows)*. **B,** Consecutive axial CT images obtained through the acetabular roof demonstrate transverse fracture line. Note sagittal orientation of fracture with involvement of anterior *(arrow)* and posterior *(arrowhead)* walls. F, top of the femoral head.

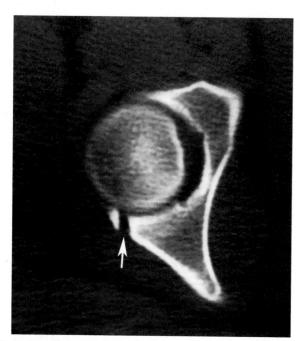

Figure 10-9   Posterior wall fracture. Axial CT performed after relocation of a posterior hip dislocation demonstrates fracture of posterior wall *(arrows)* with only minimal displacement.

(Continued)

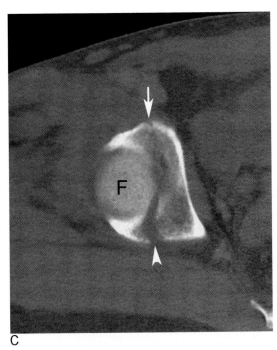

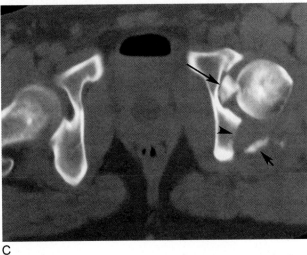

C

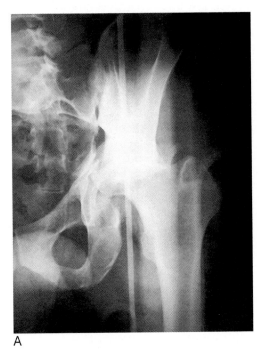

C

Figure 10-10—(Cont'd) **C,** Consecutive axial CT images obtained through the acetabular roof demonstrate transverse fracture line. Note sagittal orientation of fracture with involvement of anterior *(arrow)* and posterior *(arrowhead)* walls. F, top of the femoral head.

Figure 10-11—(Cont'd) **B,** Axial CT image obtained after hip relocation demonstrates transverse fracture line *(arrow)* and displaced posterior wall fragments *(arrowhead)*. **C,** Axial CT image caudal to image shown in part B demonstrates posterior wall fracture *(short arrow)* with blunted posterior wall margin *(arrowhead)* and displaced intra-articular fracture fragment *(long arrow)* preventing complete femoral head reduction.

Figure 10-11 Transverse-posterior wall–associated fractures. This is a transverse fracture through the superior acetabulum and a posterior wall fracture. **A,** Frontal radiograph demonstrates posterior dislocation or hip and complex fracture pattern at acetabulum.

(Continued)

Associated, or combination, fractures are those in which more than one elemental fracture is present. The five major associated fracture patterns are transverse-posterior wall (Fig. 10-11), T-shaped (Fig. 10-12), both column, posterior column-posterior wall, and anterior wall-posterior hemitransverse fractures (Fig. 10-13). Of these associated fracture patterns, the *transverse-posterior wall* fracture is most common, occurring in 19% of acetabular fractures.

Judet views are extremely useful in evaluating acetabular fractures because these oblique views allow assessment of the cortical margins both anteriorly and posteriorly at the acetabulum. A fracture line extending anteroposteriorly involving iliopectineal and ilioischial lines must be a transverse fracture. Vertical fractures arising from the sciatic

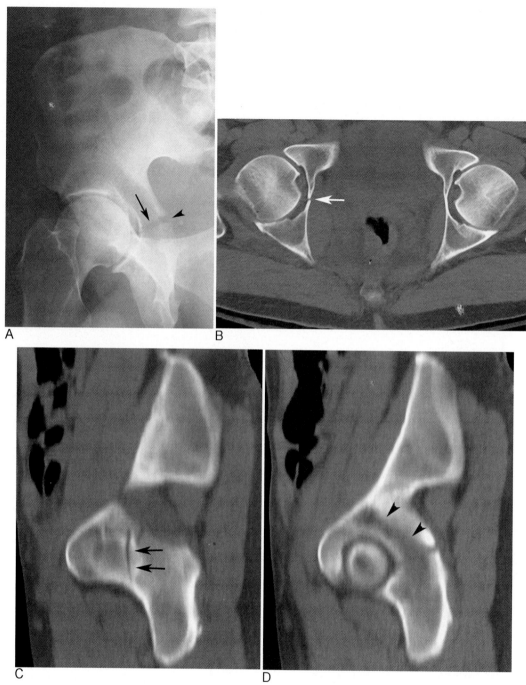

Figure 10-12   T-shaped fracture. This is a transverse fracture through the acetabulum and a coronal fracture extending inferiorly. **A,** Iliac Judet radiographic view demonstrates transverse fracture line *(arrow)* extending to ilioischial line *(arrowhead).* **B,** Axial CT image demonstrates the vertical component of T-shaped fracture in medial wall of acetabulum *(arrow).* **C and D,** Sagittal CT reformations at the medial acetabulum (part C medial to part D) demonstrate vertical *(arrows* in part C) and transverse *(arrowheads* in part D) components of T-shaped fracture in medial wall and roof of acetabulum.

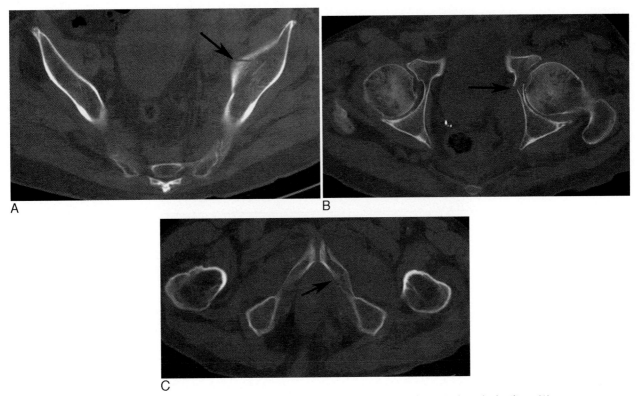

Figure 10-13 Anterior column fracture. **A–C,** Axial CT images show fractures through the ilium (A), acetabulum (B), and ischium/inferior pubic ramus (C).

notch must be posterior column fractures. Vertically oriented fractures through the iliac wing and acetabulum must be anterior column fractures. Fractures isolated to the rims of the acetabulum must be anterior or posterior wall fractures. If the obturator ring is disrupted, the acetabular fracture must be either a T-shaped fracture or a column fracture. If there is a "spur" sign, representing a spur of bone located superior and posterior to the acetabulum on the obturator oblique view, there must be a posterior column or both column fracture.

CT imaging is also extremely useful in evaluation of the acetabulum because fracture lines are more clearly demonstrated, and multiplanar and 3D reformations are possible, thus aiding fracture characterization and preoperative planning. The following are quick clues to the elemental fracture pattern. If an acetabular fracture plane is sagittal (directed anteroposteriorly), it is a transverse fracture. If the fracture plane is coronal and through the medial wall, it is either an anterior or posterior column fracture. Sagittally oriented or oblique fractures isolated to the anterior or posterior rim are wall fractures.

ANATOMY
DISLOCATION
FEMORAL NECK FRACTURES
INTERTROCHANTERIC FRACTURES
AVULSION FRACTURE OF THE LESSER TROCHANTER
SLIPPED CAPITAL FEMORAL EPIPHYSIS
FEMORAL SHAFT FRACTURE
STRESS FRACTURES OF THE FEMUR
SNAPPING HIP
FEMOROACETABULAR IMPINGEMENT
ADDITIONAL SOFT TISSUE CONDITIONS

Key Concepts	Hip Joint Anatomy
Ball-and-socket joint Normal angle between the femoral neck and shaft averages 135 degrees (range, 115–140 degrees)	

ANATOMY

The hip is a ball-and-socket joint. The joint is invested by a strong capsule and is supported by the iliofemoral, pubofemoral, and ischiofemoral ligaments, with further support from the acetabular labrum, the transverse acetabular ligament, and the ligament of the head of the femur (ligamentum teres). The vascular supply to the femoral head is tenuous. Although the artery of the ligamentum teres contributes to the vascular supply of the femoral head, most of the arterial supply is from the medial and lateral circumflex femoral arteries, which are primary branches of the common femoral artery. In the frontal plane, the normal angle between the femoral neck and shaft averages 135 degrees (range, 115 to 140 degrees). *Coxa valga* is an abnormally increased femoral neck-shaft angle. Internal or external rotation of the femur can falsely simulate coxa valga. The femoral neck is normally *anteverted* relative to the femoral shaft by approximately 15 degrees. In other words, if a femur were placed horizontally on a flat surface with the posterior aspect of both condyles touching the table, the femoral neck would angle anteriorly away from the table surface. Stated yet another way, the femoral condyles are internally rotated relative to the femoral neck. The greater trochanter and lesser trochanter are both *posterior* structures. The lesser trochanter is posteromedial in location and the greater trochanter posterolateral. Thus, when the femur is internally rotated, the greater trochanter is shown in profile and the lesser trochanter is hidden from view. When the femur is externally rotated, the lesser trochanter is in profile and the greater trochanter is hidden from view. This anatomic relationship plays an important role in assessment of hip dislocations, which will be described later in the chapter. Furthermore, the posterior positions of the greater and lesser trochanters obscure visualization of portions of the femoral neck on both frontal and frog-lateral radiographic views of the hip. These two views also foreshorten the radiographic appearance of the femoral neck. Because of these limitations, radiographic assessment of trauma to the hip requires the groin lateral (true lateral) view. This view profiles the femoral neck without superimposition of the trochanters (Fig. 11-1).

The hip joint capsule extends over the proximal femoral neck to insert on the basicervical region. Fat planes about the hip may bulge away from the hip joint in the presence of a large hip joint effusion. However, this finding lacks sensitivity and specificity for the assessment of effusion. A more reliable plain film indicator is measurement of the distance between the teardrop of the acetabulum and the medial femoral head on a well-positioned anteroposterior (AP) view, with asymmetric increase indicating the side of effusion. Ultrasonography (US) or magnetic resonance imaging (MRI) provide the most reliable imaging methods for detection of a hip joint effusion. Hip effusions are most apparent around the femoral neck.

DISLOCATION

Dislocation is an unusual complication of trauma, often overlooked because of its common association with femoral shaft fractures that dominate the clinical evaluation.

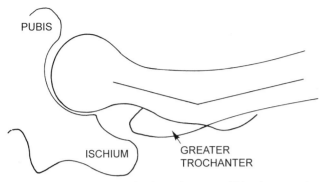

Figure 11-1 Groin lateral radiographic view of hip, demonstrating the normal anatomy and normal neck-shaft angle. Note that the trochanters project posterior to the femoral neck, allowing radiographic assessment of femoral neck fracture without superimposition of the trochanters. (Reproduced with permission from Manaster BJ: Handbook of Skeletal Radiology, ed 2. St. Louis, Mosby, 1997.)

Approximately 90% of dislocations are posterior. Posterior dislocations are especially common after motor vehicle accidents in which the flexed knee strikes the dashboard, driving the flexed hip posteriorly. Posterior hip dislocation is commonly associated with fracture of the posterior acetabular wall. With posterior dislocation, the femoral head is typically not only posteriorly positioned relative to the acetabulum, but also superiorly positioned, and the femur is in internal rotation with the greater trochanter in profile and the lesser trochanter obscured (Fig. 11-2). Clinically, the lower extremity appears

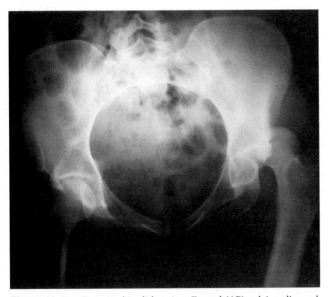

Figure 11-2 Posterior hip dislocation. Frontal (AP) pelvis radiograph demonstrates superior position of the left femoral head and internal rotation of the femur. Note also the smaller appearance of the left femoral head compared to the right. This is due to the closer positioning of the femoral head to the x-ray cassette, and thus less radiographic magnification.

adducted, extended, and internally rotated, and is shortened because of superior femoral head displacement. Radiographically, dislocations are easy to recognize if the femoral head is superior in position relative to the acetabulum. However, the degree of superior displacement may be minimal. In these situations, dislocation may be difficult to recognize on the frontal film. In such subtle cases, there may be lack of congruence of the femoral head and the acetabulum. Additionally, a dislocated femoral head appears smaller than the contralateral femoral head because the dislocated femoral head is posterior in position and closer to the film, thus less magnified.

Key Concepts	Hip Dislocation

Posterior: Most common. Femoral head posterior and superior to acetabulum, femur in internal rotation.
Anterior: Flexed position = obturator anterior dislocation. Femoral head medial and inferior, overlying the obturator foramen.
Extended thigh = Iliac dislocation. Femoral head superior to the acetabulum, like a posterior dislocation, but the femur is in external rotation.

Anterior dislocations are uncommon, and occur in the externally rotated and abducted thigh. They may present with the femur in either a flexed or extended position. In a flexed position, the dislocation is known as an obturator anterior dislocation because the femoral head is positioned medially and inferiorly, overlying the obturator foramen (Fig. 11-3). In the extended thigh, anterior dislocation is superior to the acetabulum, much like a posterior dislocation. However, this form of anterior dislocation, known as iliac dislocation, can be discriminated from a posterior dislocation because the femur is in external rotation with the lesser trochanter in profile and the greater trochanter obscured.

With both anterior and posterior dislocations, there is risk of fracture of the femoral head. This can result from impaction injury with compression of a portion of the femoral head, not unlike the Hill-Sachs and trough fractures associated with shoulder dislocations. Another form of femur fracture dislocation is shear fracture of the femoral head (Fig. 11-4). Intra-articular fragments may result from such fractures. Fragments may also result from acetabular fracture fragments. Avulsion fractures related to tension of the ligamentum teres insertion on the femur are a third cause of intra-articular loose bodies. Intra-articular loose bodies can be suspected with demonstration of widening and incongruence of the femoral head and acetabulum, and can cause increased distance between the acetabular teardrop and the medial femoral head. Computed tomography (CT)

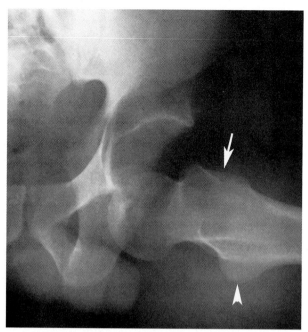

Figure 11-3   Anterior hip dislocation. AP radiographic view shows obturator anterior dislocation with inferomedial displacement of the femoral head and external rotation of the femur with profile view of lesser trochanter *(arrowhead)* and obscured greater trochanter *(arrow)*.

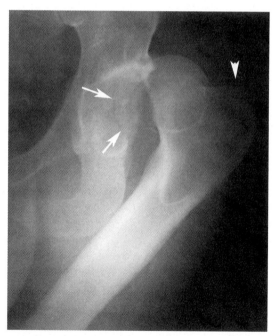

Figure 11-4   Posterior dislocation with shear fracture of femoral head *(arrows)*. Note internal rotation of femur with obscuration of lesser trochanter and profile view of greater trochanter *(arrowhead)*.

is usually definitive in detecting bone fragments. Another common complication after hip dislocation is avascular necrosis (AVN), which markedly increases in likelihood if a dislocation is not reduced within 24 hours. Approximately 50% of hip reductions delayed after 24 hours undergo subsequent AVN.

FEMORAL NECK FRACTURES

Fractures of the femur are divided into those involving the femoral head, the femoral neck, the intertrochanteric region, the shaft, and the condyles. As noted previously, femoral head fractures occur during dislocations and appear as impaction or shearing injuries. Such fractures have high risk for nonunion and AVN. Computed tomography is useful to search for intra-articular fracture fragments, which require surgical removal.

Femoral neck and intertrochanteric fractures are rare in young adults and middle-aged patients but extremely common in the elderly population. This high prevalence corresponds to the high prevalence of osteoporosis in the elderly. By age 80, 10% of white women and 5% of white men sustain a hip fracture. By age 90, the rates increase to 20% and 10%, respectively. Falls resulting in femoral neck fractures are highly associated with fractures of the distal radius and proximal humerus.

WHAT THE CLINICIAN WANTS TO KNOW:
FEMORAL NECK FRACTURES

Head, neck, intertrochanteric, or shaft
Neck: Subcapital, midcervical, or basicervical
Subcapital fractures: Garden classification

Femoral neck fractures are divided into subcapital, midcervical, and basicervical types. In general, the more proximal the fracture line and the more displaced the fracture, the higher the risk for AVN and nonunion. Basicervical and midcervical fractures are rare. The subcapital fracture is common. The *Garden classification* categorizes subcapital fractures into four stages. An important clue to identifying the correct stage is the relative orientation of the trabeculae of the femoral neck, femoral head, and acetabulum. Stage I fractures are considered incomplete fractures with lateral impaction due to external rotation of the femoral shaft, and valgus of the femoral head (Fig. 11-5). This is identified by the valgus orientation of the femoral head and neck trabeculae. Because the femoral head is in valgus, the trabeculae of the femoral head and the acetabulum are in varus alignment (i.e., the apex of the angle formed by these trabeculae is oriented laterally).

Stage II fractures are complete subcapital fractures without displacement. In this stage, there is anatomic positioning of the femoral shaft, and the femoral head shows mild varus or anatomic position. This stage is identified by mild varus orientation of the femoral head and neck trabeculae. Because the femoral head is in varus, the trabeculae of the femoral head and the acetabulum are in valgus alignment (i.e., the apex of the angle formed by these trabeculae is oriented medially).

Stage III fractures are complete fractures with partial displacement. The femoral shaft is externally rotated, and the femoral head is medially rotated and in mild varus (Fig. 11-6).

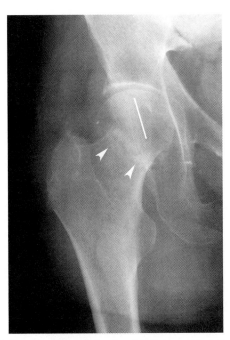

Figure 11-5   Garden stage I subcapital fracture. Note fracture line *(arrowheads)* and lateralized direction of femoral head trabecular lines (*line* marks the direction of the femoral head trabecular lines).

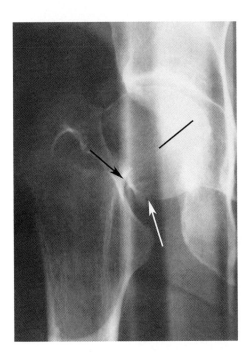

Figure 11-6   Garden stage III subcapital femoral fracture. Note medial direction of femoral head trabecular lines *(line)* and partial superior displacement of medial femoral neck *(black arrow)* compared with medial femoral head margin *(white arrow)*.

This stage is identified by more severe varus orientation of the femoral head and neck trabeculae, usually forming less than a 160-degree angle (normal, 180 degrees) The external rotation of the femoral shaft may be apparent as prominence of the lesser trochanter. As with stage II fractures, femoral head varus

alignment causes the trabeculae of the femoral head and the acetabulum to be in valgus alignment.

Stage IV fractures are complete fractures with gross proximal displacement of the shaft relative to the head. The femoral shaft is not only externally rotated but telescoped. However, the femoral head is in anatomic alignment relative to the acetabulum (Fig. 11-7). Thus, the trabeculae of the femoral head and the acetabulum are parallel.

The Garden staging system is used because it indicates the higher degree of complication with higher-stage fractures, and therefore guides therapy. Major complications after subcapital fracture are nonunion and AVN. The occurrence of both complications increases substantially with higher stages. Stage I fractures have the best prognosis and can be adequately treated with percutaneous Knowles pin or screw fixation. Among stage IV fractures there is a greater than 40% nonunion rate and a 30% rate of AVN. Thus, many orthopedic surgeons proceed directly to hemiarthroplasty when treating a stage IV fracture. Treatment of stage II and III fractures varies with the surgeon's preference.

Detection of a subcapital fracture may be extremely difficult. The bones are often demineralized and hence poorly seen on radiographs. Cortical and trabecular disruption may be minimal. Ring-like femoral head osteophytes in a setting of osteoarthritis may yield a similar appearance to fracture and give a false impression of fracture. Awareness of this pitfall may lead to underdiagnosis in patients with osteoarthritis. When the diagnosis is unclear, MRI has extremely high accuracy, even with low-field scanners, and is not affected by patient age

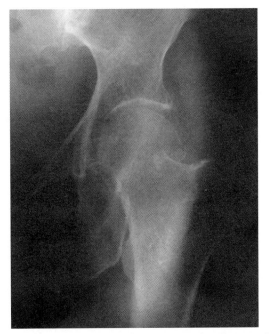

Figure 11-7   Garden stage IV fracture. Femoral neck is completely displaced. Note substantial shortening of femoral neck and anatomic femoral head alignment.

or osteoporosis (Fig. 11-8). The evaluation can be abbreviated to T1-weighted spin-echo and inversion recovery sequences, with total scan times of about 10 to 15 minutes. Magnetic resonance imaging also will demonstrate other fractures, such as fractures of the pelvic ring, soft tissue contusions, and muscle strains. In patients with contraindication to MRI, such

as a pacemaker, or if MRI is not available, radionuclide bone scanning (Fig. 11-9) is useful; however, this test is insensitive among the elderly for fracture detection in the first 72 hours. After 72 hours, the sensitivity is about 90%. CT with reformats is also used in the acute or delayed setting, but it is less sensitive than MRI.

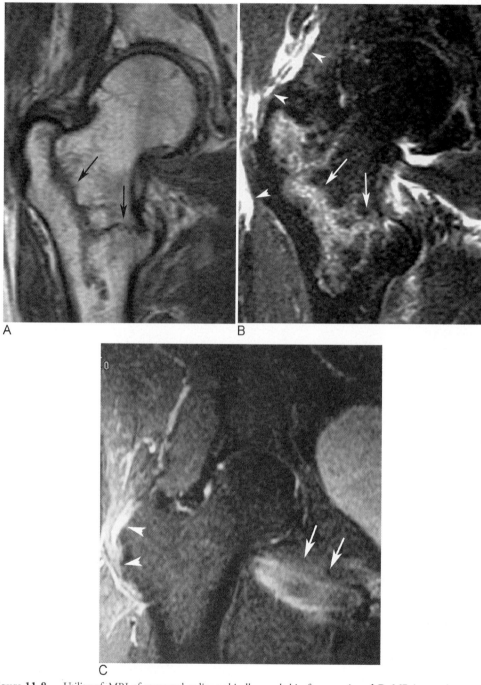

Figure 11-8   Utility of MRI of suspected radiographically occult hip fracture. **A and B,** MR images in elderly patient who fell; radiographs were normal. Coronal T1-weighted MR image (A) shows nondisplaced intertrochanteric fractures seen as an irregular low signal intensity line *(arrows)*. Coronal inversion recovery MR image (B) shows high signal along the fracture *(arrows)* due to edema. Also note high signal contusion and bursal fluid lateral to the hip *(arrowheads)*. **C,** Coronal inversion recovery MR image in a different patient shows use of MRI for the exclusion of fracture and demonstration of the cause of the patient's symptoms. Marrow signal was normal on all sequences, excluding a fracture. Note high signal in obturator externus *(arrows)*, indicating strain, and lateral contusion *(arrowheads)*.

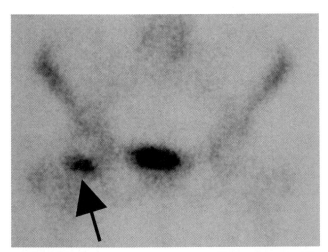

Figure 11-9   Radionuclide bone scan in an elderly patient who fell 3 days previously and had continued hip pain and negative radiographs. Diphosphate bone scan shows intense, linear tracer uptake *(arrow)* crossing the femoral neck, indicating fracture.

INTERTROCHANTERIC FRACTURES

These fractures occur in older persons than subcapital fractures do, and they are less common. They are classified as two-, three-, or four-part fractures, depending on involvement of lesser and greater trochanters. The dominant fracture is usually obliquely oriented along a line joining the greater and lesser trochanters (Fig. 11-10). The opposite obliquity is rare and unstable.

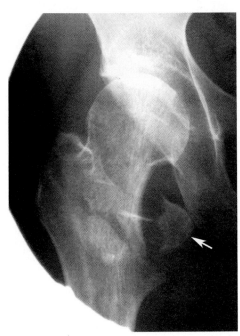

Figure 11-10   Intertrochanteric fracture. Frontal radiograph demonstrates fracture with displaced lesser trochanter fragment *(arrow)*. Traction by the iliopsoas tendon tends to displace lesser trochanter fragments superiorly and anteriorly.

Generally, intertrochanteric fractures have a good prognosis without compromise of blood supply. Avascular necrosis or nonunion as a result of such fractures is uncommon. Treatment is usually with internal fixation using a dynamic hip screw (Fig. 11-11). This device consists of a femoral diaphyseal

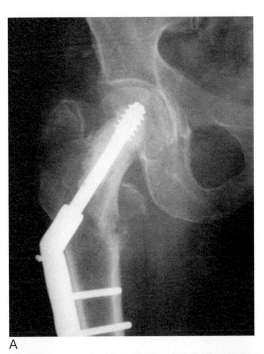

A

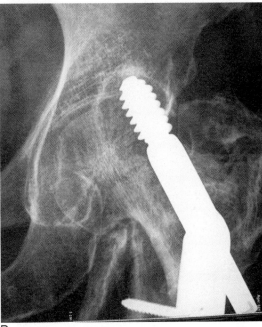

B

Figure 11-11   Dynamic hip screw. **A,** This patient with an intertrochanteric fracture has been stabilized with a dynamic screw and plate system, which allows settling at the fracture site without the screw cutting-out through the osteoporotic bone of the femoral head. **B,** Dynamic hip screw failure in a different patient. The screw head has migrated through the top of the femoral head and neck and eroded into the acetabular roof.

cortical plate with a superior hollow cylindrical shaft that is placed over a femoral head screw. There are no threads where the screw contacts the cylinder, rather only a slot on the screw to prevent rotation. Thus, the screw is restricted from transverse and torsional displacement but is free to undergo compression when the patient stands. This form of fixation allows settling at the fracture site with impaction of the fracture fragments, which accelerates healing. Occasionally there may be excessive settling, and the femoral head screw can back out of the hollow cylinder. This most commonly occurs in the setting of collapse of the fixation into a varus configuration (Fig. 11-11B).

AVULSION FRACTURE OF THE LESSER TROCHANTER

This is an occasional type of fracture in children and adolescents resulting from avulsion of the iliopsoas at the lesser trochanteric apophysis. The iliopsoas tendon pulls the fragment anteriorly and superiorly. In adults, lesser trochanter avulsion is unusual as an isolated injury, and is most commonly due to underlying pathology, notably metastatic disease (Fig. 11-12). However, this injury is a common component of an intertrochanteric fracture.

SLIPPED CAPITAL FEMORAL EPIPHYSIS

Slipped capital femoral epiphysis (SCFE) is seen during periods of rapid skeletal growth, at 10 to 16 years of age,

during a period in which body weight and muscle strength increase rapidly and the femoral neck develops greater varus. This results in increased shear loading on the capital femoral physis and predisposes the child to Salter-Harris I fracture with displacement. The injury is probably due to repetitive minor trauma and is seen more commonly in males, black persons, obese individuals, and children with delayed skeletal maturation. The disorder occurs bilaterally in 20% of children but is usually asymmetric in appearance. The capital epiphysis displaces posteromedially relative to the neck, resulting in a radiographic appearance in which the physis appears wider and with indistinct margins (Fig. 11-13). The

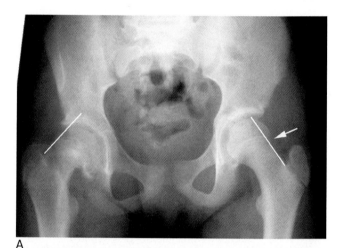

A

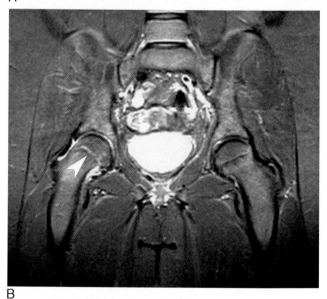

B

Figure 11-13   Slipped capital femoral epiphysis (SCFE). **A,** AP radiograph shows normal left side. Line drawn along superior cortex of left femoral neck *(arrow)* crosses the capital femoral epiphysis. Right side is abnormal: this line fails to intersect femoral capital epiphysis. Note the wider physis on the right, which is another clue to the diagnosis. **B,** Coronal inversion recovery MR image in a different child with right SCFE shows medial displacement of the right capital femoral epiphysis, a joint effusion, and edema in the physis *(arrowhead)*.

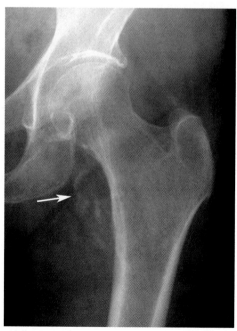

Figure 11-12   Lesser trochanter avulsion *(arrow)*, in this case due to metastatic lung cancer.

malalignment may be most evident, or indeed may be evident only on a frog-leg lateral or groin radiograph, where the head is seen to be posterior relative to the femoral neck (Fig. 11-14). The most helpful sign of SCFE on a frontal radiograph is demonstrated by drawing a line tangent to the lateral margin of the femoral neck. Ordinarily, this line should intersect a portion of the capital epiphysis. In SCFE, however, the tangent line is superior and lateral to the capital epiphysis. The disorder is treated with three-point pinning without reduction. This results in varus deformity with a short and broad femoral neck. The disorder is commonly complicated by osteoarthritis in adulthood, usually occurring after 30 years of age. In addition, AVN occurs in 10% of

individuals, especially after attempts at epiphyseal reduction (Fig. 11-15). Rarely, acute chondrolysis can occur. The surgeon may elect to pin the contralateral hip in order to prevent a SCFE from developing, and to maintain symmetric growth.

FEMORAL SHAFT FRACTURE

These fractures may be seen in isolation or in combination with other femoral fractures, including femoral neck fractures and condylar fractures. They are often comminuted with butterfly or segmental fragments. Fractures in children are usually treated with casting. Fractures in adults are usually fixed internally with an interlocking intramedullary nail. Side plate fixation is less desirable because placement of a plate requires disturbing some of the numerous muscle attachments that cover much of the

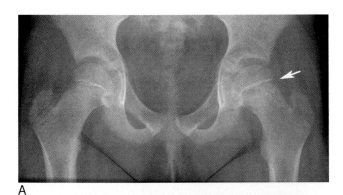

A

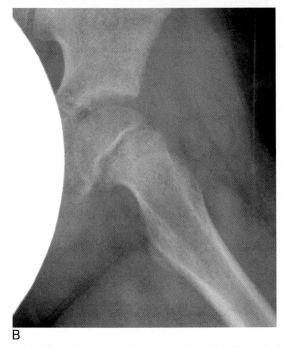

B

Figure 11-14   Slipped capital femoral epiphysis (SCFE). Right side is normal. **A,** AP radiograph shows only minimal displacement, which could easily be overlooked. Note the wide physis on the left *(arrow)*. **B,** Frog-leg lateral view of the left hip shows medial and posterior displacement of the capital femoral epiphysis. This example illustrates the need for a lateral radiograph when evaluating for suspected SCFE.

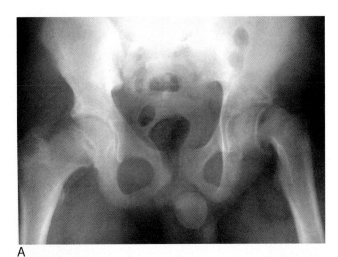

A

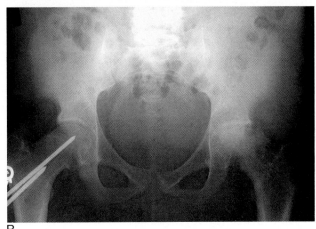

B

Figure 11-15   Bilateral slipped capital femoral epiphysis (SCFE). **A,** Note severely displaced fracture on the left. **B,** Same patient 3 years later shows collapsed left femoral head due to complication of avascular necrosis.

femoral shaft cortex. The surgeon must check for rotational deformity so that appropriate reduction may be achieved. Computed tomography can help assess for the degree of rotation (version) by obtaining only a few CT sections at the femoral neck and at the femoral condyles (Fig. 11-16). The degree of version can be measured by summing the angles of the femoral neck and condyles. This is done at each location by drawing a line parallel to the bottom edge of the film, a second line through the middle of the femoral neck, and another line at the knee tangent to the posterior margin of the femoral condyles. The two angles are summed and can be compared with the contralateral side, which should be within 5 degrees of the fractured side. For further discussion of femoral torsion, see Chapter 44.

STRESS FRACTURES OF THE FEMUR

The femur is susceptible to stress fracture, particularly involving the medial femoral neck proximal to the lesser trochanter, the medial cortex in the proximal and midshaft regions, and the posterior cortex in the distal shaft. Patients with femoral neck stress fractures usually present with vague hip or groin pain. Radiographs may reveal linear sclerosis with occasional central linear lucency or solid periosteal new bone formation, but findings may be equivocal or even normal (Fig. 11-17A). In such cases, bone scanning or MRI is useful for diagnosis of stress fracture. We prefer MRI because of its remarkable marrow contrast (Fig. 11-17).

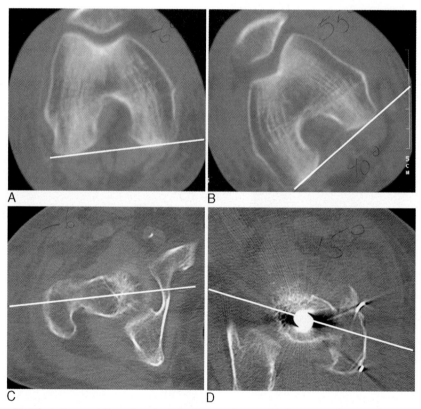

Figure 11-16   Abnormal femoral torsion after fracture fixation. Adult patient who had a left femur fracture fixed with an intramedullary rod. Limited CT sections were obtained through the knees; the couch was then moved without moving the patient and limited sections were obtained through the proximal femurs. Representative images are shown. The uninjured right side has 0 degrees of anteversion. On the left, the fragments had twisted around the rod, resulting in 55 degrees of femoral anteversion. Corrective surgery was required. A, right knee; B, left knee; C, right femoral neck; D, left femoral neck.

Stress fractures that are not treated with non–weight-bearing can result in a complete fracture requiring internal fixation. Stress fractures are usually transversely oriented to the length of the femoral neck or shaft, although vertically oriented stress fractures rarely occur. Vertical stress fractures are extremely subtle on radiographs and can produce a confusing marrow edema pattern on MRI. Computed tomography is often helpful in these situations because reformatted images reveal a vertical thin sclerotic line. "Thigh splints" is a stress reaction of the femoral shaft with clinical and imaging features similar to those of "shin splints" in the tibia (Fig. 11-18).

SNAPPING HIP

The sensation of snapping with pain may be due to many causes. These include (1) tendon snapping over the greater trochanter by the iliotibial band or the anterior margin of the gluteus maximus, often with an associated bursitis; (2) tendon snapping over the pubic tubercle by the iliopsoas tendon; (3) a local detachment or tear of the acetabular labrum; (4) intra-articular body (chondral or osteochondral fragment or synovial chondromatosis); and (5) femoroacetabular impingement. Femoroacetabular impingement is discussed later in this

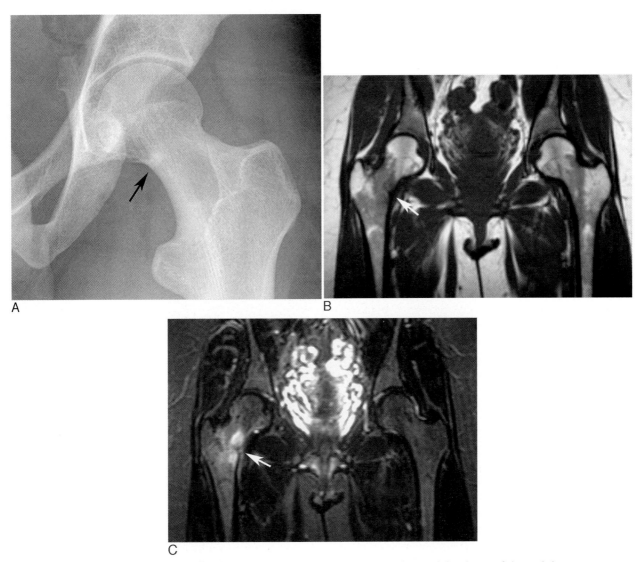

Figure 11-17 Stress fracture of femoral neck. **A,** AP radiographs shows subtle sclerosis of the medial femoral neck *(arrow)*. **B and C,** Coronal T1 (B) and inversion recovery (C) MR images in a different patient with femoral neck stress fracture show incomplete, low-signal-intensity linear fracture line at medial femoral neck cortex *(arrow)* with surrounding bone marrow edema in part C.

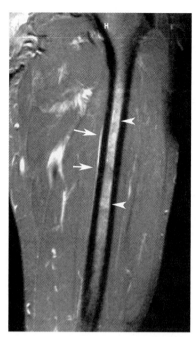

Figure 11-18 Femoral shaft stress reaction in 25-year-old female runner with left thigh pain. Coronal fat-suppressed T2-weighted MR image shows marrow edema *(arrowheads)* and periosteal edema *(arrows)* along the medial midshaft. These findings were unilateral and resolved with cessation of running.

chapter. Intra-articular bodies can be diagnosed with MRI or CT arthrography. The tendinous causes of snapping can be diagnosed clinically and confirmed with US. Associated bursitis, when present, may also be seen on MRI because of bursal distention with fluid. Iliotibial band snapping is usually diagnosed clinically because this snapping sensation is more lateral than is snapping from the iliopsoas tendon and from labral tears, which is anterior. The iliopsoas variety can be diagnosed with iliopsoas bursography as well, although US is preferred to dynamically show the tendon snapping.

Key Concepts	Snapping Hip
Iliopsoas tendon or iliotibial band	
Labral tear	
Intra-articular body	
Femoroacetabular impingement, early osteoarthritis (OA)	

Tear or detachment of the acetabular labrum is diagnosed with MR arthrography, which demonstrates contrast undermining a portion of the acetabular labrum (Fig. 11-19). The most frequent location of a labral tear is anterosuperior. A normal variant sulcus may be seen between the posteroinferior labrum and the acetabulum, which may simulate a tear. Magnetic resonance arthrography is also the most reliable test for detection of hip joint articular cartilage defects (Fig. 11-20). Additional important causes of hip pain not discussed in this chapter include AVN, transient osteoporosis, infection, and metastatic disease. These conditions are discussed in later chapters.

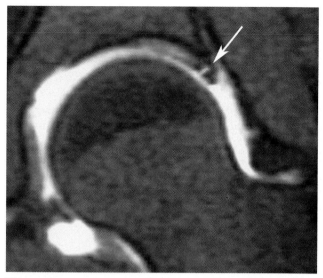

Figure 11-19 Acetabular labral tear. Coronal fat-suppressed T1-weighted MR arthrogram shows high signal intensity *(arrow)* extending into a tear in the superior labrum.

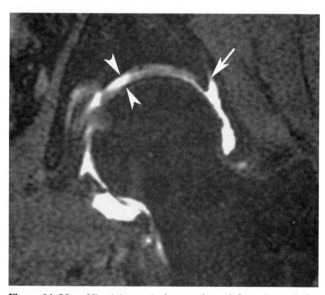

Figure 11-20 Hip joint articular cartilage defect. Coronal fat-suppressed T1-weighted MR arthrogram shows matching chondral defects in the acetabulum and femoral head *(arrowheads)*. The examination was performed for hip pain, suspected to be due to a labral tear, which was not found.

FEMOROACETABULAR IMPINGEMENT

Femoroacetabular impingement (FAI) is impingement of the acetabular labrum and adjacent articular cartilage between the femur head-neck junction and the acetabulum rim. The impingement leads to labral tear and degeneration of adjacent articular cartilage.

Understanding of FAI is evolving and is somewhat controversial. Current understanding is that the most common

Compression of labrum and cartilage between the acetabular rim and the femoral head-neck junction

Most common cause: Dysmorphic overgrowth of anterolateral head-neck junction ("cam" or "femoral" impingement)

Other causes: Excessively deep acetabulum with overgrowth of the anterior superior acetabulum rim (pincer-type impingement), excessive acetabular retroversion, or femur anteversion

Radiographs

Early: May be normal. Upsloping lateral margin of acetabular rim, acetabular ossicles, crossover sign, lateral femoral neck "bump," and herniation pits may be associated

Later: Osteoarthritis (OA)

MRI: Labral tears, cartilage loss and delamination, subchondral cysts

pattern is *femoral* impingement, also known a *cam-type* impingement, which is caused by a nonspherical femoral head or a dysmorphic bulge of bone at the anterolateral femoral head-neck junction. This abnormal bulge causes mechanical impingement of the labrum during hip flexion or internal rotation. The dysmorphic shape of the femoral head-neck junction has been likened to the mechanical engineering concept of a cam, which is a disk with an eccentric bulge that is used, for example, to open and close valves in an automobile engine as it rotates (Fig. 11-21). The offending bulge may be congenital, or acquired (e.g., due to a femoral head osteophyte or a slipped capital femoral epiphysis). Other deformities may cause FAI, including an excessively deep acetabulum, acetabular retroversion (acetabulum oriented too posteriorly), decreased femoral neck anteversion (femur too externally rotated), and femoral head osteophytes. These deformities may exist in combination. Deformity associated with old Legg-Calvé-Perthes disease (Chapter 22) or developmental dysplasia of the hip (DDH, Chapter 44) also causes FAI. The term "lateral rim syndrome" is sometimes used to describe FAI related to old DDH. Regardless of the cause, impingement may result in pain, labral degeneration and tear, articular cartilage wear and delamination, and early osteoarthritis.

Radiographic findings that have been reported to be associated with cam-type FAI include overgrowth of the anterolateral femoral head-neck junction (the cam) with associated elevated alpha angle (Figs. 11-21, 11-22B), a blunted contour of the lateral acetabular roof margin (Fig. 11-22A), and possibly small ossicles adjacent to the acetabular rim and herniation pit in the femoral neck. A herniation pit, also termed "fibrocystic change of the anterosuperior femoral neck," "synovial herniation pit" or

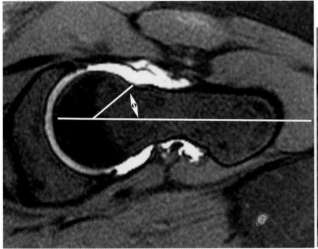

A

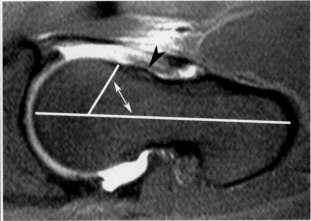

B

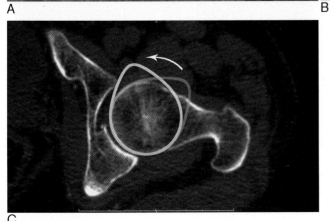

C

Figure 11-21 Femoroacetabular impingement (FAI): femoral (cam) impingement and the alpha angle. Oblique axial-sagittal fat-suppressed T1-weighted hip arthrogram obtained parallel to the femoral neck. Anterior is to the left of the image. **A,** Normal. The alpha angle (*double arrow,* not to be confused with the acetabular alpha angle used to describe developmental dysplasia of the hip) is the angle subtended between the axis of the femoral neck and the head-neck junction, with the angle apex at the center of the femoral head. Normal alpha angle is less than 50 degrees. **B,** Abnormal. Patient with FAI with dysmorphic bump at the anterior femoral head neck junction (*arrowhead*), with resulting elevated alpha angle. **C,** This image illustrates cam impingement. Diagram of a cam superimposed on a normal hip axial CT image shows how a dysmorphic, cam-like bulge of the anterior head-neck junction could impinge against the anterior acetabulum with internal rotation.

"Pitt's pit" after Michael Pitt (who described it), is a small well-circumscribed lucency with a thin sclerotic rim in the anterior or anterior superior femoral neck (Fig. 11-22B, C). These were long thought to be incidental, but it seems likely that some, perhaps most, are due to impingement on the anterior femoral neck by the anterior joint capsule, iliopsoas tendon, or

Key Concepts	Herniation Pit

Small, well-circumscribed lucency with a thin sclerotic rim
Anterior or anterior-superior femoral neck
Long thought to be incidental
Now recognized that some, perhaps most, due to
    impingement on the anterior femoral neck by the anterior
    joint capsule, iliopsoas tendon, or femoroacetabular
    impingement

FAI. This is controversial, as herniation pits are frequently encountered in asymptomatic patients, and many patients with impingement do not have a herniation pit. Another radiographic finding that has been reported to be associated with FAI is the "crossover sign" of the anterior margin of the acetabulum projecting lateral to the posterior margin of the acetabulum (Fig. 11-23). This finding is associated with FAI due to acetabular rim overgrowth that has been likened to a pincer that impinges against the femoral neck. The *alpha angle,* not to be confused with the acetabular alpha angle in developmental hip dysplasia, is the angle subtended between the axis of the femoral neck and the head-neck junction, with the angle apex at the center of the femoral head (see Fig. 11-21).

Magnetic resonance arthrography is the most sensitive test for detection of impingement changes, which include subchondral marrow edema in the lateral superior acetabulum or adjacent lateral femoral head and neck (Fig. 11-22C). Subchondral cysts, cartilage edema, loss or delamination, and an adjacent labral tear may be seen as well.

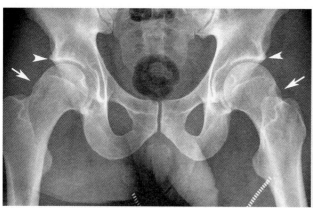

A

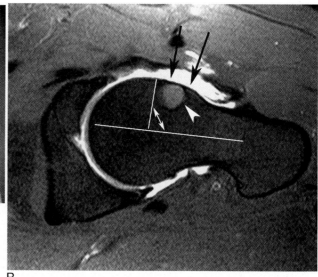

B

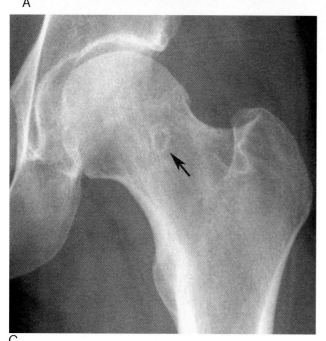

C

Figure 11-22 Femoroacetabular impingement (FAI). **A,** AP radiograph shows dysmorphic overgrowth of both anterior-superior femoral head-neck junctions *(arrows).* These act like the lobe (bulge) of a cam when the hip is flexed or internally rotated. Also note the up-sloping lateral acetabular margins *(arrowheads),* a finding that has been reported to be associated with FAI. **B,** Oblique axial fat-suppressed T1-weighted MR arthrogram in different patient. The image is parallel to the femoral neck (similar to Fig. 11-21A, B). Note the anterior cam-like bulge *(arrows).* Other images (not shown) showed an anterior-superior labral tear. Also note the intermediate-signal-intensity herniation pit *(arrowhead),* which some authors believe is associated with FAI. **C,** Herniation pit in a different patient with cam-type FAI. AP hip radiograph shows lucent region surrounded by a thin sclerotic ring in the anterior femoral neck *(arrow).*

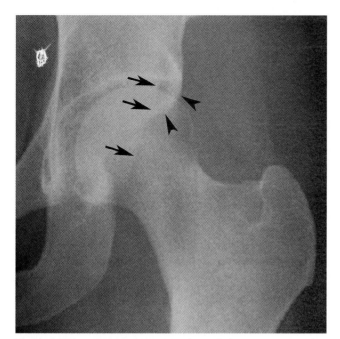

Figure 11-23   Crossover sign. AP radiograph shows anterior acetabular rim *(arrowheads)* projecting lateral to the posterior rim *(arrows)*. This finding is associated with femoroacetabular impingement due to anterior acetabular overgrowth, called "acetabular" or "pincer" impingement.

Management of FAI is a topic of great interest and some controversy. Some surgeons advocate surgical resection of the overgrown portion of the acetabulum or femoral neck. Acetabular surgery requires detaching the labrum, removing excessive bone, and then reattaching the labrum.

ADDITIONAL SOFT TISSUE CONDITIONS

The muscles of the pelvic girdle are frequent sites of muscle strain and tendon injury. The hamstrings muscles, like other muscles that undergo eccentric contraction (contract during elongation), are especially prone to strains. Hamstring and adductor origin tendon injuries can be difficult to assess clinically. Magnetic resonance imaging (and US in expert hands) can help identify and often quantify these injuries (Figs. 11-24, 11-25). The thigh is a frequent site of muscle hematoma and myositis ossificans owing to the large size of thigh muscles and frequent blunt trauma to this region (see Figs. 2-16, 2-17).

Piriformis syndrome is gluteal pain that radiates in an L5 or S1 distribution caused by irritation of the sciatic nerve as it courses between the small hip external rotator muscles posterior to the femoral neck. Causes are numerous, and include

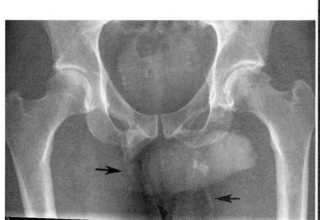

A

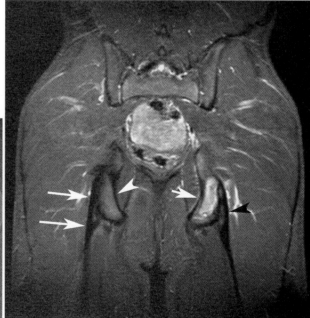

B

Figure 11-24   Chronic hamstring avulsion. **A,** AP radiograph shows mature bone formation extending inferiorly from the hamstring origins at the ischial tuberosities *(arrows)*. **B,** Coronal inversion recovery MR image in a different patient shows normal right ischium *(white arrowhead)* and hamstring tendon *(long arrows)*. Contrast with edematous left ischium *(short arrow)* and increased signal in the left hamstring *(black arrowhead)*.

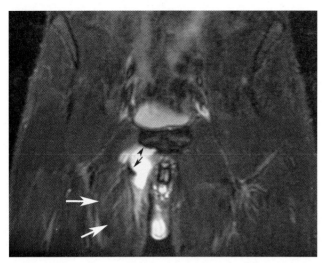

Figure 11-25   Acute hip adductor avulsion. Coronal inversion recovery MR image shows avulsed adductor tendon *(small black arrow)* and retracted, edematous adductor brevis *(white arrows)*. The *small black arrowhead* marks the pubic origin.

mass, piriformis muscle hypertrophy, trauma, and aberrant course of the sciatic nerve through or around the piriformis. Computed tomography or MRI may show a mass, asymmetric hypertrophy of the ipsilateral piriformis, or subtle inflammatory changes around the sciatic nerve.

Trochanteric bursitis is seen on MR images as fluid lateral to the greater trochanter. Iliopsoas bursitis can be difficult to detect with imaging studies. A fluid collection medial to the iliopsoas tendon, anterior to the femoral head, may be seen, suggesting a paralabral cyst.

Sports hernia, or sportsman's hernia, is an evolving and controversial concept of groin pain caused by a partial tear of the fascial structures around the inguinal ligament. Sports hernia occurs in athletes who simultaneously run and twist at the waist, such as football and hockey players, kickers, pole vaulters, and runners. The symptoms overlap with groin pain due to pubic stress injury and proximal adductor injury, adding to the confusion.

CHAPTER 12

Knee 1: Fractures and Dislocations

RADIOGRAPHIC ANATOMY
INTERCONDYLAR FRACTURES
TIBIAL PLATEAU FRACTURES
PATELLAR FRACTURES
PATELLAR DISLOCATION
AVULSION INJURIES
PHYSEAL INJURY
STRESS FRACTURE
KNEE DISLOCATION

RADIOGRAPHIC ANATOMY

The knee joint is composed of three articulations: the medial and lateral femorotibial and patellofemoral articulations. Although they share a common joint capsule, these articulations are often referred to separately as the medial, lateral, and patellofemoral compartments or joints.

An anteroposterior (AP) knee radiograph shows the condyles and tibial plateaus (Fig. 12-1). The medial and lateral compartment radiolucent "joint spaces" or "cartilage spaces" should be equal with the knee extended; asymmetry usually indicates cartilage loss, ligamentous laxity, or both. Standing views may accentuate such findings. A standing view with the knees slightly flexed can be even better to demonstrate cartilage loss not evident with the knee fully extended, because earlier and more severe cartilage loss often occurs along the posterior weight-bearing portions of the femoral condyles. Shallow oblique AP views may demonstrate a subtle fracture not visible on AP or lateral views. There is normally about 5 degrees of valgus at the adult knee, slightly greater in females because of a wider pelvis. Infants and toddlers frequently have physiologic bowlegs, with genu varum (knee varus) and lateral tibial bowing. This situation reverses by age 3 to 4 years, when genu valgum ("knock knees," knee valgus) may be seen as a normal variant.

A lateral radiograph profiles the anterior weight-bearing, mid-weight-bearing, and posterior weight-bearing surfaces of the femoral condyles, and also reveals differences between the condyles and tibial plateaus (Fig. 12-2). Some pathology may be visible only on a lateral radiograph, so awareness of these differences can be useful for localizing a lesion. The lateral femoral condyle is relatively flat along its distal (anterior weight-bearing) surface. The medial femoral condyle has a rounder contour of the distal surface. Similarly, the lateral tibial plateau has a flat surface, and the medial plateau has a subtly concave surface. The lateral femoral *condylar sulcus* is a mild concavity in the flat distal articular surface of the lateral femoral condyle. The medial condyle also has a condylar sulcus, but this sulcus is located more anteriorly, as part of the medial margin of the trochlea. The knee joint capsule extends several centimeters above the upper pole of the patella. A joint effusion or synovitis can be seen on a lateral radiograph as thickening of the

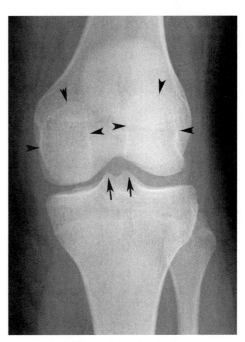

Figure 12-1　Normal knee radiographic anatomy: AP view. Note the medial and lateral tibial eminences *(arrows)* and femoral condyles *(arrowheads).*

209

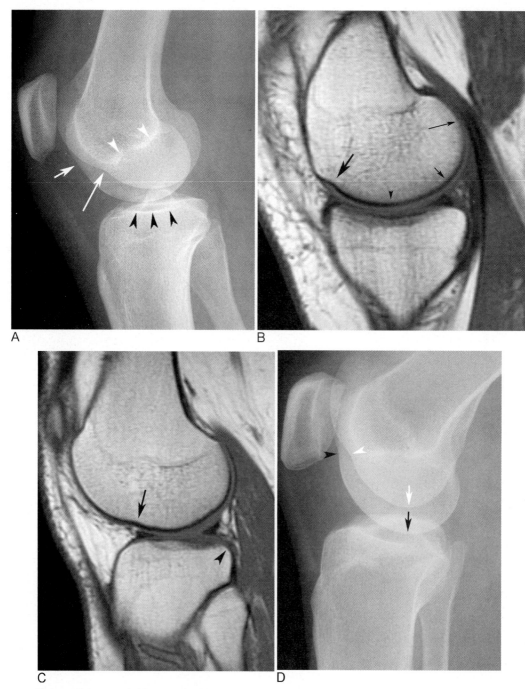

Figure 12-2   Normal knee radiographic anatomy: lateral view. **A,** This example is slightly oblique in the coronal plane, with the medial compartment projecting slightly lower, to better demonstrate the subtle differences between compartments. Note the concave medial tibial plateau *(black arrowheads)* projecting just below the straight lateral tibial plateau. Each femoral condyle has a flat or concave region termed the condylar sulcus, which is located on the anterior weight-bearing surface of the lateral condyle *(long arrow),* but more anteriorly on the medial condyle *(short arrow).* Also note the intercondylar notch roof *(white arrowheads).* **B,** Sagittal T1-weighted MR image in the medial compartment shows the concave medial condylar sulcus anteriorly *(large arrow),* and concave contour of the medial tibial plateau and matching contour of the medial femoral condyle. The articular surface of each femoral condyle may be subdivided into trochlea (anteriorly, articulates with patella) and anterior *(small arrowhead),* mid *(short small arrow),* and posterior *(long small arrow)* surfaces. **C,** Sagittal T1-weighted MR image in the lateral compartment in the same patient as in part B shows the concave lateral condylar sulcus more posterior in position, at the anterior weight-bearing surface *(arrow),* and flat contour of the lateral tibial plateau. Also note the convex contour of the posterior margin of the lateral plateau *(arrowhead),* which is also visible on radiographs. **D,** Slightly oblique lateral radiograph with the knee flexed 40 degrees shows the mid-weight-bearing surfaces of the femoral condyles *(arrows)* in contact with the tibial plateaus. Note that the articular contact is centered somewhat posteriorly, and the articular surface area of the condyles, especially the lateral condyle *(white arrow),* is smaller than at extension. This view also shows the femoral condylar sulci *(black arrowhead,* medial; *white arrowhead,* lateral).

suprapatellar joint capsule (Fig. 12-3). A cross-table lateral radiograph is used to demonstrate fluid-fluid levels within a knee joint. Hemarthrosis after knee trauma usually indicates the presence of a fracture, prominent bony contusion, or anterior cruciate ligament tear. A lipohemarthrosis indicates a fracture or prominent bony contusion (see Fig. 1-14).

A lateral radiograph also demonstrates the distal quadriceps tendon, which inserts into the anterior patellar upper pole and the patellar tendon (or ligament) that connects the anterior patel-lar lower pole and the tibial tubercle. The patellar tendon, patella, and quadriceps tendon are collectively termed the *extensor mechanism*. *Hoffa's fat pad* is located posterior to the patellar lower pole and patellar tendon and anterior to the knee joint. The *fabella* is a variably present small sesamoid in the gastrocnemius lateral head that is often best seen on the lateral view. When seen on an AP view, a fabella usually projects over the lateral femoral condyle.

A notch or tunnel view is a frontal view with the knee flexed 45 degrees and the x-ray beam parallel to the tibial

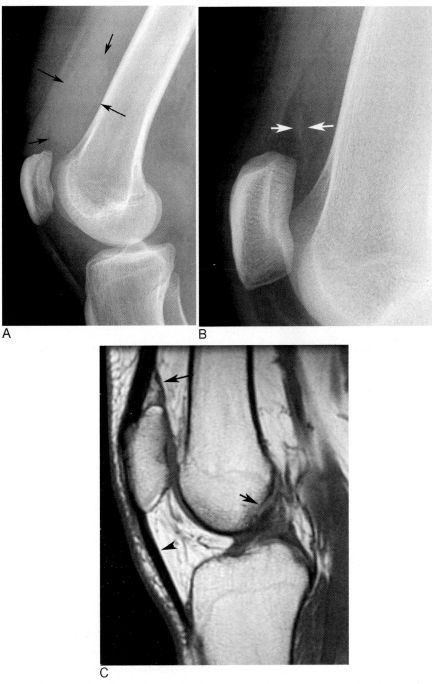

Figure 12-3 Knee joint effusion. **A,** Lateral radiograph shows distention of the superior joint capsule seen as soft tissue density *(arrows)*. **B and C,** Normal superior joint *(arrows)* shown for comparison. Part C is sagittal T1-weighted MR image. Also note notch roof *(short arrow)* and patellar tendon *(arrowhead)* in part C. See also Figure 1-14.

plateau (Fig. 12-4). This view is useful for detection of calcified intra-articular bodies, which often settle within the notch. The medial radiolucent cartilage space normally appears narrower on this view because of normally thinner cartilage at the contact points of the condyles and tibial plateaus when the knee is flexed 45 degrees.

The femoral trochlea (groove) is the anterior femoral margin between the condyles, in which the patella glides during flexion and extension. A sunrise view is an axial view tangential to this articulation (Fig. 12-5). The posterior articular surface of the patella has three facets (relatively flat surfaces): the lateral, medial, and odd facets. The lateral facet is usually the widest. The lateral and medial facets meet at the median ridge. The odd

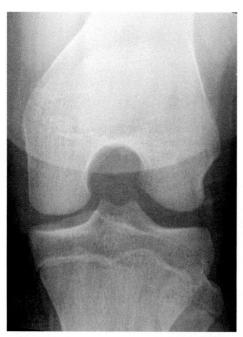

Figure 12-4   Normal knee radiographic anatomy: notch (tunnel) view.

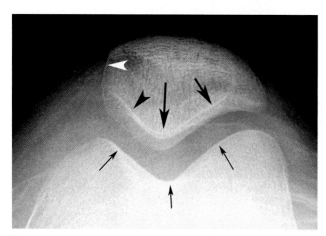

Figure 12-5   Normal knee radiographic anatomy: axial (sunrise) view. This view is optimally obtained with knee flexed about 20 degrees. Note the medial patellar facet *(black arrowhead)* separated from the wider lateral facet *(short black arrow)* by the median ridge *(long black arrow)*, odd facet *(white arrowhead)*, and femoral trochlea (groove, *small arrows*).

facet is the most medial and is often sagittal in orientation. A sunrise view is useful for assessing patellar alignment in patients with anterior knee pain. Optimally, the knee is flexed only about 20 to 25 degrees when this view is obtained (Merchant technique) because clinically significant patellofemoral malalignment may not be evident with greater flexion.

A common trauma radiographic protocol includes AP, cross-table lateral, and bilateral oblique views. Notch views are often obtained for chronic knee pain or if an intra-articular body is suspected. Sunrise views are often obtained when anterior knee pain is present. Computed tomography (CT) with coronal and sagittal reformats is frequently used in preoperative assessment of a tibial plateau fracture. The main role of magnetic resonance imaging (MRI) of the knee is soft tissue assessment, but MRI is also the most sensitive technique for fracture detection and is therefore useful when traumatic knee pain is not explained with radiographs or CT. Bone scanning can also depict occult fractures but is inferior to MRI.

INTERCONDYLAR FRACTURES

Transcondylar fractures of the distal femur usually involve metaphyseal and condylar components (Fig. 12-6). The metaphyseal component is usually transverse in orientation. The condylar component may be in sagittal or coronal planes. Coronal intra-articular fractures place the patient at risk for avascular necrosis of the condylar fragments. Coronally oriented intra-articular condylar fractures also have a worse prognosis than sagittal fractures because of the risk of displacement with joint incongruity when the patient begins weight bearing, despite frequently robust internal fixation.

TIBIAL PLATEAU FRACTURES

Tibial plateau fractures are classically seen in pedestrian-automobile accidents because the plateau is at the level of car bumpers. Most (80%) are localized to the lateral tibial plateau because most fractures result from a valgus load with impaction at the lateral tibial condyle. Tibial plateau fractures are intra-articular fractures that typically produce large hemarthroses. These fractures are classified by the location of fracture lines, articular depression, and metaphyseal extension.

Key Concepts	Tibial Plateau Fracture

80% are localized to the lateral tibial plateau
Large hemarthrosis, often with fat-fluid level
CT with reformats for presurgical planning
Describe any articular fragment depression and diastasis

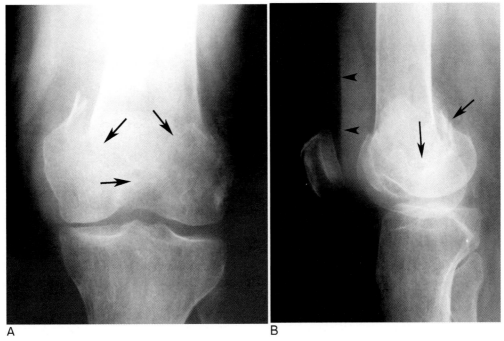

A   B

Figure 12-6   Comminuted intercondylar fracture distal femur. **A,** Frontal radiograph shows Y-shaped fracture *(arrows).* **B,** Lateral view demonstrates fracture line *(arrows)* and fluid level of lipohemarthrosis *(arrowheads).*

Although not a reflection of the severity of injury, the Schatzker classification is useful for communication of the findings and surgical planning (Figs. 1-12, 12-7). The classification is as follows: type I, cleavage fracture of the lateral tibial plateau; type II, combined cleavage and depressed fracture of the lateral tibial plateau; type III, purely depressed fracture of the lateral tibial plateau; type IV, lateral condylar tibial cleavage fracture that extends to the medial tibial condyle; type V, bicondylar fracture; and type VI, any fracture with a transmetaphyseal component.

Imaging is important in the assessment of tibial plateau fractures because the goal of surgery is restoration of congruence of the articular margin, in order to decrease the risk of eventual post-traumatic osteoarthritis. Radiographs can be confusing because the lateral tibial plateau normally downslopes slightly and thus its margins are not tangential to the knee joint on AP radiographs. Depressed fragments are easily overlooked anteriorly and are exaggerated posteriorly. The fracture line is often in an oblique plane; therefore, an AP view may completely miss a tibial plateau fracture whereas the oblique view will show the fracture. Both MRI and CT are useful in the evaluation of these fractures for presurgical planning. However, CT is particularly helpful in showing fracture fragment margins because CT with multiplanar reformations can demonstrate the degree of fracture depression and displacement. The threshold of depression or displacement at which surgery is indicated is controversial. Many centers are adopting a "zero tolerance" approach to articular depression and the need for surgical reduction. Generally, however, depression greater than 3 mm or distraction greater than 3 mm requires internal fixation. Various forms of fixation are used in tibial plateau fractures. Cleavage fractures typically are treated with transverse lateromedial lag screws. Combination depressed and cleavage fractures usually require a lateral buttress plate. Depressed fractures usually require elevation of the articular fragment with placement of subarticular bone graft. Bicondylar fractures require both medial and lateral fixation. Bicondylar fractures and fractures with metaphyseal components often require the addition of external fixation.

PATELLAR FRACTURES

Patellar fractures may be due either to direct impaction (falling on the patella) resulting in a comminuted fracture, or to sudden tension of the extensor mechanism of the thigh, resulting in transverse and often distracted fractures (Fig. 1-1). Often, both mechanisms are present, usually resulting in a transverse fracture. Sixty percent of patellar fractures are transverse. The degree of distraction depends on the integrity of the medial and lateral patellar retinacula and extensor tendon fibers that extend across the anterior patella. A patellar sleeve fracture is a nonarticular avulsion fracture at the inferior margin of the patella, located at the origin of the patellar tendon, typically in the skeletally immature (Fig. 12-8). With this injury, the patellar lower pole periosteum avulses from the bone like a shirt sleeve. It is also a result of sudden tension of the extensor mechanism of the thigh. These injuries result in an elongated patella. Osteochondral fractures of the patella may occur as well. These are usually located at the medial patellar facet and are associated with transient lateral patellar dislocation (see following discussion).

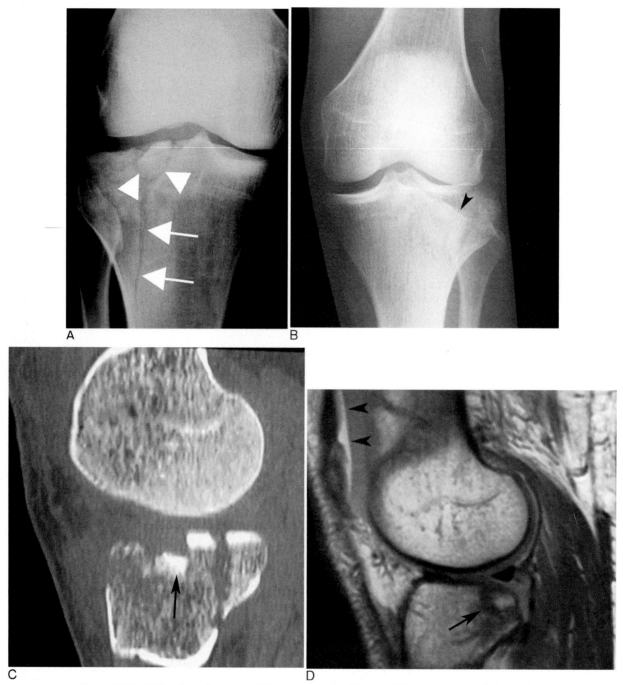

Figure 12-7 Tibial plateau fractures in different patients. **A,** Schatzker II fracture with sagittal cleavage line *(arrows)* and depressed lateral plateau fracture *(arrowheads)*. See also Figure 1-15. **B,** Schatzker III fracture with depressed lateral tibial plateau *(arrowheads)*. **C,** Sagittal CT reconstruction shows extensive comminution of the lateral plateau with fragment depression *(arrow)*. **D,** Sagittal T1-weighted MR image demonstrates lipo-hemarthrosis *(arrowheads)* and mildly depressed fracture of posterior lateral tibial condyle *(arrow)*.

(Continued)

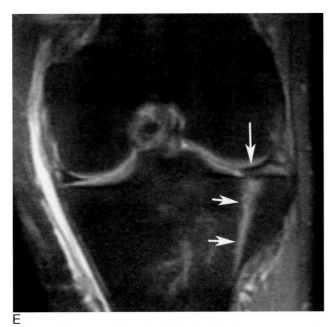

E

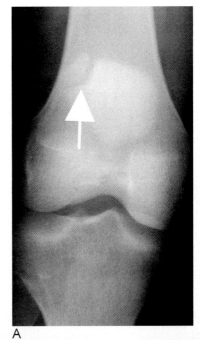

A

Figure 12-7—(Cont'd)   E, Coronal fat-suppressed proton density image shows a Schatzker I fracture *(arrowheads)*. Also note that the lateral meniscus *(arrow)* is partially trapped between the diastatic fracture fragments, potentially blocking reduction.

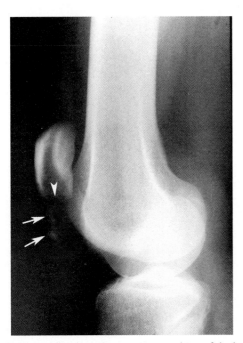

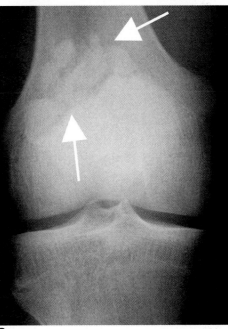

B

Figure 12-9   Normal variant patellar fragmentation **A,** Bipartite patella *(arrow)*. Note the typical superolateral location of fragment. **B,** Multipartite patella *(arrows)*.

Figure 12-8   Patellar sleeve fracture. Note avulsion of the lower pole *(arrowhead)* and small fragments more distally *(arrows)*. These fractures are often extra-articular, and this fracture had no hemarthrosis.

Patellar fractures may be confused with normal variants of the patella. *Bipartite* and *multipartite patellae* represent fragmentation of the superolateral portion of the patella with well-corticated margins (Fig. 12-9). Magnetic resonance imaging shows normal adjacent articular cartilage. They are often bilateral, and their location is a clue to their non-traumatic cause. Dorsal defect of the patella is a rounded lucency at the superolateral dorsal (articular) margin of the patella. It is also a normal variant. Osteochondritis dissecans (OCD) can occur in the patella, often superolateral as well. Clinical findings and MRI can help to distinguish OCD from a normal variant.

PATELLAR DISLOCATION

Patellar dislocation is almost always transient and is a commonly overlooked injury. In *transient patellar dislocation,* the patella briefly dislocates laterally and then relocates. Dislocations are almost always lateral because of the normal valgus alignment of the knee and the weaker mechanical properties of the medial patellar retinaculum and vastus medialis. In the process of relocating, impaction occurs between the medial pole of the patella and the anterolateral margin of the lateral femoral condyle. The medial patellar retinaculum becomes stretched or torn. Bone bruises occur at the sites of impaction at the medial patella and the lateral femoral condyle. Hemarthrosis is usually present. As noted previously, an osteochondral fracture often arises from the medial patella as a result of shearing injury at the site of impaction at the lateral femoral condyle during relocation (Fig. 12-10). The osteochondral fracture will be found either at the site of impact adjacent to the lateral femoral condyle or in situ at the medial facet of the relocated patella. Magnetic resonance imaging is the ideal modality with which to evaluate transient patellar dislocation (Fig. 12-11). At MRI, a large hemarthrosis is evident, as are the bone bruises of the medial patella and lateral femoral condyle. The disruption of the medial patellar retinaculum is clearly evident, and usually occurs at the medial patellofemoral ligament at either the femoral or patellar attachments. The osteochondral fragment is also readily demonstrated. The relocated patella usually demonstrates residual lateral patellar tilt or subluxation.

Being a sesamoid bone with a large craniocaudal excursion, the patella is prone to tracking abnormalities as it courses through the trochlear groove of the femur. Tracking abnormalities are usually laterally oriented with lateral patellar tilt and subluxation. Anterior knee pain and premature osteoarthritis may result, and some cases are associated with a greater risk of dislocation. Muscle imbalance, with a relatively weak distal vastus medialis, is one predisposing factor for tracking abnormalities. Anatomic variations also may predispose to tracking error. Patella alta is an elongated patellar tendon. This can be diagnosed on a lateral radiograph (Fig. 12-12). The ratio of the patellar tendon length (as measured from the inferior pole of the patella to the anterior tibial tubercle) to the length of the patella should yield a ratio of about 1.1 ± 0.2. A ratio greater than 1.35 of tendon to patella represents *patella alta* (i.e., "high patella"). *Patella baja* (i.e., low patella) is due to a short patellar tendon and usually is the result of scar retraction below the patella (e.g., following open knee surgery). A shallow trochlear groove, also known as trochlear dysplasia, is a second anatomic variation that is associated with abnormal patellar tracking. A sunrise radiograph or axial CT or MRI can show the shallow groove. A lateral radiograph or sagittal MR image might show a shelf-like prominence of the proximal trochlea.

Imaging evaluation of patellofemoral tracking is often done with limited, low-dose axial CT with the knees in varying degrees of flexion (Fig. 12-13). This provides a quasi-dynamic evaluation. Most lateral subluxation occurs only with shallow flexion. Orthopedic measurements of lateral patellar tilt and subluxation on static radiographs have become highly evolved

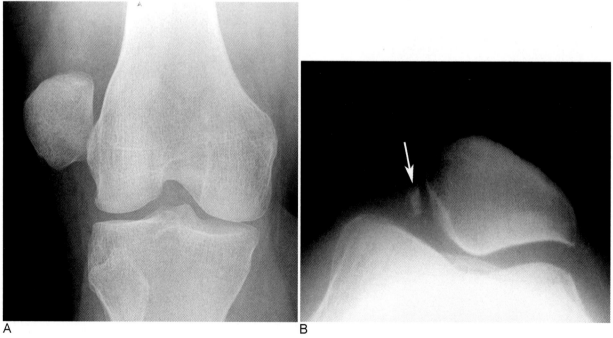

A   B

Figure 12-10   Patellar dislocation. **A,** Note lateral position of the patella. This is an unusual radiographic finding, as most cases of patellar subluxation reduce spontaneously long before radiographs are obtained. **B,** Axial view of patella in a different patient after transient patellar dislocation demonstrates medial pole patellar fragment *(arrow)* due to transient dislocation.

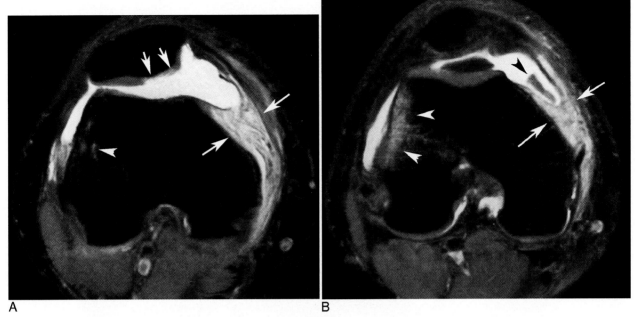

Figure 12-11   MR imaging after transient dislocation of the patella. **A and B,** Two contiguous axial fat-suppressed proton density-weighted MR images show lateral femoral bone bruise *(white arrowheads),* chondral defect at medial pole of patella *(short arrows),* and medial patellar retinaculum tear with substantial edema *(long arrows).* Note chondral fragment surrounded by joint fluid *(black arrowhead* in B).

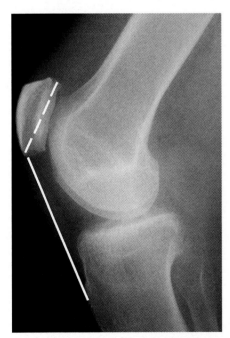

Figure 12-12   Patella alta. Note substantially greater length of patellar tendon *(solid line)* compared with length of patella *(dashed line).*

and are described here for interest. These measures are obtained from studying an axial (Merchant) radiographic view obtained with the knee flexed only 20 degrees. Ordinarily the lateral patellar facet is parallel to the lateral trochlea. Lateral tilt is present when the margins between lateral patella and lateral trochlea are no longer parallel but narrower laterally. Another angle that is useful for determining trochlear dysplasia is the *sulcus angle,* which is the angle formed by connecting the two highest points of the medial and lateral femoral trochlea with the deepest portion of the trochlear groove. This is normally 138 degrees. A third measure is the *congruence angle.* This is formed by drawing two lines to the sulcus of the trochlear groove. The first line extends to the groove from the anterior apex of the patella. The second line to the base of the trochlear groove is drawn from the posterior apex of the patella. The line formed by the posterior apex is usually lateral to that formed by the anterior apex. If lateral, it suggests lateral subluxation, particularly if the angle is greater than 16 degrees.

AVULSION INJURIES

There are numerous avulsion sites at the knee (Fig. 12-14). Common locations include the anterior cruciate ligament insertion on the intercondylar eminence of the tibia (Fig. 12-15), the posterior cruciate ligament insertion at the posterior tibia, and the lateral joint capsule at the lateral margin of the tibia (Fig. 12-16). The latter is also termed a *Segond fracture,* and is highly associated with anterior cruciate ligament injury. Other avulsions include the anterior lateral tibial margin (Gerdy's tubercle) at the site of the iliotibial band insertion, the lateral collateral ligament insertion at the proximal fibula (which is also the biceps femoris insertion), and the medial collateral ligament origin and insertion at the medial femoral and tibial condyles, respectively. The anterior tibial tubercle is another site prone to tension injury of the patellar

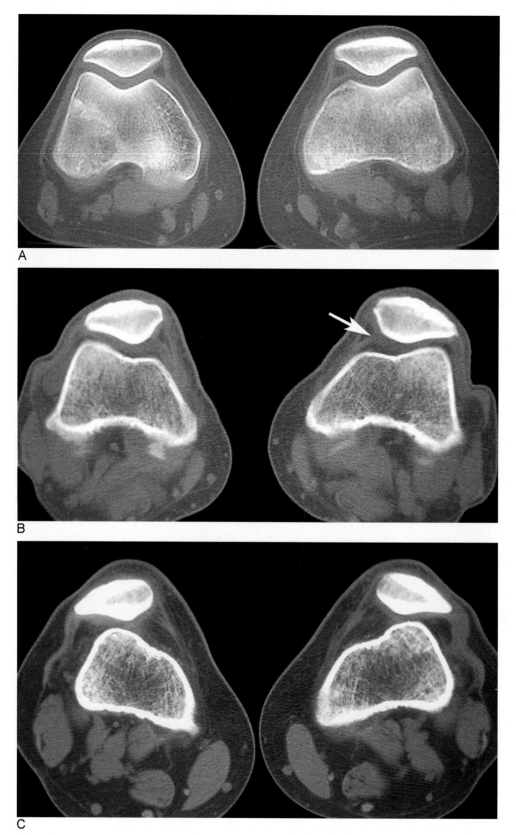

Figure 12-13 Patellofemoral tracking error in different patients. All images are axial CT images with the knees flexed 15 to 20 degrees. **A,** Normal. **B,** Lateralized left patella *(arrow)*. **C,** More severe, bilateral subluxation in a patient with patella alta.

(Continued)

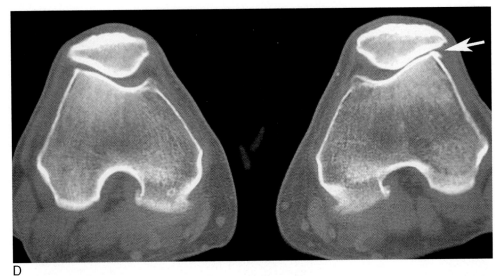

D

Figure 12-13—(Cont'd) **D,** Chronic bilateral tracking error with early osteoarthritis with joint space narrowing and osteophyte formation, more advanced on the left *(arrow)*.

tendon, which is commonly seen in children and young adolescents (Fig. 12-17). With repetitive stress, the tubercle may become fragmented, and if associated with tenderness and swelling, the disorder is termed *Osgood-Schlatter disease* (Fig. 12-18). Most cases are associated with overuse and rapid

growth and are self-limited. It is rarely complicated by either nonunion of the tibial tubercle or premature closure of the tibial tubercle physis with secondary development of genu recurvatum (posterior bowing of the knee). Adults with old Osgood-Schlatter disease often have asymptomatic or minimally symptomatic ossicles in the posterior distal patellar tendon. *Sinding-Larsen-Johansson* is a process similar to Osgood-Schlatter disease that occurs at the lower pole of the patella in the same age group (Fig. 12-19).

Figure 12-14 Avulsion sites around the knee: A, anterior cruciate ligament (ACL) origin; B, ACL insertion; C, lateral capsular attachment (Segond); D, posterior cruciate ligament (PCL) origin; E, PCL insertion; F, medial collateral ligament (MCL) origin; G, MCL deep fiber (menisco-tibial) insertion; H, MCL superficial fiber insertion; I, lateral collateral ligament (LCL) origin; J, common insertion of LCL and biceps femoris; K, Gerdy's tubercle, insertion of iliotibial band. (Reproduced with permission from Manaster BJ: Handbook of Skeletal Radiology, ed 2. St. Louis, Mosby, 1997.)

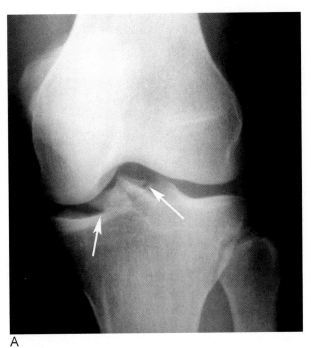

A

Figure 12-15 Avulsion of tibial insertion of anterior cruciate ligament. **A,** Frontal radiograph demonstrates fracture at medial tibial intercondylar eminence *(arrows).*

(Continued)

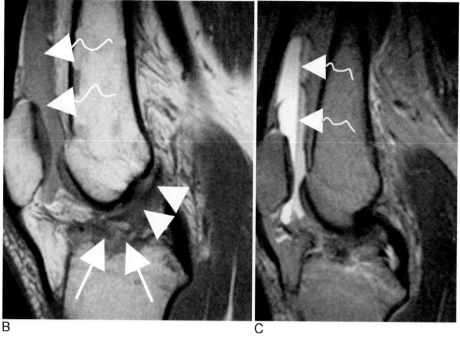

B   C

Figure 12-15—(Cont'd)   B and C, Sagittal proton density (B) and T2-weighted (C) spin-echo MR images show the avulsion fracture fragment *(straight arrows)* with adjacent marrow edema. The anterior cruciate ligament (ACL) was intact *(arrowheads)*. Also note hemarthrosis *(curved arrows)*.

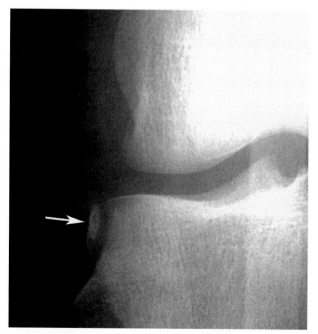

Figure 12-16   Segond fracture. Detail of AP radiograph at the lateral joint line shows small avulsion from the lateral tibia *(arrow)*. This fracture is nearly 100% associated with acute anterior cruciate ligament (ACL) tear.

PHYSEAL INJURY

Growth plate injuries at the knee are uncommon, but they are highly associated with complications, particularly growth disturbance (see Fig. 3-6). Proximal tibial epiphyseal fractures

often occur in association with patellar tendon traction (see Fig. 12-17). In the distal femur, Salter-Harris II fractures predominate, occurring in 70% of injuries; the next most common pattern is Salter-Harris III fractures, occurring in 15% of children. Most Salter-Harris III fractures of the distal femur

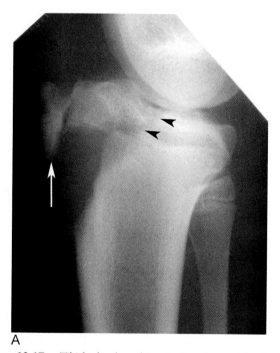

A

Figure 12-17   Tibial tubercle avulsion. **A,** Complete avulsion *(arrow)*. Also note Salter-Harris III fracture of the proximal tibial epiphysis *(arrowheads)*.

(Continued)

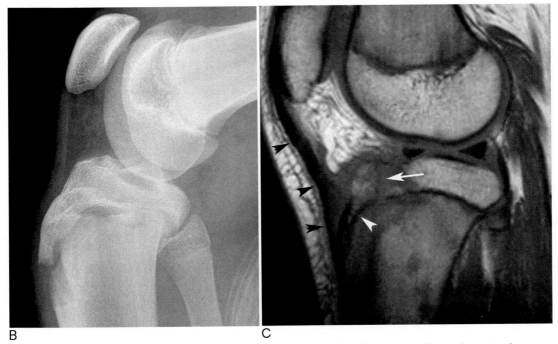

B   C

Figure 12-17—(Cont'd)   **B,** In an older child, the tibial tubercle ossification center fuses to the proximal tibial epiphysis, and traction injury may result in a Salter-Harris I injury, as in this example. **C,** Salter-Harris III fracture in an older child with fused tibial tubercle and proximal tibial epiphysis *(white arrowhead)*. Sagittal T1-weighted MR image shows the epiphyseal fracture line *(arrow)* and intact patellar tendon *(black arrowheads)*.

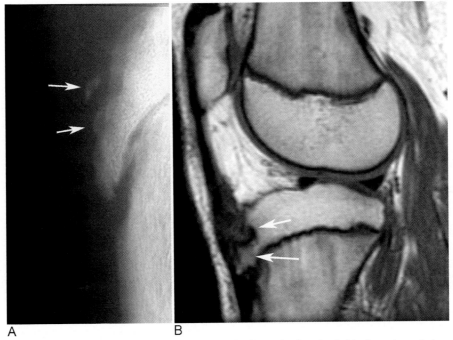

A   B

Figure 12-18   Osgood-Schlatter disease. **A,** Lateral radiograph of proximal tibia shows the typical osseous irregularity at patellar tendon insertion *(arrow)*. The child was tender at the tibial tubercle, making the diagnosis. Sagittal T1-weighted (B)

(Continued)

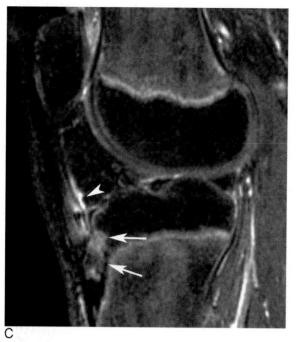

Figure 12-18—(Cont'd) and fat-suppressed T2-weighted (C) MR images in a different child with Osgood-Schlatter disease show similar findings at the tibial tubercle *(arrows)* and edema in the distal patellar tendon *(arrowhead* in part C).

involve the medial femoral condyle and are due to valgus stress. They are usually without displacement and are occult radiographically yet can be demonstrated at MRI. The knee is the most common site for Salter-Harris V fractures, which occur at the proximal tibia and have a high frequency of localized growth plate arrest with angular deformity or growth arrest. Salter-Harris I fractures can be subtle, seen only as asymmetry of the physis (Fig. 12-20).

STRESS FRACTURE

Stress fractures are common in the tibia and appear similar to stress fractures elsewhere, with an early faint transverse or oblique lucency followed by sclerosis involving the same distribution in the overlying cortex (see Figs. 1-17, 1-18). Most occur within the posterior cortex of the proximal tibial shaft, discriminated from "shin splints." Shin splints are characterized by anterior tibial shaft pain, which may have longitudinal abnormal tracer uptake in the anterior tibial cortex on bone scanning or adjacent marrow edema on MRI. Some activities, such as basketball and ballet, are associated with stress fractures in the anterior cortex of the mid-tibia. Stress fractures are usually multiple and can be radiographically detected by numerous

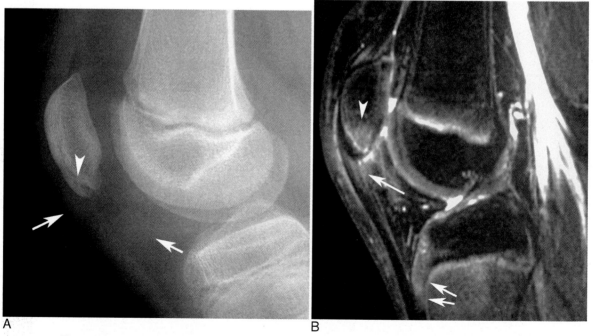

Figure 12-19 Sinding-Larsen-Johansson disease. **A and B,** Lateral radiograph (A) and sagittal fat-suppressed T2-weighted MR image (B) in a 12-year-old soccer player show fragmentation of the patellar lower pole *(arrowhead)* and adjacent soft tissue edema *(arrows)*. Also note mild marrow edema in the tibial tubercle (*short arrows* in part B) that was not symptomatic. This is a benign stress reaction.

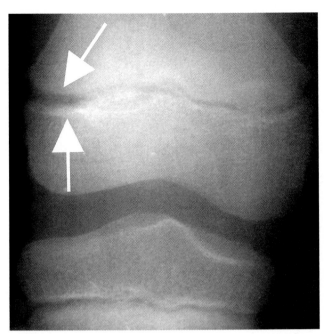

Figure 12-20   Salter-Harris I fracture of distal femur. Note slight widening of lateral distal femoral physis *(arrows)*.

small transverse partial fractures at various stages of healing. Because the radiographic detection of stress fracture lags several weeks behind clinical findings, MRI and nuclear bone scanning play an important role in the early detection of these injuries.

Bone scans will show eccentric, cortically based increased activity on the side of symptoms. Magnetic resonance imaging demonstrates the localized marrow abnormality with a linear low-signal-intensity line, centrally within the area of bone marrow edema (see Fig. 1-18).

KNEE DISLOCATION

Knee dislocations (i.e., femorotibial dislocations) can occur in any direction. A large minority of patients with knee dislocation (30%) have associated arterial injury due to the close proximity of the popiteal artery, which is fixed proximally in the adductor canal and distally at its bifurcation near the tibiofibular syndesmosis. Patients with knee dislocation are assessed for neurologic injury and distal pulses and hue at the time of injury. Any question of arterial injury requires arteriography for detection of intimal arterial disruption or pseudoaneurysm (Fig. 12-21). Other soft tissue injuries are common in the setting of knee dislocation. These include tears of the cruciate and collateral ligaments, the joint capsule, and often the articular cartilage. Peroneal nerve injury is also common in dislocation because of its tenuous course at the knee, where it runs posterior to the margin of the fibular head and lateral to the margin of the fibular neck.

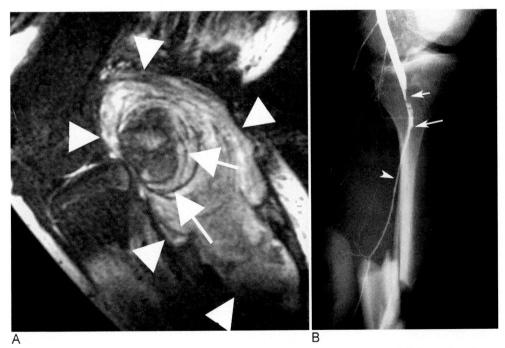

A   B

Figure 12-21   Post-traumatic popliteal artery injuries. **A,** Sagittal inversion recovery MR image shows large pseudoaneurysm *(arrowheads)*. Note concentric rings of clot *(arrows)*. **B,** AP angiogram in a different patient with comminuted tibial fracture and knee dislocation (after reduction) shows popliteal artery intimal injury with in situ thrombosis *(short arrow)* and occlusion at popliteal trifurcation *(long arrow)*. Distal runoff is limited to the peroneal artery *(arrowhead)*.

Knee 2: Soft Tissues

MENISCAL TEARS
CRUCIATE LIGAMENT INJURY
COLLATERAL LIGAMENT INJURY
ADDITIONAL TENDON AND BURSAL CONDITIONS
HYALINE CARTILAGE INJURY AND MISCELLANEOUS KNEE
  CONDITIONS

MENISCAL TEARS

The menisci of the knee are semicircular bands of fibrocartilage that line the peripheral aspects of the medial and lateral compartments and function to increase the tibiofemoral contact area, thus allowing a more evenly distributed load across the knee joint. Because the medial tibial plateau is larger, the medial meniscus is larger than the lateral meniscus, and thus the medial meniscus is slightly more C-shaped than is the more circular lateral meniscus (Fig. 13-1). The menisci taper from a height of 3 to 5 mm at the periphery to a thin, sharp, central free margin. Therefore, the menisci appear triangular in shape on coronal and sagittal magnetic resonance imaging (MRI) (Fig. 13-2). The anterior and posterior horns of the lateral meniscus are similar in size; however, the posterior horn of the medial meniscus is larger than its anterior horn. On sagittal imaging, the lateral meniscis shows a bowtie configuration with closely apposed anterior and posterior horns. Because the medial meniscus is larger, the horns are more separated from one another and on some images does not resemble a bowtie (see Fig. 13-2).

WHAT THE CLINICIAN WANTS TO KNOW:
MENISCAL TEARS

Location: Side, horn, surface(s)
Displacement
Configuration: Vertical-radial, horizontal cleavage, vertical-
  longitudinal, parrot-beak, bucket-handle, meniscocapsular
  separation
Discoid meniscus

The menisci function not only as shock absorbers but also as passive stabilizers of the knee. The menisci are firmly attached to the tibia at anterior and posterior tibial insertion sites. In addition, meniscofemoral ligaments course from the posterior horn of the lateral meniscus to the medial femoral condyle. These ligaments are variably present. If the meniscofemoral ligament is found anterior to the posterior cruciate ligament, it is called the anterior meniscofemoral ligament or the meniscofemoral ligament of Humphrey; if found posterior to the posterior cruciate ligament, it is called the posterior meniscofemoral ligament or meniscofemoral ligament of Wrisberg (Fig. 13-3C). There is also a variable presence of oblique intermeniscal ligaments that course from the posterior horn of one meniscus to the anterior horn of the other meniscus. The medial meniscus is firmly attached to the joint capsule and is mobile except at the anterior and posterior tibial insertion sites. The lateral meniscus is less intimately attached to the joint capsule than is the medial meniscus because the lateral meniscus must be loosely attached at its body and posterior horn to allow passage of the popliteus tendon (the tendon courses peripheral to the meniscus from the lateral femoral condyle to its musculotendinous junction posterior to the proximal tibial metaphysis). The lateral meniscus is attached to the joint capsule by only an inferior retinaculum at the body, by superior and inferior retinacula at the junction of the body and posterior horn, and by a superior retinaculum at the posterior horn (Fig. 13-3D). There also are variably present, small, stabilizing ligaments between the popliteus tendon and the lateral meniscus, but these are not seen reliably with routine clinical MRI (Fig. 13-3D). In contrast, most of the medial meniscus is closely and firmly attached to the joint capsule. This firm attachment makes the medial meniscus less mobile and thus at greater risk for tear.

Microscopically, the menisci consist of circumferential horizontal bundles of collagen fibers interspersed with fibers extending radially from the periphery toward the free margin. This allows stabilization of fibers with centripetal loading, which is the most common form of loading of the knee. However, this orientation yields a relative weakness in the menisci to loads in the horizontal and vertical planes. The anisotropic structure of menisci results in uniform low signal intensity on MR images.

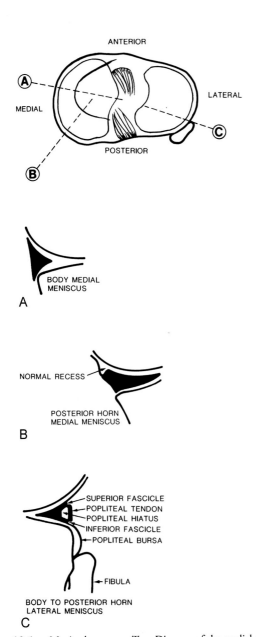

Figure 13-1   Meniscal anatomy. Top: Diagram of the medial and lateral menisci, looking down on the tibial plateau. The labeled lines represent the various planes in which MR sequences are commonly obtained. **A and B,** Radial planes through the body and posterior horns, respectively, of the medial meniscus. **C,** Radial cuts through the body and posterior horn of the lateral meniscus. (Reproduced with permission from Manaster BJ: Handbook of Skeletal Radiology, ed 2. St. Louis, Mosby, 1997.)

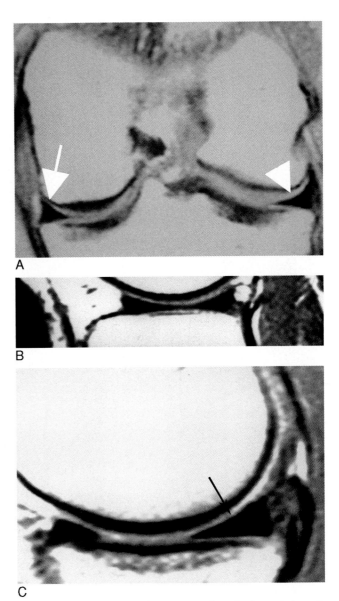

Figure 13-2   MR images showing normal meniscal morphology. **A,** Coronal T1-weighted MR image displayed at high-contrast "meniscal windows" shows triangular appearance of medial *(arrow)* and lateral *(arrowhead)* menisci. Note that height is greatest peripherally and that height tapers to a sharp central free margin. **B and C,** Sagittal proton density MR images of lateral (B) and medial (C) menisci demonstrate uniform dark signal intensity. Note equal size of anterior and posterior horns of lateral meniscus in part B compared with larger size of posterior horn of medial meniscus in part C *(arrow in C).* Also note the distinctive morphology of the medial and lateral femoral condyles and tibial plateaus (see also Fig. 12-2).

Disruptions of menisci are called meniscal tears. Meniscal tears can occur in various configurations (Figs. 13-4, 13-5). Most commonly, meniscal tears are complex, meaning that they attain multiple orientations. A *vertical-radial meniscal tear* occurs in a vertical plane extending from the periphery of the meniscus to the free margin of the meniscus, thus radially splitting a meniscus. A *horizontal cleavage tear* consists of a tear in a plane splitting the meniscus into superior and inferior portions. Tears related to underlying meniscal degeneration are often horizontal tears. A *vertical-longitudinal tear* is a circumferential tear perpendicular to the tibial plateau that extends from the superior to inferior meniscal margin and propagates around the circumference of the meniscus. These tears may be peripheral in location, or involve the free margin as a *parrot-beak tear. Bucket-handle tears* are vertical-longitudinal tears that are so extensive that the central portion displaces. The classic MRI appearance of a meniscal tear

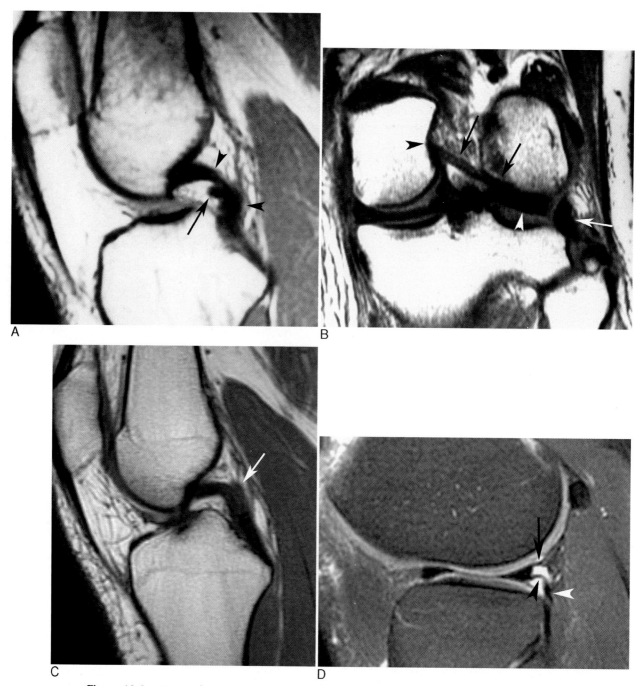

Figure 13-3   Meniscofemoral ligaments and lateral meniscus retinacula. **A and B,** Anterior meniscofemoral ligament (Humphrey). Sagittal (A) and coronal (B) proton density MR images show the obliquely
oriented ligament of Humphrey *(black arrows)* connecting the posterior horn of lateral meniscus *(white
arrowhead* in part B) to lateral margin of medial femoral condyle *(black arrowhead* in part B). The ligament
is anterior to posterior cruciate ligament (PCL) *(black arrowheads* in part A). Also note popliteus tendon
(long white arrow) adjacent to the lateral meniscus in part B. Normal fluid between this tendon and the
peripheral margin of the meniscus can be confused with a meniscal tear. Knowledge of this anatomy allows
discrimination between popliteus tendon and meniscal tear. **C,** Posterior meniscofemoral ligament
(Wrisberg). Sagittal T1-weighted MR image shows ligament in cross-section, located posterior to the PCL
(arrow). **D,** Lateral meniscus retinacula and meniscopopliteal ligament. Sagittal fat-suppressed proton
density MR image shows superior retinaculum *(black arrow)* between the posterior horn and the joint
capsule, and small ligament *(black arrowhead)* between the posterior horn and the popliteus tendon *(white
arrowhead).*

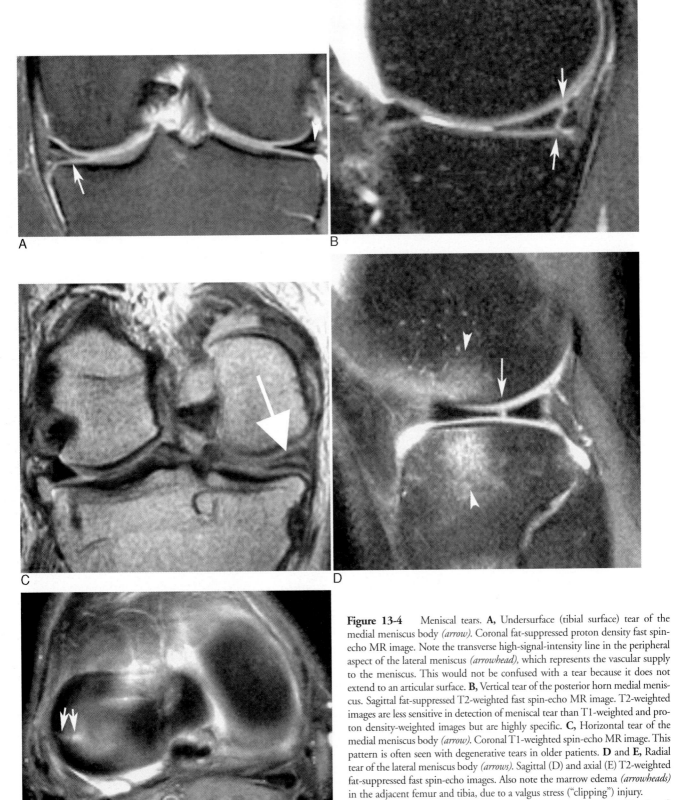

Figure 13-4   Meniscal tears. **A,** Undersurface (tibial surface) tear of the medial meniscus body *(arrow)*. Coronal fat-suppressed proton density fast spin-echo MR image. Note the transverse high-signal-intensity line in the peripheral aspect of the lateral meniscus *(arrowhead)*, which represents the vascular supply to the meniscus. This would not be confused with a tear because it does not extend to an articular surface. **B,** Vertical tear of the posterior horn medial meniscus. Sagittal fat-suppressed T2-weighted fast spin-echo MR image. T2-weighted images are less sensitive in detection of meniscal tear than T1-weighted and proton density-weighted images but are highly specific. **C,** Horizontal tear of the medial meniscus body *(arrow)*. Coronal T1-weighted spin-echo MR image. This pattern is often seen with degenerative tears in older patients. **D** and **E,** Radial tear of the lateral meniscus body *(arrows)*. Sagittal (D) and axial (E) T2-weighted fat-suppressed fast spin-echo images. Also note the marrow edema *(arrowheads)* in the adjacent femur and tibia, due to a valgus stress ("clipping") injury.

(Continued)

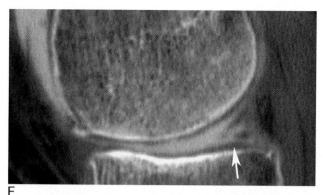

F

Figure 13-4—(Cont'd)   **F,** Meniscus tear diagnosed with CT arthrogram in patient with pacemaker (who was therefore unable to have MR imaging) and medial knee pain. Sagittal CT reformat shows tibial surface tear of the medial meniscus posterior horn.

logic separation. At other sites, bright T2 signal between the peripheral margin of the meniscus and the capsule indicates meniscocapsular separation. Additionally, the menisci should appose the tibial plateau cartilage. Peripheral displacement by 3 mm or more suggests a radial tear. Peripheral displacement may also be caused by osteophytes. Elevation of a large portion of a meniscus from the tibial plateau after a knee dislocation indicates a significant disruption of meniscal fixation that requires surgical repair. In contrast, the free edge of the medial meniscus body can elevate slightly from the tibial plateau as a normal variant, known as the "meniscal flounce." A *meniscal bruise* is a transient compressive injury, more often encountered in younger patients with lax ligaments, seen on MR images as amorphous signal. These injuries usually resolve clinically and on MR images with conservative therapy. A *meniscal root avulsion* is disruption of the fibrous "root" or insertion that fixes the posterior horn of the medial meniscus to the tibia (Fig. 13-7).

Magnetic resonance imaging criteria for meniscal tears have been extensively studied, and T1-weighted and proton density-weighted spin-echo MR have been found to have the highest accuracy in detecting meniscal tears. Fast spin-echo imaging with proton density weighting has also been shown to be accurate in meniscal tear detection. Although the exact appearance of a meniscal tear at imaging may not closely correlate with what is found at surgery, there is high accuracy for the detection of meniscal tear as well as the determination of its location. Evaluation of menisci in both sagittal and coronal

is linear or, sometimes, globular areas of increased signal within the meniscus that extends to an articular surface (tibial or femoral) on at least two adjacent images. An apparent meniscal tear seen on only one image is a highly sensitive finding but has poor specificity.

There are other, less common patterns of meniscal injury. *Meniscocapsular separation* is separation of the meniscus from the capsule (Fig. 13-6). As noted previously, there is a normal gap between the posterior horn and posterior body of the lateral meniscus and capsule, not to be confused with a patho-

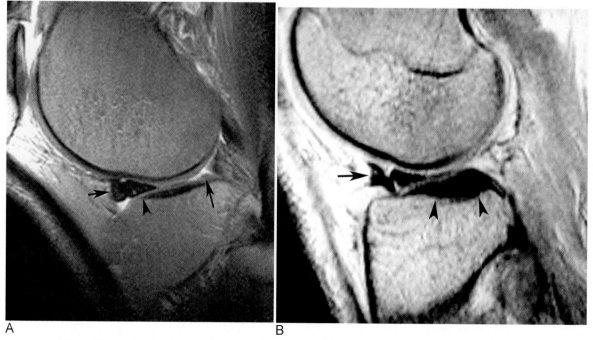

A   B

Figure 13-5   Displaced meniscal tears. **A,** Flipped posterior horn lateral meniscus. Sagittal fat-suppressed proton density fast spin-echo MR image shows normal anterior horn *(arrowhead),* fluid signal in the expected position of the posterior horn *(long arrow),* and displaced posterior horn located anterior to the anterior horn *(short arrow).* **B,** Similar injury as in part A, with posterior horn *(arrow)* anterior to anterior horn. Also note displaced lateral meniscus body *(arrowheads).* Sagittal proton density MR image.

(Continued)

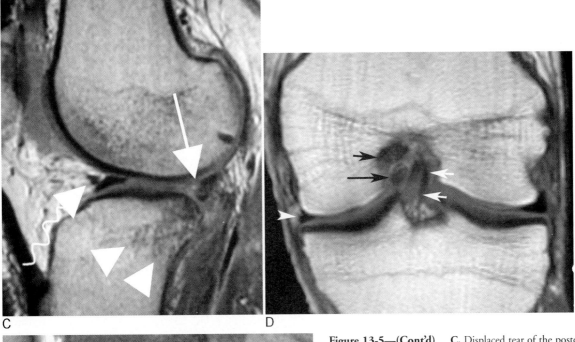

C

D

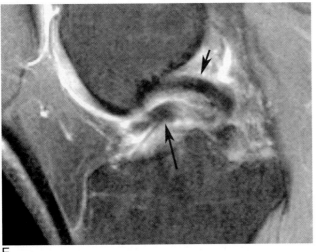

E

Figure 13-5—(Cont'd)   C, Displaced tear of the posterior horn lateral meniscus. Sagittal proton density spin-echo MR image. Note the blunted free edge *(arrow)* indicating either a tear with displaced fragment or prior partial resection; correlation with the surgical history is essential. Also note the normal transverse meniscal ligament *(curved arrow)* that connects the anterior margins of the frontal horns, which can mimic anterior horn meniscal tear. Also note indirect evidence of anterior cruciate ligament (ACL) tear (discussed later in text) with posterior lateral tibial bone bruise *(arrowheads)* and substantial anterior tibial subluxation. **D and E,** Bucket handle medial meniscus tear with double posterior cruciate ligament (PCL) sign. Coronal T1-weighted spin-echo MR image (D) shows small body of medial meniscus *(white arrowhead)*. Note normal ACL *(short white arrows)* and PCL *(short black arrow)*. The displaced meniscal fragment *(long black arrow)* represents a third intercondylar region structure, and thus is a clue to the presence of bucket handle meniscal tear. Sagittal fat-suppressed T2-weighted MR image (E) shows the normal PCL *(short black arrow)* and displaced meniscal fragment *(long black arrow)* creating the "double PCL sign."

planes is essential because the coronal plane is used to evaluate the body of the meniscus and the sagittal plane is used to evaluate the anterior and posterior horns. The signal within normal meniscus should be uniformly diminished in intensity. Many authors use the following system to grade meniscal signal alterations. Small lobular areas of increased signal within the central portion of the meniscus as demonstrated on sagittal or coronal proton density or T1-weighted spin-echo images are named grade I signal abnormalities and have no clinical significance because they do not correlate with meniscal disruption. Grade II signal abnormalities represent linear or globular increased signal in the central portion of the meniscus, which does not reach an articular surface. Grade II signal has a low association with meniscal tear. Magic angle effect can also result in diffuse or amorphous increased signal intensity as a normal finding in the posterior horns. However,

extensive areas of grade II signal have a higher association with meniscal tear. Patients with extensive intrameniscal signal are found to have a 10% to 20% incidence of meniscal tear at arthroscopy. For this reason, patients who have grade II signal in the meniscus who do not improve after 6 weeks of conservative therapy undergo arthroscopy. Grade III signal is increased signal within the meniscus that comes in contact with either the superior or inferior articular surface on at least two adjacent images. This represents direct MRI evidence of meniscal tear and has a sensitivity and specificity exceeding 90%. It is noteworthy that meniscal tears may be inapparent on T2-weighted images unless there is a fluid-like signal within the linear defects. Rarely, intrameniscal cysts can occur, which can be confused with meniscal tear. However, intrameniscal cysts are rare compared with the extremely common occurrence of meniscal tears. Grade III pathologic signal should be

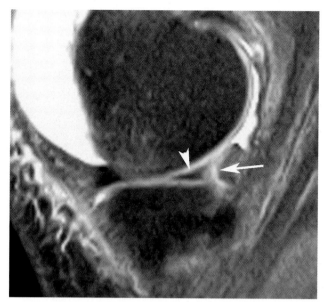

Figure 13-6   Meniscocapsular separation. Sagittal fat-suppressed T2-weighted MR image shows high signal *(arrow)* between the posterior horn of the medial meniscus *(arrowhead)* and the capsule.

distinguished from a normal finding of a linear transverse intermediate signal line in the peripheral third of the meniscus that extends to the peripheral margin. This line probably represents the tenuous meniscal blood supply and is usually apparent in children and young adults.

Menisci can also be evaluated for indirect evidence of meniscal tear (see Fig. 13-5). Indirect evidence is primarily shown morphologically. As noted previously, the menisci should appear triangular in shape. The anterior and posterior horns of the lateral meniscus are symmetric in size, whereas the posterior horn of the medial meniscus is larger and more elongated in appearance compared with the anterior horn of the medial meniscus. Therefore, the appearance of a similar size in the posterior horn of the medial meniscus as the anterior horn is abnormal, and is diagnostic of a meniscal tear or prior par-

tial resection of the posterior horn. A blunted appearance of the triangular free margin of a meniscus indicates a tear or prior resection. Finally, menisci should be uniformly diminished in signal intensity on all sequential imaging sections. If an intervening section fails to demonstrate a meniscus or shows a meniscus of substantially higher diffuse signal, this suggests the presence of a radial tear (a tear in the plane of imaging). A complete radial tear is usually associated with peripheral displacement beyond the margin of the corresponding cortical margin of the tibial plateau, often by at least 3 mm. Axial scans can be especially helpful in confirming a radial tear (see Fig. 13-4D, E).

A *bucket handle meniscal tear* is a vertical-longitudinal tear that involves all three portions of the meniscus. Part of the meniscus is displaced, like a bucket handle rotated on its hinge, often into the intercondylar notch. Or, the fragment may flip anteriorly or posteriorly, abutting the opposite meniscal horn. Bucket handle tears must be carefully sought at MRI because the sensitivity of their detection is low, around 60%, and detection will be missed unless conscious search is made for them (see Fig. 13-5D, E). On MR images in which there is intercondylar meniscal displacement, one should be able to follow the signal of meniscus along its displaced course in the intercondylar notch in a continuous fashion, connecting the anterior and posterior horns. This must be associated with a proportionately diminished size of the nondisplaced donor meniscal body and posterior horn. Because the displaced fragment is apposed adjacent to the posterior cruciate ligament, it can give the appearance of a second posterior cruciate ligament. When there is displacement adjacent to another meniscal horn, the donor meniscal site appears too small, whereas the site of displacement appears too large.

Discoid meniscus is a developmental variant in which the meniscus is more disk-shaped than semicircular and in which a portion of meniscus extends to the central portion of the tibial plateau (Fig. 13-8). This is far more common in the lateral meniscus and is clinically significant for two reasons. First, a discoid meniscus itself may be symptomatic, giving

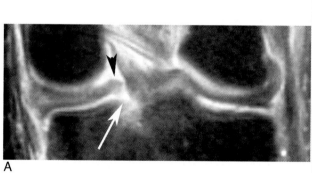
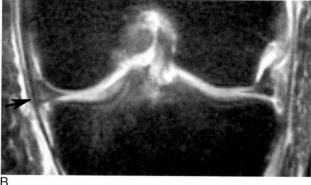

A   B

Figure 13-7   Meniscal root avulsion. Coronal fat-suppressed proton density MR images. **A,** Posterior image shows lateral margin of the medial meniscus posterior horn *(black arrowhead)* and fluid signal representing torn medial meniscal root *(white arrow)*. **B,** More anterior image shows peripheral displacement of the medial meniscus body *(arrow)*.

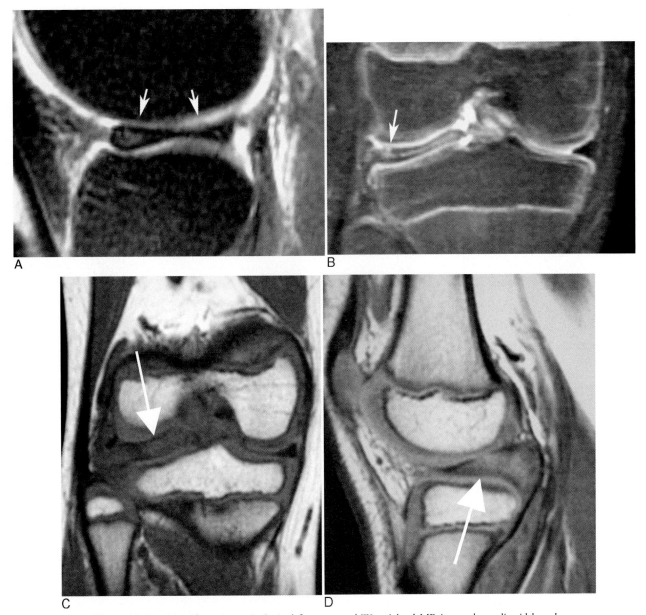

Figure 13-8   Discoid meniscus. **A,** Sagittal fat-suppressed T2-weighted MR image shows discoid lateral meniscus *(arrows)*. **B,** Torn discoid lateral meniscus. Coronal fat-suppressed proton density fast spin-echo MR image shows discoid lateral meniscus with high signal extending to the femoral surface *(arrow)* that represents a tear. **C and D,** Degenerated discoid lateral meniscus in another child. Coronal T1-weighted (C) and sagittal proton density (D) MR images demonstrate extremely prominent intrameniscal grade II signal *(arrows)*. Meniscus was found to be degenerated and torn at arthroscopy.

patients symptoms of locking and joint line pain. Second, a discoid meniscus is prone to tear because of its aberrant morphology and suboptimal biomechanical properties. A discoid meniscus is suspected when children and young adolescents present with signs of meniscal tear. Discoid meniscus is demonstrated on coronal MR images when the horizontal measurement between the free margin and periphery of the body of the meniscus is more than 1.4 cm. In addition, on sagittal images obtained at 3- to 4-mm section thickness with 1-mm interslice sections, the body of the meniscus should

not be shown on more than two to three sequential images. If shown on more than three images, discoid meniscus is diagnosed.

There are pitfalls at MRI in diagnosing meniscal tears. These are due to the presence of normal structures that are in close proximity to the periphery of the meniscus, causing signal that can be confused with grade III meniscal signal. One example is the popliteus tendon within the popliteal hiatus. Higher signal from fluid within the hiatus, located between the tendon and the periphery of the lateral meniscus, may produce signal mimicking meniscal tear. The meniscofemoral ligaments also may produce an appearance mimicking meniscal tear because they course posterior to the posterior horn of the lateral meniscus. The transverse meniscal ligament is a ligament connecting the anterior horns of the medial and lateral menisci. Like the meniscofemoral ligaments, this ligament may extend peripheral to the anterior horn of either meniscus with intervening signal mimicking that of meniscal tear. The oblique meniscal ligaments, which are found occasionally, and which connect the anterior horn of one meniscus with the posterior horn of the other meniscus, can be confused with bucket handle tears as this ligament is identified coursing through the intercondylar notch. Finally, the normal fibro-fatty meniscocapsular junction can be confused with meniscal tear or meniscocapsular separation due to its high signal.

Key Concepts	Pitfalls at MR Imaging in Diagnosing Meniscal Tears
Popliteus tendon within the popliteal hiatus Meniscofemoral ligaments Transverse meniscal ligament (anterior horns) Oblique meniscal ligaments Normal fibrofatty meniscocapsular junction Previous repair	

Parameniscal cysts are occasionally found at MRI and have a high association with meniscal tear (Fig. 13-9). These ganglia are frequently multiloculated and are located at the peripheral margin of the meniscus and are occasionally intrameniscal. They are usually located along the anterolateral margin of the meniscus and are more common in the lateral meniscus. When a parameniscal cyst is found, a careful search for the presence of a meniscal tear must be made because the likelihood of meniscal tear is greatly increased, especially horizontal tears. Occasionally, parameniscal cysts are ganglion cysts or synovial cysts whose appearance is identical except for the lack of a coincident meniscal tear.

A healed, surgically repaired meniscus can resemble a torn meniscus (Fig. 13-10). This is primarily because grade III signal persists in the meniscus after primary repair and cannot be discriminated from a meniscal retear on T1-weighted or proton density-weighted images. In other words, T1-weighted and proton density-weighted images have reduced specificity in distinguishing a healed tear from a new tear or a retear. Therefore, findings on T2-weighted images must be emphasized in the postoperative knee: look for the high signal of joint fluid within a tear. Accuracy for detection of retears is enhanced with MR arthrography: look for contrast medium within the meniscus. Multidetector CT arthrography uses the same principle: look for contrast medium in a tear. Magnetic resonance arthrography has a high accuracy in the diagnosis of

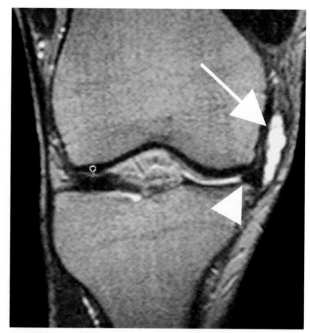

Figure 13-9 Meniscal cyst. Coronal T2-weighted spin-echo MR image shows meniscal cyst *(arrow)* in patient with meniscal tear. Note small meniscal body *(arrowhead)* with blunted free margin.

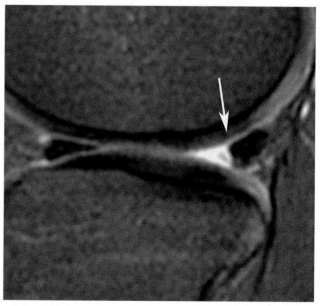

Figure 13-10 Postoperative meniscus. Fat-suppressed sagittal T2-weighted MR image shows resected free edge of the lateral meniscus posterior horn *(arrow)*. Knowledge of the surgical history is necessary to avoid mistaking this finding for a tear.

a retear, approaching 90%, compared with about 80% for plain MRI. Some authors advocate MR arthrography in any postoperative knee, but others recommend MR arthrography only if the meniscus has been partially or largely resected during the prior repair.

CRUCIATE LIGAMENT INJURY

The cruciate ligaments are crossing ligaments that are intracapsular yet extrasynovial in location. With the medial and lateral collateral ligaments, the cruciate ligaments form the major stabilizers of the knee joint. The anterior cruciate ligament (ACL) is the primary stabilizer of the knee against anterior tibial subluxation. It originates from the medial margin of the lateral femoral condyle at the intercondylar notch and courses anteriorly, medially, and inferiorly to insert at the anterior aspect of the intercondylar eminence (Fig. 13-11). The ACL is narrow medial to lateral and much wider anterior to posterior and thus is somewhat sheet-like. The ACL remains taut

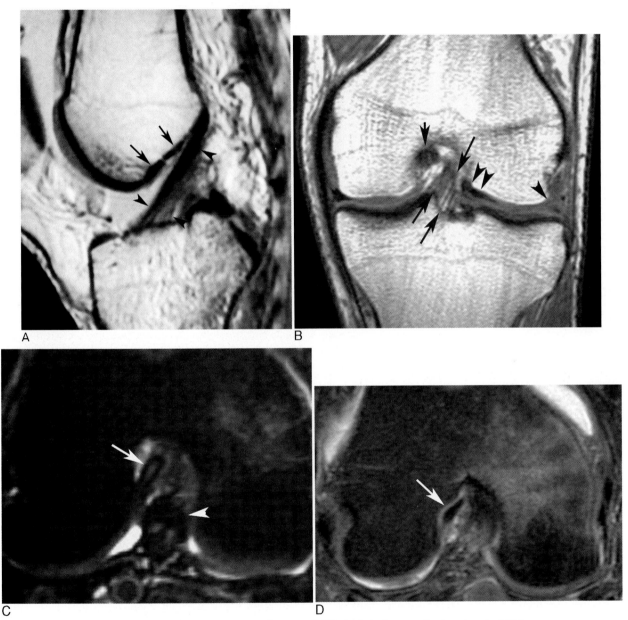

Figure 13-11   Normal anterior cruciate ligament (ACL). **A,** Sagittal proton density spin-echo MR image (ACL denoted by *arrowheads*). Note the roof of the intercondylar notch *(arrows)*. Also note the normal orientation of the ACL, which is more vertical than the notch roof. **B,** Coronal T1-weighted MR image of a left knee shows normal fan-like appearance of ACL *(long arrows)* with linear bands of dark signal interspersed with fibrofatty bands of intermediate signal. Also note normal posterior cruciate ligament (PCL) *(short arrow)* and bucket handle tear of the lateral meniscus *(arrowheads)*. **C and D,** Axial fat-suppressed T2-weighted MR images in right knees of different patients with normal ACLs show normal ovoid cross-section of the ACL *(arrows)*. The periphery of the ligament should have low signal intensity, although the central portion may have high T2 signal (as in part C) or low signal (as in part D). Also note PCL *(arrowheads)*.

through the range of knee motion. The posterior cruciate ligament is the primary restraint against posterior tibial subluxation. It originates from the lateral margin of the medial femoral condyle at the intercondylar notch to course in a posterior, lateral, and inferior direction to insert in a depression behind the intercondylar region of the tibia. The posterior cruciate ligament (PCL) is round in cross-section, and is taut only in knee flexion (assuming that the ACL is intact). On sagittal MR images with the knee in extension, the PCL appears thick and curved with its apex posterior (Fig. 13-12).

The ACL is the most commonly torn ligament at the knee, and search for ACL tear is a frequent indication for MRI. An ACL tear typically occurs in the setting of a clipping injury, in which the knee is placed in valgus, or a pivot-shift injury, in which the femur laterally rotates on the planted leg. Thus, valgus and anterolateral rotatory subluxation of the knee can lead to ACL injury. There are four primary signs of a ligament tear. These signs apply for any ligament, and for the assessment of the anterior cruciate ligament they are highly accurate. These signs are *swelling, increased signal, fiber discontinuity,* and *change in the expected ligament course* (Fig. 13-13). For ACL evaluation, these primary signs have an accuracy in excess of 90%. Lines drawn along the course of the normal ACL and the roof of the femoral notch form an angle whose apex points posteriorly. In the setting of ACL disruption, the ligament

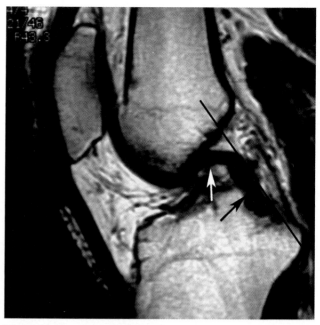

Figure 13-12 Normal posterior cruciate ligament (PCL). Sagittal proton density spin-echo MR image shows normal PCL *(arrows).* Note that a line drawn tangent to the posterior margin of the descending limb *(solid line)* intersects distal femur. This is an indirect sign of an intact anterior cruciate ligament.

Key Concepts	Anterior Cruciate Ligament (ACL) Injury

If ACL appears intact on any sequence, it probably is intact
Findings of tear: Laxity, abnormal orientation
Numerous secondary signs, most specific in adults: Bone bruises in anterior weight bearing femoral condyle(s) and posterior tibial plateau(s) (kissing lesions during subluxation)

fibers flatten to a horizontal position, and the angle formed by the torn ligament and the roof of the intercondylar notch has an apex that points anteriorly. It should be noted that ligament rupture is by far more common than ligament avulsion. The location of rupture is usually near the femoral origin. The MRI plane most useful for evaluation of the anterior cruciate ligament is the sagittal plane. This allows demonstration of fiber continuity, ACL swelling and signal changes, and ACL course. However, because the ACL is a thin and fan-like ligament, spreading transversely as it extends inferiorly toward the tibia, the sagittal plane sometimes poorly demonstrates the ACL, even though it is not torn. In this situation, coronal and axial imaging planes are extremely useful because they show the ACL in cross-section. The demonstration of a normal ACL without swelling or edema-like signal in any imaging plane excludes an ACL tear. The most useful types of imaging sequence for the evaluation of the ACL are the T2-weighted spin-echo and the

fat-suppressed proton density-weighted or T2-weighted fast spin-echo sequences. This allows the best demonstration of edema-like signal while still allowing clear visualization of soft tissue anatomy. Inversion recovery images are sensitive to the detection of edema, but anatomic resolution is diminished owing to lower signal-to-noise ratio.

Several secondary signs of ACL tear independently show high accuracy in assessment of ACL disruption (Fig. 13-14). However, these signs are only occasionally helpful in diagnosing ACL tear because they usually are present only when the ACL is obviously torn. The most specific of these secondary signs is a pattern of "kissing" subchondral bone bruises of one or both posterior tibial plateaus and the ipsilateral anterior weight-bearing femoral condyle. The presence of these bruises suggests that the ACL injury occurred within the prior 6 to 8 weeks, as bone bruises usually resolve during this time. The mechanism of such an injury is anterior subluxation of the tibia with ACL tear with bone impaction. The presence of a posterolateral tibial bone bruise itself has a high predictive value for ACL tear. An exception to this association is with pediatric patients, in whom a bone bruise in this location may occur in the absence of ACL tear. This is due to greater laxity of the ACL in children. Another sensitive secondary sign of ACL tear is the presence of a hemarthrosis. In fact, as many as 75% of acute knee hemarthroses are due to ACL rupture. Other causes of hemarthrosis in the setting of trauma are large bone bruises and intra-articular fractures. In the setting of ACL injury, the PCL can appear hyperangulated. Normally, a line drawn tangent to the posterior margin of the PCL should

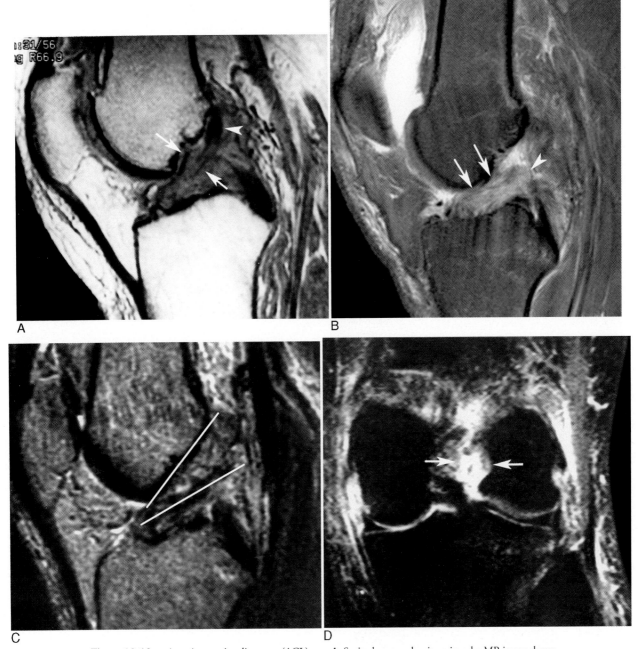

Figure 13-13   Anterior cruciate ligament (ACL) tear. **A,** Sagittal proton density spin-echo MR image shows fiber discontinuity, swelling, and increased signal of torn ACL *(arrows).* Note intact femoral origin *(arrowhead).* **B,** Sagittal fat-suppressed T2-weighted MR image shows lax, wavy, horizontally oriented ACL fibers and edema *(arrows).* Note torn tendon margin proximally *(arrowhead).* **C,** Sagittal T2-weighted spin-echo MR image in another patient shows abnormal course of anterior cruciate ligament. Note that the ACL is oriented more horizontally than the notch roof. **D,** Coronal inversion recovery MR image shows localized increased signal *(arrows)* in lateral intercondylar notch at expected location of proximal ACL. A normal ligament is not seen.

intersect the distal 4 to 6 cm of the femur. When this line fails to intersect the distal femur, there is implied ACL tear. Another sign is known as the "anterior drawer sign." This is shown when the tibia subluxes anteriorly relative to the femur. If lines are drawn vertical to the posterior margins of the lateral tibial and femoral condyles in the mid-lateral compart-ment, and the tibia is more than 7 mm anteriorly subluxed, this is considered a sign of a complete ACL rupture. A related finding is when the posterior horn of the lateral meniscus is posteriorly subluxed relative to the posterior cortical margin of the lateral tibial condyle. Such posterior meniscal displacement is also associated with ACL tear.

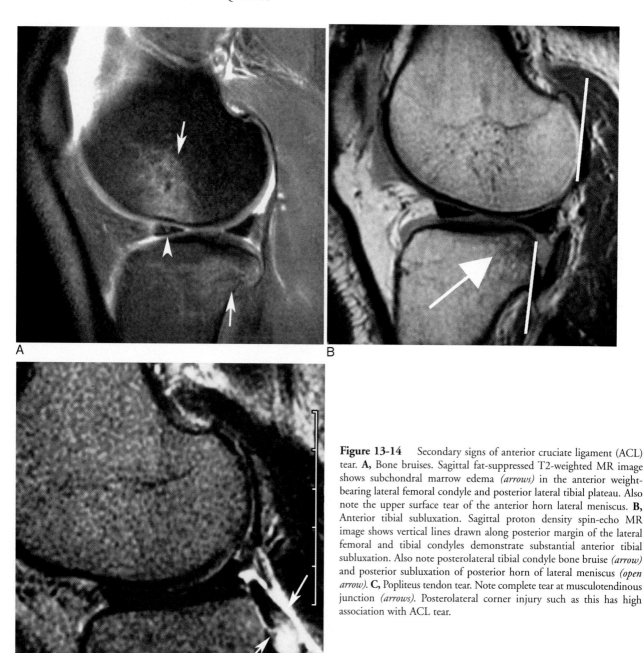

Figure 13-14   Secondary signs of anterior cruciate ligament (ACL) tear. **A,** Bone bruises. Sagittal fat-suppressed T2-weighted MR image shows subchondral marrow edema *(arrows)* in the anterior weight-bearing lateral femoral condyle and posterior lateral tibial plateau. Also note the upper surface tear of the anterior horn lateral meniscus. **B,** Anterior tibial subluxation. Sagittal proton density spin-echo MR image shows vertical lines drawn along posterior margin of the lateral femoral and tibial condyles demonstrate substantial anterior tibial subluxation. Also note posterolateral tibial condyle bone bruise *(arrow)* and posterior subluxation of posterior horn of lateral meniscus *(open arrow)*. **C,** Popliteus tendon tear. Note complete tear at musculotendinous junction *(arrows)*. Posterolateral corner injury such as this has high association with ACL tear.

An ACL injury can be associated with medial collateral ligament injury and medial meniscal tear. This association is termed *O'Donoghue's terrible triad*. In truth, however, the lateral meniscus is more commonly torn in the setting of ACL injury because of lateral impaction that occurs with clipping and pivot-shift injuries. However, sensitivity of detecting lateral meniscal tears is drastically reduced in the setting of ACL tear. Another associated injury pattern is the *Segond fracture,* which is a lateral capsule avulsion fracture at the lateral tibial plateau due to internal rotation and varus stress on a flexed knee (see Figs. 12-14, 12-16). Segond fracture is nearly 100%

associated with an ACL tear. In most of the few cases in which an ACL tear is not present, the ACL insertion is avulsed.

Posterolateral corner injury also may occur with ACL tear. Posterolateral corner structures include the lateral collateral ligament, lateral capsule, popliteus tendon, and several smaller ligaments that are poorly seen with MRI, such as the arcuate ligament, the fabellofibular ligament, and the ligament of Winslow. The occurrence of posterolateral corner injuries at MRI implies ACL tear (see Fig. 13-14C). Injuries at this location are only now being studied, and are considered an indication for early surgical repair owing to concern for delayed

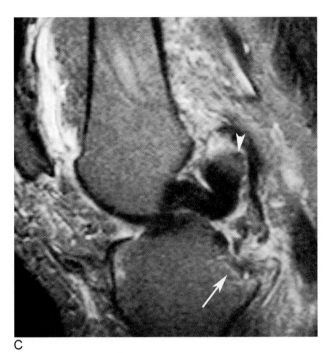

C

Figure 13-17—(Cont'd)   C, Avulsion fracture of the PCL tibial insertion. Sagittal T2-weighted spin-echo MR image shows intact but displaced PCL attached to avulsed tibial bone fragment *(arrowhead).* Note edema at the fracture donor site *(arrow).*

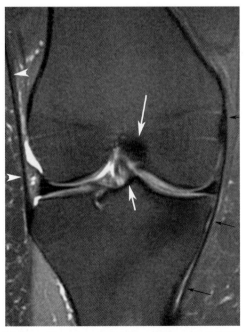

Figure 13-18   Normal medial collateral ligament (MCL). Coronal fat-suppressed proton density MR image of a right knee shows normal medial collateral ligament *(small black arrows).* This is the middle layer of the ligament. The deep layer is the joint capsule. Also note the iliotibial band *(white arrowheads)* laterally and the anterior cruciate ligament (ACL) *(short white arrow)* and posterior cruciate ligament (PCL) *(long white arrow)* in the intercondylar notch.

origin or at the posterior tibial insertion. Posterior cruciate ligament reconstructions are controversial. At many centers, PCL ruptures are not repaired because isolated PCL injury is not felt to be associated with substantial instability. One rarely encounters knees in which PCL repair has been performed.

COLLATERAL LIGAMENT INJURY

The medial and lateral collateral ligaments are the primary restraints to valgus and varus loads, respectively. The medial collateral ligament (MCL) is a large, complex structure. It is composed of three layers. The most superficial layer is the superficial fascia. The middle layer is the true ligament, which originates just distal to the adductor tubercle of the femur, coursing inferiorly to the medial tibial tubercle, inserting at a level 5 cm below the joint line (Fig. 13-18). The deep layer of the medial collateral ligament is actually the joint capsule and is intimately associated with the medial meniscus, originating and inserting on the margins of the joint.

The lateral collateral ligament (LCL, Fig. 13-19) is part of the posterolateral complex of the knee and originates in a sulcus along the lateral femoral condyle, extending distally and posteriorly to insert as a conjoint insertion with the biceps femoris tendon on the fibular head. It is a major contributor to posterolateral stability.

Injuries of the MCL and LCL usually occur in combination with other injuries. An MCL rupture is commonly associated with ACL tears and meniscal tears. Ruptures of the MCL are associated with valgus injuries and, like other ligament injuries, range from partial ligament disruptions, in which edema and hemorrhage predominate, to complete ligament disruptions, in which fiber discontinuity is evident (Fig. 13-20A). Osseous abnormalities can be associated with MCL injury and include bone bruises in the apposing lateral margins of the lateral tibial and femoral condyles at the site of impaction during valgus injury. *Pellegrini-Stieda* disease represents post-traumatic calcification around the MCL origin related to previous trauma. Ruptures of the LCL are uncommon and are rarely isolated (Fig. 13-20B). They are associated not only with ACL injury but with posterolateral corner instability. They can also be associated with peroneal nerve injury owing to the nerve's proximity to the fibular head and LCL insertion. Imaging criteria for LCL disruption are as for other ligament injuries. Associated osseous abnormalities include avulsion of the fibular head and medial bone bruises that may occur as a result of the varus injury pattern.

ADDITIONAL TENDON AND BURSAL CONDITIONS

The tendons of the knee are important to evaluate because injury of the knee may be isolated to tendon pathology. The most common tendons affected at the knee are the extensor

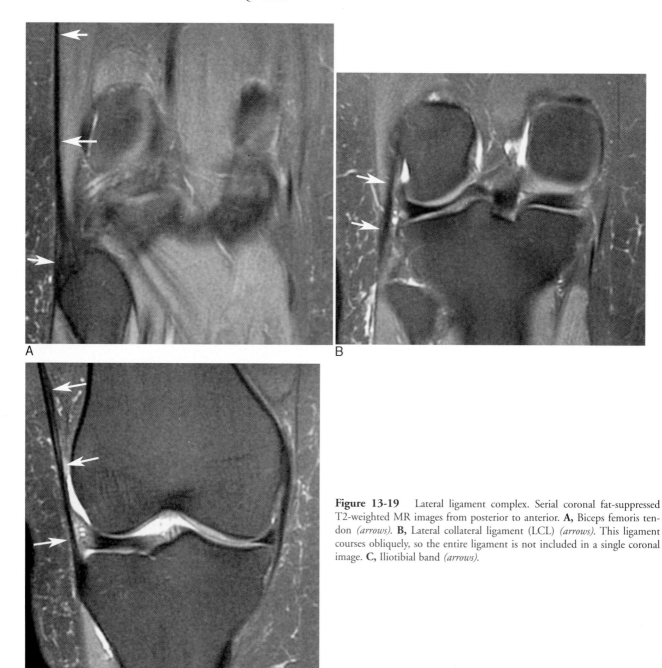

Figure 13-19   Lateral ligament complex. Serial coronal fat-suppressed T2-weighted MR images from posterior to anterior. **A,** Biceps femoris tendon *(arrows).* **B,** Lateral collateral ligament (LCL) *(arrows).* This ligament courses obliquely, so the entire ligament is not included in a single coronal image. **C,** Iliotibial band *(arrows).*

tendons (quadriceps tendon and patellar tendon), the pes anserinus (sartorius, gracilis, and semitendinosus insertions at the medial aspect of the proximal tibia), and the popliteus musculotendinous junction.

On axial images of the knee, it can be difficult to determine medial and lateral landmarks. Helpful landmarks include the patella, whose lateral facet is longer than the medial facet. Furthermore, consideration of muscle anatomy allows easy determination of geography because in the popliteal fossa, excluding the gastrocnemius muscles, there are only one muscle group laterally (the biceps femoris) but four medially (semimembranosus, semitendinosus, sartorius, and gracilis) (Fig. 13-21).

Anteriorly, the quadriceps muscles (rectus femoris, vastus lateralis, vastus intermedius, vastus medialis) join to form the quadriceps tendon in multiple layers, usually three, as noted on sagittal MR images. The superficial layer is the rectus femoris, the middle layer is the conjoint vastus lateralis and medialis, and the deep layer is the vastus intermedius. Fascial extensions of the quadriceps aponeurosis form a hood over the anterior half of the knee, known as the flexor retinaculum. It is the medial retinaculum that can stretch and tear during transient patellar dislocation.

Jumper's knee is an overuse injury associated with repetitive jumping, such as with basketball (Fig. 13-22). In jumper's

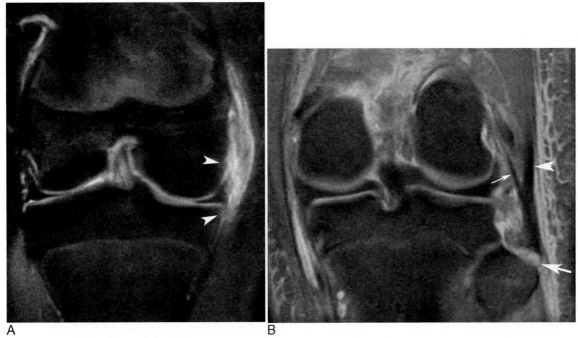

A   B

Figure 13-20   Collateral ligament injuries. **A,** Coronal fat-suppressed proton density MR image shows thick, edematous medial collateral ligament (MCL), with no intact fibers. Most MCL tears are proximal. Also note subtle marrow edema at the insertion sites of the deep MCL (i.e., the joint capsule, *arrowheads*). In contrast with the conspicuous marrow edema associated with most traumatic bone injuries, the marrow edema associated with ligament and capsular avulsion injuries can be extremely subtle. **B,** Fibular avulsion *(large arrow)* of the biceps femoris tendon *(arrowhead)* and lateral collateral ligament (LCL) *(small arrow).*

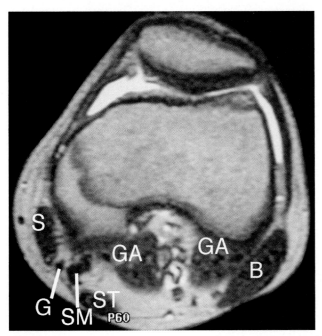

Figure 13-21   Normal muscle anatomy of popliteal fossa. Axial T2-weighted fast spin-echo MR image. B, biceps femoris muscle; G, gracilis tendon; GA, gastrocnemius muscles; S, sartorius muscle; SM, semimembranosus tendon; ST, semitendinosus tendon.

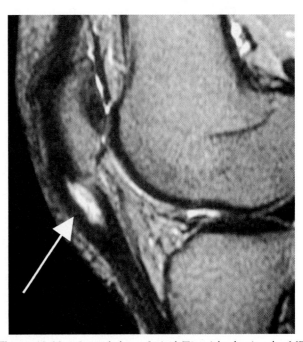

Figure 13-22   Jumper's knee. Sagittal T2-weighted spin-echo MR image shows high signal within the posterior proximal patellar tendon adjacent to the patella *(arrow).*

knee, findings predominate in the proximal patellar tendon and appear at MRI as increased transverse dimension and increased signal on T2-weighted images, particularly in the posterior midline fibers. Marrow edema may be present in the adjacent patella. The childhood conditions Sinding-Larsen-Johansson and Osgood-Schlatter diseases, discussed in Chapter 12, also include varying degrees of adjacent patellar tendonitis. Patellar tendon disorders are prone to healing with irregular ossicles within or partly within the substance of the patellar tendon. Tears of the distal quadriceps are fairly common, and imaging is occasionally requested, especially if clini-

cal findings are equivocal (Fig. 13-23). Patients with rheumatoid arthritis who are taking corticosteroids are prone to quadriceps tendon tears.

The poorly named *cortical desmoid* is bony irregularity and excavation in the posteromedial aspect of the distal femoral diametaphysis, at the site of insertion of the adductor magnus muscle or origin of the medial head of the gastrocnemius muscle (Fig. 13-24). A technically more accurate name for this finding is "avulsive cortical irregularity." However, "cortical desmoid" is easier to say, so this term has endured. A similar lesion may occur at the gastrocnemius lateral head origin. This

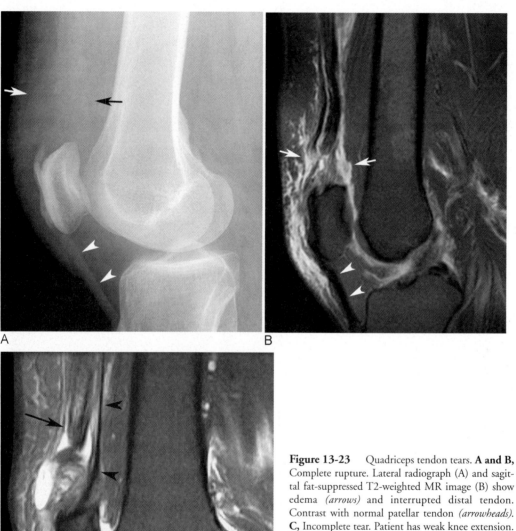

Figure 13-23   Quadriceps tendon tears. **A and B,** Complete rupture. Lateral radiograph (A) and sagittal fat-suppressed T2-weighted MR image (B) show edema *(arrows)* and interrupted distal tendon. Contrast with normal patellar tendon *(arrowheads).* **C,** Incomplete tear. Patient has weak knee extension. The superficial layer (rectus femoris) and middle layer (vastus medialis and lateralis) fibers are ruptured *(arrow),* but the deepest layer *(arrowheads,* vastus intermedius) is intact.

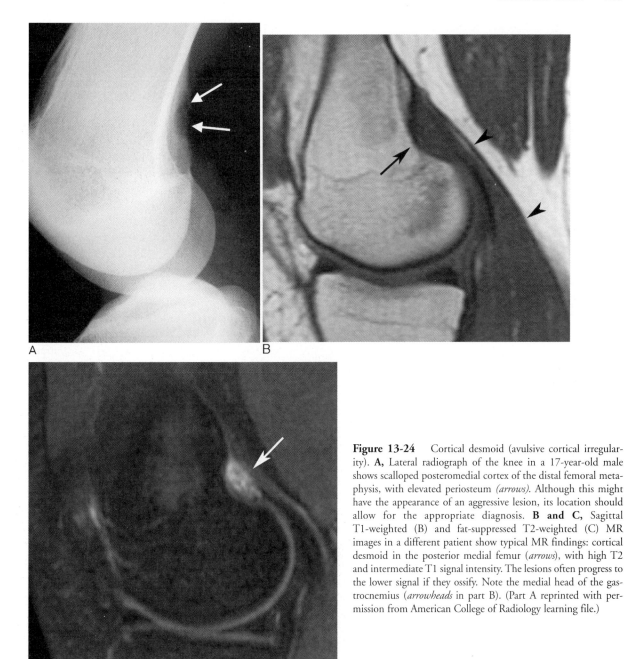

Figure 13-24   Cortical desmoid (avulsive cortical irregularity). **A,** Lateral radiograph of the knee in a 17-year-old male shows scalloped posteromedial cortex of the distal femoral metaphysis, with elevated periosteum *(arrows)*. Although this might have the appearance of an aggressive lesion, its location should allow for the appropriate diagnosis. **B and C,** Sagittal T1-weighted (B) and fat-suppressed T2-weighted (C) MR images in a different patient show typical MR findings: cortical desmoid in the posterior medial femur *(arrows)*, with high T2 and intermediate T1 signal intensity. The lesions often progress to the lower signal if they ossify. Note the medial head of the gastrocnemius *(arrowheads* in part B). (Part A reprinted with permission from American College of Radiology learning file.)

fairly common finding in older children usually is a normal variant, but can be associated with overuse. The lesion is a mixture of connective tissue and usually vanishes during adulthood. A cortical desmoid may mimic osseous neoplasia on radiographs. The defect is often filled with fibrocartilaginous tissue that is seen on MRI as a parosteal area of fairly high T2 signal. Marrow edema is variably present. This appearance at the muscle attachment site allows neoplasia to be excluded.

Patients may present with pain at the pes anserinus insertion related to a bursitis, which can be documented at MRI with the demonstration of a fluid collection surrounding the tendons as they insert on the medial aspect of the proximal tibia (Fig. 13-25). Other sites of bursal fluid accumulation in the knee include the gastrocnemius-semimembranosus bursa, which may extend to form a Baker's cyst (Fig. 13-26), the prepatellar bursa (see Fig. 2-4), and the superficial and deep infrapatellar bursae. The Baker's cyst deserves special mention because it is so common and may become multiloculated and very large, and contain osteochondral bodies and other debris (Fig. 13-27). Most Baker's cysts are initiated by a chronic knee effusion, but they may persist after the knee effusion resolves.

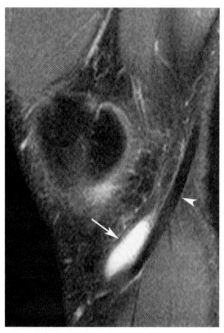

Figure 13-25   Pes anserinus bursitis. Sagittal fat-suppressed T2-weighted MR image obtained through the medial knee shows well-circumscribed bursal fluid collection *(arrow)* adjacent to the semitendinosus tendon *(arrowhead).*

A final area of tendon and bursal pain occurs around the insertion of the iliotibial band with symptoms anterolaterally at the knee. At MRI, altered signal in the fat deep to the iliotibial band is shown, and represents the occurrence of an adventitial bursal fluid collection.

Ganglion cysts are common around the knee. As noted previously, many originate from meniscal tears (meniscal cyst). Ganglia also may develop within tendons, often the ACL (Fig. 13-28) or PCL, and may cause mechanical impingement on the surrounding tendon.

HYALINE CARTILAGE INJURY AND MISCELLANEOUS KNEE CONDITIONS

Knee articular cartilage defects are most common at the medial femoral and the patellar surfaces (see Figs. 2-27–2-30). Injuries to articular cartilage range from chondral to osteochondral injury, and associated injuries are common. In particular, there is association of articular cartilage injury with meniscal tears. These associated injuries are usually in close proximity to one another. If a meniscal tear is found, a careful search for associated articular cartilage tear should be undertaken.

Osteochondritis dissecans was discussed in Chapter 3. *Spontaneous osteonecrosis of the knee* (SONK) is a rapid, painful subchondral collapse of the anterior weightbearing femoral condyle. It is almost always medial, is almost always associated with medial meniscal tear, and almost always occurs in the elderly (Fig. 13-29). This condition may occur after seemingly minor trauma, such as knee arthroscopy, or after a knee injection, but most cases are idiopathic. Initial MRI shows only subchondral marrow edema, or may show a subchondral fracture that resembles avascular necrosis. Over 2 to 3 months, there can be rapid progression to painful subchondral collapse and osteoarthritis requiring joint replacement. This condition was originally

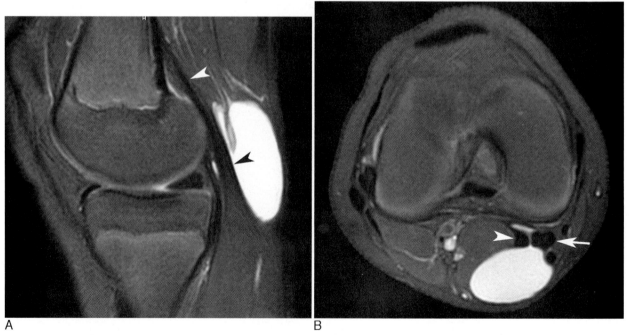

A   B

Figure 13-26   Baker's cyst. Uncomplicated cyst. **A and B,** Sagittal (A) and axial (B) fat-suppressed T2-weighted MR images show distended gastrocnemius-semimembranosus bursa. Note tendons of the gastrocnemius medial head *(arrowheads)* and semimembranosus *(arrow in part B).*

(Continued)

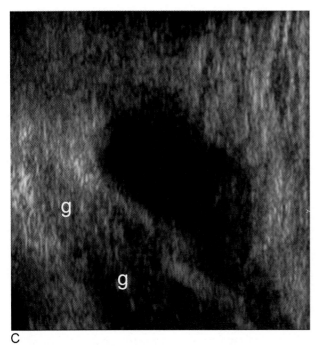

C

Figure 13-26—(Cont'd) **C,** Sagittal ultrasonogram in a different patient oriented similar to an MR image (with superior at the top of the image) shows anechoic Baker's cyst with enhanced through sound transmission. g, gastrocnemius medial head.

thought to be due to spontaneous or traumatic avascular necrosis, but it is now recognized to be a post-traumatic condition initiated by a subchondral insufficiency fracture. Because of this, the term SONK is falling out of favor and being replaced by a variety of terms, including subcondral insufficiency fracture or subchondral impaction fracture.

Popliteal artery entrapment is anomalous course of the popliteal artery relative to the proximal gastrocnemius muscle, most often with the artery coursing through or around the medial head. Patients present in their 20s or 30s with a syndrome of calf claudication when standing or with exercise. Definitive diagnosis can be made with MR or conventional angiography, or with ultrasonography.

The peroneal nerve is vulnerable to injury as it courses around the fibular neck. A mass such as an osteochondroma or trauma to this region can result in peroneal nerve dysfunction with foot drop and evidence of denervation of lateral leg musculature on MR images (Table 13-1).

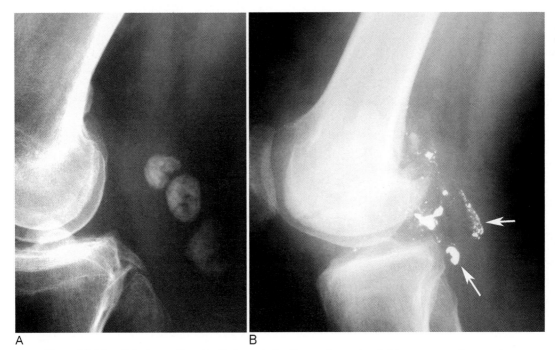

A B

Figure 13-27 Baker's cyst. Complex findings. **A,** Cartilage and osteochondral fragments are often seen in chronic Baker's cysts in patients with osteoarthritis. **B,** More exotic debris, bullet fragments in this example *(arrows),* may also be seen.

(Continued)

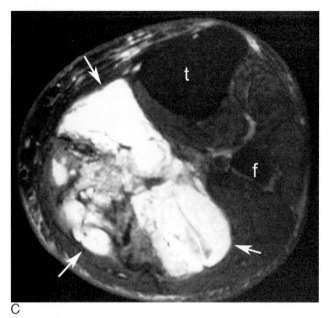

C

Figure 13-27—(Cont'd)   C, Cysts may become very large, and may contain bizarre signal due to internal hemorrhage. Axial fat-suppressed T2-weighted MR image in the proximal left leg shows mass with mixed signal intensity that more superior images showed was continuous with the gastrocnemius-semimembranosus bursa. Surgical biopsy yielded old blood. f, fibula; t, tibia.

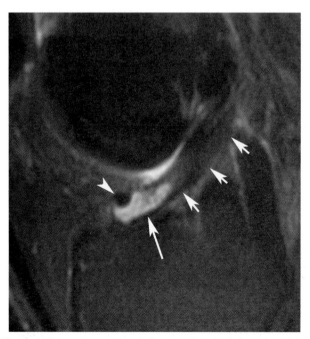

Figure 13-28   Anterior cruciate ligament (ACL) ganglion. Sagittal fat-suppressed T2-weighted MR image shows well-circumscribed ganglion *(long arrow)* in the distal ACL *(short arrows).* Note the transverse ligament *(arrowhead)* that connects the anterior horns of the menisci.

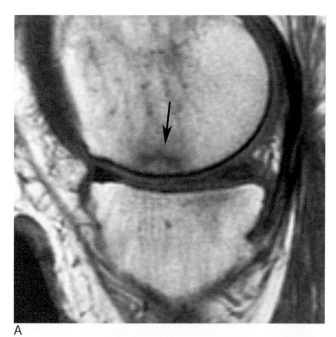

A

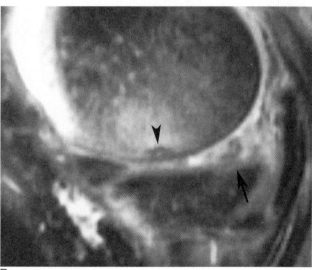

B

Figure 13-29   Medial femoral condyle subchondral insufficiency fracture, early findings. Neither patient had a known history of trauma, and after these studies they both developed rapidly progressive medial compartment knee osteoarthritis. **A,** Sagittal T1-weighted MR image obtained through the medial compartment shows irregular low signal fracture line *(arrow)* suggestive of avascular necrosis. Surrounding marrow edema is seen as vague reduced signal intensity. **B,** Sagittal fat-suppressed T2-weighted MR image in a different patient with early SONK shows the fracture line *(arrow)* and a posterior horn medial meniscal tear *(arrowhead).*

The suprapatellar, mediopatellar, and infrapatellar plicae are variably present synovial infoldings of the knee joint capsule that are remnants of normal embryologic development (Fig. 13-30). The most commonly identified on imaging studies is the medial plica, which is a coronally oriented band medial to the patella. Most medial plicae are incidental, but, occasionally, a thickened medial plica can cause joint effusion, anteromedial knee pain, and snapping (Fig. 13-31). The suprapatellar plica is

Table 13-1   Anterior Knee Pain Causes

Frequent:
    Patellofemoral malalignment
    Patellar cartilage defect/chondromalacia
    Patellar tendinitis
Less frequent:
    Medial plica
    Impingement on Hoffa's fat pad

in an oblique axial plane in the suprapatellar portion of the joint space. Rarely, a superior plica can entrap synovium or intra-articular debris in the superior joint space. The infrapatellar plica (also termed the ligamentum mucosum) extends in the sagittal plane through the mid and lower portion of Hoffa's fat pad to the intercondylar notch, where it may attach to the ACL. Rarely, inferior plicae can become thickened and inflamed. A more frequent cause of abnormal MRI findings and symptoms in Hoffa's fat pad is *Hoffa's disease,* which is inflammation or hemorrhage within Hoffa's fat pad, usually due to trauma and impingement, which may progress to chronic fibrosis and hyalinization with chronic pain (Fig. 13-32).

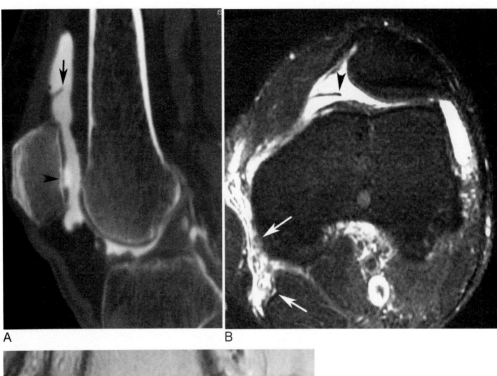

A   B

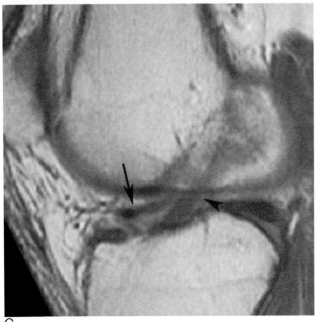

C

Figure 13-30 Normal knee plicae. **A,** Superior plica *(arrow)* oriented transversely in the superior joint recess. Sagittal CT arthrogram reformat. Also note high-grade patellar cartilage defect *(arrowhead).* **B,** Medial plica *(arrow)* oriented coronally in the medial joint. Axial fat-suppressed T2-weighted MR image. Also note the ruptured Baker's cyst *(arrows).* **C,** Infrapatellar plica *(arrow)* extending from the anterior intercondylar notch anteriorly into Hoffa's fat pad. Oblique sagittal T1-weighted MR image. Also note anterior cruciate ligament (ACL) *(arrowhead).*

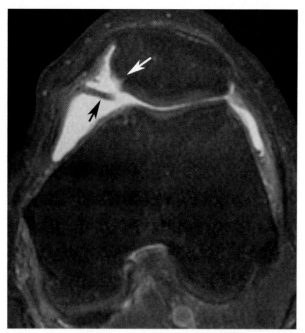

Figure 13-31 Pathologic medial plica. Axial fat-suppressed T2-weighted MR image in a 22-year-old woman with anterior left knee pain shows a thick medial plica *(black arrow)* with associated articular cartilage defect in the medial patellar facet *(white arrow)* and joint effusion.

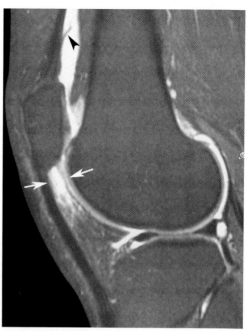

Figure 13-32 Hoffa's fat pad trauma in a 29-year-old woman with patella alta and anterior knee pain. Sagittal fat-suppressed T2-weighted MR image shows focal edema *(arrows)* in lateral superior Hoffa's fat pad due to impingement. Also note incidental superior plica *(arrowhead)*.

ANATOMY
TRAUMA PATTERNS
TENDON INJURY
LIGAMENT INJURY
ANKLE IMPINGEMENT SYNDROMES
TARSAL TUNNEL SYNDROME

ANATOMY

The ankle is formed by the tibia, the fibula, and the talus, creating a hinge joint. The tibial articular margin is called the tibial *plafond* (ceiling). The lateral malleolus is positioned 1 cm distal and posterior to the medial malleolus (Fig. 14-1A). The medial and lateral articular margins of the ankle joint are formed by the talus and medial malleolus, and by the talus and lateral malleolus, which are obliquely oriented such that a 15- to 20-degree internal oblique view *(mortise view)* allows visualization of the articular margins in profile (Fig. 14-1B, C). The talar dome has a complex shape, semicircular when viewed from the side but subtly saddle-shaped when viewed anteriorly (Fig. 14-1D). It fits snugly within the articulation formed by the tibia and fibula, such that there is a symmetric 3- to 4-mm margin between the entire talar surface and the apposing plafond and malleolar margins. The tibiotalar joint frequently communicates with the posterior subtalar facet as a normal variant.

The ankle is supported by a complex array of ligaments (Fig. 14-2). A syndesmosis is present between the tibia and fibula, the distal aspect of which forms the strong anterior and posterior distal tibiofibular ligaments. The anterior and posterior distal tibiofibular ligaments are the most superior set of ankle ligaments, seen on axial magnetic resonance imaging (MRI) immediately above the ankle joint. These appear as uniform, thin, low-signal structures on all imaging sequences, passing between anterior and posterior margins of the tibia and the apposing fibula. The medial margin of the fibula is convex or straight at this level. Below the anterior and posterior distal

tibiofibular ligaments, the lateral collateral ligaments are found. This ligament complex is composed of three structures (see Fig. 14-2). The anterior talofibular ligament extends from the anterior fibula to the lateral talar neck, shown best on the axial plane at the level where the medial aspect of the fibula is con-

Key Concepts	Ankle Ligaments

Distal tibiofibular syndesmosis: Strong anterior and posterior distal tibiofibular ligaments
Lateral:
    Anterior talofibular ligament (most frequently torn ankle ligament)
    Calcaneofibular ligament (most difficult to see at MRI)
    Posterior talofibular ligament (strongest lateral ligament)
Medial:
    Deltoid complex

cave. The anterior talofibular ligament is the most frequently torn ankle ligament. The posterior talofibular ligament is a large fan-shaped ligament extending from the distal aspect of the lateral malleolar fossa to the lateral tubercle of the posterior talar process. The ligament is seen at the same level on axial MR images as the anterior talofibular ligament but appears more inhomogeneous because of the fan-shaped ligament fibers. The third ligament of the lateral collateral ligaments is the calcaneofibular ligament, which extends from the tip of the lateral malleolus to the lateral aspect of the calcaneus. This is the most difficult of the lateral ankle ligaments to see at MRI; it can be seen partially on either coronal or axial images but is best shown on oblique axial images with the foot in plantar flexion.

The medial collateral ligament is also known as the deltoid ligament or deltoid complex and consists of five overlapping parts. The medial collateral ligament is a much stronger ligament complex than the lateral collateral ligaments and is less

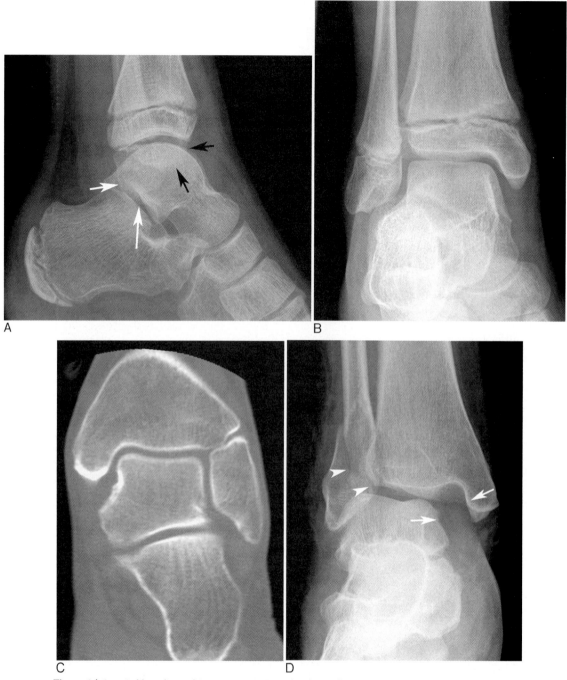

Figure 14-1 Ankle radiographic anatomy. **A,** Lateral radiograph. Note that the lateral malleolus *(white arrows)* is posterior to the medial malleolus *(black arrows).* **B and C,** Mortise views. **D,** Mortise view of fracture subluxation shows the saddle shape of the talar dome and matching contour of the tibial plafond. Note the oblique fracture *(arrowheads)* in distal fibula at the level of the tibiotalar joint and widened ankle joint at medial mortise *(arrows)* indicating deltoid ligament tear. C, coronal CT reformat.

commonly torn. Located deep to the flexor tendons, the deltoid ligament consists of superficial and deep components. The superficial ligaments are the tibiocalcaneal, tibiospring, and tibionavicular ligaments, which course from the tibia to the calcaneus, spring ligament, and navicular bone. The deep ligaments are the anterior and posterior tibiotalar ligaments. Of all the deltoid ligaments, the tibionavicular ligament is the weakest.

The largest of the tendons found at the ankle is the Achilles tendon, which is the tendon formed by the gastrocnemius and soleus muscles that merge to form a thick tendon that inserts on the posterior calcaneus. The flexor tendons of the ankle are found posteromedially at the ankle and are, from medial to lateral, the tibialis posterior, the flexor digitorum longus, and the flexor hallucis longus tendons (Fig. 14-3). These three tendons

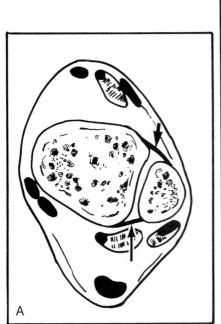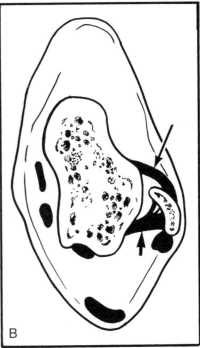

Figure 14-2   Lateral ligaments at the ankle. **A,** Axial diagram immediately superior to the ankle joint demonstrates the anterior and posterior tibiofibular ligaments (*short and long arrows,* respectively). Note the convex medial fibular shape at this level. **B,** Axial diagram demonstrating the anterior talofibular *(long arrow)* and posterior talofibular *(short arrow)* ligaments. Note that the fibular shape is concave at its medial aspect at this level. (Reproduced with permission from Manaster BJ: Handbook of Skeletal Radiology, ed 2. St. Louis, Mosby, 1997.)

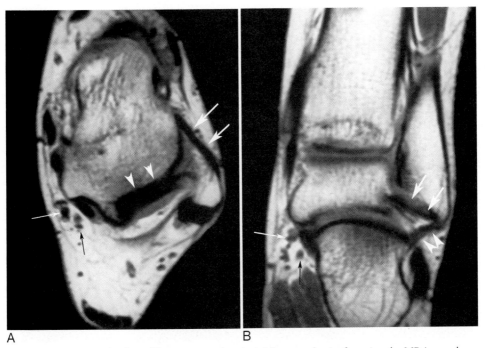

Figure 14-3   Lateral collateral ligament complex. **A,** Axial proton density fast spin-echo MR image shows anterior talofibular ligament (ATF, *arrows*) and posterior talofibular ligament (PTF, *arrowheads*). **B,** Coronal T1-weighted MR image shows ATF *(arrows)* and calcaneofibular ligament *(arrowheads)*. In parts A and B note the medial *(small white arrow)* and lateral *(small black arrow)* plantar arteries, veins, and nerves. These represent the distal extension of the tibial nerve and the posterior tibial artery and veins.

course through the tarsal tunnel, which is a fibro-osseous space confined by the flexor retinaculum, in which are also found the posterior tibial nerve and its branches, posterior tibial artery, veins, and lymphatics. The mnemonic for the relative position of these structures from anterior medial to posterior lateral is "Tom, Dick, AN (posterior tibial Artery and Nerve) Harry." The posterior tibial tendon is found in a groove along the medial malleolus, and continues through the tarsal tunnel to insert on the navicular bone with continuation of the tendon to the plantar aspect of the medial and middle cuneiform bones and the second through fourth metatarsal bases. It is the principle inverter of the foot and helps maintain the longitudinal arch. As a rule of thumb, the normal posterior tibial tendon should be no greater than twice the diameter of the other tendons at the ankle, with the exception of the Achilles tendon. The flexor digitorum longus tendon also courses in the groove found in the medial malleolus, and acts as a pulley continuing through the tarsal tunnel to insert on the second to fifth distal phalanges. The flexor hallucis longus passes beneath the sustentaculum tali of the calcaneus using its groove as a pulley and continues between the two sesamoid bones of the hallux to insert on the base of the first distal phalanx. The muscle and musculotendinous junction of the flexor hallucis longus is found more distally than the other flexor tendons, and can usually be found at the level of the ankle joint line. The peroneal tendons are found posterolaterally at the ankle. Both tendons pass behind the lateral malleolus within a groove, where they are confined by the peroneal retinaculum. The peroneus longus is found posteromedial to the peroneus

brevis. The peroneus brevis inserts on the fifth metatarsal base, and the peroneus longus extends beneath the midfoot to insert on the first metatarsal base. The peroneus longus contributes to maintaining the longitudinal arch of the foot. The extensor tendons are found anteriorly at the ankle, and from medial to lateral consist of the tibialis anterior, extensor hallucis longus, extensor digitorum longus (pneumonic: Tom, Harry, and Dick), and peroneus tertius tendons (Fig. 14-4). These tendons are confined by the anterior extensor retinaculum. The tibialis anterior inserts on the medial and inferomedial base of the first metatarsal bone. The extensor hallucis longus inserts on the dorsal base of the distal phalanx of the hallux (great toe). The extensor digitorum longus inserts on the dorsal bases of the second through fifth distal phalanges, and the peroneus tertius inserts on the dorsal base of the fifth metatarsal.

TRAUMA PATTERNS

Ankle injuries are extremely common and the most common cause for trauma-associated radiographic evaluation in emergency departments in the United States. In general, the presence of an ankle joint effusion or soft tissue swelling should prompt a search for underlying fracture, particularly if the patient is unable to bear weight. In the ankle, effusion is seen on the lateral film as an anteriorly convex soft tissue density at the ankle joint (Fig. 14-5). Soft tissue swelling may be evident over the medial and lateral malleoli as well as in the fat posterior

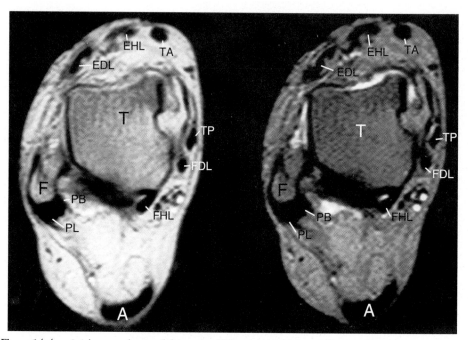

Figure 14-4   Axial proton density *(left image)* and T2-weighted *(right image)* spin-echo MR images of ankle show the tibialis posterior (TP), flexor digitorum longus (FDL), and flexor hallucis longus (FHL) tendons of the posterior compartment. The anterior compartment tendons are the tibialis anterior (TA), extensor hallucis longus (EHL), and extensor digitorum longus (EDL) tendons. Note also peroneus brevis (PB) and peroneus longus (PL) tendons and Achilles tendon (A). T, talus; F, fibula.

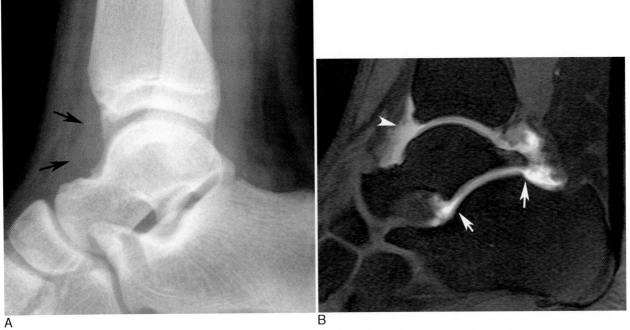

Figure 14-5   **A,** Lateral radiograph shows soft tissue density in shape of teardrop *(arrows)* anterior to ankle joint, indicating an ankle effusion. This may be the only finding of an intra-articular fracture. **B,** MR arthrogram shows similar findings with ankle joint distention. Sagittal fat-suppressed T1-weighted MR image also shows contrast medium injected into the ankle joint *(arrowhead)* communicates freely with the posterior subtalar facet joint *(arrows).* This is a common normal variant.

to the ankle. This posterior fat is known as the pre-Achilles triangle and is usually sharply circumscribed at its margin with the Achilles tendon. Obscuration of the margins of the fat triangle in the setting of trauma indicates soft tissue swelling.

Several classifications are used in the assessment of ankle fractures. The *Weber (AO) classification* is simple to use and correlates well with treatment and prognosis. It is based on determining the level of fibular fracture to deduce the injury to the tibiofibular ligaments. A Weber A injury is a transverse avulsion fracture of the lateral malleolus at or distal to the ankle joint (see Fig. 1-13A). There may be associated fracture of the medial malleolus. In type A injury, the tibiofibular ligaments and syndesmosis are intact. This fracture is caused by ankle supination, with avulsion of the tip of the lateral malleolus. Weber B injury represents oblique fractures of the lateral malleolus beginning at the level of the ankle joint. This injury pattern is usually caused by supination–external rotation or pronation. The important point with type B injury is that the tibiofibular ligaments are partially disrupted. These injuries may be associated with fractures of the medial malleolus below the ankle joint or with deltoid ligament rupture (see Fig. 14-1D). Weber C injury represents fibular fracture proximal to the level of the ankle joint. This involves tear of the tibiofibular ligaments and tibiofibular syndesmosis. This injury is usually due to pronation–external rotation. A proximal fibular fracture indicates a *Maisonneuve fracture* with syndesmosis tear to the level of the fracture (Fig. 14-6).

Key Concepts	Ankle Fractures: Weber (AO) Classification

Based on location of distal fibular fracture relative to tibiotalar joint.

Weber A:
    Transverse fracture distal to the ankle joint.
    Usual mechanism: Supination.
    Major ligaments usually intact.

Weber B:
    Oblique fracture at level of ankle joint.
    Usual mechanism: Supination–external rotation or pronation.
    Partial disruption of the tibiofibular ligaments.
    May require surgery.

Weber C:
    Proximal to the level of ankle joint.
    Usual mechanism: pronation–external rotation.
    More extensive ligament disruption.
    Usually requires surgery.

The more sophisticated *Lauge-Hansen classification* is based on the mechanism of forces that result in fractures at the ankle. This consideration is useful because an understanding of the forces producing injury indicates the direction of forces required for fracture reduction (reverse of the mechanism of

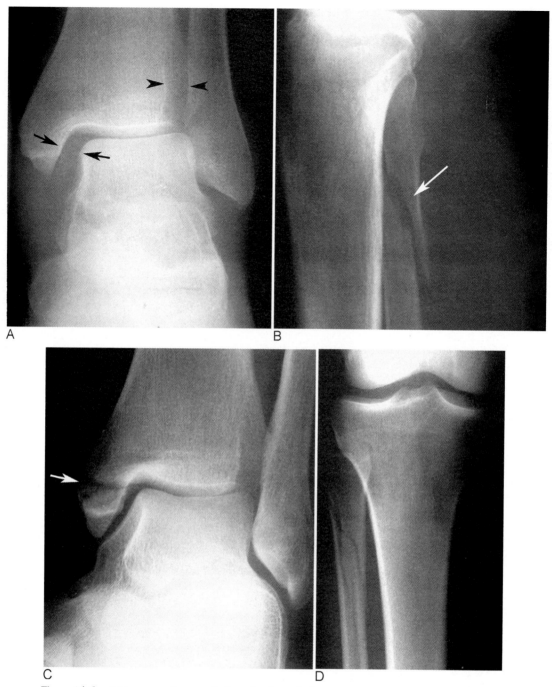

Figure 14-6   Maisonneuve fractures. **A,** Frontal radiograph demonstrates widening of ankle joint space at medial ankle mortise *(arrows),* indicating deltoid ligament tear. Also note widened tibia-fibula syndesmosis (between *arrowheads*). **B,** Lateral view of proximal leg demonstrates oblique fracture of proximal fibular diametaphysis *(arrow).* **C and D,** Different patient with a slightly different pattern of Maisonneuve fracture, with transverse fracture of the medial malleolus *(arrow* in part C), but still with characteristic widening of the distal tibia-fibula syndesmosis and proximal fibular shaft fracture (shown in part D).

injury). Five basic patterns of force can result in ankle fracture: axial loading, supination, supination–external rotation, pronation, and pronation–external rotation. Supination refers to plantar flexion of the ankle, inversion of the hindfoot, and adduction of the foot, whereas pronation refers to dorsiflexion of the ankle, eversion of the hindfoot, and abduction of the

foot. Either supination or pronation may be isolated or associated with external rotation. It is useful to be mindful of the fracture pattern in the fibula in each of these injury patterns because the fibular fracture pattern in each injury will be unique. For each fracture pattern, the ankle mortise is carefully assessed for any evidence of loss of parallel margins because this implies extensive ligament and osseous disruption resulting in ankle instability. In considering the Lauge-Hansen classification, injury stages are sequential with lowest-stage injury patterns being found before the higher-stage injuries; with a higher stage of injury, there is increasing severity of bone and/or ligament injury, along with instability.

In pure *supination,* tension is placed on the fibula resulting in either a tear of the lateral collateral ligament or a low transverse avulsion fracture of the lateral malleolus (Fig. 1-13A). This is considered a stage 1 injury. Stage 2 injury includes the findings at stage 1 injury, with the addition of a vertically oriented fracture of the medial malleolus.

Supination–external rotation is the most common injury pattern at the ankle, accounting for nearly three fourths of all ankle injuries. In supination–external rotation, the lateral wall of the distal talar pole impacts the anterior wall of the lateral malleolus, driving it posteriorly. This results in an oblique fracture oriented in the coronal plane that is best seen on the lateral view of the ankle (Fig. 14-7). Stage 1 supination–external rotation injury represents disruption of the anterior distal tibiofibular ligament. Stage 2 injury includes stage 1 findings plus the distal fibular fracture. Stage 3 findings include findings from stages 1 and 2 plus a tear of the posterior distal tibiofibular ligament versus fracture of the posterior malleolus (avulsion of posterior distal tibiofibular ligament insertion). Stage 4 injury represents findings at stages 1 to 3 plus transverse fracture of the medial malleolus.

In *pronation,* the lateral wall of the proximal talar pole impacts the medial wall of the lateral malleolus, driving it laterally. This results in an oblique fracture of the lateral malleolus oriented in the sagittal plane, which is best shown on the frontal view of the ankle (Fig. 14-1D). There are three stages of pronation injury. Stage 1 is that of an avulsion of the medial malleolus versus a tear of the deltoid ligaments. Stage 2 represents stage 1 findings plus rupture of the anterior and posterior distal tibiofibular ligaments. Stage 3 represents stage 1 and 2 findings plus the fibular fracture. Thus, demonstration of a sagittally oriented oblique fracture of the fibula indicates the most severe form of pronation injury.

In *pronation–external rotation,* talar impaction at both lateral and anterior fibular surfaces results in a spiraling force through the tibiofibular syndesmosis with forces exiting through the fibula at a point more proximal to the ankle joint (see Fig. 14-6). There are four stages of pronation-external rotation injury. Stage 1 injury involves avulsion of the medial malleolus or a deltoid ligament tear. Stage 2 represents stage 1 findings plus tear of the anterior distal tibiofibular ligament and the tibiofibular syndesmosis. Stage 3 represents stage 1 and 2 findings plus the fibular fracture. Stage 4 injury represents the findings from stages 1 to 3 plus tear of the posterior distal tibiofibular ligament versus posterior malleolar fracture. Therefore, if medial malleolar swelling is demonstrated and there is posterior malleolar fracture, absence of visualization of a fibular fracture on an ankle film implies a more proximal fibular fracture, prompting search with leg radiography.

In the skeletally immature, fusion of the distal tibial epiphysis begins at 12 to 13 years of age, beginning at a superior convexity in the growth plate known as *Kump's bump* (or the Bump of Kump if you prefer Dr. Seuss; Fig. 14-8), which is located in the anterior-medial quadrant of the physis, and proceeding medially and laterally. Children in this age range are prone to lateral Salter-Harris fractures during physeal closure. One such

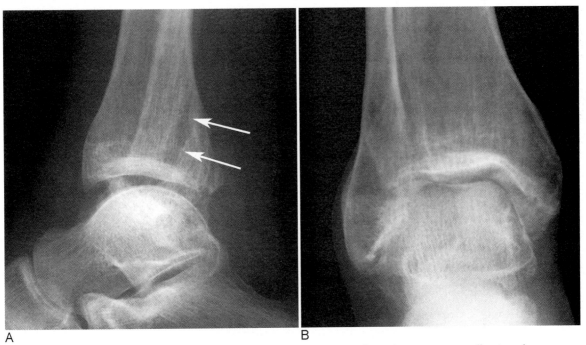

A   B

Figure 14-7 Supination–external rotation injury at ankle. **A,** Lateral view demonstrates coronally oriented oblique fracture of distal fibula. **B,** Note absence of visualization of fracture on frontal view.

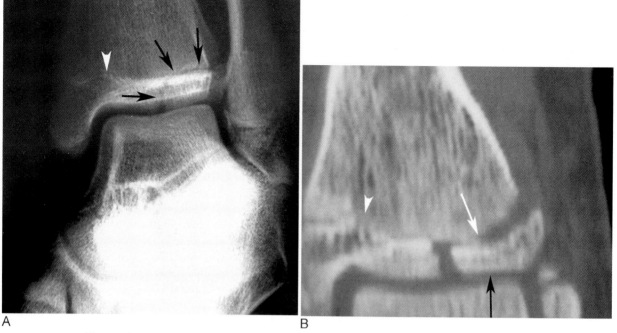

Figure 14-8   Tillaux fracture. **A,** Frontal radiograph demonstrates Salter-Harris III (epiphyseal) fracture of lateral tibial plafond *(arrows)*. **B,** Coronally reformatted CT image shows same fracture *(arrows)*. Note the articular surface diastasis, which required surgical reduction. In both images, note Kump's bump medially *(arrowhead)*, a proximal undulation of the distal tibial physis that fuses before the remainder of the physis.

fracture is known as the *juvenile Tillaux fracture,* or simply Tillaux fracture, which is a Salter-Harris III fracture of the lateral portion of the distal tibial epiphysis, sparing the fused medial portion of the epiphysis (see Fig. 14-8). It relates to avulsion of the anterior and posterior distal tibiofibular ligaments. Fracture displacement of more than 2 mm or articular incongruence indicates the need for surgical intervention. A *triplane fracture* is the other growth plate fracture at the ankle, and involves the lateral half of the distal tibial epiphysis and a posterior triangular metaphyseal fragment. This is a Salter-Harris IV fracture. The term "triplane" indicates the three planes of the fracture, coronal-oblique through the posterior distal tibial metaphysis, horizontal through the tibial growth plate, and sagittal through the tibial epiphysis (Fig. 14-9). There are two types. If a triplane fracture occurs after the medial portion of the epiphysis has fused, the medial malleolus remains intact and a two-fragment triplane fracture results. If the triplane fracture occurs before the epiphysis begins to fuse, there may be a three-fragment fracture. With either type, the appearance of a triplane fracture consists of a combination of a Tillaux fracture and Salter-Harris II fracture. Other growth plate injury patterns at the ankle occur, including Salter-Harris II and other Salter-Harris IV fractures of the distal tibia and fibula (Fig. 14-10). Salter-Harris V fractures are uncommon and a result of axial loading.

It is important to include the base of the fifth metatarsal on images of the ankle because metatarsal fractures may clinically mimic ankle fractures (Fig. 14-11). Fractures at the base of the

fifth metatarsal are due to avulsion of the insertion of the peroneus brevis tendon. There is variable distraction of the avulsed fracture fragment, with retraction occasionally extending to the level of ankle and lateral ankle pain. Lateral and frontal views are both useful for detection of fifth metatarsal base fractures. It is also useful to observe the anterior process of the calcaneus, as this is a site of missed fractures.

Axial loading results in intra-articular fractures of the tibial plafond. The talar dome acts like a wedge, driving the fragments apart. These are called *pilon* fractures (Fig. 14-12). Axial forces result in severe distal tibial comminution, while the malleoli usually maintain an anatomic relationship with the talus. Talar fractures may coexist. Pilon fractures are classified as type 1 (nondisplaced), type 2 (moderately displaced), and type 3 (severely displaced and impacted).

Fatigue fractures may occur at the ankle, especially among skeletally immature runners, seen occasionally as Salter I injuries with widening and irregular contour of the distal fibular growth plate (Fig. 14-13), or in adults as linear bands of lucency or sclerosis (depending on the age of healing) in the distal tibial metaphysis 3 to 4 cm proximal to the level of the tibial plafond (Fig. 14-14) or distal fibula 3 to 7 cm from the tip of the lateral malleolus (Fig. 14-15). Insufficiency fractures may simultaneously occur in the distal tibia and fibula.

Instability is a common complication of ankle injury. Stress films with varus and valgus force applied to the calcaneus and anterior drawer stress (which is anterior force applied to the calcaneal tuberosity) are useful for determining laxity in the

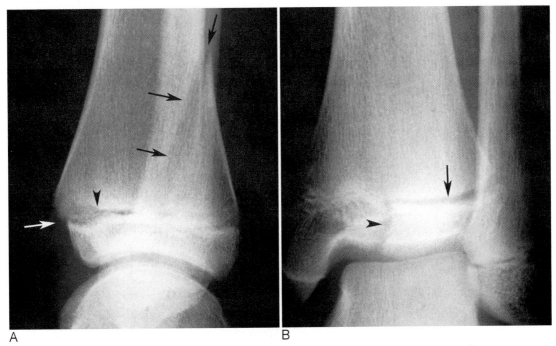

Figure 14-9   Triplane fracture. **A,** Lateral ankle radiograph shows coronally oriented fracture of posterior aspect of distal tibial metaphysis *(black arrows)* and transverse fracture through anterior growth plate *(arrowhead).* Note posterior displacement of the distal fragment, seen as a stepoff anteriorly at the physeal fracture line *(white arrow).* **B,** Frontal radiograph demonstrates sagittally oriented epiphyseal fracture *(arrowhead)* and transversely oriented physeal fracture *(arrow).*

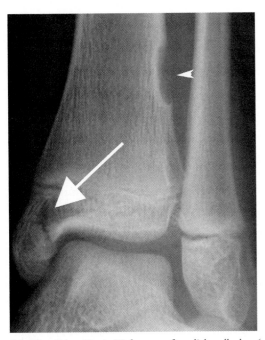

Figure 14-10   Salter-Harris III fracture of medial malleolus *(arrow).* Note the well-circumscribed lytic lesion in the lateral tibial cortex *(arrowhead).* This is an incidental fibrous cortical defect, also termed a fibroxanthoma or nonossifying fibroma (see Chapter 33 for further discussion of this lesion).

ankle joint (see Fig. 2-2). Medial talar tilt (varus) on stress radiographs is normally less than 10 to 12 degrees, and anterior drawer is usually less than 1 cm. However, it is important to compare with the contralateral side because congenital laxity is sometimes present. In general, varus greater than 15 degrees strongly suggests lateral collateral ligament injury, and anterior talar displacement greater than 1 cm indicates injury to the anterior talofibular ligament.

Although rarely used, conventional arthrography is helpful for detecting ligament injury. Ordinarily, contrast medium opacifies the ankle joint, the posterior subtalar joint, and occasionally the tendon sheath of the flexor hallucis longus. If contrast medium extends around the tip of the fibula, a tear of the anterior talofibular ligament is present. Filling of the peroneal tendon sheath indicates a tear of the calcaneofibular ligament. If contrast medium is found in the tibiofibular syndesmosis above the level of the ankle joint, a tear of the anterior distal tibiofibular ligament is suggested. It should be noted that anterior talofibular ligament tears precede other lateral collateral ligament injuries in supination–external rotation and supination.

A final fracture of the ankle to consider is osteochondral injury (see Fig. 1-16). Osteochondral injury may involve the medial or lateral talar dome, especially in patients with ligament laxity, and is sometimes considered a form of osteochondritis dissecans. As discussed in Chapter 3, the critical diagnostic

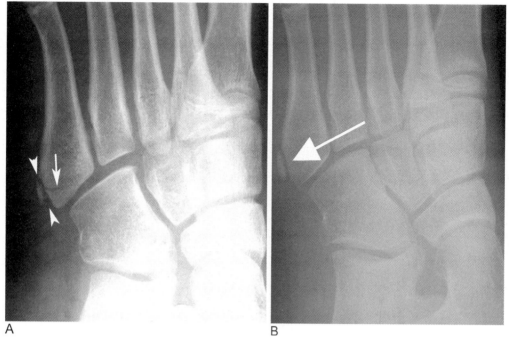

Figure 14-11   Fracture at base of fifth metatarsal. **A,** Oblique foot radiograph demonstrates transverse fracture *(arrow)*. Fractures at this site are *transverse,* not to be confused with the *sagittally* oriented physis for the lateral apophysis *(arrowheads),* which is a normal finding. **B,** Normal apophysis and associated growth plate *(arrow).*

consideration with such fractures is the grade of injury and the stability of the osteochondral fragment. This is assessed by determining the integrity of the overlying articular cartilage and signal characteristics of the junction of the osteochondritis dissecans fragment and the underlying bone, which can be

performed with MR sequences sensitive to imaging articular cartilage or with MR arthrography.

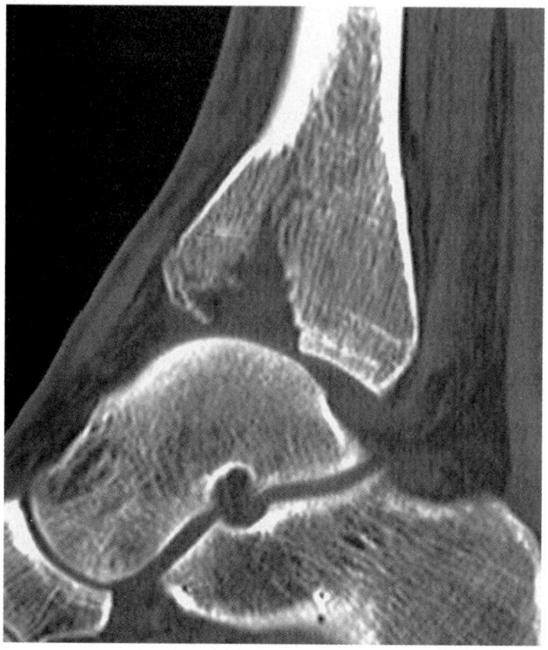

The ankle mortise may be widened by ligament injuries, fractures, or both. Most often, the talus maintains a normal anatomic relation with the lateral malleolus. Because of the saddle shape of the talar dome, even minimal lateral subluxation of the talus relative to the tibial plafond can significantly reduce the articular contact area of the tibiotalar joint. Pain and early osteoarthritis can result.

Figure 14-12   Pilon fracture. Sagittal CT reconstruction shows coronally oriented intra-articular fracture of the distal tibia with diastasis.

TENDON INJURY

Tendon abnormalities at the ankle and hindfoot are primarily degenerative disorders of multifactorial origin. Age, chronic repetitive overuse injury, and certain congenital predispositions such as anomalous muscle insertions and bone dysplasias each play a role. With repetitive injury and repair, tendons undergo mucoid degeneration and hyalinization, which eventually can result in tendon rupture.

The Achilles tendon is the most commonly injured tendon at the ankle. Normally, its anteroposterior (AP) dimension is no more than 8-mm thick, and its anterior margins are concave or flat. Achilles tendinitis is common among runners and jumpers. Acutely, the tendon margins are inflamed, resulting in blurring on radiography between the anterior Achilles tendon margin and the adjacent pre-Achilles fat. The Achilles tendon does not have a tendon sheath. The surface of the tendon is covered with peritenon, which may become inflamed if the tendon is injured. At MRI, peritendinitis is shown by fluid-

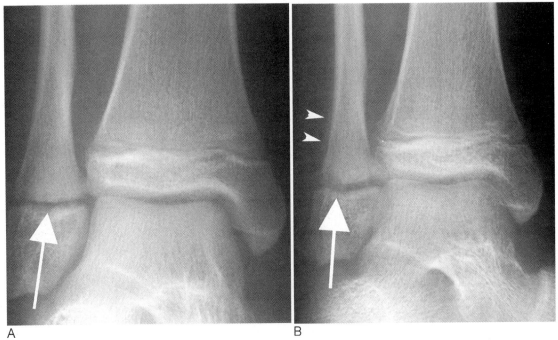

Figure 14-13   Stress fracture of distal fibular physis. **A,** Initial radiograph demonstrates only minimal irregularity of distal fibular growth plate *(arrow)*. **B,** Radiograph obtained 3 weeks later demonstrates interval widening and irregularity of growth plate of distal fibula *(arrow),* indicating partial healing. Note periosteal new bone along distal fibular shaft *(arrowheads)*.

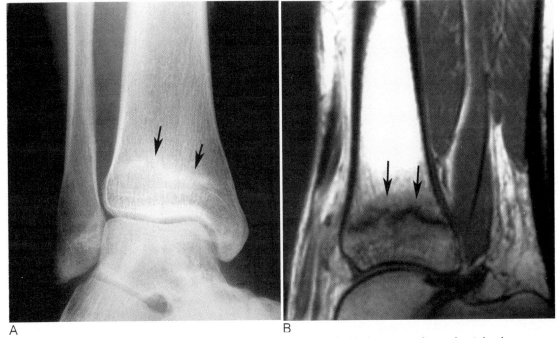

Figure 14-14   Distal tibial stress fractures. **A,** Oblique radiograph of ankle demonstrates linear sclerotic band *(arrows)* related to healing stress fracture. **B,** Sagittal T1-weighted MR image demonstrates linear band of low signal intensity representing fracture line *(arrows),* surrounded by poorly defined zone of low-signal-intensity edema *(arrowheads)*. (Part B adapted and reproduced with permission from Aerts P, Disler DG: Abnormalities of the foot and ankle: MR imaging findings. AJR 165:119–124, 1995.)

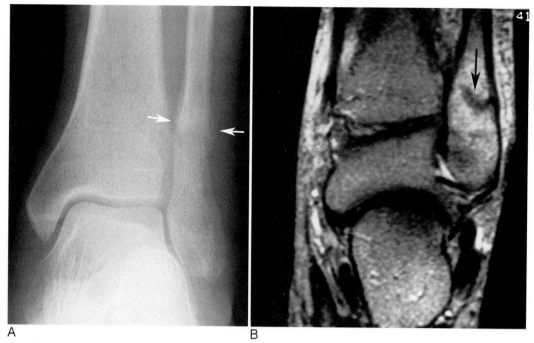

Figure 14-15   Distal fibular stress fractures **A,** AP radiograph shows transverse sclerosis of the distal fibular diaphysis with solid periosteal reaction *(arrows)*. **B,** Coronal T2-weighted spin-echo MR image in another patient demonstrates incomplete, curved, low-signal-intensity stress fracture *(arrow)* with surrounding marrow edema.

like signal in the peritendinous region (Fig. 14-16). Recurrent bouts of tendinitis and peritendinitis result in enlargement of the tendon (Fig. 14-17). Acute ruptures are superimposed on chronic tendinopathy, occurring most commonly in middle-aged men who are involved in sporadic exercise (the weekend

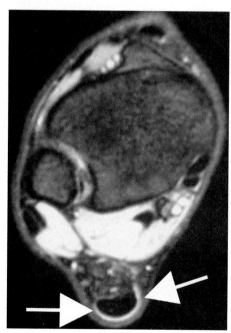

Figure 14-16   Achilles peritendinitis. Axial fat-suppressed T2-weighted MR image shows high signal intensity *(arrows)* surrounding Achilles tendon due to peritendinous edema.

warrior), or sports involving running or jumping (Fig. 14-18). Rupture also may be seen in individuals with weakened tendons as a result of systemic diseases such as rheumatoid arthritis, renal disease, and diabetes, or as a result of long-term steroid use. The most typical location of partial or complete Achilles tendon rupture is 2 to 6 cm proximal to the calcaneal insertion. This is a relatively avascular zone. Partial ruptures may be either within the substance or marginal in location, and may be either transverse or longitudinal in orientation. Chronic overuse may also manifest as dystrophic calcification or ossification within the distal tendon, occasionally requiring surgical debridement in high-level athletes.

The plantaris tendon, which originates from the lateral femoral condyle, and which inserts anterior to the Achilles tendon on the calcaneal tuberosity, is important to know about for two reasons. First, an intact plantaris tendon in the setting of a complete Achilles tear may mimic a partially intact Achilles tendon on both clinical and radiologic grounds. Clinically, with an intact plantaris tendon, the patient may still be able to plantarflex the ankle, suggesting a partially intact Achilles tendon. Radiologically, the plantaris tendon may mimic intact anteromedial Achilles tendon fibers by its similar anatomic course, although the anteromedial location of the plantaris tendon at the calcaneus should provide a clue to its origin. Plantaris tear may be seen more proximally on MR images as edema or hemorrhage between the gastrocnemius medial head and the medial soleus in the proximal leg (Fig. 14-19).

Nontraumatic causes of thickening of the Achilles tendon may also occur. An accessory soleus muscle may mimic

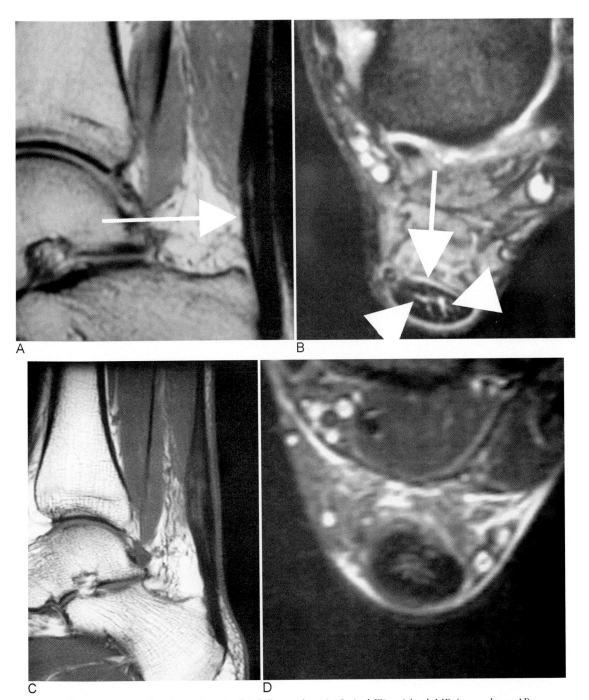

Figure 14-17 Chronic tendinosis of Achilles tendon. **A,** Sagittal T1-weighted MR image shows AP thickening of Achilles tendon *(arrow)* with central vertically oriented increased signal, indicating longitudinal interstitial tear. **B,** Axial gradient-echo MR image shows convex anterior margin of Achilles tendon with mild peritendinous increased signal *(arrow)* and central tendinous increased signal *(arrowheads)* related to interstitial tear. **C and D,** Sagittal T1-weighted (C) and axial inversion recovery (D) MR images in another patient with chronic tendinosis of the Achilles tendon show substantial thickening of the tendon, convex anterior margin of tendon, and substantial intratendinous signal. Note the characteristic longitudinal location of the tendinopathy in both cases, centered in the midportion of the tendon.

(Continued)

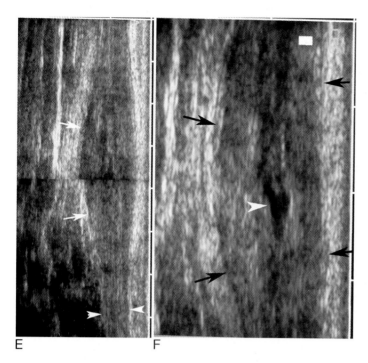

E   F

Figure 14-17—(Cont'd) **E,** US findings. Sagittal composite image oriented to match sagittal MR imaging (MRI) orientation, with anterior to the viewer's left, shows thickened tendon *(arrows)* with areas of hypoechogenicity. Note normal distal tendon *(arrowheads)*. **F,** More severe tendinopathy in a different patient, with thick tendon *(arrows)* and anechoic fluid collection in the tendon *(white arrowhead)*.

Achilles tendon thickening, although the signal at MRI of the accessory soleus is that of muscle and not of tendon. After surgery, the Achilles tendon may appear thickened and retain areas of high signal. A thickened Achilles tendon may also be seen with xanthomas, which occur in the setting of familial hyperlipidemias. The appearance is of marked tendon enlargement; heterogeneously mixed low- and intermediate-signal masses; and stippled, linear areas of central low signal intensity (Fig. 14-20). Multiple tendons may be affected, although the Achilles is the most common.

Peritendinous edema, retrocalcaneal bursitis, and thickening with heterogeneous signal in the distal Achilles are seen in *Haglund's disease* (Fig. 14-21). This disorder is often caused by

Figure 14-18 Achilles tendon rupture. Sagittal fat-suppressed T2-weighted MR image in a rugby player with an acute Achilles rupture *(arrow)*. Note the marrow edema at the anterior ankle due to hyperextension at the time of the Achilles rupture *(arrowheads)*. See also Figure 2-10A.

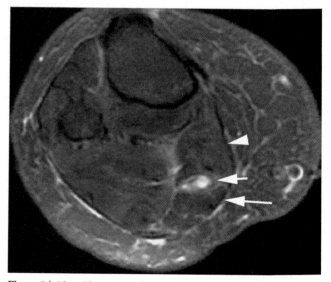

Figure 14-19 Plantaris tendon tear. Axial fat-suppressed T2-weighted MR image in the proximal leg shows high signal intensity at the tear *(short arrow)* between gastrocnemius medial head *(arrowhead)* and medial soleus *(long arrow)*. (Courtesy of William Pommersheim, MD.)

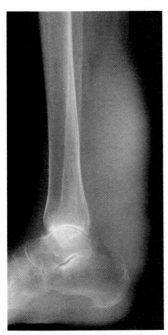

Figure 14-20   Xanthomatosis of the Achilles tendon due to familial hyperlipidemia. Note the extraordinary tendon enlargement.

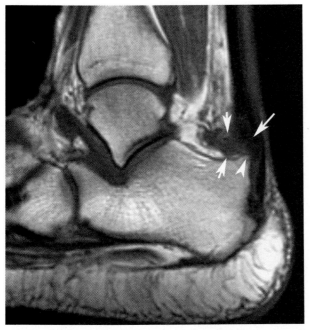

Figure 14-21   Haglund's disease. Sagittal T1-weighted MR image shows overgrowth of the proximal calcaneus *(arrowhead)* with tear of the adjacent Achilles tendon *(long arrow)* and retrocalcaneal bursal distention *(short arrows)*.

ill-fitting shoes that compress the distal Achilles tendon. Bony overgrowth of the proximal posterior calcaneus also is associated with this condition.

The second most common site of ankle tendinosis is the posterior tibial tendon (PTT). The PTT contributes to maintaining the longitudinal and transverse arches of the foot.

Posterior tibial tendinopathy is most common among women older than 50 years of age, usually with a clinical picture of an acute painful flatfoot that progressively worsens. The pathologic process is slow stretching of the PTT due to accumulated microtears. Plain radiographs may reveal flatfoot and lateral subluxation of the navicular, exposing the medial distal articular surface of the talar head. A clinician standing behind the patient can observe the "too many toes sign," which is seeing most of the patient's toes due to lateral subluxation of the navicular and forefoot. As with other tendinopathies, predisposing conditions include rheumatoid arthritis, renal failure, diabetes, steroid use, and chronic overuse. Ultrasonography (US) may show tendon thickening, tendon sheath fluid, or loss of the normal tendon echogenicity. The equivalent MRI findings are tendon thickening, tendon sheath fluid, and increased tendon signal on T2-weighted images. As noted previously, the PTT should not have more than twice the cross-sectional area of the adjacent flexor digitorum longus tendon. Another useful guide is that the thickness of the PTT should be no more than the combined thicknesses of the peroneus longus and brevis tendons (Fig. 14-22).

There are several pitfalls in diagnosis of PTT tendinosis. The tendon normally broadens at the PTT insertion, where it may normally be larger than the guidelines noted previously. The tendon may falsely appear thickened on T1-weighted images because of fluid in the tendon sheath. Review of T2-weighted images will avoid this pitfall. Magic angle effect can cause heterogeneous signal within any tendon on short echo time sequences (e.g., gradient echo, T1, and proton density) at the locations where the tendon is aligned at approximately 55 degrees relative to the main magnetic field. This often occurs where ankle tendons curve around the malleoli at the ankle. Thus, when one is unsure of magic angle versus tendinopathy on a T1-weighted or a proton density-weighted sequence, rely on a T2-weighted sequence or change the angle of the foot in the scanner. The echogenicity of the tendon on US is highly dependent on transducer position, and subtle changes in transducer position can falsely suggest tendinosis as the tendon curves around the medial malleolus (Fig. 14-23, 14-24).

Anomalies of the navicular insertion site can predispose to posterior tibial tendinosis. These include the presence of an *accessory navicular (os tibiale externum)*. An accessory navicular is a large ossicle closely apposed to the medial pole of the navicular bone. With an accessory navicular, the posterior tibial tendon often inserts solely on the ossicle without continuing distally to insert on the plantar surfaces of the cuneiforms and the metatarsal bases. An associated pain syndrome may be caused by traction between the ossicle and the navicular bone. Classic findings include a jagged, edematous pseudoarticulation between the ossicle and the navicular bone, best seen at MRI (Fig. 14-25).

Among the other flexors of the ankle, injury is rare with the exception of the flexor hallucis longus (Fig. 14-26), where occasionally injury may be seen in ballet dancers as a result of

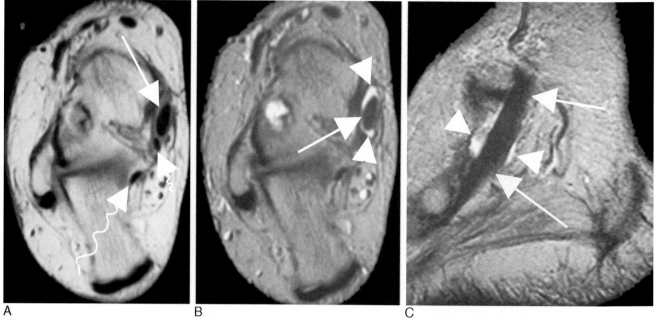

Figure 14-22   Posterior tibialis tendon mild tendinosis. **A and B,** Axial proton density (A) and T2-weighted (B) spin-echo MR images show enlargement of inframalleolar posterior tibial tendon *(arrow)* and tendon sheath fluid *(arrowheads)*. Note the substantial degree of enlargement of the posterior tibialis tendon relative to other tendons at the ankle. Curved long arrow points to flexor hallucis longus tendon, and curved short arrow points to flexor digitorum longus tendon. **C,** Sagittal T2-weighted MR image shows thickened posterior tibialis tendon *(arrows)* and tendon sheath fluid *(arrowheads)*. (Parts A and C adapted and reproduced with permission from Aerts P, Disler DG: Abnormalities of the foot and ankle: MR imaging findings. AJR 165:119–124, 1995.)

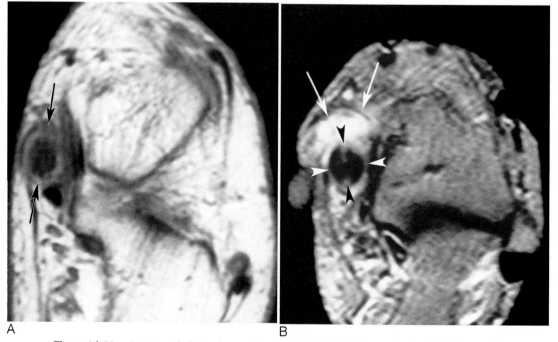

Figure 14-23   Posterior tibialis tendon: moderate tendinosis. **A,** Axial proton density MR image shows marked thickening of tendon *(arrows)*. **B,** T2-weighted spin-echo MR image shows that a great deal of the appearance of tendon thickening in part A is actually due to tendon sheath fluid *(arrows)*. However, substantial tendon thickening *(white arrowheads)* is still shown. Also note the cleft *(black arrowheads)* in the tendon, indicating a longitudinal tear.

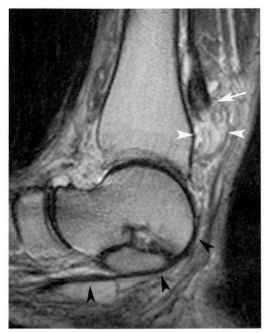

Figure 14-24   Posterior tibialis tendon: complete tear. Sagittal T2-weighted MR image shows retracted torn tendon posterior to the distal tibial metaphysis *(arrow)*. Note fluid around the tendon margin *(white arrowheads)*. Also note normal flexor hallucis longus coursing below the sustentaculum tali *(black arrowheads)*. See also Figure 2-10B.

the repetitive pushoff from the forefoot or from impingement against the os trigonum (see Fig. 15-3). Fluid within the tendon sheath of the flexor hallucis longus does not necessarily indicate the presence to tenosynovitis, because in 20% of the population there is normally free communication of joint fluid between the ankle joint and the flexor hallucis longus tendon sheath. However, disproportionately increased fluid within the tendon sheath helps make the diagnosis.

The peroneal tendons are the third most commonly injured tendons at the ankle. The peroneus quartus is an occasionally demonstrated accessory muscle that originates from the muscular portion of the peroneus brevis, the peroneus longus, or the fibula, and inserts on the peroneal tubercle of the calcaneus, which is located laterally along the calcaneal tuberosity. Tendinopathy is more common in the peroneus brevis, and is most commonly affected with a pattern known as *split peroneus brevis syndrome,* which refers to longitudinal tearing of this tendon. The term "peroneal splits" is also used to describe this finding. With this disorder, the peroneus brevis, which is normally the more anteriorly located tendon, is impinged between the peroneus longus and the fibula (Figs. 14-27, 14-28). In extreme cases, the peroneus brevis splits longitudinally, with the nearly parallel peroneus longus positioned between the split halves of the peroneus brevis. In milder cases, the peroneus brevis tendon may assume a boomerang or U-shaped cross-sectional contour (Fig. 14-28B).

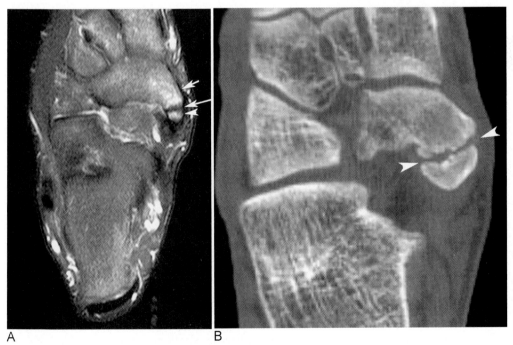

A   B

Figure 14-25   Symptomatic accessory navicular. **A,** Axial inversion recovery MR image shows marrow edema in an os naviculare *(arrowhead)* and adjacent navicular bone *(short arrow)*, with irregular margin between the two *(long arrow)*. **B,** Axial CT image in a different patient shows irregular margin *(arrowheads)* between the os and the navicular.

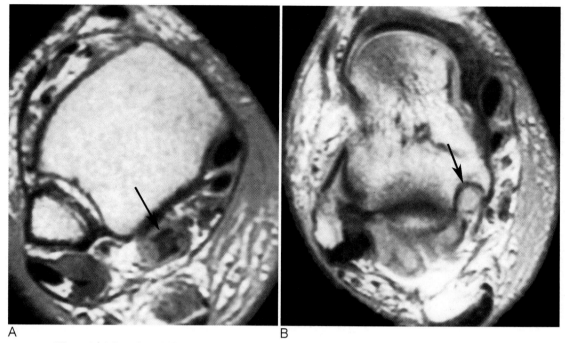

Figure 14-26   Flexor hallucis longus tendon tear. **A,** Axial proton density MR image shows marked tendon thickening at level of distal tibial epiphysis *(arrow)*. **B,** More distal image shows only fluid signal intensity and absence of tendon in expected groove in the posterolateral talus *(arrow)*. Findings indicate grade III tendinosis (tendon rupture).

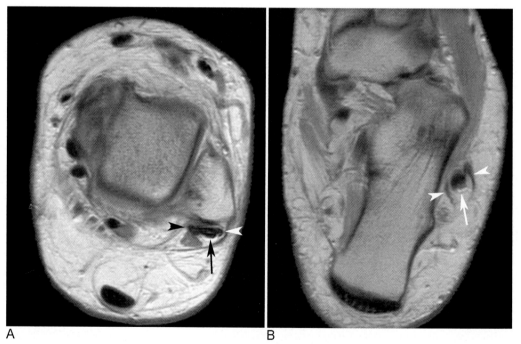

Figure 14-27   Peroneus brevis tendon tears. **A,** Axial proton density MR image at the level of the lateral malleolus shows flat peroneus brevis tendon *(arrowheads)*. Note peroneus longus tendon *(arrow)*. Also note the convex posterior margin of the lateral malleolus, which increases the risk of peroneal tendon subluxation. **B,** More distal image shows peroneus longus tendon *(arrow)* between longitudinally split peroneus brevis tendon *(arrowheads)*.

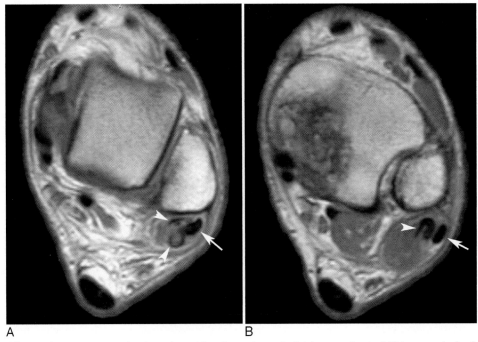

Figure 14-28   Peroneus brevis tendon subluxation and tear. **A,** Axial proton density MR image at the level of the lateral malleolus shows torn brevis tendon *(arrowheads)*, with one portion posterior to the peroneus longus tendon *(arrow)*. **B,** More proximal image shows U-shaped peroneus brevis tendon *(arrowheads)* medial to the peroneus longus tendon *(arrow)*.

This syndrome may develop on account of several factors, among them a tight compartment resulting from an accessory muscle, an abnormally distal position of the peroneus longus or brevis muscle bellies, dysplasia of the adjacent fibula, or peroneal subluxation (Fig. 14-29). Normally, the posterior

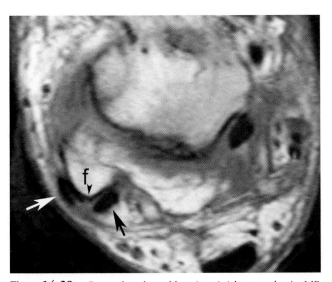

Figure 14-29   Peroneal tendon subluxation. Axial proton density MR image shows longitudinally torn peroneus brevis *(white arrow)* subluxed laterally and anteriorly from its normal position adjacent to the peroneus longus *(black arrow)*. Note that the distal fibula has a rounded contour *(small black arrowhead)*, a finding that can be associated with peroneal subluxation. f, fibula.

margin of the fibula is concave and forms a retromalleolar groove where it contacts the peroneal tendons. If the posterior margin is convex, the tendons are prone to sublux laterally during plantar flexion of the ankle. Occasionally, a hook may be seen posterolaterally in the fibula, which further predisposes to split peroneus brevis. The overlying peroneal retinaculum may avulse during forced plantar flexion, further leading to tendon subluxation or dislocation.

The peroneal tendons are prone to stenosing tenosynovitis, which is difficult to diagnose radiologically unless tendon sheath contrast medium is administered. In this disorder, contrast within the tendon sheath appears cut off or beaded rather than continuous.

It is important to recognize the occasional presence of the peroneus quartus muscle. This muscle and tendon can give an appearance suggesting a peroneus tendon longitudinal tear because fat is present between the accessory structure and the adjacent normal peroneus tendons. It can be recognized by following the course of the accessory tendon to its insertion at the peroneal tubercle of the calcaneal tuberosity rather than continuing into the midfoot as do the peroneus longus and brevis. The peroneus quartus may be responsible for peroneus longus and brevis tendinopathy because the accessory muscle and tendon cause impingement. Accessory muscles at the ankle are very common, occurring in 8% of the population. They are important to recognize because they may mimic tendinopathy, occasionally cause impingement within compartments, and may become symptomatic with exercise because of tenuous blood supply.

Extensor tendon injury is quite rare, and is usually diagnosed clinically because the anteriorly positioned extensor tendons are more easily assessed with physical examination than are the posterior and peroneal tendons. The anterior tibial tendon is occasionally injured in downhill runners and hikers but rarely progresses to complete rupture.

LIGAMENT INJURY

Ankle ligament injury is far more common than tendon injury. It is typically a result of acute ankle trauma, unlike tendon injury, which is usually a result of chronic repetitive microtrauma. Ligament injuries were extensively discussed under the Lauge-Hansen classification of ankle trauma, but a few points are discussed here. First, as supination–external rotation is the most common injury at the ankle, the most commonly injured ligaments are the lateral collateral ligaments. Among the lateral collateral ligaments, the anterior talofibular (ATF) ligament is most commonly torn. In fact, if the ATF is intact, then the other lateral collateral ligaments are almost always intact as well. The ATF ligament is often the best-shown ligament on MRI and US. Nonvisualization of this ligament on MR images or wavy, lax fibers with surrounding edema usually indicate the presence of ligament sprain, particularly if supporting findings of injury, such as ankle effusion, lateral edema, and swelling, are seen acutely (Fig. 14-30). Tears of the ATF ligament frequently heal, but with thickening and irregular margins due to surrounding fibrosis. Findings on US

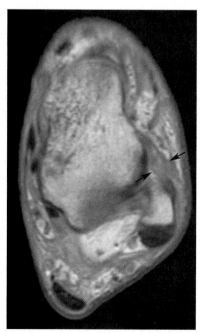

Figure 14-30   Anterior talofibular ligament sprain. Axial proton density MR image shows thick, edematous ligament (between *arrows*) due to partial tear.

are similar. The calcaneofibular and posterior talofibular ligaments are less frequently torn. These injuries may also be diagnosed with MRI and US.

The distal tibiofibular ligaments, along with the syndesmosis, stabilize the distal tibiofibular joint. Syndesmosis sprains, also called "high ankle sprains," range from mild distal tibiofibular ligament injuries to syndesmotic diastasis, as for example in a Maisonneuve fracture. The mechanism of injury is usually dorsiflexion, abduction, and external rotation. These mechanisms cause the talus to pry apart the malleoli. Nondisplaced sprains may show only edema between the distal tibial and fibula or isolated tear of the anterior tibiofibular ligament, and may be easily overlooked on MRI (Fig. 14-31).

The *spring ligament,* also termed the *plantar calcaneonavicular ligament,* is perhaps the most important ligament in the hindfoot because it helps to support the longitudinal arch, along with the tibialis posterior tendon, plantar fascia, and several other ligaments, and to a lesser degree the peroneus longus tendon. The spring ligament is located between the talus, medial calcaneus, and navicular bone. This ligament is difficult to image, and the reliability of MRI in diagnosing injury is under investigation but has not been established.

ANKLE IMPINGEMENT SYNDROMES

Anterior ankle impingement with dorsiflexion may be caused by anterior tibial osteophytes and traction spurs on the dorsal talar neck (Fig. 14-32). *Anterolateral impingement,* also termed *anterolateral gutter impingement,* is anterolateral ankle pain exacerbated by dorsiflexion due to soft tissue fibrosis, synovitis, and cartilage injury at the anterolateral margin of the tibiotalar joint. The condition usually is initiated by trauma. A subset of patients develop hyalinization of anterolateral soft tissues that becomes firm, hence the term "meniscoid syndrome." Magnetic resonance imaging shows soft tissue and possible marrow edema centered at the anterolateral tibiotalar joint. An intermediate-signal mass representing hyalinized tissue and cartilage loss may also be seen. The hyalinized tissue may undergo metaplasia to bone, which may be visible on radiographs.

Posterior ankle impingement during plantar flexion may occur with posterior tibial osteophytes or in association with an os trigonum. The os trigonum is a classic example of a normal variant that may be symptomatic, in a condition known as *os trigonum syndrome.* The os trigonum is usually attached to the underlying posterior process of the talus by a synchondrosis. During skeletal growth, the apophysis usually fuses with the talus; however, in approximately 10% to 14% of individuals it remains as a separate ossicle. In some cases, os trigonum may be a chronic fracture. An asymptomatic os trigonum is likely to have the following features: smooth contour, a uniform cortical margin, and a gap of a few millimeters or more between the os and the talus. A

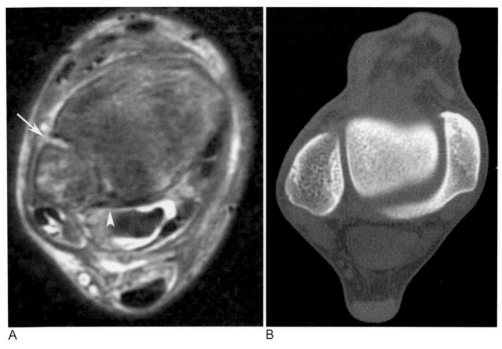

A   B

Figure 14-31   Syndesmosis sprain (high ankle sprain) with anterior distal tibiofibular ligament tear. **A,** Axial inversion recovery magnetic resonance (MR) image shows interrupted ligament *(arrow)*. Note intact posterior ligament *(arrowhead)*. **B,** Axial CT image at the level of the talar dome in an uninjured patient shows one mechanism of this injury. Note that the talar dome is slightly wider anteriorly than posteriorly. Because of this wedge-like anatomy, forced ankle dorsiflexion can pry apart the anterior mortise.

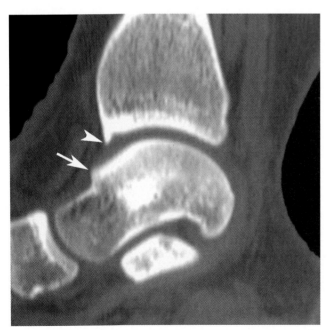

Figure 14-32   Anterior ankle impingement. Sagittal CT reformat shows spurs at the anterior medial distal tibia *(arrowhead)* and dorsal medial talar neck *(arrow)* in a patient with medial anterior ankle pain with dorsiflexion.

painful os trigonum is likely to have the following features: irregular contour, sclerosis and subcortical cysts along the margin that closely abuts the talus, and marrow edema and adjacent fluid on MR images. These features are similar to a symptomatic accessory navicular (Fig. 14-25). Bone scanning demonstrates intensely increased activity in the posterolateral talus with this syndrome. In other words, the appearance on all imaging studies may simulate or may be a result of ununited fracture of the posterior process of the talus. Symptomatic os trigonum is more common in ballet dancers and soccer players. These activities involve repetitive, forceful plantar flexion. Posterior ankle impingement pain may also be due to a large os trigonum or posterolateral process of the talus, which is compressed between the calcaneus and posterior tibia in extreme plantar flexion. The flexor hallucis longus tendon lies medial to the os trigonum. Tenosynovitis of the flexor hallucis longus may thus produce symptoms in this region. As noted in Chapter 13, some fluid in the flexor hallucis longus tendon sheath may be seen as a normal finding, but markedly increased fluid indicates tenosynovitis. A distinct syndrome with similar clinical features is associated with an MRI finding of edema in the posterior talofibular ligament.

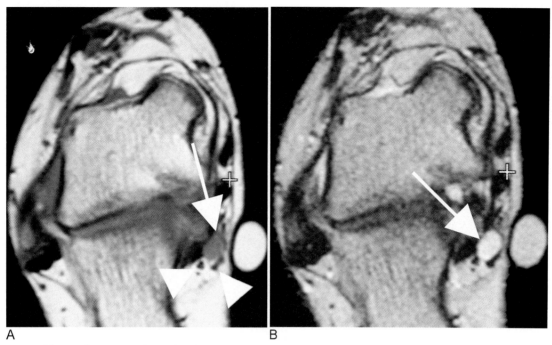

Figure 14-33 Tarsal tunnel syndrome. **A and B,** Axial proton density-weighted (A) and T2-weighted spin-echo (B) MR images show ganglion cyst *(arrow)* in tarsal tunnel. Note adjacent medial and lateral plantar vessels and nerves *(arrowheads)*. High-signal-intensity skin marker is present.

TARSAL TUNNEL SYNDROME

The tarsal tunnel represents the soft tissues invested by the flexor retinaculum at the ankle. As noted previously, the flexor tendons, fat, lymphatic tissues, and the medial and lateral plantar arteries, veins, and nerves lie within the tarsal tunnel. The medial margin of the tunnel is the flexor retinaculum, whereas the lateral margin consists of the talus and calcaneus. Pressure on the medial and lateral plantar nerves results in the syndrome that is analogous to carpal tunnel syndrome, and consists of tingling, pain, and burning in the sole and the medial toes. Half of the cases of tarsal tunnel syndrome will not have a morphologic abnormality identified on MR images. However, abnormalities that can be shown are space-occupying lesions that produce mass effect on the medial and lateral plantar nerves. Abnormalities include such common pathologies as flexor tendon tenosynovitis, an abnormally distal extent of the abductor hallucis muscle, thickening of the flexor retinaculum, and ganglion cysts (Fig. 14-33). Uncommon causes include neurogenic tumors, lymphangiomas or hemangiomas, varices, or other masses.

ANATOMY
CALCANEUS FRACTURE
TALUS FRACTURE
NAVICULAR BONE FRACTURE
LISFRANC'S FRACTURE-DISLOCATION
FOREFOOT FRACTURES
SOFT TISSUE INJURY

ANATOMY

In addition to the 28 bones in the foot, accessory ossicles are extremely common and are often bilateral in occurrence. Accessory ossicles normally are corticated and smoothly contoured, which helps differentiate them from fracture fragments. The most common accessory ossicles are the os trigonum (shown posterior to the talus on the lateral view of the foot), os peroneum (lateral to the cuboid), and os tibiale externum (adjacent to the proximal medial navicular bone on the frontal foot film). Radiologists usually refer to atlases of normal variants, and a good source is the *Atlas of Normal Roentgen Variants That May Simulate Disease* by Theodore Keats and Mark Anderson. Not all accessory ossicles are incidental. The os trigonum and os naviculare can be associated with pain syndromes, as discussed in Chapter 14.

The foot is divided into the hindfoot (calcaneus and talus), midfoot (cuboid, navicular, and cuneiforms), and forefoot (metatarsals and phalanges). The articulation between the hindfoot and midfoot is termed *Chopart's joint*. The articulation between the midfoot and forefoot is termed *Lisfranc's joint*.

Key Concepts	Foot Anatomy
Hindfoot (calcaneus and talus)	
Midfoot (cuboid, navicular, and cuneiforms)	
Forefoot (metatarsals and phalanges)	
Hindfoot and midfoot articulation: *Chopart's joint*	
Midfoot and forefoot articulation: *Lisfranc's joint*	

The calcaneus is the largest bone of the foot and is a tent-shaped bone consisting of a nonarticulating tuberosity posteriorly and an articulating anterior process. The talus articulates with the calcaneus at the posterior, middle, and anterior facet, in combination known as the subtalar joints, which form a tripod-like support for the talus (Fig. 15-1). The medial sustentaculum talus extends to the middle facet and may be seen on an oblique frontal radiograph known as a Harris or skier's view (Fig. 15-1B). The posterior facet is the largest. The cone-shaped sinus tarsi is interposed between the talus and calcaneus. The cuboid articulates with the calcaneus at the calcaneocuboid joint, and it spans the midfoot between two rows of tarsals. The first row consists of the navicular bone and the second row consists of the medial, middle, and lateral cuneiform bones. The cuboid articulates with the fourth and fifth metatarsals, whereas the medial, middle, and lateral cuneiforms articulate with the first, second, and third metatarsals, respectively. The foot then terminates with the phalanges.

It is extremely important to study the tarsal-metatarsal articulations carefully on frontal, oblique, and lateral radiographs because subtle malalignment may indicate the presence of midfoot-forefoot (Lisfranc) fracture-dislocation, which is discussed later. The frontal film will show the lateral border of the first metatarsal aligning with lateral border of the medial cuneiform, and will also show the medial border of the second metatarsal aligning with the medial margin of the middle cuneiform (Fig. 15-2). The oblique radiograph will show the alignment of the lateral margins of the lateral cuneiform and third metatarsal and the medial margins of the fourth metatarsal and the cuboid. The fifth metatarsal should be parallel in alignment proximally with its articulation with the distal-lateral margin of the cuboid. The lateral margins of the cuboid and fifth metatarsal do not align because the lateral margin of the fifth metatarsal base extends proximally and laterally relative to the cuboid bone. The second metatarsal base lies proximal and dorsal to the bases of the other metatarsal bones. Its function is similar to that of a keystone in a Roman arch. Its anatomic position assures the proper position of the other metatarsal

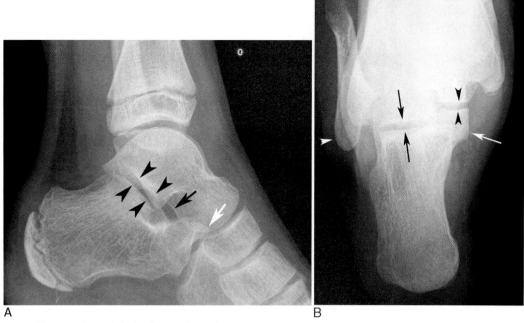

Figure 15-1 Subtalar facets radiographic anatomy. **A,** Lateral radiograph shows posterior *(black arrowheads)* and middle *(black arrow)* facet joints and the calcaneus anterior process *(white arrow).* **B,** Harris (skier's) view of the right hindfoot shows posterior facet *(black arrows),* middle facet *(black arrowheads),* sustentaculum *(white arrow),* and base of fifth metatarsal *(white arrowhead).* See also Figure 14-5C.

bones. The second metatarsal base is supported by a strong ligament, named *Lisfranc's ligament,* connecting the lateral-distal margin of the medial cuneiform with the adjacent medial-proximal margin of the second metatarsal bone (Fig. 15-2B).

In the skeletally immature, there are two secondary centers of ossification to be aware of. The first is at the apophysis of the calcaneal tuberosity. In the skeletally immature, the apophysis is normally dense and frequently fragmented. This is a normal appearance and does not represent avascular necrosis (AVN) or fracture. The second ossification center of which to be aware is the apophysis at the lateral base of the fifth metatarsal, which is longitudinally oriented (see Fig. 14-11). This must not be mistaken for an avulsion fracture. Avulsion fractures are transverse in orientation.

The anatomic position of the lower extremity is with the ankle plantar-flexed and the forefoot and toes pointed inferiorly. This can lead to confusion when cross-sectional imaging studies of the foot and ankle are performed because many radiologists, clinicians, and technologists visualize the patient in the standing position on a flat surface. Suggested terminology to avoid confusion is "short axis" for the anatomic axial plane and "footprint" for the plane parallel to the sole of the foot.

CALCANEUS FRACTURE

Calcaneus fractures usually occur after falls from heights. Because a jump from a balcony to escape the unexpected arrival of a spouse can cause these fractures, they are known as

"lover's" fractures or "Don Juan" fractures. In patients with calcaneus fractures and a history of falling from a height, evaluation of the thoracic and lumbar spine is indicated to assess for associated thoracolumbar spine compression fracture. Ten percent of calcaneus fractures are bilateral. The most common method for classifying these fractures is the Rowe classification scheme, with five types. Type I fractures occur in 21% of cases and are fractures of the calcaneal tuberosity, sustentaculum tali, or anterior process (Fig. 15-3). Type II fractures occur in approximately 4% of cases and are horizontal fractures of the

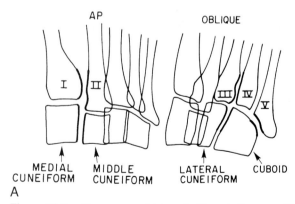

Figure 15-2 Tarsometatarsal joints. **A,** Normal alignment. The first and second metatarsals are evaluated on the AP radiograph. The third, fourth, and fifth metatarsals are evaluated on the oblique film. The bold lines indicate which surfaces of the tarsals and metatarsals must align with one another on each view. The alignment must be precise.

(Continued)

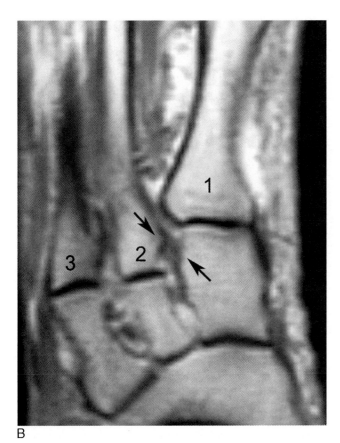

B

Figure 15-2—(Cont'd) **B,** Lisfranc's ligament. Footprint (AP equivalent) proton density MR image shows the obliquely oriented ligament *(arrows)* between the medial cuneiform bone and the base of the second metatarsal. There is no ligament between the proximal first and second metatarsals, so Lisfranc's ligament is an essential midfoot-forefoot stabilizer. (Part A reproduced with permission from Manaster BJ: Handbook of Skeletal Radiology, ed 2. St. Louis, Mosby, 1997.)

calcaneal tuberosity. Type III fractures occur in approximately 20% of cases and are oblique fractures without extension to the subtalar joint. Type IV fractures occur in approximately 25% of cases and extend to the subtalar joints. Type V fractures occur in 31% of cases and are intra-articular fractures with depression of the posterior subtalar joint or substantial comminution (Fig. 15-4). In assessing radiographs of the calcaneus, the degree of the osseous depression is important to ascertain. *Boehler's angle* is measured from two lines off the lateral film (Fig. 15-4A). One line connects the superior margin of the anterior process and the posterior margin of the posterior articular facet of the calcaneus. The other line connects the posterior margin of the posterior articular facet of the calcaneus and the posterosuperior margin of the calcaneal tuberosity. The angles subtended by these two lines should be between 28 and 48 degrees. With depression of the posterior articular facet in type V fractures, the angle can diminish substantially. Both articular depression and the degree of comminution of the lateral margin of the calcaneus are important to assess on radiographs; plate fixation is usually placed along the lateral calcaneus. Excessive comminution of the lateral calcaneus lim-

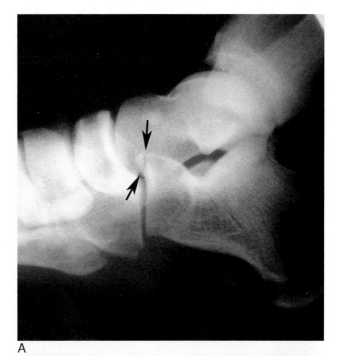

A

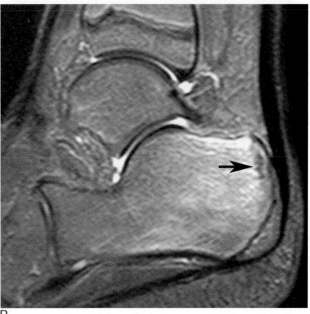

B

Figure 15-3 Calcaneus fractures. **A,** Anterior process fracture *(arrows).* **B,** Stress fracture in an older child. Sagittal inversion recovery MR image shows marrow edema in the posterior calcaneus and a low-signal stress fracture line *(arrow)* in typical coronal orientation and location anterior to the physis.

its placement of hardware plates. Computed tomography (CT) is extremely useful for evaluation of calcaneal fractures. Both coronal and axial imaging planes are useful, as are sagittal reformations, in determining the degree of comminution of the lateral margin of the calcaneus and the degree of depression of the posterior calcaneal facet.

Stress fractures of the calcaneus are often seen within the calcaneal tuberosity, which occur by 10 to 14 days after

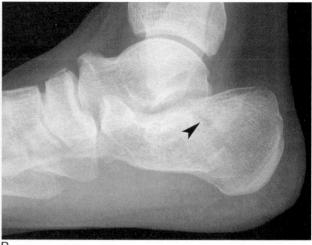

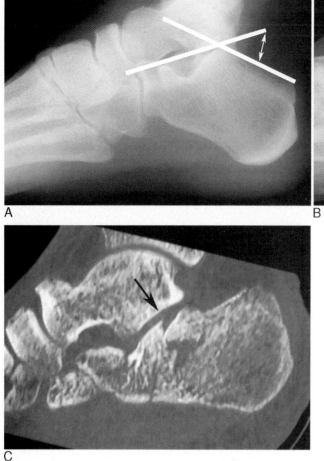

Figure 15-4 Calcaneus fracture and Boehler's angle. **A,** Lateral radiograph of normal foot demonstrates Boehler's angle with line drawn along superior-anterior margin of anterior process and superior-posterior margin of posterior facet, and line drawn between posterior-superior margin of posterior facet and posterior-superior margin of calcaneal tuberosity. Angle subtended by these two lines should be between 28 and 48 degrees. **B,** Lateral radiograph demonstrates comminution of calcaneus with flattened Boehler's angle. Note fracture extension to posterior subtalar joint *(arrowhead)*. **C,** Sagittal CT reconstruction better demonstrates the fractures. Note articular stepoff at the posterior facet *(arrow)*.

the onset of symptoms. They usually run perpendicular to the major trabeculae of the calcaneal tuberosity and are seen as vertically oriented linear densities on the lateral radiographic view (see Fig. 1-17E) with similar magnetic resonance imaging (MRI) findings (Fig. 15-3B). An avulsion at the Achilles insertion can occur as an insufficiency fracture, especially among diabetic patients (see Fig. 40-7B). Both MRI and bone scanning are useful in assessing for radiographically or clinically suspected calcaneal stress fractures.

Avulsion of the extensor digitorum brevis origin is an uncommon injury. This muscle originates at the anterolateral calcaneus. It is best shown on the frontal view of the ankle with the fragment located adjacent to the lateral margin of the calcaneus, 2 cm distal to the lateral malleolus. It may also be seen on the frontal foot film lateral to the anterior calcaneus.

TALUS FRACTURE

Talus fractures are less common than calcaneal fractures. Three fourths of fractures occur in the neck and body of the talus. The remainder are avulsion fractures or chip fractures. Talar neck fractures may be associated with talar dislocations (Fig. 15-5). Owing to the precarious vascular supply of the proximal talar pole, fractures at and proximal to the midpole of the talus are highly susceptible to AVN within the proximal pole (Fig. 15-6). Avulsion fractures are most common in the anterior-superior surface of the midtalar neck, which is the ankle capsule attachment site. Other avulsion fractures are seen along the lateral process of the talus ("snowboarder's fracture"), and along the superomedial margin of the talus. Osteochondral fractures and osteochondritis dissecans of the talar dome occur laterally or medially (see Fig. 1-16). The medial lesions are found posteriorly along the talar dome, whereas the lateral lesions are found mostly in the midportion. Fracture of the posterior process may resemble an os trigonum. Stress fractures also can occur in the talus (Fig. 15-7).

NAVICULAR BONE FRACTURE

Stress fractures of the navicular bone are uncommon but may occur in joggers and basketball players. Patients present with pain that is usually poorly localized in the medial arch of the foot. Fractures are usually sagittally oriented at the junction of the middle and lateral thirds of the navicular bone (Fig. 15-8). Although they are usually occult on radiographs, these are well shown on CT and MRI in the true axial and coronal planes.

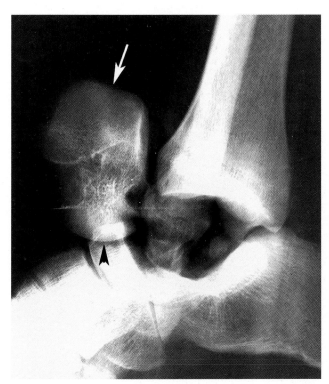

Figure 15-5 Lateral radiograph demonstrates anterior talar dislocation. Talar dome is denoted by arrow and talar head (navicular articular margin) by arrowhead.

Bone scanning will show localized activity in the navicular bone and is thus sensitive but not specific. Avascular necrosis of the lateral fragment is a potential complication of complete navicular fracture. Avulsion fractures of the navicular bone also occur, at the talonavicular capsule insertion. They present as a dorsal

bone fragment at the proximal navicular margin. Rarely, fractures of the medial tuberosity of the navicular bone may occur at the insertion site of the posterior tibialis tendon and the tibionavicular ligament of the deltoid ligament complex.

Os naviculare (accessory navicular, os tibiale externum) may be symptomatic. As discussed in Chapter 14, os naviculare often have an anomalous insertion of the posterior tibialis tendon solely on the os naviculare without continuation to cuneiform and metatarsal based insertions. These patients are prone to flatfoot deformity and hindfoot valgus. Magnetic resonance imaging will show edema-like signal within the ossicle and adjacent navicular bone.

LISFRANC'S FRACTURE-DISLOCATION

Lisfranc's fracture-dislocation typically occurs in the setting of axial loading of the plantar-flexed foot. This can occur with minimal trauma (e.g., misstepping when coming down stairs or foot entrapment on an automobile break pedal) and as a sports injury (e.g., when an opponent falls on the heel of a plantar-flexed foot). These injuries involve rupture of the major supporting ligaments of the tarsal-metatarsal articulations, especially Lisfranc's ligament. Alternatively, Lisfranc's ligament may remain intact even though an avulsion occurs at either the medial cuneiform or second metatarsal base insertions. With this injury, stability of the tarsal-metatarsal articulations is disrupted and lateral subluxation of the second through fifth metatarsals ensues (Fig. 15-9A). There is usually dorsal subluxation or dislocation of the tarsal-metatarsal joints, which may appear quite subtle on the lateral views (Fig. 15-9C). Two types of subluxation occur. One is the *homolateral*

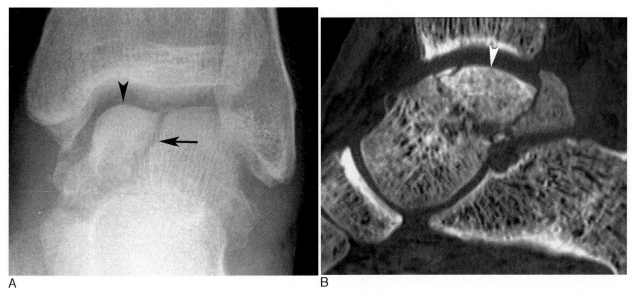

A   B

Figure 15-6 Talus fracture and post-traumatic talar dome avascular necrosis (AVN). **A and B,** AP view (A) and sagittal CT reformat (B) show a talus fracture (*arrow* in part A) that occurred 6 weeks previously. Note the sclerosis and lack of subchondral bone resorption in the medial fragment (*arrowhead*).

(Continued)

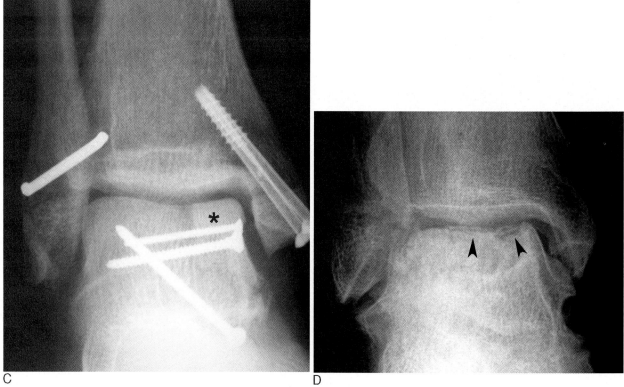

C

D

Figure 15-6—(Cont'd)   C, Frontal radiograph of ankle in a different patient shows medial malleolar, lateral malleolar, and talar fixation. AVN of medial talar bone fragment *(asterisk)* is shown as increased density, related to lack of hyperemic healing response. **D,** AP radiograph of the ankle in a different patient, a 22-year-old man who sustained a talar neck fracture several months previously, shows late-stage findings of AVN. The talar dome sclerotic and the subchondral bone has fragmented and collapsed *(arrowheads).*

(convergent) subluxation in which all five metatarsal bones are subluxed laterally (Fig. 15-9B). The other is *divergent* subluxation, in which there is lateral subluxation of the second through fifth metatarsals and variable medial subluxation of the first metatarsal (Fig. 15-9). There are usually associated

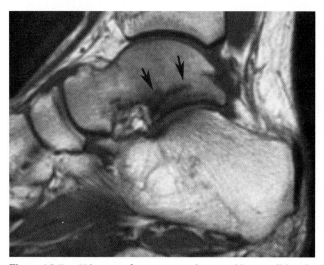

Figure 15-7   Talus stress fracture seen as low-signal line parallel to the posterior facet *(arrows)* in this T1-weighted sagittal MR image.

fractures of the metatarsal bones, although these may be radiographically occult. The degree of subluxation may be extremely subtle and in suspected cases CT or MRI will prove useful for detecting radiographically occult fracture and subluxation at the tarsal-metatarsal articulations. Slight widening of the interspace between the first and second metatarsals may be the only clue to the appropriate diagnosis on radiographs and should prompt additional imaging with CT or MRI. Lisfranc's fracture-dislocations are also common complications of diabetic neuropathic arthropathy. However, the findings in

Key Concepts	**Lisfranc's Fracture-Dislocation**
Homolateral (convergent): All five metatarsal bones subluxed laterally	
Divergent: Lateral subluxation of the second through fifth metatarsals away from first metatarsal	
CT or MRI	
Slight widening of interspace between first and second metatarsals may be only clue	
Common in diabetic neuropathic arthropathy	

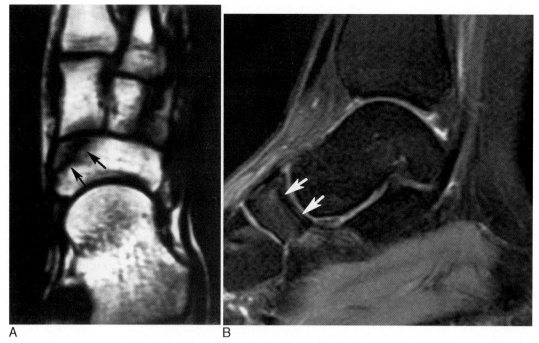

Figure 15-8   Navicular stress fracture. **A,** Axial T1-weighted MR image shows stress fracture of medial pole of navicular bone *(arrows).* **B,** Sagittal fat-suppressed proton density-weighted MR image in a different patient shows low-signal fracture line *(arrows)* with diffuse mild navicular marrow edema.

the setting of neuropathic arthropathy are usually not subtle and usually do not carry the same urgency for surgical intervention as do those of traumatic cause. Lisfranc's fracture-dislocations have a poor prognosis. The likelihood of eventual osteoarthritis is high. For this reason, subluxation and intra-articular fractures that demonstrate any degree of displacement undergo surgical reduction and fixation.

FOREFOOT FRACTURES

Jones fracture is a fracture through the fifth metatarsal 1.5–2 cm distal to the tuberosity (Fig. 15-10). The true Jones fracture is a different fracture than avulsion of the peroneus brevis insertion at the proximal tip of the fifth metatarsal bone (see Fig. 14-11). The latter articular fracture results from tension of the peroneus brevis tendon insertion, whereas the Jones fracture is an impaction injury that usually develops as a stress fracture. The differentiation is important because the proximal fractures usually heal readily, whereas the Jones fracture is prone to delayed union and nonunion and therefore requires more aggressive therapy, often with internal fixation.

Metatarsal stress fractures are common stress fractures that usually occur in the second or third metatarsal shafts. The synonym "March fracture" refers to a classic etiology of extended marches by new military recruits. These fractures are usually nondisplaced and become radiographically apparent 7 to 10 days after the onset of symptoms, with the appearance of ill-defined periosteal new bone formation at the site of fracture (see Fig. 1-17D). Eventually a sclerotic healed fracture line will appear.

Stubbing one's toe is a common injury. Such injuries may be occasionally associated with nail bed injuries or with fractures of the distal phalangeal tuft. In the skeletally immature, Salter-Harris I or II fractures may result from a stubbed toe because the nail bed of the toe is attached to the periosteum of the distal phalanx at the level of the proximal metaphysis. Because the nail bed is often disrupted, patients are prone to osteomyelitis. This concern particularly applies to the great toe.

The plantar (tarsal) plate is a fibrocartilaginous structure on the plantar aspect of the metatarsophalangeal and proximal interphalangeal joints, analogous to the volar plate in the hand. Tarsal plate injury may result in a planter proximal avulsion fracture. *Turf toe* is a chronic great toe tarsal plate injury associated with repetitive forced dorsiflexion while under load. It is more frequent in athletes who play football and soccer on unyielding artificial surfaces. Also similar to the hand, avulsion of a toe extensor tendon may result in a dorsal chip fracture of the proximal dorsal aspect of a toe phalanx.

SOFT TISSUE INJURY

The ligaments and tendons of the ankle and hindfoot are discussed in Chapter 14.

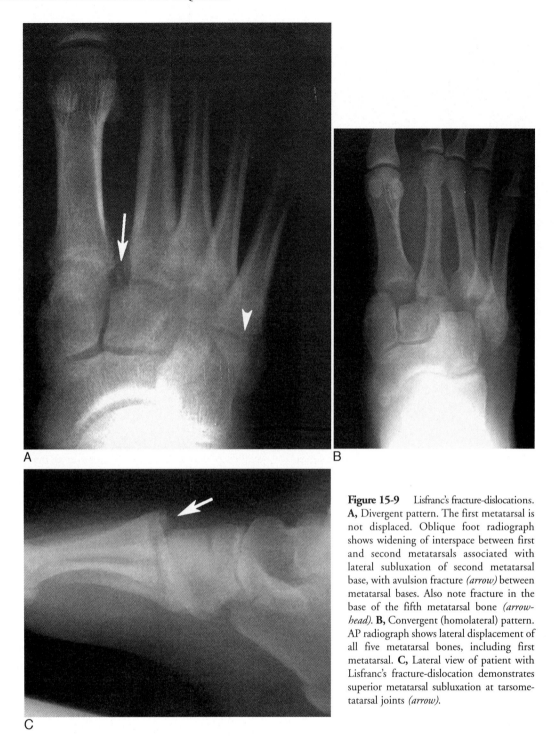

Figure 15-9 Lisfranc's fracture-dislocations. **A,** Divergent pattern. The first metatarsal is not displaced. Oblique foot radiograph shows widening of interspace between first and second metatarsals associated with lateral subluxation of second metatarsal base, with avulsion fracture *(arrow)* between metatarsal bases. Also note fracture in the base of the fifth metatarsal bone *(arrowhead)*. **B,** Convergent (homolateral) pattern. AP radiograph shows lateral displacement of all five metatarsal bones, including first metatarsal. **C,** Lateral view of patient with Lisfranc's fracture-dislocation demonstrates superior metatarsal subluxation at tarsometatarsal joints *(arrow)*.

Another anatomic compartment at the ankle and hindfoot is the sinus tarsi, which is the cone-shaped central and lateral space between the midpole of the talus and the anterior process of the calcaneus, located between the posterior subtalar joint and the talocalcaneonavicular joint. This space is occupied by fat, a small neurovascular bundle, and talocalcaneal ligaments, which provide lateral stability to the lateral ankle. Sinus tarsi syndrome results from inflammation or hemorrhage within this site and leads to lateral foot pain.

Causes include ankle inversion injury and rheumatoid arthritis. On MR images, the abnormal sinus tarsi does not show signal compatible with fat (Fig. 15-11). It may show signal consistent with edema, fibrosis, and synovial cysts arising from the adjacent posterior subtalar and talocalcaneonavicular joints. Although subtalar ligament tears may be present, they are not shown reliably with MRI. As this disorder usually arises after supination injury, many patients have lateral collateral ligament tears of the ankle.

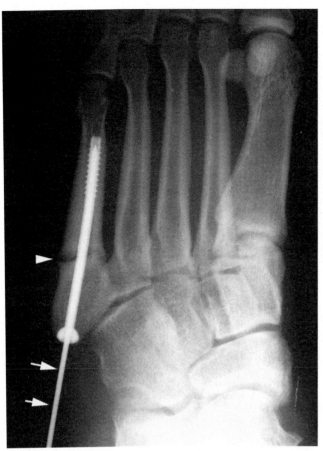

Figure 15-10   Oblique radiograph of foot shows Jones fracture *(arrowhead)* in a collegiate basketball player. Note cannulated screw placed over a guide pin *(arrows)* in this intraoperative film.

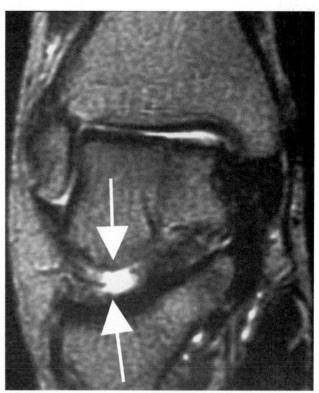

Figure 15-11   Sinus tarsi syndrome. Coronal T2-weighted spin-echo MR image demonstrates fluid-like signal *(arrows)* in sinus tarsi in patient with sinus tarsi syndrome. (Adapted and reproduced with permission from Aerts P, Disler DG: Abnormalities of the foot and ankle: MR imaging findings. AJR 165:119–124, 1995.)

The *plantar fascia* (plantar aponeurosis) arises from two cords at the plantar aspect of the calcaneal tuberosity. The medial cord is the flexor digitorum brevis, and the lateral cord is the abductor digiti minimi. Chronic repetitive trauma may result in tear or tendinopathy and inflammation at of the origin of the plantar aponeurosis known as *plantar fasciitis*, resulting in extreme tenderness as well as pain with ambulation at the plantar calcaneal tuberosity (Fig. 15-12). At MRI, one may see heterogeneous signal in the origin of the plantar aponeurosis and adjacent subtle bone marrow and soft tissue signal changes. There is variable thickening of the plantar aponeurosis. Occasionally, one may see atrophy with fatty infiltration in either the flexor digitorum brevis or abductor digiti minimi. Heel spurs may result from plantar fasciitis but are entirely nonspecific, as chronic asymptomatic traction at the origin of the plantar aponeurosis similarly may produce heel spurs. Furthermore, heel spurs may result from inflammatory enthesitis, which is commonly at the origin of the plantar aponeurosis in the setting of chronic reactive arthritis or psoriatic arthropathy.

Ainhum is hyperkeratosis of the tip of a toe (occasionally a finger) with progressive bone resorption. Ulceration and spontaneous amputation may ensue. This condition occurs in middle-aged men of West African descent.

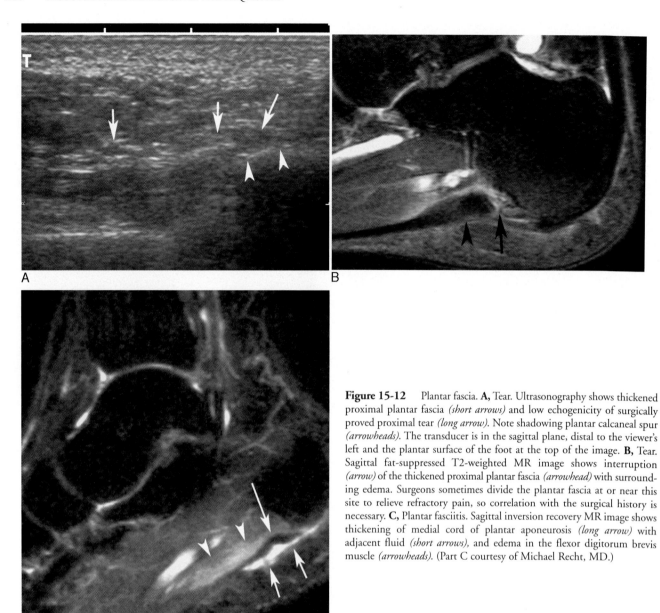

Figure 15-12 Plantar fascia. **A,** Tear. Ultrasonography shows thickened proximal plantar fascia *(short arrows)* and low echogenicity of surgically proved proximal tear *(long arrow)*. Note shadowing plantar calcaneal spur *(arrowheads)*. The transducer is in the sagittal plane, distal to the viewer's left and the plantar surface of the foot at the top of the image. **B,** Tear. Sagittal fat-suppressed T2-weighted MR image shows interruption *(arrow)* of the thickened proximal plantar fascia *(arrowhead)* with surrounding edema. Surgeons sometimes divide the plantar fascia at or near this site to relieve refractory pain, so correlation with the surgical history is necessary. **C,** Plantar fasciitis. Sagittal inversion recovery MR image shows thickening of medial cord of plantar aponeurosis *(long arrow)* with adjacent fluid *(short arrows)*, and edema in the flexor digitorum brevis muscle *(arrowheads)*. (Part C courtesy of Michael Recht, MD.)

Part III Sources and Suggested Readings

Affram P: An epidemiologic study of cervical and trochanteric fractures of the femur in an urban population. Analysis of 1664 cases with special reference to etiologic factors. Acta Orthop Scand Suppl 64:11, 1964.

Allen W, Cope R: Coxa saltans: The snapping hip revisited. J Am Acad Orthop Surg 3:303–308, 1995.

Applegate GR, Flannigan BD, Fox T, Del Pizzo W: MR diagnosis of recurrent tears of the knee: Value of intraarticular contrast material. AJR 161:821–825, 1993.

Bayliss A, Davidson J: Traumatic osteonecrosis of the femoral head following intracapsular fracture. Incidence and earliest radiological features. Clin Radiol 28:407–414, 1977.

Beall DP, Sweet CF, Martin HD, et al: Imaging findings of femoroacetabular impingement syndrome. Skeletal Radiology 34:691–701, 2005.

Ben-Menachem Y, Coldwell D, Young J, Burgess A: Hemorrhage associated with pelvic fractures: Causes, diagnosis, and emergent management. AJR 157:1005–1014, 1991.

Bikkina RS, Tujo CA, Schraner AB, Major NM: The "floating" meniscus: MRI in knee trauma and implications for surgery. AJR 184:200–204, 2005

Chien AJ, Jacobson JA, Jamadar DA, et al: Imaging appearances of lateral ankle ligament reconstruction. Radiographics 24:999–1008, 2004.

Costa CR, Morrison WB, Carrino JA: Medial meniscus extrusion on knee MRI: Is extent associated with severity of degeneration or type of tear? AJR 183:17–23, 2004.

Delfaut EM, Demondion X, Dieganski A, et al: Imaging of foot and ankle nerve entrapment syndromes: From well-demonstrated to unfamiliar sites. Radiographics 23:613–623, 2003.

DeSmet A, Fisher D, Burnstein M, et al: Value of MR imaging in staging osteochondral lesions of the talus (osteochondritis dissecans): Results in 14 patients. AJR 154:555–558, 1990.

Deutsch A, Mink J, Fox F, et al: Peripheral meniscal tears: MR findings after conservative treatment or arthroscopic repair. Radiology 176:485–488, 1990.

Deutsch A, Mink J, Fox J, et al: The postoperative knee. Mag Reson 8:23–54, 1992.

Disler DG: Fat-suppressed 3-D spoiled gradient-recalled MR imaging: Assessment of articular and physeal hyaline cartilage. AJR 169:1117–1123, 1997

Dussault R, Kaplan P, Roederer G: MR imaging of Achilles tendon in patients with familial hyperlipidemia. AJR 164:403–407, 1995.

Escobedo EM, Mills WJ, Hunter JC: The "reverse Segond" fracture: Association with a tear of the PCL and medial meniscus. AJR 178:979–983, 2002.

Fisher S, Fox J, Del Pizzo W, et al: Accuracy of diagnoses from magnetic resonance imaging of the knee. J Bone Joint Surg 73A:2–10, 1991.

Ganz R, Parvizi J, Beck M, et al: Femoroacetabular impingement: A cause for osteoarthritis of the hip. Clin Orthop Relat Res 417: 112–120, 2003.

Garden RS: Stability and union of subcapital fractures of the femour. J Bone Joint Surg 46b:630–712, 1964.

Gill K, Bucholz R: The role of CT scanning in the evaluation of major pelvic fractures. J Bone Joint Surg Am 66A:34–39, 1984.

Holder J, Yu J, Goodwin D, et al: MR arthrography of the hip: Improved imaging of the acetabular labrum with histologic correlation in cadavers. AJR 165:887–891, 1995.

Ito K, Minka-II MA, Leunig S, et al: Femoroacetabular impingement and the cam-effect. J Bone Joint Surg 83B:171–176, 2001.

Judet R, Judet J, Letournel E: Fractures of the acetabulum: Classification and surgical approaches to reduction. J Bone Joint Surg 46a:1615–1646, 1964.

Karasick D, Schweitzer M: The os trigonum syndrome: Imaging features. AJR 166:125–129, 1996.

Koulouris G, Connell D: Hamstring muscle complex: An imaging review. Radiographics 25:571–586, 2005.

Lauge-Hansen N: Fractures of the ankle: Genetic roentgenologic diagnosis of fractures of the ankle. AJR 71:456–471, 1954.

Laurin C, Dussault R, Levesque H: The tangential x-ray investigation of the patellofemoral joint. Clin Orthop 144:16–26, 1979.

Leunig M, Beck M, Kalhor M, et al: Fibrocystic changes at the anterosuperior femoral neck: Prevalence in hips with femoroacetabular impingement. Radiology 236:237–246, 2005.

Mainwaring B, Daffner R, Reiner B: Pylon fractures of the ankle: A distinct clinical and radiographic entity. Radiology 168: 215–218, 1998.

Manaster BJ: Imaging knee ligament reconstructions. RSNA Categorical course in Musculoskeletal Radiology 211–218, 1993.

McCauley TR: MR imaging evaluation of the postoperative knee. Radiology 234:53–61, 2005.

Mirvis SE, Shanmuganathan K (eds): Imaging in Trauma and Critical Care, 2nd ed. Philadelphia, WB Saunders, 2003.

Notzli HP, Wyss TF, Stoecklin CH, et al: The contour of the femoral head-neck junction as a predictor for the risk of anterior impingement. J Bone Joint Surg 84B:556–560, 2002.

Prince J, Laor T, Bean J. MRI of ACL injuries and associated findings in the pediatric knee: Changes with skeletal maturation. AJR 185:756–762, 2005.

Resnick C, Stackhouse D, Shanmuganathan K, Young J: Diagnosis of pelvic fractures with acute pelvic trauma: Efficacy of plain radiographs. AJR 158:109–112, 1992.

Rowe CR, Sakellarides HT, Freeman PA, Sorbie C: Fractures of the os calcis: A long term follow-up study of 146 patients. JAMA 184:920, 1963.

Schwappach J, Murphey M, Kokmayer S, et al: Subcapital fractures of the femoral neck: Prevalence and cause of radiographic appearance simulating pathologic fractures. AJR 162:651–654, 1994.

Siebenrock KA, Wahab KHA, Werlen S, et al: Abnormal epiphyseal extension of the femoral head as a cause of femoro-acetabular impingement. Clin Orthop 418:54–60, 2004.

Schmid M, Notzli H, Anetti M, et al: Cartilage lesions in the hip: diagnostic effectiveness of MR arthrography. Radiology 226:383–386, 2003.

Smith D: Imaging of sports injuries of the ankle and foot. Oper Tech Sports Med 3:47–70, 1995.

Smith D, May D, Phillips P: MR imaging of the anterior cruciate ligament: Frequency of discordant findings on sagittal-oblique images and correlations with arthroscopic findings. AJR 166:411–413, 1996.

Steinbach L, Tirmon P: MRI of the ankle. Radiologist 2:111–124, 1995.

Toye LR, Helms CA, Hoffman BD, et al: MRI of spring ligament tears. AJR 184:1475–1480, 2005.

White LM, Schweitzer ME, Weishaupt D, et al: Diagnosis of recurrent meniscal tears: Prospective evaluation of conventional MR imaging, indirect MR arthrography, and direct MR arthrography. Radiology 222:421–429, 2002.

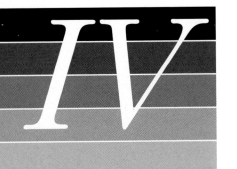

IV   ARTHRITIS

RADIOGRAPHIC ASSESSMENT OF ARTHRITIS:
   AN INTEGRATED APPROACH
RADIOGRAPHIC ASSESSMENT OF ARTHRITIS: THE ABCDE'S
   Alignment
   Bone
   Cartilage
   Distribution
   Erosions
   Soft Tissues
FUTURE DIRECTIONS

Classic cases of arthritis are generally seen in their chronic stages, which makes them relatively easy to distinguish radiographically. However, early arthritic processes may be much more subtle. The radiologist therefore needs to be able to distinguish among similar-appearing joint processes. Many arthropathies have overlapping individual features, but the overall constellation of clinical and laboratory features combined with the radiographic findings will usually lead to a single correct diagnosis. Radiographic diagnosis of arthritis is based on regional and global joint assessment. The goals are disease classification and differentiation of early versus late changes. Regardless of the imaging modality, the radiologic findings reflect the underlying pathophysiology.

Experienced radiologists and clinicians may be able to use a global pattern recognition approach to interpret arthritis studies, but this is not recommended for residents. It's just too complicated. The key to reading arthritis radiographs, especially when one is learning, is to have an organized approach that dissects the radiographic findings into manageable components. We thus offer two such approaches in the following paragraphs: the "ABCDE'S" approach, and an integrated approach that is discussed first.

RADIOGRAPHIC ASSESSMENT OF ARTHRITIS: AN INTEGRATED APPROACH

Important considerations in evaluation of arthritis radiographs include clinical evaluation, age and sex of the patient, laboratory values, distribution of the joints involved, joint deformities, and the general appearance of inflammatory erosive versus productive bony change. Of all these parameters, the radiologist is generally provided only with the patient's age and gender and must rely on the location of involvement and the general appearance of the arthritic process to render a diagnosis. Almost all arthritic processes have a preferential joint distribution, as well as a specific distribution within a joint. As with both real estate and tumor evaluation, "location" is of prime importance in distinguishing among the arthritides. Throughout this section, you will find that "location" (i.e., distribution) is stressed as a vital piece of information.

Another important parameter in evaluation of an arthritic process is the determination of whether it is primarily erosive, productive of bone, or mixed. In general, erosive arthropathies have an initial inflammatory stage that produces pannus (inflammatory granulation tissue). The pannus destroys cartilage and bone by means of lytic enzymes and by direct interference with movement of nutrients across the joint surface. Rheumatoid arthritis is an example of a purely erosive arthritic process (Fig. 16-1). Osteoarthritis (degenerative joint disease) is at the other end of the spectrum, with productive rather than erosive manifestations. Although osteoarthritis also involves cartilage and subchondral bone destruction, abnormal mechanical forces combine with host reactive processes to produce these changes, including osteophyte formation, subchondral sclerosis, and cortical buttressing (Fig. 16-2). As you will note, most of the other arthropathies generally fall between the erosive and productive ends of the spectrum, often demonstrating both erosive and productive changes (Fig. 16-3).

Regarding laboratory values, *rheumatoid factor* (RF) refers to the presence of serum antibodies that are anti-IgG. Rheumatoid factor is not specific for rheumatoid arthritis but is strongly associated, especially with more severe active disease. *Seronegative* specifically means normal serum RF, but the term is used more generally to refer to inflammatory arthritides that usually do not cause elevated RF, such as reactive arthritis, psoriasis, and ankylosing spondylitis.

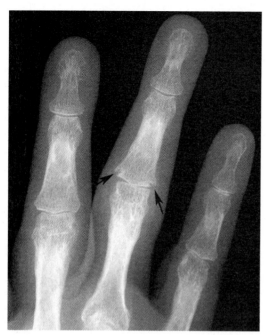

Figure 16-1   Marginal erosions. Note the fourth PIP marginal erosions in this patient with rheumatoid arthritis *(arrows)*. Also note cartilage space narrowing in all of the IP joints pictured on this AP radiograph. (Reprinted with permission of the American College of Radiology learning file.)

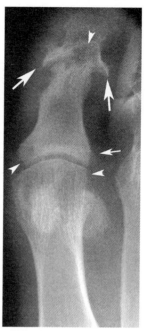

Figure 16-3   Mixed erosive and destructive arthritis. AP radiograph of the foot in a 50-year-old man with psoriatic arthritis demonstrates multiple erosions *(arrowheads)* and new bone production *(arrows)*.

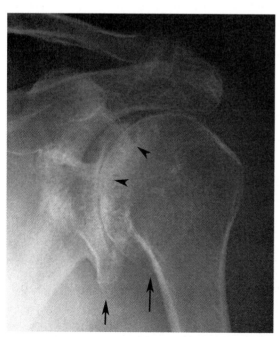

Figure 16-2   Purely productive arthritis: osteoarthritis. AP shoulder radiograph shows osteophytes *(arrows)* and subchondral sclerosis *(arrowheads)*.

RADIOGRAPHIC ASSESSMENT OF ARTHRITIS: THE ABCDE'S

The "ABCDE'S" stands for alignment, bone, cartilage, distribution, erosions, and soft tissues. This approach maximally dissects the radiographic findings into individual components. You may choose to evaluate these features in any order, as long as all are covered.

Key Concepts	Radiographic Assessment of Arthritis: The ABCDE'S
Alignment Bone: Density, new bone production Cartilage Distribution Erosions Soft tissues	

Alignment

Deformities can occur secondary to ligamentous laxity without erosion, as in lupus or Jaccoud's arthropathy. Deformities related to osteoarthritis include varus or valgus caused by asymmetric cartilage wear. Classic deformities of rheumatoid arthritis are discussed in Chapter 17. These include the swan neck and boutonnière deformities, varus subluxations, and deformities related to severe erosion. The pencil-in-cup deformity is associated with psoriatic arthritis.

Bone

Inflammation and associated hyperemia induce osteoclast activation with bone resorption, which can be periarticular or regional. The pattern of osteopenia reflects pattern of active inflammation in inflammatory arthropathies. Periarticular osteopenia can be extremely subtle.

Bone density may become locally increased in reactive, reparative processes. Classic examples are subchondral sclerosis and osteophyte formation in osteoarthritis. The pattern of bone formation indicates distribution of disease in noninflammatory arthropathies.

"Enthesophyte" refers to new bone formation at an enthesis. Large, bulky enthesophytes are associated with reactive arthritis, psoriasis, and diffuse idiopathic skeletal hyperostosis (DISH). Fine, delicate ossification of annular disc fibers are termed "syndesmophytes" and are a classic finding in ankylosing spondylitis.

Cartilage

Hyaline cartilage destruction causes joint space narrowing (Fig. 16-4). In inflammatory arthritis, pannus produces proteolytic enzymes and interferes with nutrient diffusion, causing uniform cartilage loss throughout the joint. In noninflammatory arthritis, especially osteoarthritis, cartilage loss occurs along lines of force, and thus tends to be asymmetrically greater at load-bearing surfaces. Crystal deposition disease

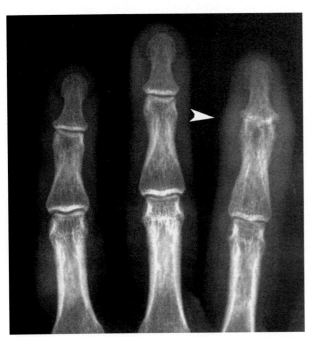

Figure 16-4   Soft tissue swelling and joint space narrowing without periarticular demineralization. Another patient with psoriatic arthritis.

such as calcium pyrophosphate deposition (CPPD) often results in uniform joint space loss because of the systemic nature of the process.

Some arthritides are associated with preservation of articular cartilage, at least until late in the disease (Table 16-1).

Ankylosis is fibrous, cartilaginous, or osseous fusion across a joint. Ankylosis is associated with ankylosing spondylitis (sacroiliac [SI] joints and spine), late-stage juvenile rheumatoid arthritis (wrists and cervical facet joints), reactive arthritis and psoriasis (hand), rheumatoid arthritis (wrist), and can be seen following any process that utterly destroys a joint's cartilage. Ankylosis distal to wrist is most likely in trauma, infection, or seronegative spondyloarthropathy.

Distribution

Distribution refers to the geographic pattern of radiographic findings. Arthritis may be *monoarticular* (one joint involved), *oligoarticular* (just a few joints), or *polyarticular* (multiple joints). Polyarticular disease virtually excludes infection because septic arthritis usually is a monoarticular disease, and only rarely is oligoarticular. Monoarticular and oligoarticular involvement is unusual for rheumatoid arthritis, but is more typical of seronegative arthritis, infection, pigmented villonodular synovitis, synovial chondromatosis, crystal deposition disease, and hemophilic arthropathy.

Although it sometimes is important to provide a catalogue of specific joints involved in oligoarticular and polyarticular disease, more generalized terms are helpful in describing the pattern of distribution. Arthritis may be symmetric vs. asymmetric with regard to right sided vs. left sided. Symmetry favors rheumatoid arthritis and CPPD. Asymmetry is seen in osteoarthritis, seronegative spondyloarthropathies, and gout. Reactive arthritis and psoriasis are often polyarticular and involve entire rays, but rarely show symmetry.

Arthritis in the hands and feet can occur in a distal (involves the distal interphalangeal [DIP] and proximal interphalangeal [PIP] joints) or proximal (metacarpophalangeal [MCP] and wrist) pattern. Proximal disease favors rheumatoid arthritis and crystal deposition diseases. Distal and first-ray disease favors osteoarthritis. Either pattern can be seen with seronegative arthritis. Distal inflammatory disease favors seronegative arthritis.

Some arthritides may primarily involve the axial skeleton. *Spondyloarthropathy* means arthritis with spine involvement.

Table 16-1   Arthritis with Preserved Cartilage Space
Infection with low virulence organisms (fungus, tuberculosis)
Amyloid
Silastic arthropathy
Gout
Any arthritis in early stages
Avascular necrosis (AVN) (not a type of arthritis but may lead to osteoarthritis)

Symmetric SI joint disease favors ankylosing spondylitis and enteropathic arthropathy. Reactive arthritis and psoriatic arthritis may have symmetric or asymmetric SI joint involvement. Rheumatoid arthritis rarely involves the SI joints, in which case it is usually asymmetric. Ankylosing spondylitis ascends the spine continuously, especially in males. Reactive arthritis and psoriatic arthritis skip levels. Disk involvement indicates enthesitis (i.e., involvement of the peripheral annular fibers of the disk vertebral bodies, which excludes rheumatoid arthritis).

As noted previously, osteoarthritis often involves weight-bearing joints and, within a joint, tends to involve load-bearing surfaces.

Erosions

Erosion is focal subcortical loss of bone. Erosions are classified as *marginal, nonmarginal,* and *subchondral.* Marginal erosions occur along the periphery of the joint space in "bare areas" of bone that are within the joint capsule but are not covered with articular cartilage (see Fig. 16-1). Marginal erosions occur in inflammatory arthritis. The borders of acute or active erosions are indistinct. One must look at the edges of erosions for evidence of bone proliferation because such production, as well as capsular enthesophytes, is associated with seronegative arthropathy. Nonmarginal erosions are further removed from the joint margin and usually show sharp, sclerotic borders. Overhanging edges may result from reactive bone formation. These erosions are associated with crystal deposition diseases.

Subchondral erosions occur in subchondral bone and can overlap in appearance with subchondral cysts of osteoarthritis. Subchondral erosions can be due to inflammatory or noninflammatory joint disease. Subchondral cysts caused by inflammatory joint disease are due to pannus intrusion in subchondral bone. Subchondral cysts caused by noninflammatory joint disease are due to liquefaction of subchondral bone following pressure necrosis, or synovial intrusion at joint surfaces worn down to bone. Sharp, sclerotic borders suggest a noninflammatory process, or an inactive inflammatory process.

Soft Tissues

Fusiform swelling centered at a joint is an indicator of inflammatory pannus or effusion (Figs. 16-4, 16-5). This is the pattern most associated with rheumatoid arthritis and septic arthritis. Diffuse swelling (e.g., involving an entire digit) suggests inflammation beyond the joint, as can occur in enthesitis. This pattern is most typical of psoriatic arthritis and reactive arthritis. Tophaceous deposits in gout tend to be eccentric (i.e., centered near but not at the joint). Thus, soft tissue swelling due to gout tends to be asymmetric and lumpy-bumpy in appearance. This matches the nonmarginal pattern of erosions associated with gout.

Periarticular soft tissue calcification may be due to crystals, enthesophytes, and dystrophic and vascular calcifications.

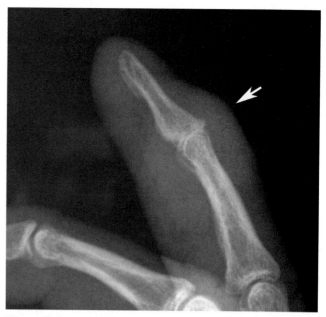

Figure 16-5 Single joint involvement in a different patient with psoriatic arthritis. Note the soft tissue swelling and joint space narrowing of the second DIP joint *(arrow).*

Tophaceous calcium urate deposits in gout tend to be radiographically mildly dense, in addition to eccentric as noted previously. Hydroxyapatite deposits occur in tendons and bursae. These tend to be uniformly dense and amorphous. Crystals of CPPD are seen as fine linear deposits in articular cartilage, capsule, synovium, and entheses.

FUTURE DIRECTIONS

The role of imaging in arthritis is evolving as disease-modifying drugs that reduce the prevalence of classic radiographic findings are developed. Radiography certainly remains a first-line diagnostic test, but several factors have reduced (although certainly not eliminated) the role of radiography in diagnosis and assessment of disease activity in several types of arthritis. Laboratory diagnosis and clinical understanding are constantly advancing.

Key Concepts	Cross-Sectional Imaging in Arthritis
US: Synovium, effusion, small joint erosions CT: Large and small joint erosions and productive change, synovium, effusion, cartilage (with arthrography) MRI: Cartilage, synovium, effusion, erosions, earliest changes of inflammatory arthritis (including marrow edema)	

Numerous avenues of research are demonstrating that magnetic resonance imaging (MRI) is more sensitive in detecting early changes of arthritis, quantifying arthritic changes, and assessing response to medication. The new anti–tumor necrosis factor drugs are revolutionizing therapy for inflammatory arthritides such as rheumatoid arthritis, psoriatic arthritis, reactive arthritis, and ankylosing spondylitis, such that classic, advanced cases may someday become a historical curiosity. Rheumatologists will probably be requesting advanced imaging techniques, especially MRI, with greater frequency. This test allows direct visualization and quantification of enhancing pannus as well as articular cartilage defects and overall cartilage volume. Physical properties of cartilage relating to degeneration may be measurable by MR spectroscopy or T2 mapping (assessment of cartilage properties on a voxel by voxel basis). Contrast-enhanced MRI and ultrasonography (US) can be used to assess synovium volume and vascularity. Magnetic resonance imaging, US, and computed tomography (CT) can depict erosions with greater sensitivity than can radiography. In general, CT and radiography are superior to MRI in depiction of productive changes such as enthesophytes, whereas MRI is more sensitive in depiction of the earliest changes if inflammatory arthritis.

CHAPTER 17

Rheumatoid Arthritis and Juvenile Rheumatoid Arthritis

RHEUMATOID ARTHRITIS
  Hand and Wrist
  Elbow
  Shoulder Girdle
  Feet
  Knee
  Hip
  Spine
  Robust Rheumatoid Arthritis
  Adult Still's Disease
  Differential Diagnosis
JUVENILE RHEUMATOID ARTHRITIS

RHEUMATOID ARTHRITIS

Rheumatoid arthritis (RA) is the most common purely erosive inflammatory arthropathy. It results from immune-mediated synovial inflammation, initiated by an attack on an unknown antigen. The resulting inflammatory synovial proliferation is termed *pannus,* which is responsible for the articular destruction found in this disease. Joint disease is invariably polyarticular and typically symmetric, involving the axial as well as appendicular skeleton, the upper and lower extremities, and the large and small joints. RA can first develop in either young or middle-aged adults. There is a distinct sex preference, with females affected more frequently than males (2:1 or 3:1 ratio). It is a multi-system disease, but the joint symptoms generally predominate.

Joint symptoms may be continuous or episodic. These symptoms include early morning stiffness, pain, boggy synovial swelling, tendon contractures and ruptures, and eventually several characteristic deformities. Rheumatoid factor (RF) is not entirely specific; it may be negative early in the disease process, but does eventually become positive in 90% to 95% of cases. It may, however, be falsely positive in older individuals.

Key Concepts	Rheumatoid Arthritis

Purely erosive
Fusiform soft tissue swelling
Periarticular osteoporosis
Uniform cartilage destruction
Bilaterally symmetric
Wrist: Radiocarpal joint, distal radioulnar joint; deformities
Hand: Proximal (MCP and PIP); deformities
Foot: Metatarsophalangeal (MTP) and retrocalcaneal bursa
Shoulder: Rotator cuff tear, erosion of distal clavicle
Knee: Valgus deformity
Hips: Uniform cartilage loss, protrusion
Upper cervical spine: Facet erosions, atlantoaxial impaction, atlantoaxial subluxation

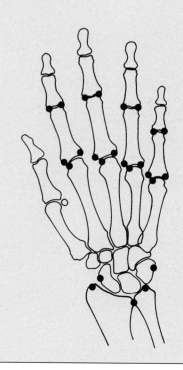

Patients with RA may have extra-articular manifestations, including nodules in tendon sheaths or subcutaneous locations, tenosynovitis (Fig. 17-1) or bursitis, pleural or pericardial effusion, rheumatoid pulmonary nodules, and diffuse interstitial pneumonitis.

Key Concepts	Rheumatoid Arthritis (RA): Extra-articular Manifestations

Skin: Subcutaneous nodules on extensor surfaces of extremities

General musculoskeletal: Osteoporosis, muscle weakness and atrophy, joint infections

Lung: Unilateral effusion, basilar intersitial disease, nodules (frequent cavitation), infections

Heart: Pericarditis, arrhythmia

Vascular: Aortitis, small vessel inflammation, pulmonary hypertension

Neurologic: Peripheral neuropathy, nerve compression by giant effusions

Lymphadenopathy

Felty syndrome: Long-standing RA, splenomegaly, neutropenia, weight loss, leg ulcers, abnormal skin pigmentation

Sjögren syndrome

Initial radiographic characteristics of a joint involved with RA include fusiform swelling secondary to effusion and synovitis.

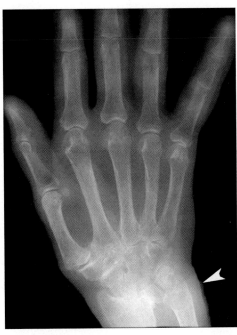

Figure 17-1   Rheumatoid arthritis. PA view of the hand demonstrates the typical findings of rheumatoid arthritis, with diffuse osteopenia, soft tissue swelling at the MCP joints, loss of cartilage width at the radiocarpal joint, erosions at the distal radioulnar joint and ulnar styloid, and carpal instability with ulnar translocation of the entire carpus. Note the only productive change is around the ulna, termed "ulnar capping" *(arrowhead).*

Periarticular osteoporosis occurs early in the disease as a result of hyperemia, but later becomes generalized due to disuse. The earliest hint of erosive change may be a "dot dash" pattern of the articular cortex. Bone erosion initially is marginal (i.e., at the bare areas of bone that are within the joint capsule but not protected by overlying cartilage). Subsequent cartilage destruction is uniform within a joint. Following cartilage destruction, subchondral erosions occur, along with subchondral cysts (see Fig. 17-1). Small-volume, indistensible joints such as the joints of the hands and feet tend to develop erosions earlier and more extensively than more distensible joints such as the knee and shoulder, which can accommodate comparatively large pannus volume before bone erosion occurs.

It is important to note that productive bone of any type is extremely unusual in RA; specifically, periositis and enthesopathy do not occur. Ankylosis of a joint is extraordinarily rare and limited to fibrous ankylosis carpal and tarsal bones. Osteophytes are not seen in the absence of secondary degenerative joint disease. The exception to this rule is found in the distal ulna, where bone formation may be seen in a minority of patients with long-term RA. This productive change is termed "ulnar capping" (see Fig. 17-1).

Rheumatoid arthritis is remarkable for its symmetry. Although most synovial joints in the body can be affected by RA, survey films for the disease should include posteroanterior (PA) and ball catcher's *(Norgaard)* views of the hand, which is an AP oblique view with the hands internally rotated as if holding a large ball; AP and lateral views of the feet; and a lateral cervical spine, as these are the most frequent or clinically relevant sites.

Hand and Wrist

Proximal disease is the hallmark of RA of the hand and wrist, and the wrist demonstrates some of the earliest findings in RA. Early erosions are found in the distal radioulnar joint, pisotriquetral joint, ulnar styloid, radial styloid, and scaphoid waist (Figs. 17-2, 17-3). Early erosions in the triquetrum and pisiform are best seen on the Norgaard view (see Fig. 17-3). Thus, although RA eventually involves the midcarpal row and the carpal-metacarpal joints, its initial involvement in the hand and wrist is in the distal radioulnar joint and radiocarpal joint. In addition to the erosive change, ligamentous rupture can result in instability patterns and deformities (Figs. 17-4, 17-5), including ulnar translocation in which the entire carpus translates in an ulnar direction, scapholunate dissociation, distal radioulnar subluxation or dislocation, and dorsal as well as volar flexion carpal instability patterns. More distally, the early erosive ·pattern is seen in the metacarpophalangeal (MCP) joints. Although MCP erosions can be seen on the usual PA view, they sometimes are better seen on the Norgaard view (Fig. 17-6). Involvement of the MCP joints is usually followed by proximal interphalangeal (PIP) involvement (see Fig. 16-1). Distal interphalangeal (DIP) joints are spared early in the disease but may be involved once the disease becomes diffuse.

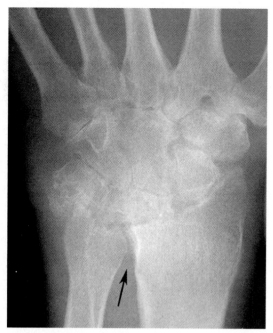

Figure 17-2   Rheumatoid arthritis, wrist. PA radiograph demonstrates osteopenia, complete loss of cartilage width in the radiocarpal as well as intercarpal joints, soft tissue swelling, and typical erosions of the distal radioulnar joint *(arrow)*, ulnar styloid, radiocarpal structures, and intercarpals. Note also that the entire carpus is slightly translocated in the ulnar direction.

Tendon ruptures are frequent, resulting in characteristic deformities. At the MCP joints, ulnar deviation and volar subluxations or dislocations are frequent, often with associated pressure erosions (see Figs. 17-4, 17-5). Swan neck deformities (PIP hyperextension and DIP hyperflexion) as well as boutonnière deformities (PIP hyperflexion and DIP hyperextension) are frequent. Hitchhiker's thumb (MCP flexion and IP extension) is seen frequently as well.

Elbow

The elbow is frequently involved in RA. The entire articulation is involved, with a positive fat pad sign indicating synovitis and/or effusion, and prominent erosions of the distal humerus, radial head and neck, and coronoid process (Fig. 17-7). Olecranon bursitis may be seen as a "mass" at the olecranon bursa, without joint involvement necessarily being associated.

Shoulder Girdle

The acromioclavicular joint is frequently involved with RA, with early changes seen as lysis of the distal clavicle and erosion of the coracoclavicular ligament insertion (Fig. 17-8). Although the sternomanubrial and sternoclavicular joints frequently have erosions, they are infrequently imaged. Marginal erosions can be

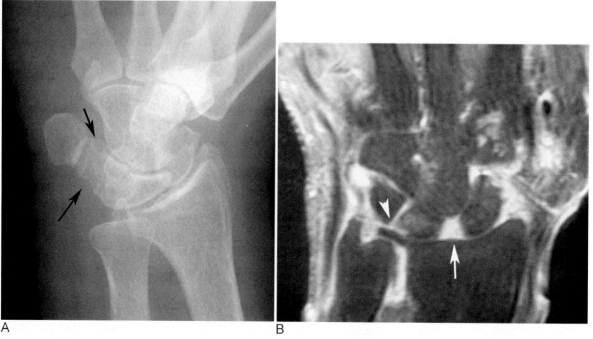

A   B

Figure 17-3   Rheumatoid arthritis, wrist. **A,** Norgaard (ball catcher's) view of the wrist demonstrates an erosion in the triquetrum *(arrows)*, which was not demonstrated on the PA view. There were no other abnormalities on this patient's hand, but this single erosion in this typical location allows for a diagnosis of rheumatoid arthritis. **B,** Coronal contrast-enhanced fat-suppressed T1-weighted MR image shows diffuse synovial enhancement, lunotriquetral interosseous ligament tear *(arrowhead)*, and scapholunate interosseous ligament tear with separation of these bones *(arrow)*. Rheumatoid arthritis pannus destroys carpal ligaments and thus is associated with carpal instability, discussed further in Chapter 7. (Part A reprinted with permission of the American College of Radiology learning file.)

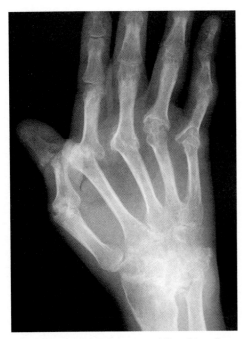

Figure 17-4   Rheumatoid arthritis, instability. PA radiographic view demonstrates the instability that can be seen in late rheumatoid arthritis, with ulnar translocation of the carpus, a "hitchhiker's thumb," volar subluxation, ulnar deviation of the MCP joints, and a boutonnière deformity of the fifth finger. A lateral view (not shown) might show dorsal or volar flexion instability patterns of the carpus. (Reprinted with permission of the American College of Radiology learning file.)

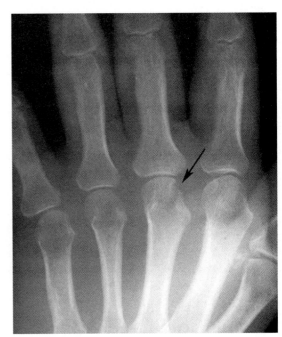

Figure 17-6   Rheumatoid arthritis, MCP joints. Ball catcher's radiographic view demonstrates periarticular osteopenia, soft tissue swelling at the MCP joints, and a solitary erosion at the head of the third metacarpal *(arrow)*. This was the only erosion seen in this patient, and the only view in which it was discernible. (Reprinted with permission of the American College of Radiology learning file.)

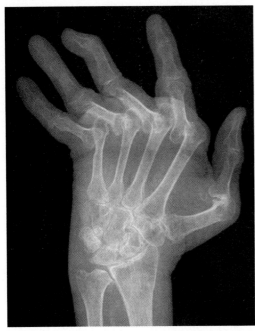

Figure 17-5   Rheumatoid arthritis, instability. PA view shows MCP dislocations and ulnar deviation of the second through fifth fingers, swan neck deformity of the third finger, as well as carpal and MCP erosions.

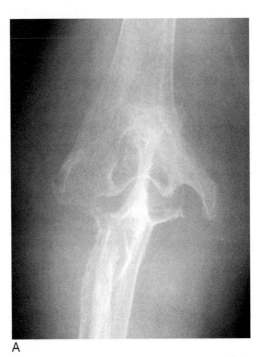

A

Figure 17-7   Rheumatoid arthritis, elbow. AP (A) and lateral (B) radiographs of the elbow in a patient with advanced rheumatoid arthritis demonstrate the diffuse and uniform erosive change that can be seen in this disease process.

(Continued)

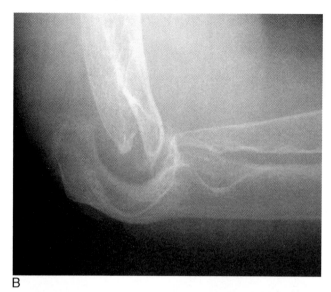

B

Figure 17-7—(Cont'd)   B, Radiographs of the elbow in a patient with advanced rheumatoid arthritis demonstrates the diffuse and uniform erosive change that can be seen in this disease process.

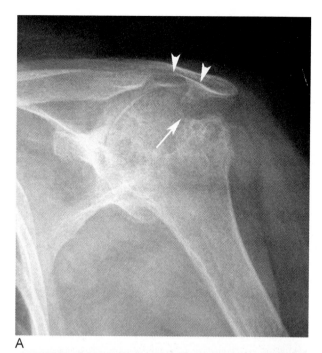

A

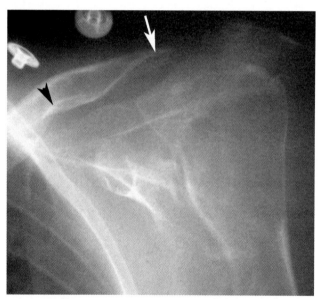

Figure 17-8   Rheumatoid arthritis, shoulder and acromioclavicular joint. AP radiograph of the acromioclavicular joint demonstrates elevation of the humeral head due to chronic rotator cuff tear, as well as erosions involving both the distal end of the clavicle *(arrow)* and the insertion of the coracoclavicular ligament *(arrowhead).*

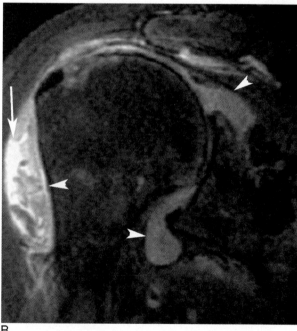

B

Figure 17-9   Rheumatoid arthritis, shoulder. **A,** AP radiograph shows osteopenia. The humeral head articulates with the undersurface of the acromion due to a chronic complete rotator cuff tear with retraction. Note the eroded undersurface of the acromion *(arrowheads)* and erosion in the greater tuberosity *(arrow).* **B,** Coronal fat-suppressed T2-weighted MR image shows intermediate-signal-intensity pannus *(arrowheads)* distending the joint, but only a small high-signal-intensity effusion. Also note high riding humeral head and thin rotator cuff. Other images (not shown) revealed cuff tears and muscle atrophy.

found at the humeral head adjacent to the greater tuberosity, at the capsular insertion on the anatomic neck of the humerus. As with other joints, tendons are frequently disrupted. In the case of the shoulder, the rotator cuff is frequently torn. These tears of course can be diagnosed on MRI or at arthrography. However, the chronicity of the rotator cuff tear is so prominent in patients with RA that they often develop the elevated humeral head and mechanical erosion at the undersurface of the acromion, which make the diagnosis obvious by radiography (Fig. 17-9). With the

elevation of the humeral head due to rotator cuff tear, mechanical erosion of the medial surgical neck of the humerus by the inferior glenoid can occur, occasionally resulting in a pathologic surgical neck fracture.

Feet

The metatarsophalangeal (MTP) joints commonly show early erosive changes, particularly at the fifth digit (Fig. 17-10). Interphalangeal and intertarsal erosions occur later in the disease. Associated deformities in the digits include lateral deviation at the MTP joints, hammer toe deformities (flexion of the PIP and DIP joints), and cock-up deformities (hyperextended MTP joints). Lateral foot films may demonstrate a retrocalcaneal bursitis, which may obliterate the normal pre-Achilles fat triangle, occasionally associated with erosive change at the posterior calcaneus (Fig. 17-11). This posterior calcaneal inflammatory and erosive change is also seen in psoriatic arthritis and reactive arthritis.

Knee

The knee is very frequently involved in RA, with joint effusion and popliteal synovial cysts seen early in the disease (Fig. 17-12). The latter may present as a large mass lesion. Once erosive change begins, all three compartments of the knee demonstrate uniform cartilage loss, erosions, and subchondral cyst formation. Valgus deformity most often occurs. Patellar tendon ruptures occasionally occur, and the distal femoral shaft can develop anterior mechanical erosion from patellar pressure.

Hip

Rheumatoid involvement in the hip results in a *concentric decrease in joint space* with axial migration of the femoral

head (i.e., relative to the axis of the femoral neck). Combined with acetabular remodeling, this can result in *protrusio acetabuli deformity* (medial displacement of the femoral head such that the medial femoral head cortex lies medial to the ilioischial line) (Fig. 17-13). These two characteristics can help to distinguish RA from osteoarthritis of the hip, which

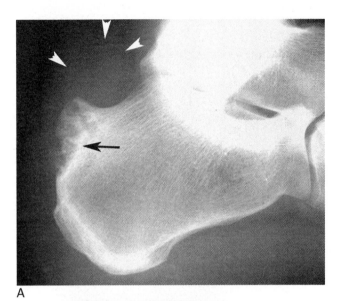

A

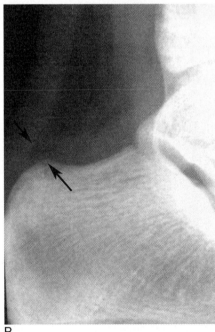

B

Figure 17-11   Rheumatoid arthritis, calcaneus. **A,** Lateral radiograph of the calcaneus demonstrates erosions at the posterior calcaneus *(arrow),* and retrocalcaneal bursitis seen as soft tissue density in the pre-Achilles fat triangle *(arrowheads).* These findings also can be associated with psoriasis and reactive arthritis. Most cases of retrocalcaneal bursitis are more subtle, and without erosion. **B,** Normal retrocalcaneal bursa for comparison. Note normal finding of inverted triangle fat between the distal Achilles tendon and the superior-posterior calcaneus (between *arrows).* (Part A reprinted with permission of the American College of Radiology learning file.)

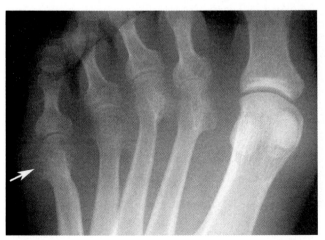

Figure 17-10   Rheumatoid arthritis, metatarsophalangeal (MTP) joints. AP radiograph of the foot demonstrates soft tissue swelling at the MTP joints and prominent metatarsal head erosions at the second, third, and fifth metatarsals *(arrow).* Erosions at the MTP joints are a frequent finding in rheumatoid arthritis. (Reprinted with permission of the American College of Radiology learning file.)

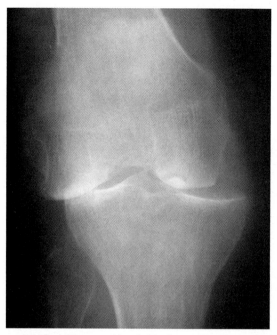

Figure 17-12 Rheumatoid arthritis, knee. AP radiograph shows diffuse osteopenia, uniform loss of cartilage space, and medial subluxation of the tibia with valgus angulation. This is a typical alignment and appearance of advanced RA involving the knee. (Reprinted with permission of the American College of Radiology learning file.)

shows preferential decrease in joint space width at the weight-bearing region, usually with superolateral subluxation. However, up to 20% of cases of osteoarthritis show protrusio. Even with protrusio, osteoarthritis shows osteophytes and normal bone density, whereas RA shows erosions and osteoporosis; these findings differentiate the two.

Soft tissue abnormalities may occur around hips in patients with RA. A soft tissue mass may develop anterior to the hip joint; in a patient with RA this almost invariably represents decompression of a large synovial effusion into the iliopsoas bursa. This is seen as a fluid collection elevating the neurovascular bundle on computed tomography (CT) (Fig. 17-14) as well as magnetic resonance imaging (MRI) (Fig. 17-15). Pannus and effusion also can decompress in other directions, notably inferiorly. Tendon ruptures occasionally occur around the hip. These are best diagnosed with MRI (see Fig. 17-15).

Spine

Involvement of the thoracic spine, lumbar spine, and sacroiliac joints by RA is usually mild and infrequently noted. The cervical region, however, is commonly involved. Abnormalities at C1–C2 are particularly important to diagnose because devastating neurologic deficits can result. The most frequently noted complication

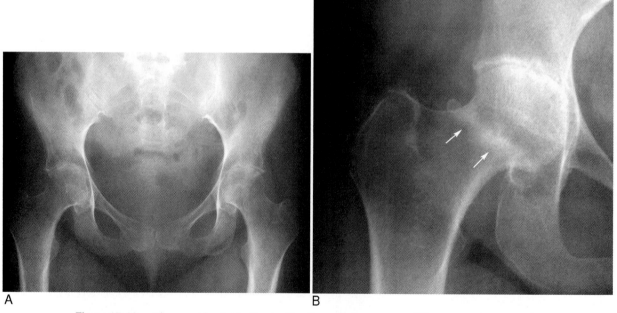

A   B

Figure 17-13 Rheumatoid arthritis, hip. **A,** AP radiograph demonstrates diffuse osteopenia, symmetric loss of cartilage width ("axial" migration of the femoral heads, in contrast with osteoarthritis, which may have superior migration of the femoral heads due to greater cartilage loss in the weight-bearing portion of the joint), small erosions, and mild protrusio of both hips. The appearance is typical of long-standing rheumatoid arthritis. **B,** Similar findings in a different patient, who also has a stress fracture of the femoral neck *(arrows).* The osteopenia associated with rheumatoid arthritis and steroid therapy increases the risk of stress and insufficiency fractures. (Part A reprinted with permission of the American College of Radiology learning file.)

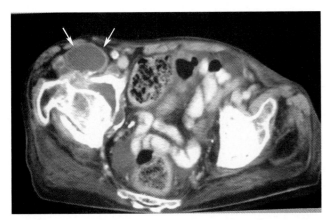

Figure 17-14   Rheumatoid arthritis, hip. Axial CT demonstrates a water density mass in the right iliopsoas bursa *(arrows)*, displacing the femoral neurovascular bundle medially. Note that the hip shows severe protrusio and erosive disease. The combination of the erosive disease in the hip with this mass makes the diagnosis of rheumatoid arthritis with decompression of synovial fluid into the iliopsoas bursa. (Reprinted with permission of the American College of Radiology learning file.)

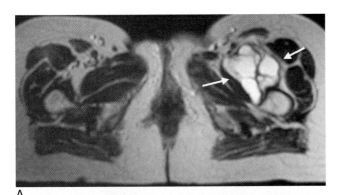

A

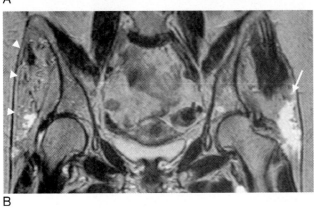

B

Figure 17-15   Rheumatoid arthritis, hip. **A,** Axial T2-weighted MR image in a 35-year-old woman with rheumatoid arthritis demonstrates a multiloculated cystic mass located within the iliopsoas bursa *(arrows)*. Like the mass seen in Figure 17-14, this represents decompression of synovial fluid from the hip into the iliopsoas bursa through the relatively weak anterior hip capsule. **B,** Coronal T2-weighted MR image in the same patient demonstrates bilateral gluteal tendon ruptures. On the left, note the high signal intensity at the site of the rupture *(arrow)*. The left rupture is relatively recent, as the musculature is not atrophic. On the right side, the gluteal musculature shows complete fatty atrophy, indicating a chronic tendon rupture *(arrowheads)*.

of RA in the C1–C2 region is atlantoaxial subluxation. In this process, pannus around the dens causes transverse atlantoaxial ligament laxity or disruption, resulting in the atlantoaxial distance measuring greater than 2.5 mm. Atlantoaxial subluxation often increases in flexion and reduces in extension (Fig. 17-16). Further-

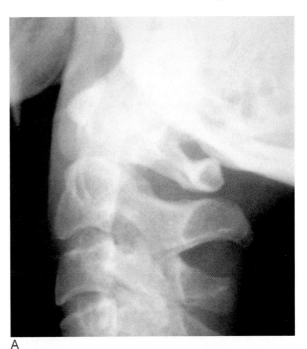

A

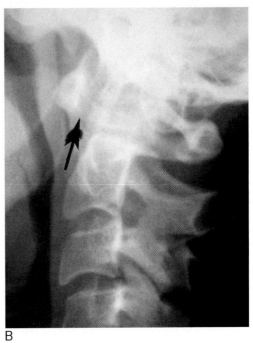

B

Figure 17-16   Rheumatoid arthritis, cervical spine. Atlantoaxial subluxation can be prominently seen, especially in flexion of the cervical spine. Note that in this case with extension (A), there is no evidence of atlantoaxial subluxation. However, in flexion (B), atlantoaxial subluxation of 8 mm is seen *(arrow)*. Even if it is difficult to see the odontoid process through the mastoids, the disruption of the spinal laminar line at C1–C2 indicates atlantoaxial subluxation. The other finding of rheumatoid arthritis in this patient is the lack of cortical distinctness of the facets of C3, C4, and C5.

more, mass effect due to the pannus around the odontoid process can decrease canal width; this can be diagnosed by MRI. Although atlantoaxial subluxation is diagnosed with an atlantoaxial measurement greater than 2.5 mm, it is often not symptomatic until subluxation approaches 9 mm.

Another important complication of RA at C1–C2 is atlantoaxial impaction. This impaction is due to C1–C2 facet erosion and subsequent collapse of the facets. With the facet collapse, the odontoid process protrudes into the foramen magnum. As the odontoid itself can be difficult to observe in patients with RA owing to superimposed mastoids and generalized osteopenia, atlantoaxial impaction is perhaps best detected by observation of the relationship of the anterior arch of the atlas with the odontoid process. On the lateral film, the atlas usually is aligned with the cranial portion of the odontoid. With impaction, the anterior arch of the atlas aligns with the body of C2 (Fig. 17-17). This relationship is important to detect, as neurologic symptoms are more often associated with atlantoaxial impaction than with subluxation.

Other abnormalities of RA involving the cervical spine include odontoid erosion, unilateral facet erosion that may result in torticollis, erosions at the facets and joints of Luschka, mechanical erosion of the spinal processes, and the appearance of "discitis" at several levels. This appearance is thought to be due to a combination of osteoporosis and posterior ligament laxity that results in decreased disk height, irregularity of the endplates, and a "stair-step" deformity is seen on the lateral film.

Robust Rheumatoid Arthritis

Robust RA features large subchondral cysts and normal bone density. The distribution of abnormalities is identical to that of RA, and the abnormality seems predominantly erosive, without productive change. It is generally seen in men who maintain normal activity, thus retaining their normal bone density and forcing decompression of synovial fluid into enlarging subchondral cysts (Fig. 17-18).

Adult Still's Disease

Adult Still's disease is clinically similar to the systemic form of juvenile chronic arthritis, with intermittent fever, skin rash, pleuritis, pericarditis, lymphadenopathy, and hepatosplenomegaly. Radiographically, carpal disease predominates. Pericapitate erosions and ankylosis are seen more frequently than radiocarpal disease (Fig. 17-19).

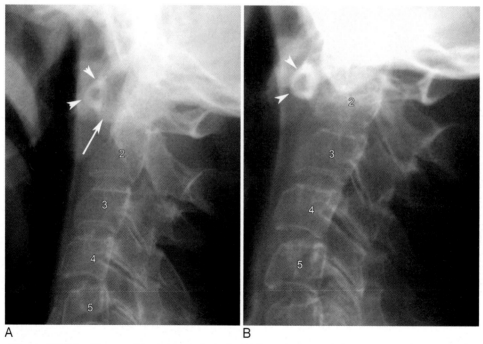

A   B

Figure 17-17 Rheumatoid arthritis, cervical spine. **A,** Lateral radiograph demonstrating atlantoaxial subluxation *(arrow)* and osteopenia. Note that the anterior arch of the atlas *(arrowheads)* is located at the level of the odontoid process and that at this point there is no evidence of atlantoaxial impaction. **B,** A film taken 2 years later demonstrates that severe atlantoaxial impaction has occurred, with the anterior arch of the atlas *(arrowheads)* now located opposite the inferior portion of the body of C2. Although you cannot actually see the odontoid process, it must be presumed to have impacted into the foramen magnum. Note the severe constriction of the spinal canal between the posterior aspect of the body of C2 and the anterior aspect of the spinous process of C1. Atlantoaxial impaction can be even more devastating to the patient's neurologic status than atlantoaxial subluxation. (Reprinted with permission of the American College of Radiology learning file.)

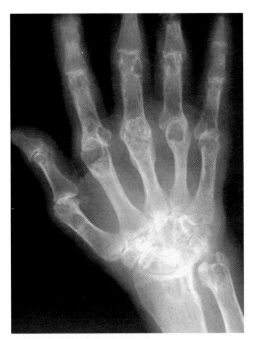

Figure 17-18   Robust rheumatoid arthritis. PA radiograph of the hand in a 47-year-old man demonstrates tremendous subchondral cyst formation as well as erosive change in the distribution of rheumatoid arthritis. The bone density is decreased, but not as much as one might expect for the severity of disease. This is a carpenter who has continued working in his profession despite his severe rheumatoid arthritis, leading to these changes of robust rheumatoid arthritis. (Reprinted with permission of the American College of Radiology learning file.)

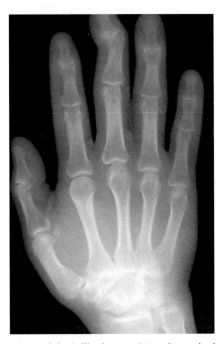

Figure 17-19   Adult Still's disease. PA radiograph demonstrates carpal and DIP disease. The pericapitate distribution of the carpal disease is typical for adult Still's disease. (Reprinted with permission of the American College of Radiology learning file.)

Differential Diagnosis

The distribution of abnormalities and pure erosive character of RA usually distinguish it from other arthritides. Occasionally, psoriatic arthritis may appear similar in the hand or foot, but the combination of proximal and distal disease and lack of symmetric distribution can allow a diagnosis of psoriatic arthritis. Retrocalcaneal bursitis and erosion of the adjacent calcaneus may appear identical in RA and reactive arthritis, but the latter may have superimposed enthesophyte formation and often has characteristic additional joint distribution (sacroiliac joints; foot findings predominating over those of the hand). The deformities seen so frequently in RA are mimicked with systemic lupus erythematosus (SLE), but the latter disease process is rarely erosive, and SLE deformities are reducible. Finally, spondyloarthropathy of hemodialysis may have discovertebral junction abnormalities similar to those found in the cervical spine in RA. However, C1–C2 and the facet joints are usually normal in spondyloarthropathy of hemodialysis, in which disk and endplate changes predominate, distinguishing this from RA.

JUVENILE RHEUMATOID ARTHRITIS

Juvenile RA is a group of related diseases of unknown cause arising in childhood. Juvenile chronic arthritis is basically a synonymous term for juvenile RA that is used in the United Kingdom. Juvenile RA symptom complexes have been divided into the following categories:

1. *Still's disease.* Twenty percent of patients with juvenile RA have Still's disease, which presents as an acute systemic process occurring in children under 5 years of age. Patients with Still's disease present with high fever, anemia, polymorphonuclear leukocytosis, hepatosplenomegaly, lymphadenopathy, and polyarthritis. They do not have iridocyclitis. Radiographic findings are often mild and erosions may not be present; however, 25% of patients with Still's disease can have chronic, destructive arthritis, which can be monoarticular or oligoarticular.

2. *Pauciarticular disease.* This is the most common type of juvenile RA, seen in 40% of patients. One fourth of such patients have chronic iridocyclitis, and they are RF negative. This type is most frequently seen in young girls. Inflammation is typically seen in one to three joints (usually large joints such as the knee, ankle, or elbow) and is rarely severe.

3. *Seronegative polyarticular disease.* Twenty-five percent of patients with juvenile RA have seronegative polyarticular disease. There is a female preponderance, the disease may occur at any age, and the patient remains RF negative. These patients show synovitis with the adult type of symmetric and widespread distribution involving both large and small joints.

4. *Seropositive polyarticular disease* (juvenile-onset adult RA). This makes up only 5% of patients with juvenile

RA. These patients show polyarticular changes typical of RA with severe erosive changes, and distribution similar to that of RA. Most patients become RA positive. This disease generally starts in the second decade of life.

5. *Juvenile ankylosing spondylitis (AS).* Juvenile AS is an inflammatory arthropathy with a strong male predominance (7:1) and strong HLA B27 positivity. These patients usually present with extra-axial arthritis and only rarely present with the classic signs and symptoms of sacroiliitis and spondylitis, which are more typical of the adult form of AS. Radiographically, sacroiliac joint abnormalities in these patients may be underdiagnosed because adolescent sacroiliac joints are normally wide, with indistinct cortices. Symptoms of pain at the symphysis pubis, ischial tuberosities, and costochondral junction are uncommon but strongly support the diagnosis. It should be remembered that juvenile AS is often misdiagnosed as juvenile RA because the abnormalities are not typical of those of adult AS and the sacroiliac joint abnormalities are particularly difficult to detect in adolescents.

Key Concepts	Juvenile Rheumatoid Arthritis (RA)

Variable clinical manifestations

Oligoarticular (pauciarticular) more frequent than polyarticular

Knee, elbow, hip most common sites

Minority of cases are early-onset RA or ankylosing spondylitis (AS)

Periarticular osteopenia

Cartilage destruction and erosions are late manifestations.

Joint contractures

Large joints: Effusions and synovitis, epiphyseal overgrowth, early growth plate closure

Hip: Valgus, protrusio acetabuli

Hand: MCP and PIP; ankylosis

Wrist: Midcarpal joint; ankylosis

Cervical spine: Atlantoaxial subluxation, odontoid erosions, ankylosis

Whatever the clinical symptom complex may be, the radiographic changes of the arthropathy of juvenile RA are similar among the various categories, particularly Still's and pauciarticular disease. Patients with juvenile RA have a radiologic appearance distinct from that of adult RA. The articular bones are usually osteoporotic, but cartilage destruction and erosive change occur only as late manifestations. Subchondral cysts are rarely present. Periosteal reaction may be seen in early juvenile RA (Fig. 17-20), and ankylosis is more common in juvenile RA than adult RA. Joint contractures are common. One very distinctive feature of juvenile RA is growth abnormalities. With hyperemia in the skeletally immature patient, there is overgrowth of the involved epiphyses. This leads to "ballooning" of joints clinically, and radiography demonstrates epiphyseal overgrowth and advanced skeletal maturation with premature physeal fusion in the involved joints. Therefore, asymmetry in epiphyseal size and maturation may suggest juvenile RA as a diagnosis (Fig. 17-21). With premature fusion, one may find a shortened limb on the affected side.

The distribution of joint involvement in juvenile RA can be similar to that in adult RA. However, there is generally a predilection for large joints rather than small joints. Thus, the knee and the elbow are commonly and distinctively involved. The knee shows an effusion, widened intercondylar notch, metaphyseal and epiphyseal flaring, overgrowth relating to the hyperemia, and uniform cartilage destructive change (Fig. 17-22). The elbow also shows effusion, enlargement of the trochlear notch, radial head enlargement due to overgrowth from hyperemia, and uniform cartilage destructive change (Fig. 17-23). The hip also shows common distinctive involvement, with femoral head enlargement, a short neck with valgus, and significant protrusio acetabuli (Fig. 17-24). The iliac wings are often

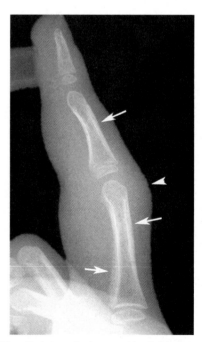

Figure 17-20   Early juvenile rheumatoid arthritis. Lateral radiograph of the index finger in a 6-year-old girl demonstrates soft tissue swelling and dense periosteal reaction *(arrows)* and mild soft tissue swelling *(arrowhead)*. Although these changes are not pathognomonic for juvenile rheumatoid arthritis (they could be seen in a bone infarct in a young patient with sickle cell disease, or infection), they are typical as the first manifestation of juvenile rheumatoid arthritis.

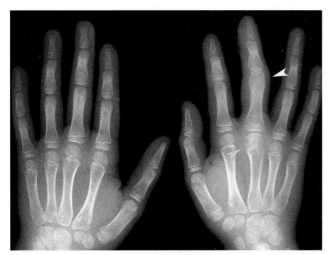

Figure 17-21   Pauciarticular juvenile rheumatoid arthritis with focal overgrowth. PA radiograph of the hands in this 8-year-old girl demonstrates soft tissue swelling and bone overgrowth *(arrows)* of the right third ray (metacarpal and finger) compared with the opposite normal left side. This focal acceleration of skeletal maturation results from chronic hyperemia at this site with pauciarticular juvenile rheumatoid arthritis.

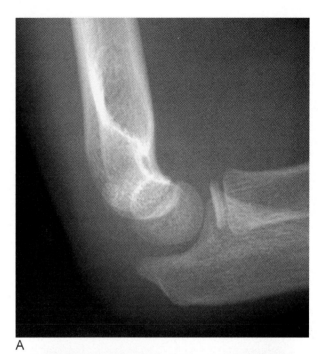

A

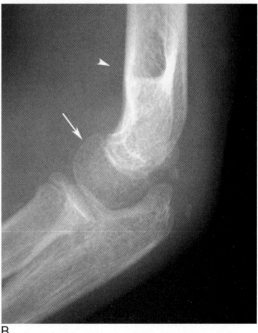

B

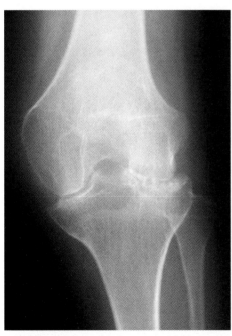

Figure 17-22   Juvenile rheumatoid arthritis, knee. AP radiograph of the knee in this 23-year-old patient demonstrates typical findings of long-standing juvenile rheumatoid arthritis, with overgrown epiphyses and metaphyses, normal size of the diaphyses, wide intercondylar notch, and subchondral erosions with cartilage loss. The relative enlargement of the bones at the joint compared with the diaphyses is seen in juvenile rheumatoid arthritis because of the chronic hyperemia occurring during skeletal growth. (Reprinted with permission of the American College of Radiology learning file.)

Figure 17-23   Juvenile rheumatoid arthritis, elbow. Left (A) and right (B) elbow lateral radiographs in this child with juvenile rheumatoid arthritis demonstrate relative overgrowth of the capitellum and radial head on the right side *(arrows)*. Additionally, the right elbow shows ossification of the olecranon apophysis and an AP radiograph (not shown) demonstrated asymmetric early ossification of the lateral epicondyle on the right compared with ossification of that structure not yet occurring on the left. This advancement of skeletal maturation is typical in a joint affected by juvenile rheumatoid arthritis. The adult elbow will show relative enlargement compared with the left, particularly of the radial head.

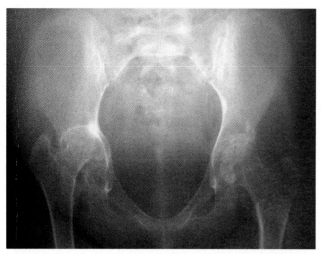

Figure 17-24 Juvenile rheumatoid arthritis, pelvis. AP radiograph of the pelvis of a 20-year-old woman with juvenile rheumatoid arthritis demonstrates the small stature and gracile diaphyses typically seen in these patients. It also shows severe erosive change involving both hips, with protrusio particularly on the right side. This particular case does not show the valgus deformity that can occur in the femoral necks. (Reprinted with permission of the American College of Radiology learning file.)

hypoplastic and the femoral shaft can be gracile. The small bones combined with the coxa valga abnormality can make joint replacement difficult.

The hand and wrist in juvenile RA shows MCP and PIP involvement similar to adult RA. However, in the wrist the radio-carpal joint may be spared and the midcarpal joint involved, particularly in the pericapitate region. This may distinguish juvenile RA from adult RA. Adult Still's disease is similar to juvenile RA in this aspect. Ankylosis is very common in the hand and wrist in juvenile RA (Fig. 17-25).

In addition to early physeal closure, the ankle may show unilateral or bilateral valgus alignment due to growth disturbance, sometimes called "tibial-talar tilt" (Fig. 17-26). Other conditions may also result in this abnormal alignment, which also may be remembered with the mnemonic "Sure Does Hurt To Jog": sickle cell anemia, skeletal dysplasias, hemophilia, and traumatic physeal injury, in addition to juvenile RA.

As in adult RA, the cervical spine is commonly affected in juvenile RA, but the pattern is different. Atlantoaxial subluxation and odontoid erosions are prominent findings. Facet erosions are seen as well. However, with juvenile RA, cervical spine ankylosis is common, especially of the facet joints. This ankylosis is thought to protect these patients from developing the discovertebral junction abnormalities seen so often in adult RA. If cervical spine ankylosis occurs before skeletal maturation, there is vertebral body hypoplasia both in height and in AP dimension, resulting in the appearance of "waisting" of the bodies (Fig. 17-27). This is a very distinctive appearance for juvenile RA.

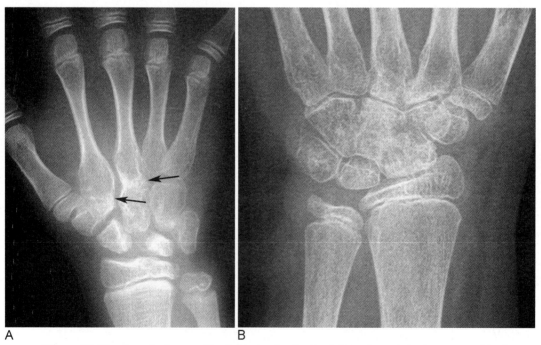

A   B

Figure 17-25 Juvenile rheumatoid arthritis, hand and wrist. **A,** PA radiograph in this 11-year-old girl demonstrates little loss of cartilage width in the wrist or MCP joints but abnormal fusion between the capitate and third metacarpal, as well as between the trapezium and second metacarpal and trapezoid *(arrows).* Early fusion in the absence of substantial erosive change or loss of cartilage is typical finding in juvenile rheumatoid arthritis. **B,** PA wrist radiograph in a different child with juvenile rheumatoid arthritis shows fusion of multiple carpal bones.

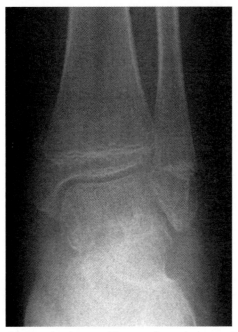

Figure 17-26 Juvenile rheumatoid arthritis, ankle. PA radiograph shows valgus alignment at the distal tibia due to growth disturbance.

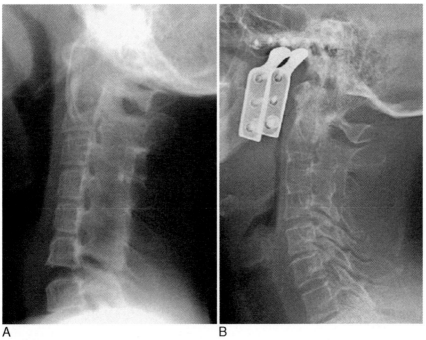

A   B

Figure 17-27 Juvenile rheumatoid arthritis, cervical spine. **A,** Lateral radiograph of the cervical spine demonstrates complete fusion of the facets of C2 through C6. This fusion protects the endplates and disk spaces from the deterioration that is seen in advanced adult rheumatoid arthritis. Fusion at an early age also results in restriction of growth of the vertebral bodies in an AP dimension (note how much smaller the bodies of C3, C4, and C5 are than C2, C6, and C7 in the AP diameter). This appearance has been termed "waisting" of the cervical bodies. **B,** Lateral CT localizer image in a different patient with juvenile rheumatoid arthritis shows congenital fusion C2–C4 and bilateral temporomandibular joint (TMJ) arthroplasties. Temporomandibular joint arthropathy occurs with both juvenile and adult rheumatoid arthritis. (Part A reprinted with permission of the American College of Radiology learning file.)

CHAPTER 18

Productive Arthritis

OSTEOARTHRITIS
NEUROPATHIC (CHARCOT'S) ARTHROPATHY
DIFFUSE IDIOPATHIC SKELETAL HYPEROSTOSIS
   (FORESTIER'S DISEASE)

OSTEOARTHRITIS

Osteoarthritis (OA) is by far the most common arthropathy and the most common cause of disability in the United States. The condition may be primary or secondary. *Secondary OA* can be caused by abnormal mechanical forces (joint deformity, obesity, occupational stresses) or as an end-stage consequence of a preceding joint insult, such as an injury, chronic rheumatoid arthritis, loose bodies, osteochondral fracture, or meniscal tear. *Primary OA* presents without such antecedent insult. Primary OA is less common and in most cases is probably due to a genetic defect in articular cartilage synthesis. As noted in Chapter 2, articular cartilage is one of the few tissues of the musculoskeletal system that is incapable of regeneration. Damaged cartilage inadequately cushions the subjacent subchondral bone, which results in adaptive changes in the subchondral bone, including osteophyte formation and subchondral fibrosis and sclerosis. These changes make the subchondral bone less compliant; as a result, the remaining cartilage is subjected to greater stress, which accelerates further cartilage loss. Adaptive remodeling of subchondral bone may lead to articular surface or joint alignment deformity, further accelerating the degenerative process. In addition to these mechanisms of cartilage destruction, synovial fluid biochemistry is altered in OA, with elevated catabolic factors. Because OA is not primarily an inflammatory process, some authors use the synonymous term *osteoarthrosis*.

Osteoarthritis affects males and females equally, with incidence increasing with age. The clinical signs of OA include pain with weight bearing, limited range of motion, crepitus, and subluxation. The radiographic severity of disease does not always correlate with the amount of pain. The radiographic

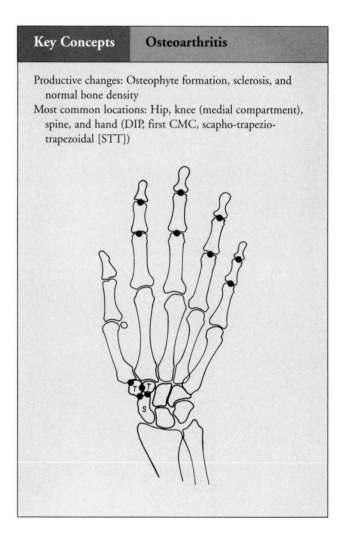

Key Concepts	Osteoarthritis

Productive changes: Osteophyte formation, sclerosis, and
   normal bone density
Most common locations: Hip, knee (medial compartment),
   spine, and hand (DIP, first CMC, scapho-trapezio-
   trapezoidal [STT])

manifestations include cartilage destruction in the weight-bearing portions of the joint, lack of erosions, subchondral cyst formation, and bone productive change. Bone production consists of osteophyte formation, which may be marginated or central. Productive change is also seen as subchondral sclerosis and cortical buttressing, which is a response to abnormal mechanical forces. In the hip, this is seen particularly well on the medial and lateral aspects of the femoral neck. Bone density is normal, or at least is not decreased around the affected joints compared to other sites. Subchondral cysts are common because of microfractures in the subchondral bone and synovial fluid pressure. The cysts tend to occur in weight-bearing areas and generally have a sclerotic margin. Traction enthesophytes are another common productive process, relating to shifts in biomechanical loading, seen particularly on the anterior aspect of the patella and at the hip and pelvic apophyses. This enthesopathy is not distinguishable from that seen in ankylosing spondylitis and the other seronegative rheumatoid variants. Ankylosis is rare in the absence of trauma. Ligament abnormalities are commonly seen in OA. Focal cartilage loss leads to joint deformity, which in turn promotes ligamentous contractures and laxity. This ligamentous abnormality in turn promotes further arthropathy because of shifts in mechanical loading and further wear.

Primary OA most frequently involves the hand, wrist, acromioclavicular joint, hip, knee, foot, and spine. Within each of these, specific sites of involvement are expected for OA. Thus, location, nonuniform joint space loss, and the purely productive nature of the process help to secure the diagnosis. In the hand, several interphalangeal joints are often involved with nonuniform cartilage narrowing, subchondral sclerosis, and osteophyte formation. The metacarpophalangeal (MCP) joints are less commonly involved than the interphalangeal (IP) joints, and almost never are involved in the absence of findings

of OA in the IP joints. The diagnosis of OA in the hand can be substantiated by typical findings of sclerosis, osteophyte formation, and cartilage loss in the first carpometacarpal joint. The second most common site of involvement in the wrist is the scaphoid-trapezium-trapezoid complex (STT) (Fig. 18-1). Osteoarthritis involving the radiocarpal or distal radioulnar joint is almost always secondary to prior trauma (e.g., a distal radial fracture that has healed with deformity).

The acromioclavicular joint frequently shows typical changes of OA. On the other hand, OA is unusual in the glenohumeral joint in the absence of previous trauma. When OA is present in the glenohumeral joint, the marginal osteophytes form around the glenoid and ring osteophytes form around the anatomic neck of the humerus, with the largest found inferiorly. Chronic rotator cuff tear and shoulder instability may predispose to OA of the glenohumeral joint.

The hip is an extremely common site of OA. Early signs include subchondral cyst formation in the acetabulum and calcar buttressing (Fig. 18-2). Recall that the calcar is the medial femoral neck cortex. Later changes show typical signs of focal cartilage narrowing in the superior weight-bearing portion, sclerosis, and osteophyte formation. Osteophytes are seen ringing the subcapital femoral neck, but can be particularly prominent medially. In 80% of patients, the hip migrates superolaterally (Fig. 18-3A). However, in 20% of patients with OA, the hip migrates in a medial direction. This may result in protrusio acetabuli (Fig. 18-3B).

Hip OA can overlap in appearance with other arthropathies. Rheumatoid arthritis also can result in protrusio

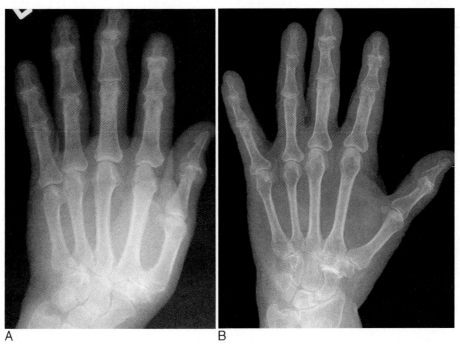

A   B

Figure 18-1   Osteoarthritis: hands. **A,** PA radiograph demonstrates the typical appearance of osteoarthritis, with normal bone density, and loss of cartilage width in the presence of osteophyte formation in the typical locations of the first carpometacarpal joint and scapho-trapezio-trapezoidal joint, as well as the DIP joints. **B,** Similar findings in a different patient.

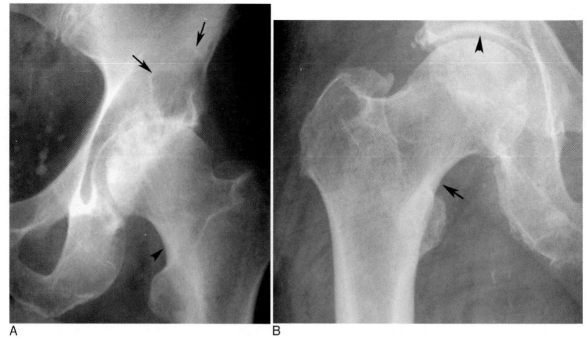

Figure 18-2   Osteoarthritis: hip. **A,** AP radiograph demonstrates typical osteoarthritis with loss of cartilage width in the weight-bearing portion of the hip (superior migration of the femoral head), osteophyte formation, normal bone density, and a large subchondral cyst located in the acetabulum *(arrows)*. Also note the calcar buttressing (thick cortex of the medial femoral neck cortex). **B,** Different patient with osteoarthritis, subchondral sclerosis of the acetabular roof *(arrowhead),* and calcar buttressing *(arrow).*

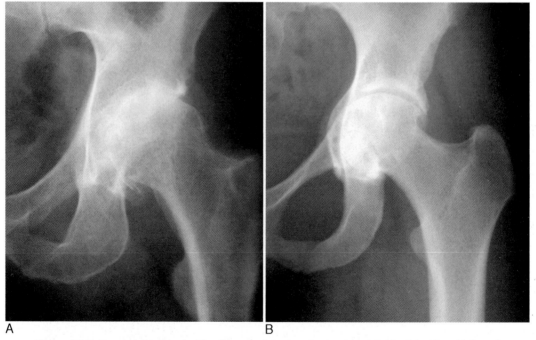

Figure 18-3 Osteoarthritis: hip. **A,** AP radiograph of classic-appearing osteoarthritis of the hip, with loss of cartilage width, osteophyte formation, mild superolateral subluxation of the femoral head, and buttressing along the femoral neck and calcar *(arrows).* **B,** AP radiograph in a different patient, also demonstrating osteoarthritis. Osteophytes are present, but this time the hip is moving into a protrusio position. Approximately 20% of patients with osteoarthritis develop circumferential cartilage loss, a pattern similar to inflammatory arthritis, rather than the more common superolateral subluxation. Protrusio acetabuli develops in some of these cases due to bone remodeling. (Reprinted with permission of the American College of Radiology learning file.)

acetabuli but will not demonstrate productive changes. Late-stage hip OA may develop large inferomedial femoral head osteophytes, which may simulate superior flattening of the head because of old, healed avascular necrosis with secondary OA. This distinction is usually not clinically significant. Focal subchondral avascular necrosis can occur in degenerative joint disease, with appearance similar to a subchondral fracture on magnetic resonance imaging (MRI) and bone scanning. Again, however, the distinction is usually not important to patient care. If large cysts are present, OA may resemble calcium pyrophosphate dihydrate deposition (CPPD; see Chapter 21) or pigmented villonodular synovitis. An early femoral head ring osteophyte in an osteoporotic hip may simulate an impacted subcapital fracture line. Magnetic resonance imaging can be useful to exclude a fracture when suspected. Finally, an unusual variant of OA in the hip is rapidly destructive hip disease. This process is seen mostly in elderly women and results in rapid destructive changes in the femoral head and acetabulum, suggestive of infection or Charcot's joint.

The knee is a common site of involvement of OA (Figs. 18-4, 18-5). It may involve one, two, or all three compartments. If a patient has single-compartment disease, it is likely to be medial, although a patellar tracking abnormality can result in predominately patellofemoral compartment disease. With medial compartment predominance, one sees a typical varus deformity of the knee and lateral subluxation of the tibia. Single-compartment disease should be specifically commented on in a report because treatment may be with a unicompartmental prosthesis or a high tibial osteotomy (Fig. 18-6). The osteophyte formation in the knee tends to be marginal in all three compartments, and can be found on the tibial spines. Enthesopathy is particularly prominent on the nonarticular surface of the patella at the quadriceps insertion. Differential diagnosis of OA of the knee includes pyrophosphate arthropathy (CPPD) or pigmented villonodular synovitis if subchon-

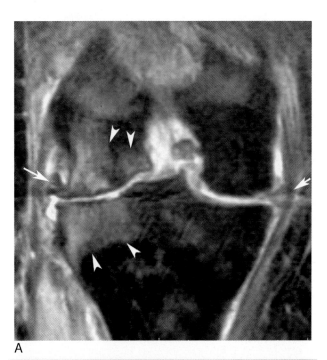

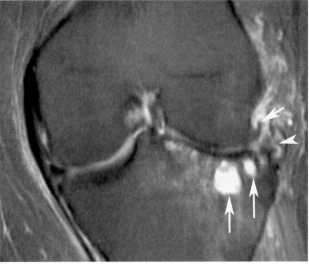

Figure 18-5   Osteoarthritis: knee. **A,** Coronal fat-suppressed proton density-weighted MR image shows peripheral extrusion of both menisci *(arrows),* complete loss of medial compartment cartilage, and edema-like signal in medial compartment subchondral bone *(arrowheads).* The marrow edema may represent trabecular microfractures or vascular fibrous ingrowth, and corresponds to some degree with the degree of symptoms. **B,** Coronal fat-suppressed proton density-weighted image in a different patient shows lateral compartment osteoarthritis with subchondral cysts *(long arrows),* surrounding marrow edema, osteophytes *(short arrow),* and peripherally extruded and macerated medial meniscus body *(arrowhead).*

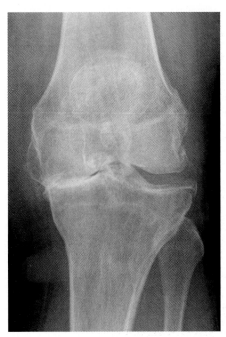

Figure 18-4   Osteoarthritis: knee. AP left knee radiograph shows osteophytes and medial compartment narrowing with varus alignment.

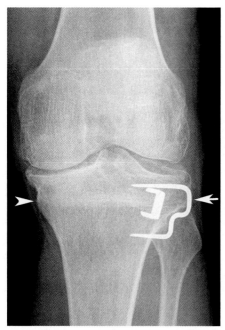

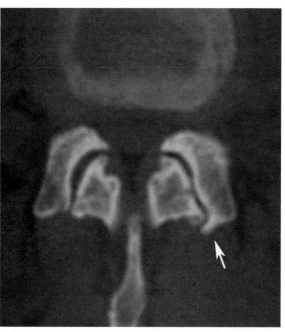

Figure 18-6 High tibial osteotomy for knee osteoarthritis. This patient had knee osteoarthritis with varus alignment. A wedge of bone was removed from the proximal tibia. The apex of the wedge was at the medial cortex *(arrowhead)*. After the wedge of bone was removed, the defect was closed, correcting the varus alignment. The osteotomy is fixed with two lateral staples. Note the Coventry staple *(arrow)*, which matches the stepoff of the lateral tibial cortex created by the osteotomy. This procedure rebalances forces across the knee, delaying or sometimes avoiding the need for arthroplasty.

Figure 18-7 Facet osteoarthritis. Axial CT shows osteophytes at the left L3–L4 facet *(arrow)*. Such osteophytes can make direct injection into the joint by using fluoroscopic guidance difficult.

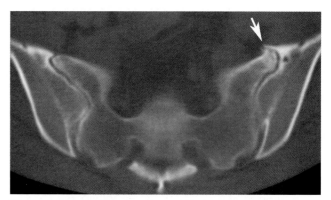

Figure 18-8 Sacroiliac joint osteoarthritis. Axial CT shows anterior osteophytes *(arrow)* at the left sacroiliac joint. Such osteophytes frequently bridge across the joint, not to be confused with ankylosis due to seronegative spondyloarthropathy.

dral cysts are especially prominent. Particularly if patellofemoral disease is prominent, one should consider CPPD and seek the presence of chondrocalcinosis for confirmation.

Osteoarthritis of the axial skeleton is extremely common. The sacroiliac joints manifest this disease with subchondral sclerosis and osteophytes, which are usually marginal in nature (Fig. 18-7). Remember that only the inferior portion of the sacroiliac joints are synovial and therefore vulnerable to OA. Large osteophytes bridge the joint anteriorly. These bridging osteophytes may be misdiagnosed as focal osteoblastic metastases on a radiograph but should be properly identified as osteophytes based on location. If confirmation is needed, computed tomography (CT) shows the bridging osteophytes. Osteoarthritis of the sacroiliac joint should be differentiated from ankylosing spondylitis. It also should not be confused with osteitis condensans ilii, which is a triangular sclerotic lesion found on the iliac side of the inferior sacroiliac joint, seen most often in multiparous women as a reactive change likely related to acquired sacroiliac ligamentous laxity.

Osteoarthritis may involve the facet (apophyseal) joints of the spine (Fig. 18-8). Facet joint OA is seen most commonly at the C5–C7 and L4–S1 levels, but any level may be involved and the process may be asymmetric. The severity of facet degenerative change is best judged with CT or MRI, with

which direct observation of foraminal stenosis can also be made. If the OA of the facets is prominent, it can result in a spondylolisthesis without spondylolysis, which also contributes to foraminal and canal stenosis. Osteoarthritis also affects the cervical uncovertebral joints (also termed uncinate joints and joints of Luschka, Fig. 18-9). These joints are found only at C3–C7 and are located posterolaterally at the vertebral bodies. In the cervical spine, these can contribute to neuroforaminal and central stenosis.

Because OA is a disease of synovial joints, degenerative disk changes are not truly OA; however, the adaptive and degenerative changes are somewhat similar. A complete

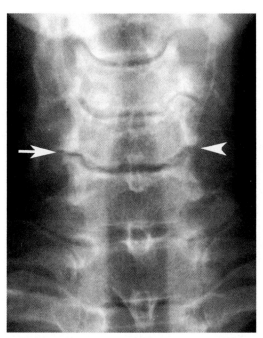

Figure 18-9 Cervical spine uncinate osteoarthritis. AP cervical spine radiograph shows right side spurs and joint space narrowing at C6–C7 *(arrow),* compared with the normal left side *(arrowhead).*

discussion of disk disease is beyond the scope of this book. This discussion of disk degeneration emphasizes the association of disk degeneration with marrow signal changes that might be confused with more serious disease, such as discitis or vertebral metastases. Degenerated disks show decreased disk height, sharply demarcated endplate signal on MRI, and possibly disk vacuum sign by radiography and CT. Bulges and protrusions are frequent. Marrow adjacent to the endplates usually shows signal alterations that are termed *Modic changes* in honor of the radiologist Michael Modic, who described them in the 1980s. Type 1 Modic change is decreased T1 and increased T2 signal intensity due to fibrovascular infiltration. Type 2 change is increased T1 and T2 signal due to fibrofatty infiltration. These changes are visible only on MRI (Figs. 18-10, 18-11). Type 3 change is low T1 and T2 signal due to reactive bone sclerosis ("discogenic sclerosis"), which may also be visible on CT or radiography (Fig. 18-10B). Modic changes are significant because first, they indicate degenerative disk disease and may themselves contribute to back pain and, second, they are otherwise incidental and should not be confused with marrow changes due to infection, tumor, or trauma. This distinction is not always easy. For example, discitis can cause Modic type 1 and 3–like changes, but with discitis the endplate is abnormal or destroyed. In addition, discogenic sclerosis of the superior endplate may be distinctive, being triangular shaped in the anterior portion of the vertebral

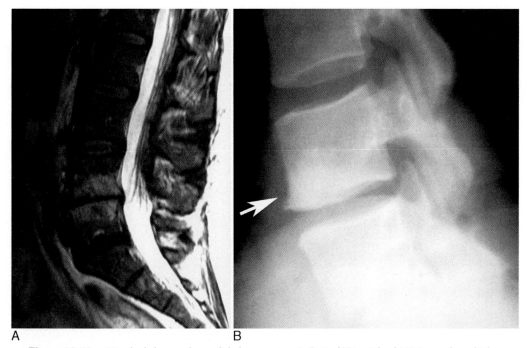

A   B

Figure 18-10 Vertebral changes due to disk degeneration. **A,** Sagittal T2-weighted MR image shows high signal intensity centered on the narrowed L4–L5 disk. This finding may be associated with low or high T1 signal intensity. **B,** Lateral radiograph. MRI is more sensitive to vertebral changes related to disk degeneration, but reactive bone sclerosis (discogenic sclerosis) can be seen on radiographs. Note the disk space narrowing at L4–L5, with sclerosis seen at the anterior inferior endplate at L4 *(arrows).*

(Continued)

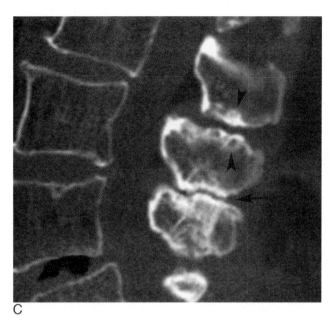

C

Figure 18-10—(Cont'd) C, Another consequence of disk degeneration is impaction of adjacent spinous processes with secondary osteoarthritis-like degenerative changes, shown on this sagittal CT reconstruction, also known as Baastrup's disease. Note subcortical "cysts" *(arrowheads),* cortical sclerosis, and impaction of adjacent spinous processes *(arrow).*

body (Fig. 18-10B). This distinctive shape may help distinguish discogenic sclerosis from a blastic metastatic tumor.

Loss of disc height contributes to facet OA and neural impingement, and may also cause impaction of adjacent spinous processes resulting in pain and OA-like radiographic changes (Fig. 18-10C) known as Baastrup's disease.

A *Schmorl's node* is intraosseous disk herniation through a weakened vertebral end plate, or metaplasia of a degenerated endplate and adjacent bone into cartilage and fibrous tissue (Fig. 18-11). An intraosseous herniation that occurs peripherally in the growing spine may separate the ring apophysis from the vertebral body, resulting in a *limbus vertebra.* This is seen on a lateral radiograph as a triangular ossicle located at the anterosuperior border of the vertebral body (Fig. 18-12). This is an incidental finding generally thought to be of no significance other than the possibility that it could mimic an ununited fracture.

Endplate spurs related to disk degeneration can occasionally be confused with the syndesmophytes of seronegative spondyloarthropathies. These spurs are sometimes called spinal osteophytes or traction spurs. Degenerative endplate spurs begin close to the endplate and extend horizontally away from the vertebral body, although they may curve around the bulging disk and may fuse with a spur from and adjacent level (Fig. 18-13). In contrast, the syndesmophytes of reactive arthritis and psoriasis originate closer to the midportion of the vertebral body and do not extend horizontally (see Fig. 19-12). *Spondylosis deformans* is an older term that describes advanced spine degeneration with prominent endplate spurs and subluxations.

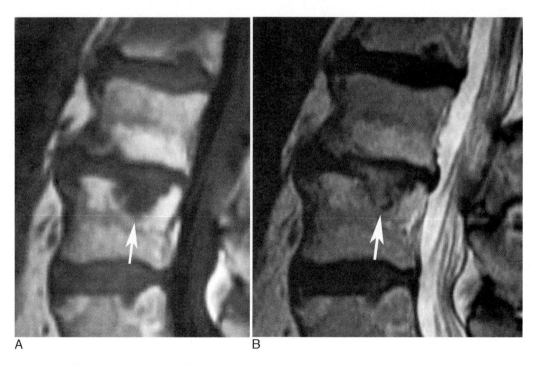

A   B

Figure 18-11 Schmorl's nodes. Sagittal T1-weighted (A) and T2-weighted (B) MR images show Modic type 1 changes (high signal on both sequences) and disk extension into an adjacent vertebral body *(arrow).*

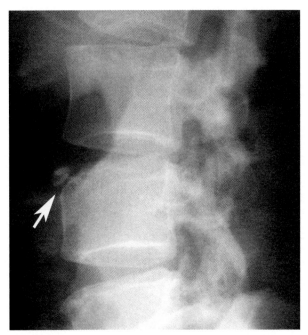

Figure 18-12   Limbus vertebra. Note the normal variant limbus vertebra, with a separated triangular fragment from the anterior superior endplate of L4 *(arrow)*.

NEUROPATHIC (CHARCOT'S) ARTHROPATHY

Neuropathic arthropathy is a severely destructive process, usually but not invariably monostotic, with several possible causes. Progression may be extremely rapid. The location of the neuropathic joint usually indicates its specific underlying cause. The most common causes of neuropathic arthropathy are diabetes, tabes dorsalis, syringomyelia, and spinal cord injury. Less frequent causes include multiple sclerosis, alcoholism, amyloidosis, intra-articular steroid use, congenital insensitivity to pain, congenital indifference to pain, and neurologic conditions such as Charcot-Marie-Tooth disease and dysautonomia (Riley-Day syndrome). The primary pathogenesis is uncertain, but most investigators agree that there is an initial alteration in sympathetic nerve control of osseous blood flow, which leads to hyperemia and active bone resorption. Secondarily, there seems to be a neurotraumatic mechanism resulting in a destructive cycle that consists first of blunted pain sensation and proprioception. This is followed by relaxation of skeletal supporting structures and chronic instability, leading to recurrent injury by normal biomechanical stresses but abnormal joint loading, resulting in bony fragmentation and joint disorganization. Mineralization may be normal at this stage.

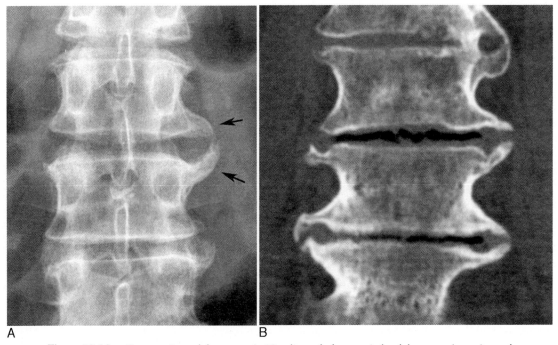

A   B

Figure 18-13   Degenerative endplate spurs. **A,** AP radiograph shows typical endplate spurs *(arrows)* caused by disk bulges with stretching of annular fibers. Note that the spurs initially extend horizontally away from the vertebral body. **B,** Coronal CT reconstruction in a different patient shows similar findings. Other terms for these bony excrescences include "spinal osteophytes," "traction spurs," and "claw osteophytes." Contrast with the nearly vertical fine marginal syndesmophytes of ankylosing spondylitis (see Fig. 19-4) and the syndesmophytes of psoriasis and reactive arthritis that do not extend horizontally (see Fig. 19-12). Also note the vacuum phenomenon seen as air density in the disks that are not fused by bridging spurs in part B.

Key Concepts	Neuropathic Arthropathy

Severe, destructive

Hypertrophic or atrophic

Consistently present: Large effusions

Ligamentous laxity: Subluxation, dislocation

Hypertrophic: Five Ds: bony debris, cartilage destruction, normal bone density, joint distention, joint disorganization (or dislocation or deformity)

Charcot's feet: Usually diabetes mellitus

Charcot's knee: Tabes dorsalis, diabetes, or congenital insensitivity/indifference to pain

Charcot's shoulder: Syringomyelia

Charcot's spine: Diabetes or instrumented spinal trauma in paraplegic patients

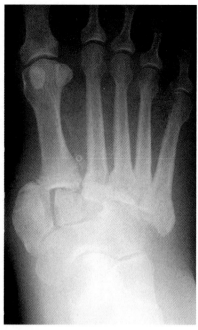

Figure 18-14 Neuropathic foot. AP radiograph demonstrates convergent Lisfranc's dislocation. Note the vascular calcification, a clue to the presence of diabetes. There is no history of significant trauma. This is a common location for a neuropathic joint in the diabetic foot. (Reprinted with permission of the American College of Radiology learning file.)

Clinically, the patient presents with a swollen unstable joint. The diagnosis of a neuropathic joint may not be clinically obvious because proprioception may be only decreased rather than eliminated in up to 30% of patients, thus allowing them to present before gross deformity has developed, and the neurologic changes may be difficult to elicit.

The classic radiographic description of neuropathic arthropathy is that of the "five Ds": normal bone density, joint distention, bony debris, joint disorganization, and dislocation. These five Ds describe the hypertrophic variety of neuropathic arthropathy well, but only 20% are purely hypertrophic. Forty percent are primarily atrophic, with such severe bone resorption that there is little or no debris and often a sharp transverse margin of an involved long bone in the metadiaphysis, which may appear almost surgically created. Another 40% of neuropathic joints are combined hypertrophic and atrophic. Regardless of the bone density, all cases invariably include large effusions. If debris is present, the effusions may decompress along fascial planes, carrying bony debris far from the joint. The bone density is typically normal, except when the underlying density is decreased, as in elderly or diabetic patients. Cartilage destruction occurs early, and erosive and productive changes coexist. Subchondral cysts may be present. Ligamentous laxity is a prominent finding, often associated with joint subluxation or dislocation. Ankylosis is rare, and in fact surgical attempts at arthrodesis often fail owing to the lack of a protective proprioceptive mechanism.

The ankle and foot are the most common areas affected by neuropathic arthropathy, related almost exclusively to diabetic arthropathy. In addition, alcoholism has been implicated as a source of neuropathic arthropathy of the foot. Diabetic Charcot's joints are usually atrophic or of mixed density. In the foot, the most frequent location for a diabetic Charcot's joint is the tarsometatarsal (Lisfranc's) joints. Subluxation of the first and second tarsometatarsal joints is evaluated on an anteroposterior (AP) film of the foot (Fig. 18-14), whereas subluxa-

tion at the third through fifth tarsometatarsal joints is evaluated on a pronated oblique foot film. Although Lisfranc's joint is the most frequently involved in diabetic Charcot's foot, other joints may be involved as well, including the talonavicular, subtalar, and intertarsal joints (Fig. 18-15).

Because neuropathic arthropathy of the foot is frequently related to diabetes as the underlying cause, superimposed infection may pose a diagnostic dilemma. Even with

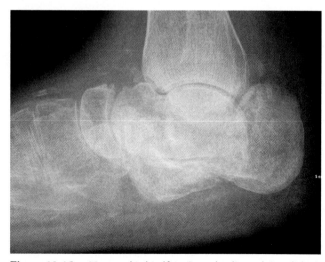

Figure 18-15 Neuropathic hindfoot. Lateral radiograph in a diabetic patient shows calcaneus fracture with collapse. Bone density in the hindfoot is preserved.

gadolinium-enhanced MRI, the difference between Charcot's and infected joints is not always clear. Important clues to the presence of infection are sinus tracts and soft tissue abscesses. This is discussed further in Chapter 40.

Charcot's arthropathy of the knee has historically implied tabes dorsalis as its prime cause. However, it is also seen in patients with diabetes, congenital insensitivity to pain, or congenital indifference to pain. The changes are usually at least partly hypertrophic. Tremendous distention of the knee with prominent debris and disorganization of the joint is the hallmark in these cases.

Shoulder neuropathic arthropathy seems to be frequently misdiagnosed. A neuropathic shoulder joint most commonly develops secondary to syringomyelia (Fig. 18-16) and in advanced cases is almost always atrophic. Thus, one sees resorption of most or all of the humeral head and neck, which may give the appearance of surgical resection of the humeral head. One should watch particularly for the location of subtle collections of debris, which may be superimposed in the expected location of shoulder bursae, such as the axillary, subscapularis or subdeltoid (Fig. 18-16B, C). Unfortunately, the debris can be misidentified as chondroid tumor matrix, and with the destruction of the humeral head, a provisional diagnosis of chondrosarcoma might be made. The true nature of the process should be recognized with MRI (Fig. 18-16B, C), where the entire process is seen to be articular, and with the "mass" simply being an enormous

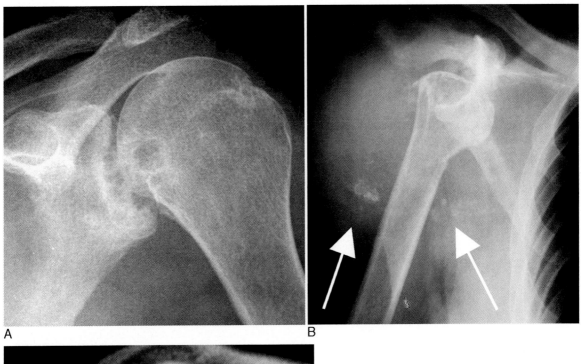

Figure 18-16 Neuropathic shoulder. **A,** Early findings. AP radiograph of the shoulder of a 40-year-old man with a cervical cord syrinx shows painless destruction of the glenohumeral joint. **B and C,** Late findings in a different patient. The diagnosis should be based on the radiograph (B) in this case, which shows all the elements necessary to diagnose neuropathic shoulder. The glenohumeral joint is dislocated, there is an enormous effusion, and debris is seen floating in the effusion *(arrows)*. If confirmation is needed, MRI demonstrates the entire abnormality, including the debris, to be intra-articular. Coronal T2-weighted MR image (C) demonstrates the destroyed and dislocated humeral head surrounded by a large joint effusion, with more fluid and debris settling into the distended subdeltoid bursa *(arrows)*. With this much destruction and a confirmed intra-articular process, the only logical diagnosis is neuropathic joint. Syringomyelia as the cause would be confirmed with MRI of the cervical spine.

effusion. Confirmation of syringomyelia as the cause is made with MRI of the cervical spine.

Spinal neuropathic arthropathy today is most frequently associated with diabetes or paraplegia. In patients with spinal cord trauma who have undergone instrumentation and fusion, the mobile segments adjacent to the fusion are most commonly involved. The appearance is similar to that of other Charcot's joints, with disorganization, ligamentous instability, and bony debris (Fig. 18-17). The disk space is narrowed, and there may be a paraspinal soft tissue mass. Discitis may have identical findings. This is a problem because the two common causes of neuropathic arthropathy in the spine (diabetes and paraplegia with spinal fusion) are also associated with increased risk for development of disk space infection. Radiologists must be aware of both the possible infectious cause and neuropathic cause of the radiographic appearance in these patients. The presence of vacuum disk, debris, spondylolisthesis, and facet involvement can help suggest that the diagnosis is spinal neuropathic arthropathy. On the other hand, findings that do not differentiate between neuropathic and infectious arthropathy include endplate sclerosis and erosions, osteophytes, decreased disk height, and paraspinal soft tissue mass. Patients undergoing long-term hemodialysis may develop a destructive process with an identical appearance, often related to aluminum toxicity or amyloid. This is discussed further in Chapter 21. Infectious discitis is usually associated with elevated markers of inflammation such as erythrocyte sedimentation rate. A paravertebral abscess indicates discitis rather than neuropathic change or hemodialysis-related disk destruc-

tion. Blood cultures may reveal the organism when discitis is present. Disk aspiration and biopsy may be necessary, yet frequently do not reveal the organism even when discitis is present.

DIFFUSE IDIOPATHIC SKELETAL HYPEROSTOSIS (FORESTIER'S DISEASE)

Diffuse idiopathic skeletal hyperostosis (DISH) results in profound ossification of spinal soft tissues, including the annulus fibrosis, anterior longitudinal ligament (ALL), and paravertebral connective tissues. Ossification of ALL results in the classic "flowing" mature ossification along the anterolateral aspect of the spine. There is usually relative preservation of disk height of the involved segments. Degenerative disk disease, as well as facet productive change, is not as prominent as the anterior ossification (Fig. 18-18). The superior (nonarticular) portions of the sacroiliac joints are often bridged by ligamentous calcification, but the lower (articular) two thirds of the sacroiliac joints are rarely affected. Moreover, the ALL ossification is a few millimeters thick, in contrast with the delicate annular calcification in the bamboo spine of ankylosing spondylitis. Therefore, DISH is usually easily differentiated from ankylosing spondylitis. The patient may also show prominent enthesophyte formation, especially in the pelvis, calcaneus, and anterior surface of the patella. Additionally, the sacrotuberous and sacrospinous pelvic ligaments may become calcified. Advanced DISH results in spine immobility, placing the patient at risk for spine fracture and neurologic injury (Fig. 18-19).

This condition occurs most frequently in middle-aged and elderly persons, males more frequently than females. It is seen most commonly in the thoracic spine, although the cervical spine is frequently involved. Interestingly, while ossification of the posterior longitudinal ligament may be seen in association with DISH, there is a separate disease entity *(ossification of the posterior longitudinal ligament [OPLL])* that shows predominately posterior longitudinal ligament ossification, often with some bulky anterior osteophyte formation (Fig. 18-20). The two disease processes overlap. Whereas OPLL predominately involves the cervical spine, DISH more frequently is thoracic in location. The former causes spinal canal stenosis and is especially common in Japan.

Differential considerations in DISH include *retinoid arthropathy,* which may be a consideration in patients using retinoic acid for skin diseases and who develop skeletal

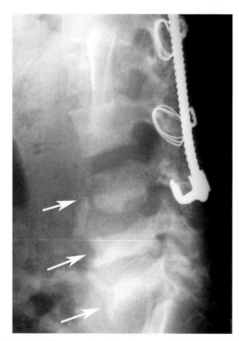

Figure 18-17 Neuropathic spine in a paraplegic patient. This patient had a burst fracture at the level of L1 and has had an anterior partial corpectomy with strut graft placement and posterior rodding from the levels of T10–L3. Below the level of the instrumentation, note subluxation and destruction of the vertebral bodies and endplates (L3 inferior endplate, L4, and L5, *arrows*). With this much destruction in a paraplegic patient, neuropathic process must be considered.

Key Concepts	Diffuse Idiopathic Skeletal Hyperostosis (DISH)

Dense ossification of anterior longitudinal ligament (versus fine calcification of the annulus fibrosis in ankylosing spondylitis)
Ossification of superior portion of sacroiliac (SI) joint, pelvic ligaments, posterior longitudinal ligament

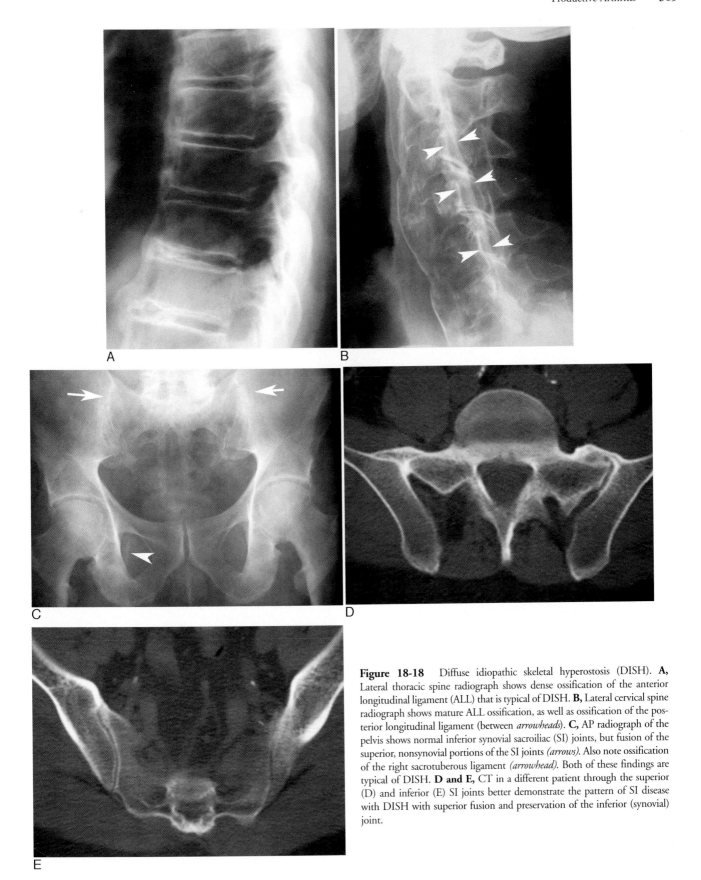

Figure 18-18 Diffuse idiopathic skeletal hyperostosis (DISH). **A,** Lateral thoracic spine radiograph shows dense ossification of the anterior longitudinal ligament (ALL) that is typical of DISH. **B,** Lateral cervical spine radiograph shows mature ALL ossification, as well as ossification of the posterior longitudinal ligament (between *arrowheads*). **C,** AP radiograph of the pelvis shows normal inferior synovial sacroiliac (SI) joints, but fusion of the superior, nonsynovial portions of the SI joints *(arrows)*. Also note ossification of the right sacrotuberous ligament *(arrowhead)*. Both of these findings are typical of DISH. **D and E,** CT in a different patient through the superior (D) and inferior (E) SI joints better demonstrate the pattern of SI disease with DISH with superior fusion and preservation of the inferior (synovial) joint.

hyperostoses similar to those seen in DISH. In retinoid arthropathy, the cervical spine is the most common site of involvement, but thoracic and lumbar involvement is seen as well (see Fig. 26-3). Eventually, along with the anterior osteophyte formation, anterior and posterior longitudinal ligament calcification may be seen. *Fluorosis* (fluoride intox-ication due to long-term ingestion) also can cause bulky paraspinous ligament calcification similar to DISH. Bones affected by fluorosis may be diffusely osteopenic or sclerotic in a patchy or "chalky" pattern. Vertebral osteophytes are frequent, as are dental abnormalities such as mottled tooth enamel.

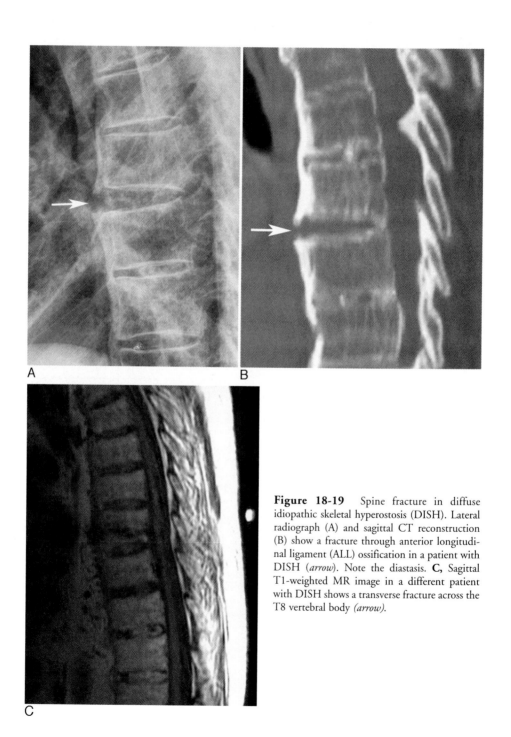

Figure 18-19 Spine fracture in diffuse idiopathic skeletal hyperostosis (DISH). Lateral radiograph (A) and sagittal CT reconstruction (B) show a fracture through anterior longitudinal ligament (ALL) ossification in a patient with DISH *(arrow)*. Note the diastasis. **C,** Sagittal T1-weighted MR image in a different patient with DISH shows a transverse fracture across the T8 vertebral body *(arrow).*

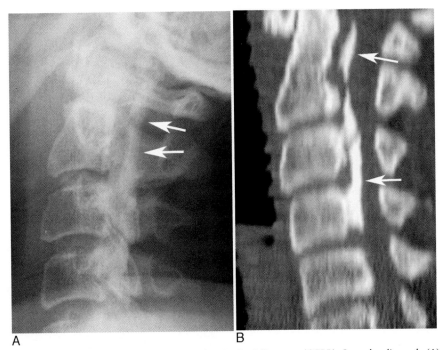

A   B

Figure 18-20   Ossification of the posterior longitudinal ligament (OPLL). Lateral radiograph (A) and sagittal CT reconstruction (B) show OPLL *(arrows)* of the cervical spine. There is associated spinal stenosis.

CHAPTER *19* Mixed Productive and Erosive Arthritis

ANKYLOSING SPONDYLITIS AND SPONDYLITIS OF
   INFLAMMATORY BOWEL DISEASE
PSORIATIC ARTHRITIS
REACTIVE ARTHRITIS
EROSIVE OSTEOARTHRITIS
SAPHO

ANKYLOSING SPONDYLITIS AND SPONDYLITIS OF INFLAMMATORY BOWEL DISEASE

Ankylosing spondylitis (AS) is the most common of the seronegative (rheumatoid factor negative) spondyloarthropathies. It is of unknown cause and is characterized by being a mixed erosive and osseous productive disease with a dominant productive component that involves predominately the axial skeleton and large proximal joints.

Ankylosing spondylitis has a strikingly higher incidence in males than females, with a male-to-female ratio of 4:1 to 10:1. The onset occurs either in adolescence or young adulthood, ranging between 15 and 35 years of age. Clinical signs are low back pain and limited chest expansion. As the disease progresses, stiffness of the spine can progress to distinct postural changes, with prominent thoracic kyphosis and limited lumbar lordosis. Laboratory testing can be helpful in the diagnosis; more than 90% of patients with ankylosing spondylitis are HLA B27 positive. This is not a specific finding because 6% to 8% of the normal population are HLA B27 positive and 50% to 80% of patients with reactive arthritis and psoriatic arthritis are positive as well.

A key feature of AS is its distribution of disease. The sacroiliac joints are classically the site of initial involvement. The first changes that can be noted radiographically are the loss of cortical definition (Fig. 19-1), followed by erosions and joint widening. These findings initially may be more prominent on the iliac side of the joint as the cartilage is normally thinner on that side; both sides are eventually involved. Magnetic resonance

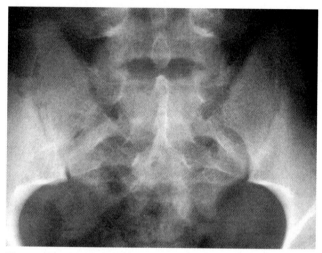

Figure 19-1   Ankylosing spondylitis, sacroiliac (SI) joints, early radiographic findings. AP radiograph of the SI joints demonstrates very early changes that can be found in the spondyloarthropathy of ankylosing spondylitis. The cortices of the SI joints are symmetrically "fuzzy" or poorly defined, although no radiographically discrete erosion is visible. MRI at this early stage will show mild marrow edema and enhancement along the SI joints.

imaging (MRI) and computed tomography (CT) can show these changes earlier than radiography. Later in the disease process sclerosis and ankylosis of the synovial (anterior inferior) portion of the sacroiliac joints develop. Although the abnormalities may initially be asymmetric, they eventually become symmetric. Thus, the hallmark of late disease is bilateral sacroiliac joint fusion, which can be easily identified on a radiograph (Fig. 19-2).

Recall that only the synovial (inferior) portion of the sacroiliac joint is involved in the erosive disease. The posterosuperior portions of the sacroiliac joints are syndesmoses without hyaline cartilage, synovium, or capsule. They are joined together by interosseous ligaments that may ossify in some disorders without representing true sacroiliitis. These bridging enthesophytes should not be confused with fusion of the true

Key Concepts	Ankylosing Spondylitis

Frequently positive for HLA-B27

Occurs more frequently in males than females

Presents in adolescents or young adults

Bilateral sacroiliac (SI) disease hallmark; erosive early, ankylosis quickly follows

Bamboo spine

Affects large proximal appendicular joints more often than distal joints

Spine fracture at C–T and T–L junction with pseudarthrosis

sacroiliac joints in AS. Ankylosing spondylitis produces enthesitis that can result in ossification of the sacroiliac syndesmosis, as can diffuse idiopathic skeletal hyperostosis, chronic reactive arthritis, psoriatic arthritis, vitamin D toxicity, and fluorosis.

In AS, involvement of the thoracolumbar spine classically follows sacroiliac abnormalities. It usually begins at the thoracolumbar and lumbosacral junctions and extends continuously, without skip areas, in a cranial direction. It should be noted that skips and asymmetry may be seen, but are far less common in AS than in reactive arthritis or psoriatic arthropathy. Vertebral involvement in ankylosing spondylitis begins with osteitis, related to erosive enthesitis at the peripheral corners of the vertebral bodies. Reactive sclerosis at the sites of osteitis may result in the "shiny corner" sign of subtle sclerosis of the peripheral corners of the vertebral bodies. Magnetic resonance imaging can depict changes at this location earlier than radiography. Inversion recovery or fat-suppressed T2-weighted MR images show marrow edema in the superior and inferior anterior corners of the vertebral bodies that precedes radiographic changes. The osteitis, in turn, leads to erosion, and thus to loss of the normal concavity of the anterior vertebral body, giving it a characteristic "squared" appearance on a lateral radiograph (Fig. 19-3). Eventually, ossifications form in the annulus fibrosis at the discovertebral junction, seen as thin vertical ossifications, termed *syndesmophytes* (also called *marginal syndesmophytes* by some authors). These are distinct in appearance from the bulky *nonmarginal osteophytes* (also called *nonmarginal syndesmophytes* or *parasyndesmophytes* by some authors) that arise from the side of the vertebral body, seen in reactive arthritis and psoriatic arthritis. By the end stage of AS, several segments will show ankylosis with an appearance that is likened to bamboo (Fig. 19-4), with undulating fusion of the vertebral bodies,

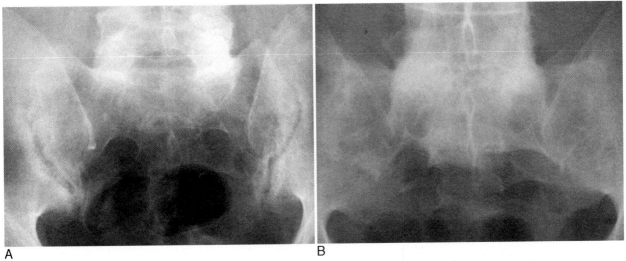

A   B

Figure 19-2   Ankylosing spondylitis, sacroiliac (SI) joints. **A,** Intermediate phase of sacroiliitis in ankylosing spondylitis, with symmetric findings of slight widening of the SI joints, sclerosis, and erosions that are more extensive in the inferior (synovial) portion of the joints. **B,** End-stage complete SI joint fusion. AP radiograph shows SI joints that are completely fused bilaterally.

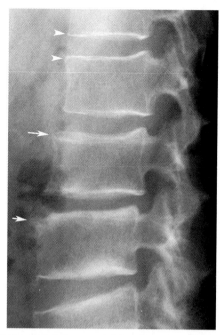

Figure 19-3 Ankylosing spondylitis, spine, early disease. This lateral radiograph demonstrates different early findings in the earlier stages of ankylosing spondylitis. Note the squaring of some of the vertebral bodies with mild sclerosis at the corners ("shiny corners," *arrowheads*), and the later finding of irregular new bone production at the corners of more inferior bodies *(arrows)*. A single vertical syndesmophyte is beginning to form at the inferior endplate of the lowest body seen on this image *(short arrow)*. The osteitis and resultant squaring are the first vertebral body abnormalities seen in ankylosing spondylitis, followed by formation of the syndesmophytes.

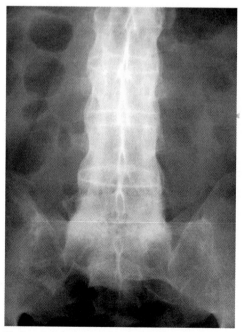

Figure 19-4 Ankylosing spondylitis, spine. AP radiograph demonstrates advanced ankylosing spondylitis, with complete fusion of the SI joints as well as fusion of the lumbar vertebral bodies. The thin vertical syndesmophytes seen at all levels of the lumbar spine outline the relatively dense endplates, giving the spine its "bamboo" appearance.

fusion of the facet (apophyseal) joints, and interspinous enthesophytes. Although initially bone density is normal in patients with AS, disuse osteoporosis ensues. This can be very significant late in the disease, leaving the fused osteoporotic spine vulnerable to fracture, much more so than in diffuse idiopathic skeletal hyperostosis (DISH). Such fractures may result from minor trauma and be extremely subtle on radiographs, yet must be sought because of the instability and risk of sudden death or paralysis that accompanies such fractures. Spine fractures in AS occur most frequently at the cervicothoracic and thoracolumbar junctions. The fracture usually extends through the disk space and the posterior elements (Fig. 19-5). Magnetic resonance imaging is useful in detection of the fracture, as well as cord injury or epidural hematoma. If the fracture goes undetected, instability across this segment of osteoporotic bone results in osseous breakdown with an appearance similar to neuropathic arthropathy.

Key Concepts	Differential Diagnosis of Ligamentous Ossification (in the Spine)

Diffuse idiopathic skeletal hyperostosis (DISH, diagnosis of exclusion)
Ankylosing spondylitis
Severe spondylosis
Vitamin A toxicity
Fluorosis

The hip is the most common appendicular joint involved in AS, with abnormalities seen in up to 50% of patients. The hip usually shows a combination of erosive and productive change, with concentric joint narrowing, mild erosions, protrusio acetabuli, and, later, ring osteophytes (Fig. 19-6). In any young adult, such radiographic appearances alone should suggest a diagnosis of ankylosing spondylitis and lead to careful scrutiny of the sacroiliac joints because they are the earliest site of involvement in AS. As with the sacroiliac joints, involvement of the hips is often bilateral but may be asymmetric.

After the hip, the glenohumeral joint is the next most commonly involved appendicular joint in AS. The symphysis pubis, sternomanubrial, and costochondral joints are commonly involved, with eventual ankylosis. The knees, ankles, hands, and feet are much less commonly involved than the large proximal joints.

Subchondral cysts, periostitis, and ligament disruption are not common features in AS. Enthesitis with productive ossification, however, is usually seen, especially in the pelvis, calcaneus, and patella.

Although AS is less common in women, the diagnosis should not be excluded on the basis of female gender. The radiographic findings tend to be neither as severe nor as typical

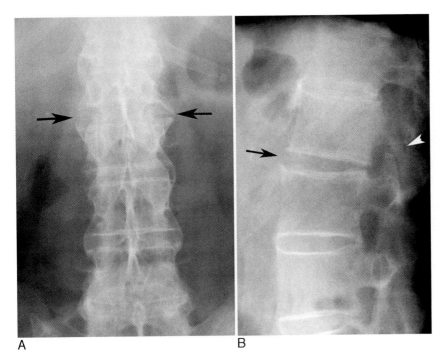

Figure 19-5 Ankylosing spondylitis, pseudarthrosis. **A,** AP radiograph of the lumbar spine in a patient with advanced ankylosing spondylitis, with fused SI joints and the "bamboo" appearance of the spine. Note interruption in the bamboo spine at the level of L1–L2, with fractures of the syndesmophytes *(arrows)*. **B,** Lateral view at the same level demonstrates the thin syndesmophytes at all levels except the L1–L2 site *(arrow)*. A very subtle fracture is seen through the pars interarticularis *(arrowhead),* completing the fracture across this disk. Pseudarthroses such as this are seen typically at the cervicothoracic or thoracolumbar junctions, and may be very subtle radiographically. These are unstable injuries with risk of paralysis.

in distribution as in male patients. The disease can present later in females and skip levels in the spine.

The arthropathy of inflammatory bowel disease can be seen in two forms. One form occurs as a result of *Salmonella, Shigella,* or *Yersinia* infections. These diseases may produce a self-limited polyarthritis, occasionally with sacroiliac joint symptoms, but usually without radiographic findings. A more pronounced spondyloarthropathy may occur with ulcerative colitis and less frequently with Crohn's disease and Whipple's disease. As many as 10% to 15% of these patients develop chronic arthropathy. Most of these patients present with mild peripheral arthralgias, but one third may develop sacroiliitis that is clinically and radiographically identical to that of ankylosing spondylitis (Fig 19-7). These patients are often positive for HLA-B27.

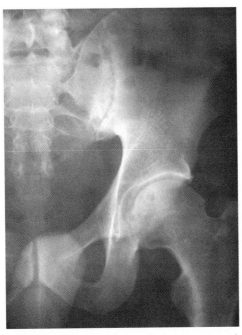

Figure 19-6 Ankylosing spondylitis, hip. Large joint involvement is typical in ankylosing spondylitis. This 25-year-old man has degenerative-appearing changes of the left hip, with osteophytes and subchondral cyst formation in the femoral head. Such degenerative change is distinctly unusual in a 25-year-old, but a glance at the sacroiliac (SI) joint demonstrates erosions with sclerosis, confirming the diagnosis of ankylosing spondylitis.

Key Concepts	Spondylitis of Inflammatory Bowel Disease
Most severe manifestations are identical to ankylosing spondylitis (AS) Most frequent in ulcerative colitis	

PSORIATIC ARTHRITIS

Psoriatic arthritis occurs in 0.5% to 25% of patients with psoriasis. Five distinct manifestations have been described: oligoarthritis, polyarthritis (predominately distal interphalangeal [DIP] joints), symmetric type (resembling rheumatoid arthritis [RA]), arthritis mutilans (deforming type), and spondyloarthropathy (spine and joint disease). Of the patients with psoriatic arthritis, 30% to 50% will develop spondyloarthropathy.

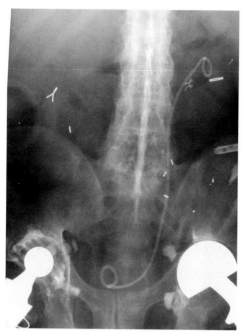

Figure 19-7 Spondylitis of inflammatory bowel disease. Abdomen radiograph in a patient with long-standing ankylosing spondylitis shows bilateral hip arthroplasties (large joint arthritis), left ureteral stent (urolithiasis), surgical clips in the right upper quadrant (cholecystectomy for cholelithiasis), right ostomy (total colectomy for ulcerative colitis), and drain in the left abdomen (increased vulnerability to infection, in this case an abdominal abscess). Other extra-articular complications of ankylosing spondylitis include iritis, aortic valve insufficiency and aortic root aneurysm, cardiac conduction abnormalities, and upper lung interstitial disease.

Patients who develop psoriatic arthritis are generally young adults. Unlike AS, psoriatic arthritis affects males and females equally. Although skin disease is usually present before the arthropathy, arthritis may predate skin findings in up to 20% of cases. The lack of skin findings can obscure the clinical diagnosis.

Clinically, the patients present with soft tissue swelling, particularly in the small joints of the hands and feet. The swelling may involve the entire digit and be so extreme as to be termed a "sausage digit." There is pain and reduced range of motion. Patients may report low back pain. Nail changes, including thickening, pitting, or discoloration, are common and are highly correlated with the severity of the arthropathy. Serum in these patients is negative for rheumatoid factor and positive for HLA B27 in 25% to 60% of the cases (usually patients with spondyloarthropathy).

The characteristic radiographic distribution of psoriatic arthritis involves the small joints of the hands and feet, with or without spondyloarthropathy. In the hand, tuft resorption and DIP erosive disease are usually seen early and involvement tends to be found in the DIP joints as well as in the proximal interphalangeal (PIP) or metacarpophalangeal (MCP) joints. This pattern helps to differentiate psoriatic

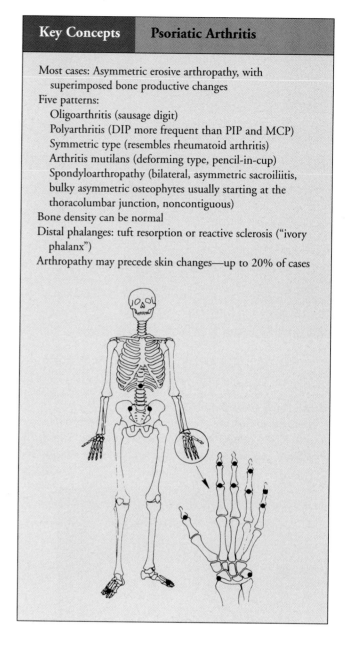

Key Concepts | **Psoriatic Arthritis**

Most cases: Asymmetric erosive arthropathy, with superimposed bone productive changes

Five patterns:
  Oligoarthritis (sausage digit)
  Polyarthritis (DIP more frequent than PIP and MCP)
  Symmetric type (resembles rheumatoid arthritis)
  Arthritis mutilans (deforming type, pencil-in-cup)
  Spondyloarthropathy (bilateral, asymmetric sacroiliitis, bulky asymmetric osteophytes usually starting at the thoracolumbar junction, noncontiguous)

Bone density can be normal

Distal phalanges: tuft resorption or reactive sclerosis ("ivory phalanx")

Arthropathy may precede skin changes—up to 20% of cases

arthritis from RA, which is rarely found in the DIP joints. In addition, asymmetric involvement is far more common in psoriatic arthritis than in RA. The erosions seen in these joints begin marginally, as in RA, but often progress to severe subchondral erosions, occasionally resulting in pencil-in-cup deformity (Fig. 19-8). Once severe erosive change has developed, the clinical "telescoping" of the joint can be observed. Although erosive changes predominate, bone productive changes are usually seen as well, frequently in the form of subtle bone excrescences at and around the joint; occasionally, dense bone proliferation can be seen in the tuft of the phalanx, producing an "ivory phalanx." This is another feature allowing differentiation from RA. Also unlike RA, subchondral cysts are uncommon.

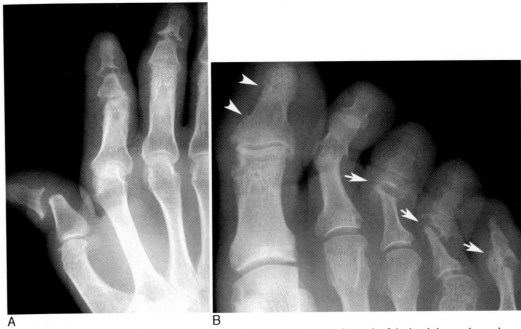

Figure 19-8   Psoriatic arthritis, arthritis mutilans pattern. **A,** AP radiograph of the hand shows advanced psoriatic arthritis changes, with so much destruction at the DIP joints of digits 1, 2, and 3 that they have developed a "pencil-in-cup" appearance. **B,** Similar findings in a different patient, showing not only the "pencil-in-cup" appearance of the third and fourth PIP joints *(arrows)* but also the new bone production ("periostitis") at the distal phalanx of the great toe *(arrowheads)*. (Part A reprinted with permission of the American College of Radiology learning file.)

Other features that differentiate psoriatic arthritis from RA are the character of the soft tissue swelling, which in psoriatic arthritis may be fusiform around a joint or involve the entire digit (sausage digit). In addition, periosteal reaction and small enthesophytes are often seen in the phalanges (Figs. 19-9, 19-10). Such findings are not seen in patients with RA, except those with juvenile RA. Ankylosis is common in the hands and feet of patients with psoriatic arthritis, a feature that also differentiates this disease from RA. In addition, the bone density can be normal in psoriatic arthritis and the joint distribution in the hands is asymmetric and can include DIP involvement.

The wrists are not as frequently involved in psoriatic arthritis as in RA; if there is wrist involvement, any compartment may be abnormal and, as with the hands, symmetry is far less common in psoriatic arthritis than in RA. In the foot, IP and metatarsophalangeal (MTP) erosive disease is common. A retrocalcaneal bursitis with erosions at the site of the Achilles tendon insertion may be seen, indistinguishable from that in RA or reactive arthritis. Enthesitis is common at the origin of plantar aponeurosis and along the plantar aspect of the calcaneus, where erosions and subsequent enthesophyte formation is found. Magnetic resonance imaging is particularly sensitive in the detection of enthesitis and underlying bony changes. Large joint involvement (ankle, knee, hip, shoulder) is much less common but does occur. If large joints are affected, the distal small joints are almost invariably involved as well.

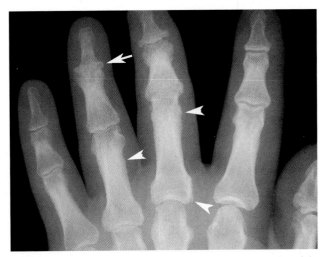

Figure 19-9   Psoriatic arthritis, polyarthritis pattern. PA view of the hand demonstrating predominately DIP disease, with fusion at the fourth DIP *(arrow)*. Note also the subtle periostitis at the proximal phalanges of the third and fourth digits *(arrowheads)*. Fusion and periostitis are hallmarks of psoriatic arthritis. Also note the small erosions at the third DIP joint. (Reprinted with permission of the American College of Radiology learning file.)

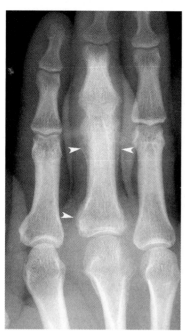

Figure 19-10   Psoriatic arthritis, oligoarticular pattern. PA radiograph of the hand demonstrates swelling in the form of a "sausage digit" in the third ray, with prominent periostitis along the metacarpal and proximal phalanx of the third ray *(arrowheads)*.

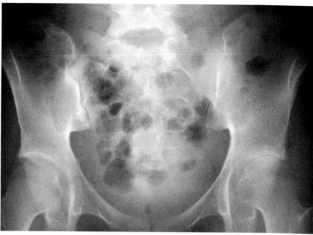

Figure 19-11   Psoriatic arthritis, hips and sacroiliac (SI) joints. AP radiograph of the pelvis in this 17-year-old female demonstrates an erosive process involving the left hip and unilateral sacroiliitis, with prominent sclerosis seen in the right SI joint. Note that the spondyloarthropathy seen in psoriatic arthritis tends to have unilateral, or at least asymmetric, involvement of the SI joints. (Reprinted with permission of the American College of Radiology learning file.)

When present, the character of the sacroiliitis seen in these patients follows the same pattern as that seen in AS, with initial subchondral marrow edema and enhancement followed by radiographic findings of cortical indistinctness, erosions, widening, sclerosis, and, eventually, fusion. However, involvement of the sacroiliac joints usually remains asymmetric (Fig. 19-11). Although sacroiliitis is usually adequately assessed with radiographs, occasionally cross-section imaging is used. Computed tomography is more sensitive than radiography in detection of small, early erosions. Magnetic resonance imaging can depict very early changes of sacroiliitis, which are seen as subcortical edema and enhancement.

The thoracolumbar spine involvement in psoriatic arthritis usually appears quite distinct from that of AS, with bulky asymmetric nonmarginal osteophytes (Fig. 19-12), also termed parasyndesmophytes, rather than the delicate syndesmophytes of AS or the relatively horizontal endplate spurs of degenerative disk disease. The syndesmophytes of psoriasis generally start in the thoracolumbar junction region, usually skip levels, and show asymmetry in the size and side of osteophyte formation.

The diagnosis of psoriatic arthritis can occasionally be difficult. Early psoriatic arthritis is occasionally indistinguishable from RA, but the involvement of DIP joints in psoriatic arthritis usually leads to the correct diagnosis. Any periostitis differentiates the two because it is not seen with RA. Adult Still's disease, with its DIP distribution, may be indistinguishable from psoriatic arthritis. Erosive osteoarthritis (OA, discussed

later in this chapter) may be confused with psoriatic arthritis because of the DIP erosions. However, features of OA are found in erosive OA, and erosive OA shows a distribution typical for OA. The spondyloarthropathy of psoriatic arthritis is indistinguishable from that of reactive arthritis. In these cases, the clinical scenario is relied upon. Psoriatic arthritis is usually associated with the psoriatic rash; reactive arthritis is associated with urethritis and uveitis. Foot disease is more prevalent in reactive arthritis, and hand disease is more prevalent in psoriatic arthritis. Finally, as noted previously, the asymmetry of the sacroiliac joint disease in psoriatic arthritis and reactive arthritis usually is distinguished from the symmetric findings in AS. The spine disease is clearly different, as is the small joint distribution.

REACTIVE ARTHRITIS

Reactive arthritis (chronic reactive arthritis), formerly known as *Reiter syndrome,* is a syndrome consisting of the triad of conjunctivitis, urethritis (cervicitis in females), and arthritis. A mnemonic is "can't see, can't pee, can't bend the knee." Reactive arthritis occurs most frequently in young men between the ages of 20 and 40 years. Clinical signs of the arthropathy include low back pain and polyarticular arthritis, particularly with heel pain predominating. As with the other spondyloarthropathies, patients with reactive arthritis are rheumatoid factor negative, and 80% are HLA B27 positive. (Recall that only 6% of the general population is HLA B27 positive.) Reactive arthritis is far less common than AS or psoriatic arthritis. Reactive arthritis usually occurs 1 to 3 weeks following a genitourinary infection with *Chlamydia trachomatis* or gastrointestinal tract infection with *Salmonella, Shigella, Yersinia,* or *Campylobacter* species, and lasts for several months. The exact mechanism of the arthritic "reaction" to these infections is not known, but is speculated to be related to antigenic similarity between the infectious agent and an antigen in synovial joints of susceptible individuals. Direct joint infection also has been hypothesized, but seems less likely. The other seronegative spondyloarthropathies, as well as rheumatoid arthritis and Behçet's syndrome, also may be initiated by an unfortunate immune cross-reaction to an unknown antigen, and thus also may be reactive, although such a connection is less clearly established.

The spondyloarthropathy seen in reactive arthritis is identical to that seen in psoriatic arthritis (see Fig. 19-12), except for differences in distribution in the extremities. As with psoriatic arthritis, sacroiliitis may be unilateral, but if bilateral is asymmetric in appearance. Bulky asymmetric nonmarginal osteophytes are seen in the thoracolumbar spine, often with skip areas, and are better seen on anteroposterior (AP) than on lateral radiographs. In reactive arthritis, the distal lower extremity, particularly the MTP

Key Concepts | **Reactive Arthritis**

Formerly known as Reiter syndrome
Least common spondyloarthropathy
Occurs more frequently in males than females
Radiographically identical to psoriasis but usually favors foot over hand
Calcaneal erosive disease and spur formation are prominent features

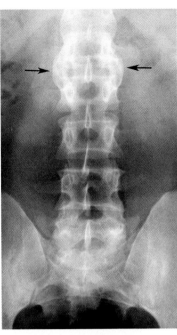

Figure 19-12 Seronegative spondyloarthropathy of psoriasis and reactive arthritis. AP radiograph of the lumbar spine demonstrates bilateral but somewhat asymmetric sacroiliitis, along with bulky syndesmophytes involving only the L1–L2 level *(arrows)*. This patient also had calcaneal erosive disease. Reactive arthritis and psoriatic arthritis have an identical-appearing spondyloarthropathy, with asymmetric sacroiliitis and bulky asymmetric syndesmophytes. Contrast with the degenerative spurs in Figure 18-13 and the fine annulus fibrosis calcification in ankylosing spondylitis in Figure 19-4.

joints, calcaneus, ankle, and knee (Fig. 19-13), are likely to be involved, but the upper extremity is usually spared. Although the distribution of distal arthropathy is different from that of psoriatic, the radiographic appearance is similar. Soft tissue swelling may be fusiform about the involved joint but may also give the appearance of a sausage digit. Involved digits may show periostitis. Erosive changes predominate, but may be seen in conjunction with mild productive bony changes. Retrocalcaneal bursitis is particularly common, along with prominent enthesitis at the Achilles tendon and plantar aponeurosis origin.

Reactive arthritis may also be confused clinically with septic arthritis, most notably gonococcal arthritis because urethritis is also present.

EROSIVE OSTEOARTHRITIS

Erosive (or inflammatory) OA is a variant of OA. Erosive OA is found primarily in middle-aged women who experience distinct inflammatory episodes, similar to those of RA, with swollen, red IP joints. Overall, erosive OA resembles OA but with soft tissue swelling and central erosions. The DIP and PIP joints are most frequently involved, with loss of cartilage, sclerosis, and combined erosive and productive bony changes. The erosions on the proximal side of the joint tend to be central

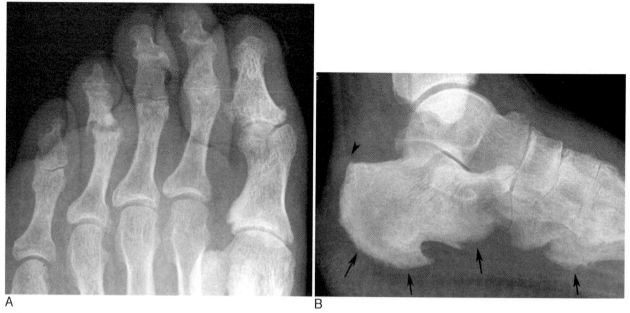

A

B

Figure 19-13   Reactive arthritis. **A,** PA radiograph of the toes shows erosions with new bone formation at the fourth PIP joint. **B,** Lateral radiograph of the hindfoot in the same patient shows extensive new bone formation along the plantar calcaneus and fifth tarsometatarsal joint *(arrows),* mixed erosions and new bone formation at the posterior calcaneus, and swelling of the retrocalcaneal bursa (arrowhead). These findings also suggest psoriatic arthritis, which is more common, but clinical evaluation and absence of arthritis elsewhere in this patient confirmed the diagnosis of reactive arthritis.

and the osteophytes, marginal, which can give a distinctive "gull-wing" appearance (Figs. 19-14, 19-15). The major differential diagnosis of erosive OA is psoriatic arthritis. In most cases of erosive OA, the first carpometacarpal joint or scaphoid-trapezoid and scaphoid-trapezium joints show typical OA changes. This location of carpal involvement is typical for OA and helpful in arriving at the correct diagnosis.

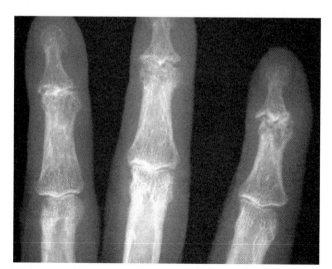

Figure 19-14   Erosive osteoarthritis. PA radiograph of the distal phalanges in a 72-year-old woman shows erosive change at the DIP joints in the shape of a gull-wing. Although erosive change of the DIP joint may be more reminiscent of psoriatic arthritis than of osteoarthritis (OA), when it is combined with erosive or productive change at the first carpal metacarpal joint, the diagnosis of OA is secure.

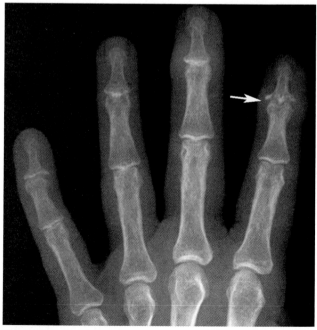

Figure 19-15   Erosive osteoarthritis. PA radiograph of the fingers shows the spectrum of findings in erosive osteoarthritis, including the classic gull-wing erosion in the second DIP joint *(arrow).* The third DIP shows soft tissue swelling and joint space narrowing that may progress to the gull-wing pattern. The fourth and fifth DIP findings are compatible with routine osteoarthritis.

SAPHO

SAPHO (synovitis, acne, pustulosis, hyperostosis, osteitis) is an uncommon form of spondyloarthropathy in which patients can have various osteoarticular manifestations, the most common being osteitis of the anterior chest wall. This is seen as frequently painful hyperostosis and soft tissue ossification between the medial clavicle, anterior portion of the upper ribs, and manubrium (Fig. 19-16). In addition to the anterior chest wall, the axial skeleton may be involved and, rarely, extra-axial tumor-simulating bone lesions are seen. Pustulosis, psoriatic lesions, and spondyloarthropathy may also be seen. SAPHO is associated with propionibacterium acne and is more frequent in HLA-B27–positive patients. The variety of manifestations exhibited by psoriatic arthritis leads to confusion, resulting in several other names being applied to this process (e.g., sternoclavicular hyperostosis). Chronic recurrent multifocal osteomyelitis, discussed in Chapter 40, shares some

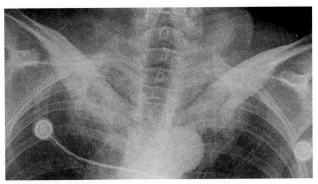

Figure 19-16   SAPHO (synovitis, acne, pustulosis, hyperostosis, osteitis). Detail from a chest radiograph shows massive thickening of the medial clavicles and manubrium with fusion. (Courtesy of William Pommersheim, MD.)

features with SAPHO, notably clavicle sclerosis and pustulosis of the palms and soles.

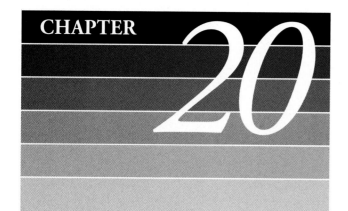

SYSTEMIC LUPUS ERYTHEMATOSUS
SCLERODERMA
POLYMYOSITIS AND DERMATOMYOSITIS

The connective tissue disorders, also known as collagen vascular diseases, are a loosely related group of multisystem diseases that have in common vasculitis, a likely autoimmune cause, a predilection for connective tissue involvement (although not specifically collagen), and related laboratory abnormalities such as immune complexes and antinuclear antibodies. Rheumatoid arthritis and polyarteritis nodosa may be included in this group.

SYSTEMIC LUPUS ERYTHEMATOSUS

Systemic lupus erythematosus (SLE) is a multisystem autoimmune disease with a variable course and potential for severe tissue injury. The musculoskeletal system is most commonly involved with polyarthritis that is generally nonerosive but often deforming. Despite the destructive processes seen radiographically, the musculoskeletal clinical symptoms are mild.

Key Concepts	Systemic Lupus Erythematosus

Multisystem inflammation
Young adults
Occurs more frequently in females than males
Occurs more frequently in African-American than white persons
Musculoskeletal: Polyarthritis with reversible deformities
Hand and wrist most commonly affected
Usually nonerosive (in contrast with rheumatoid arthritis [RA])
Avascular necrosis (AVN) (due to steroid therapy and vasculitis)
Soft tissue calcification in 10% of cases, usually lower extremity

There is a distinct sex distribution, with females more commonly affected than males (ratio ranging from 5:1 to 10:1). In addition, African-American persons are more commonly affected than white persons. The disease is usually manifested in young adults. The patients present clinically with constitutional symptoms (weakness, malaise, fever) and a skin rash such as the characteristic butterfly rash on the face. Organ system involvement includes myositis, various neurologic abnormalities, pulmonary vasculitis, pulmonary fibrosis, pleural effusions, pericarditis, cardiomyopathy, and nephritis. Patients have positive results on the lupus erythematosus cell prep test and the test for antinuclear antibody and may be positive for rheumatoid factor.

The joints most frequently affected are those of the hand and wrist, although the foot may show similar abnormalities. These joints show classic deformities of ligamentous laxity, including reducible ulnar subluxation of the metacarpophalangeal (MCP) joints and of the first carpometacarpal joint, and variable flexion or extension deformities of the interphalangeal joints. The prominent feature of these deformities is their reducibility. Because of this feature, the deformities are evident when the hands are unsupported by the film cassette while being radiographed; this results in the deformities appearing much more severe on the Norgaard (ball catcher's) view than on the posteroanterior (PA) view (Fig. 20-1). The disease is usually nonerosive. This feature helps to distinguish rheumatoid arthritis from SLE, as the alignment deformities are similar in appearance.

Streaky, linear, nodular, or amorphous subcutaneous calcifications are seen in approximately 10% of patients with SLE, usually in the lower extremities (Fig. 20-2). This incidence is much less frequent than in dermatomyositis, but can lead to some diagnostic confusion.

Another radiographic feature of SLE is the remarkably high incidence of osteonecrosis. Up to one third of patients with SLE may show avascular necrosis (AVN) at magnetic resonance imaging (MRI), although only 8% are symptomatic. Steroid therapy is felt to be the major etiologic factor, but the vasculitis due to the disease process also predisposes to AVN. The femoral head, humeral head, and knee are common sites (see Fig. 20-2). Avascular necrosis found in unusual sites should suggest the diagnosis of SLE.

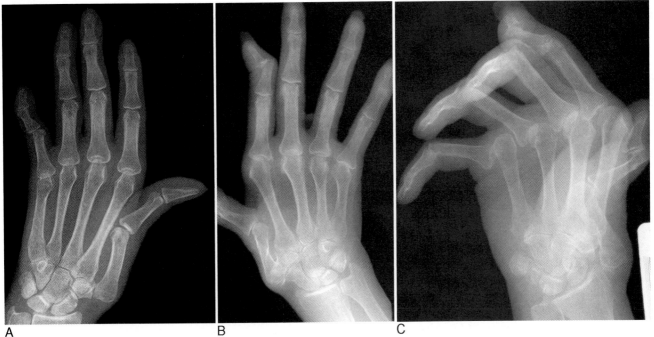

Figure 20-1   Systemic lupus erythematosus (SLE). **A,** PA radiograph of the hand shows multiple subluxations, including the "hitchhiker's thumb" **B and C,** Reversible deformities. PA (B) and Norgaard (C) views in a patient with SLE demonstrate multiple subluxations, which appear worsened in the Norgaard view because the hand is not supported on the cassette. The bones are diffusely osteoporotic, and erosions are not seen. The findings are typical of the nonerosive but deforming arthropathy of SLE. (Part A courtesy of William Pommersheim, MD.)

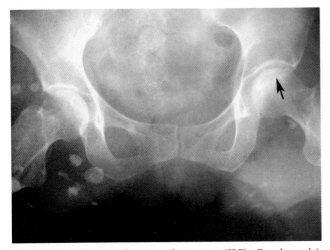

Figure 20-2   Systemic lupus erythematosus (SLE). Frog-leg pelvis radiograph demonstrates multifocal dense soft tissue calcification and left hip avascular necrosis with subchondral fracture and flattening *(arrow).* This patient is known to have SLE, and it is not at all uncommon to develop avascular necrosis with this disease process and the associated steroid use. Soft tissue calcification is uncommon but well described in patients with SLE. (Reprinted with permission of the American College of Radiology learning file.)

SCLERODERMA

Scleroderma is an umbrella term for a family of autoimmune conditions that have in common hardening of the skin. The process may be confined to the skin, or may involve several organ systems (kidneys, heart, lung, gastrointestinal, and musculoskeletal), hence the term *systemic sclerosis*. Vascular features such as Raynaud's phenomenon (episodic digital ischemia precipitated by cold or emotional stress) are common. Some authors classify scleroderma as diffuse or limited. Diffuse scleroderma involves the distal extremities and the trunk, whereas limited scleroderma involves the fingers, hands, and face. The *CREST syndrome* (skin calcinosis, Raynaud's phenomenon, esophageal dysmotility, sclerodactyly, and telangiectasia) is a common type of limited scleroderma. Scleroderma affects females more frequently than males, in a 3:1 ratio, and is most often diagnosed in the third to fifth decades of life. Laboratory tests are not specific. Most patients have elevated erythrocyte sedimentation rate, and up to 40% are positive for rheumatoid factor.

Key Concepts	Scleroderma

Often multisystem disease (systemic sclerosis)
Localized form includes CREST syndrome: Skin calcinosis,
   Raynaud's phenomenon, esophageal dysmotility,
   sclerodactyly, and telangiectasia
Acral soft tissue atrophy
Acro-osteolysis
Soft tissue calcification
Erosions, but arthritis not a prominent feature

Patients with scleroderma may have coexisting SLE or polymyositis/dermatomyositis. Many features of scleroderma are also found in *mixed connective tissue disease* (MCTD), which is a collagen vascular disease with overlapping clinical features of scleroderma, SLE, dermatomyositis, and rheumatoid arthritis. Arthritis is frequent in MCTD, with the small joints of the hands and feet and the wrist most commonly affected.

Patients with scleroderma may present with Raynaud's phenomenon; skin changes on the hands, feet, or face; distal joint pain and stiffness; dysphagia; and proximal myopathy. Esophageal atrophy and fibrosis lead to dysmotility, reflux, and reflux stricture, which may be noted as air fluid levels within the esophagus on a chest film. The dysmotility, as well as the "hidebound," thickened, squared small bowel folds and pseudosacculations of the small intestine and colon are seen with barium studies.

Soft tissue abnormalities are extremely common, seen clinically at first as edema but eventually resulting in taut, shiny, and atrophic soft tissues. In the hands, vasculitis and Raynaud's phenomenon lead to progressive distal phalangeal tapering. Radiographically, the acral (distal) tapering of the digits is seen both in the soft tissues and distal phalanges (Fig. 20-3, 20-4). This acro-osteolysis may be seen in up to 80% of patients. Acro-osteolysis is nonspecific, as it may be seen in other disorders (Table 20-1). Resorption of bone, although most commonly seen in the phalangeal tufts, may also be severe at the first carpometacarpal joint, resulting in radial subluxation of the first metacarpal. This feature is thought to be distinctive for scleroderma. Bone resorption can also be seen at the angle of the mandible and at the posterior ribs, particularly ribs 3 to 6, and diffusely about the wrist.

Other than distal resorption, the other distinctive radiographic feature in scleroderma is that of soft tissue calcification. Calcification is seen in 25% of cases, and may be subcutaneous, extra-articular, intra-articular, or even punctate within the terminal phalanx (Figs. 20-3–20-5). However, soft tissue calcification in conjunction with acro-osteolysis is not specific for scleroderma (see Tables 20-1 and 20-2 and Figs. 20-6, 20-7).

Although acro-osteolysis and soft tissue calcification are the most frequent features of scleroderma, cartilage destruction and erosive changes are occasionally seen. It may be difficult to attribute erosive change only to scleroderma because many patients have MCTD with coexisting features of rheumatoid

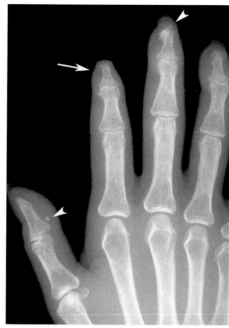

Figure 20-3   Scleroderma. PA radiograph of the hand demonstrates the tapering of the fingers of digits 2 and 3, with acro-osteolysis seen at digit 2 *(arrow)*. Soft-tissue calcification is seen both at the thumb and digit 3 *(arrowheads)*. This combination is typical for scleroderma. (Reprinted with permission of the American College of Radiology learning file.)

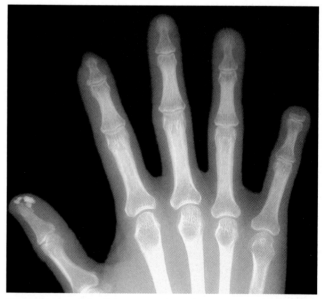

Figure 20-4   Scleroderma. More advanced example than in Figure 20-3, with amputation of the distal fifth finger.

arthritis or other overlap syndromes that might explain the presence of erosions. Overall, joint abnormalities eventually occur in nearly 50% of patients with scleroderma. These joint abnormalities are usually erosive, but relatively mild, and typically lack subchondral cyst formation. Mild bone productive changes and flexion contractures may be seen as well.

Table 20-1   Acro-osteolysis

1. Thermal injury (Fig. 20-6)
   a. Burn: May have contracture and soft tissue calcifications
   b. Frostbite: Usually spares the thumb (Fig. 2-42)
2. Environmental: Polyvinylchloride (PVC)
3. Metabolic
   a. Hyperparathyroidism: Tuft resorption, often accompanied by other signs of subperiosteal resorption, vascular calcification, or brown tumors
   b. Lesch-Nyhan disease
4. Arthritis
   a. Psoriatic: There should be associated DIP erosive disease
   b. Neuroarthropathy, especially diabetic
5. Connective tissue disease
   a. Scleroderma: Often associated with soft tissue calcification
   b. Other causes of vasculitis
6. Infection: Leprosy, associated with linear calcifications of the digital nerves (Fig. 2-43)
7. Congenital
   a. Pyknodysostosis: associated with dense bones and transverse fractures
   b. Hajdu-Cheney syndrome
   c. Epidermolysis bullosa

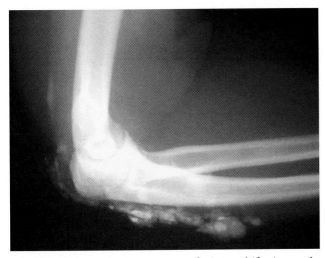

Figure 20-5   Scleroderma. Extensive soft tissue calcification at the extensor surface of the elbow and proximal forearm.

POLYMYOSITIS AND DERMATOMYOSITIS

Polymyositis and dermatomyositis are autoimmune diseases of unknown cause that produce inflammation and muscle degeneration. In polymyositis, the symptoms of proximal muscle weakness and arthralgias predominate. With dermatomyositis, a typical diffuse erythematous rash is an additional finding.

Table 20-2   Soft Tissue Calcification

1. Trauma
   a. Myositis ossificans: Has characteristic timing, maturation, and zoning phenomenon
   b. Burns: Often associated with contractures and acro-osteolysis
   c. Frostbite: Thumb is often spared; acro-osteolysis
   d. Head injury
   e. Paraplegia or quadriplegia: especially about the hips
2. Tumor: Any soft tissue tumor may have dystrophic calcification
   a. Synovial cell sarcoma
   b. Liposarcoma
   c. Fibrosarcoma/MFH
   d. Soft tissue osteosarcoma
   e. Phleboliths in vascular tumors
3. Collagen vascular diseases
   a. Scleroderma: Usually subcutaneous, with other changes (e.g., acro-osteolysis)
   b. Dermatomyositis: Sheet-like in muscle or fascial planes, but other calcification patterns are also seen
   c. SLE: Calcification is uncommon, but may occur, especially in lower extremities; consider when AVN is also seen
   d. CREST syndrome: Calcinosis cutis, Raynaud's phenomenon, esophageal dysmotility, scleroderma, telangiectasias
   e. Calcinosis cutis
4. Arthritis
   a. CPPD arthropathy: TFCC, menisci, pubic symphysis, hyaline cartilage
   b. HADD: Especially calcific bursitis, tendonitis, juxta-articular
   c. Gout: Tophus is usually juxta-articular
   d. Synovial chondromatosis: Intra-articular
5. Congenital
   a. Tumoral calcinosis: Periarticular
   b. Myositis ossificans progressiva: Usually axial, bridging between bones of the thorax
   c. Pseudohypoparathyroidism, pseudo-pseudohypoparathyroidism
   d. Progeria
   e. Ehlers-Danlos disease
6. Metabolic
   a. Hyperparathyroidism (primary or secondary)
   b. Hypoparathyroidism
   c. Renal dialysis sequela: Periarticular
7. Infectious
   a. Granulomatous: Tuberculosis, brucellosis, coccidioidomycosis
   b. Dystrophic calcification in abscesses
   c. Leprosy: Linear calcification in digital nerves
   d. Cysticercosis: Small calcified oval bodies in muscle
   e. *Echinococcus:* Usually liver or bone, but occasionally in soft tissue
8. Drugs
   a. Hypervitaminosis D
   b. Milk-alkali syndrome

AVN, avascular necrosis; CPPD, calcium pyrophosphate dihydrate deposition; HADD, hydroxyapatite deposition disease; MFH, malignant fibrous histiocytoma; SLE, systemic lupus erythematosus; TFCC, triangular fibrocartilage complex.

Polymyositis and dermatomyositis usually present in the third through fifth decades of life, and females are more frequently affected than males. Dermatomyositis may also be seen in children, associated with very severe systemic symptoms. Patients with this disease show muscle weakness and tenderness with eventual contracture and atrophy. The muscles involved are usually

Key Concepts	Polymyositis and Dermatomyositis

Active disease: MRI shows muscle edema
Late stage: Fatty atrophy, eventual soft tissue calcifications, either subcutaneous or sheet-like in fascial or muscle planes
MRI to guide biopsy: Look for sites of active inflammation
Avascular necrosis (AVN) can result from corticosteroid therapy
Arthralgias, but erosions rare

proximal muscles. Early in the disease, the muscles develop edema, followed later by atrophy and calcification (Fig. 20-8). The early muscle disease may be identified on MRI with edema-like signal intensity in muscle, seen best with fat-saturated T2-weighted or inversion recovery sequences. Late-stage disease shows fatty atrophy. The calcifications that develop late in the disease are seen on radiographs. The most common calcification pattern is a nonspecific subcutaneous calcification. "Sheet-like" calcifications along fascial or muscle planes are less common but thought to be pathognomonic for the disease. Classically, these sheet-like calcifications are seen in the proximal large muscles. Occasionally,

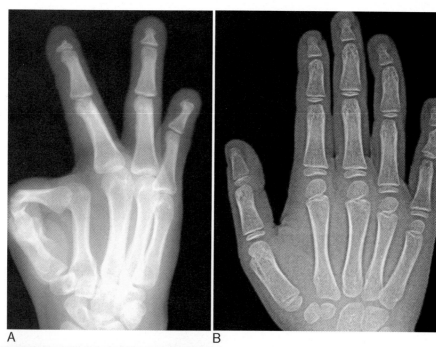

A B

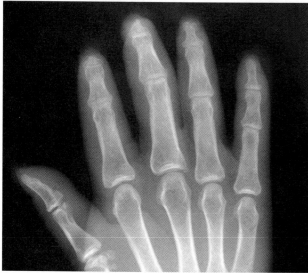

C

Figure 20-6 Acro-osteolysis due to thermal injuries. **A,** Burn. Oblique radiograph demonstrates severe acro-osteolysis at digits 3, 4, and 5, with a contracture of digits 1 and 2. The combination is typical of burn. Soft tissue calcifications are sometimes seen as well, although not in this case. **B,** Sequela of frostbite in a 7-year-old child. Note that the physes of the distal phalanges of digits 2 to 5 have closed prematurely *(arrowheads)*, whereas that at the thumb is normal. The growth centers are most at risk for thermal injury, and this patient's distal phalanges will not grow further. As an adult, this patient will have short distal phalanges. Note also that the thumb is normal in size and morphology. This is typical of frostbite because the thumb is protected by the cupped hand when one is cold. **C,** Frostbite, more severe case. PA radiograph of the hand in an adult shows amputations of the distal second and third fingers and short distal phalanx of the fourth finger. Even the thumb shows some tissue loss. (Part A reprinted with permission of the American College of Radiology learning file.)

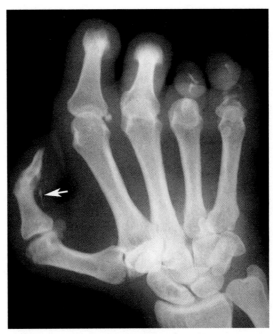

Figure 20-7   Acro-osteolysis: leprosy. This patient has tremendous acro-osteolysis, involving all the digits, and has the added feature of a calcified digital nerve *(arrow)*. This feature is typical of leprosy.

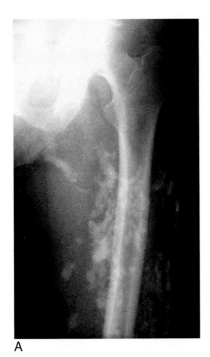

A

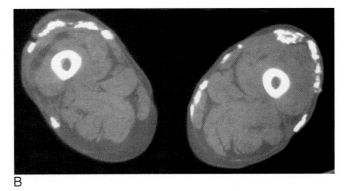

B

Figure 20-8   Dermatomyositis, late-stage findings. **A,** AP radiograph demonstrates sheet-like calcifications in the soft tissues of the thigh of this 50-year-old woman. **B,** CT confirms the location of the calcifications to be both within the muscle and fascial planes. Sheet-like calcifications are typically described with late-stage dermatomyositis, but the calcifications may assume other configurations. (Reprinted with permission of the American College of Radiology learning file.)

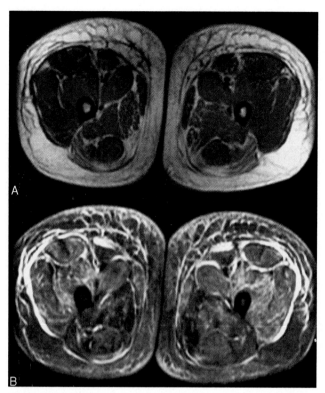

Figure 20-9   Dermatomyositis, MRI of active disease. Axial T1-weighted (A) and inversion recovery (B) MR images of the thighs in a 35-year-old woman with new-onset dermatomyositis show extensive edema in thigh musculature and subcutaneous tissues (B). An optimal biopsy site shows edema but no fatty infiltration, as the latter indicates irreversible disease and provides nonspecific biopsy findings. Potential biopsy sites abound in this patient because there is little fatty infiltration.

periarticular calcification may occur. As noted in Chapter 2, MRI is useful in guiding a biopsy when polymyositis or dermatomyositis is suspected because an optimal biopsy site should not show nonspecific end-stage fatty atrophy, but rather edema related to active inflammatory cell infiltration (Fig. 20-9).

Although the hands, wrists, and knees are affected with arthralgias, radiographic bone or joint abnormalities are rare. However, because these patients are treated with corticosteroids, they may develop AVN and osteoporosis as a complication of therapy.

Arthritis Due to Biochemical Disorders and Depositional Disease

21

GOUT
CALCIUM PYROPHOSPHATE DIHYDRATE CRYSTAL
   DEPOSITION DISEASE (PYROPHOSPHATE
   ARTHROPATHY)
HEMOCHROMATOSIS ARTHROPATHY
WILSON'S DISEASE
CALCIUM HYDROXYAPATITE DEPOSITION DISEASE
ALCAPTONURIA (OCHRONOSIS)
AMYLOIDOSIS

The arthritides reviewed in this chapter are due to systemic biochemical disorders that result in deposition of crystals or other pathogenic material in joints.

GOUT

Gout is a sodium urate crystal–induced deposition disorder that may be limited to occasional acute attacks or may be associated with a chronic arthropathy, with crystal deposition in capsular and synovial tissues, periarticular soft tissues, articular cartilage, and subchondral bone. This crystal deposition provokes very specific degenerative changes. Gout may occur secondary to chronic disease processes that cause elevated serum urate production or decreased renal clearance, such as myeloproliferative disorders, renal disease, hyperparathyroidism, hypoparathyroidism, psoriasis, diuretic therapy, enzyme defects, or long-term moonshine ingestion. However, most patients have idiopathic gout, with no associated condition. Gout typically occurs in middle-aged or elderly men and is extremely rare in premenopausal women unless they have one of the predisposing factors outlined above. White persons are more commonly affected than African Americans. Gout is also seen relatively frequently in young Polynesian males.

Key Concepts	Gout

Sodium urate crystal–induced arthropathy
Middle-aged to elderly men
Chronic disease processes may predispose to gout
Normal bone density
Cartilage often intact
Erosions: Sharply marginated and may be intra-articular or para-articular ("nonmarginal")
Overhanging edge of a para-articular erosion is virtually pathognomonic
First MTP, DIP, and PIP joints and patella most frequent joints
Gouty tophus radiographs: May show amorphus calcification (calcium urate)
Gouty tophus MRI: Low signal intensity on T1, variably high or low signal on T2, enhances with gadolinium

Gout presents with acute episodes of red, swollen, and extremely painful joints. The episodes are so severe as to be termed "attacks." The attacks may be separated by weeks, months, or years. Recurrent attacks can lead to chronic tophaceous gout. Laboratory abnormalities include hyperuricemia and sodium urate crystals in synovial fluid. The crystals are needle-or rod-shaped and negatively birefringent when viewed with polarized light microscopy. One theory of the pathogenesis suggests that acute gout results when unsuccessful ingestion of urate crystals by leukocytes leads to release of inflammatory factors.

Recurrent attacks may occur for several years before radiographic abnormalities appear. A monoarticular or oligoarticular arthropathy can develop with secondary osteoarthritis due to either chronic chondral deposition of crystals or recurrent bouts of acute arthritis. The bone density usually remains normal. Gouty *tophi* are monosodium urate deposits that may be seen radiographically as eccentric soft tissue nodules either in a bursa or in the periarticular soft tissues (Figs. 21-1–21-4). Gouty tophi often contain subtle amorphous calcification (Figs. 21-1C, 21-2B). In the setting of tophaceous disease, the joint width and thus articular cartilage remains intact, even late in the disease process, and even with large articular tophi and subchondral erosions. This can be an important discrimi-

nating feature. Subchondral cysts are usually not present, but occasionally may be quite large (Figs. 21-1, 21-3, 21-5). Ligamentous laxity is uncommon.

The erosions in gout tend to have a sclerotic margin and productive change. Once erosions occur, they may be intra-articular (often marginal) or para-articular (also termed *non-marginal*, often beneath tophi). The para-articular erosions are pathognomonic for gout and may show the additional feature of an *overhanging edge* (see Figs. 21-1, 21-3). The overhanging edge is a bony excrescence that extends out

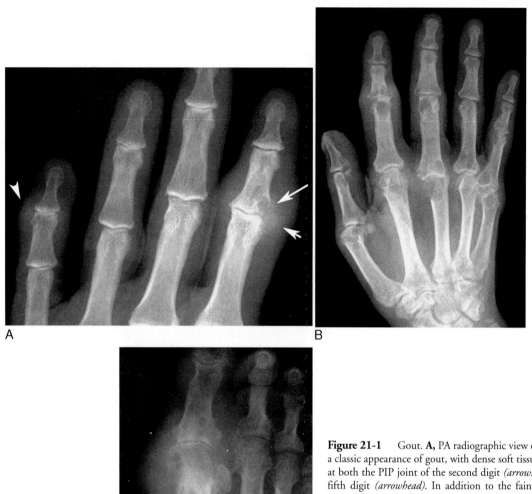

A   B

C

Figure 21-1   Gout. **A,** PA radiographic view of the fingers demonstrates a classic appearance of gout, with dense soft tissue swelling with tophi seen at both the PIP joint of the second digit *(arrows)* and the DIP joint of the fifth digit *(arrowhead)*. In addition to the faintly calcified tophus at the second PIP joint *(short arrow)*, there is a well-defined erosion with a "overhanging edge" at the base of the middle phalanx of the second digit *(long arrow)*. Note the normal bone density and preserved cartilage space in the second PIP joint. **B,** Similar, but more extensive gout in a different patient. **C,** Foot radiograph in another patient with gout shows juxta-articular erosions and calcified tophi.

toward the tophus, beyond the normal bony margin. It has an appearance of the tophus undermining the bone, but is due to new bone production.

In general, gout more frequently affects the lower extremity than the upper extremity, and small joints more often than large joints. The first metatarsophalangeal (MTP) joint is most frequently involved, but other MTPs and interphalangeal joints, as well as the midfoot and hindfoot, may also be involved. In the knee, the patellofemoral compartment is more frequently involved than the medial or lateral

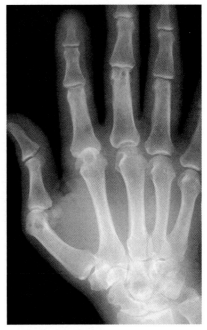

Figure 21-3 Gout simulating rheumatoid arthritis (RA). PA radiograph of the hand in a 50-year-old man shows erosions in a proximal distribution suggestive of RA. However, the normal bone density and the distinctness of the erosions suggest gout as a diagnosis, even in the absence of tophus formation. Aspiration proved gout in this case.

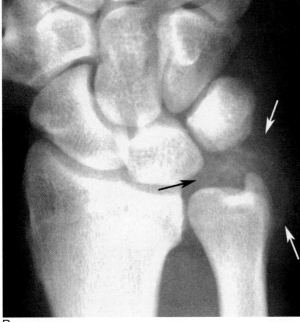

Figure 21-2 Gout. **A,** Oblique hand radiograph in an early case shows only eccentric juxta-articular soft tissue swelling *(arrowheads)*. Joint aspiration showed urate crystals. **B,** AP radiograph of a wrist in a 44-year-old male shows a faintly calcified soft-tissue mass adjacent to the ulnar styloid *(arrows)*. Bones appear normal. Differential diagnosis includes gouty tophus, but calcified neoplasm, such as synovial cell sarcoma or juxtacortical chondroma, is also a possibility.

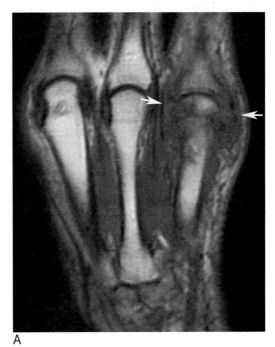

Figure 21-4 Gout, MRI. **A–C,** Coronal T1 (A),

(Continued)

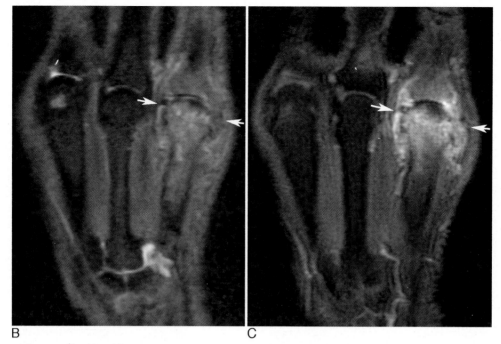

B   C

Figure 21-4—(Cont'd) inversion recovery (B), and fat-suppressed contrast-enhanced T1-weighted (C) MR images in a patient with tophaceous gout of the fifth MTP joint show the mass to have intermediate to low signal intensity on parts A and B *(arrows)*, and intense enhancement in part C *(arrows)*, which are typical MR findings in gout.

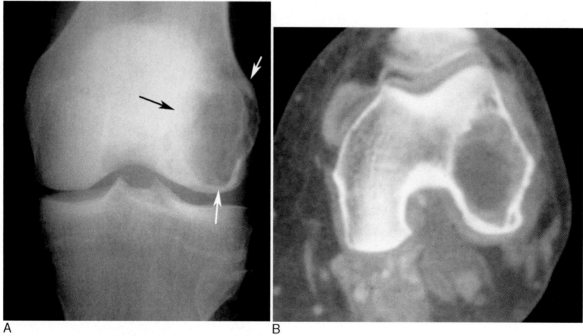

A   B

Figure 21-5 Gout, unusual presentation as large lytic lesion. **A,** AP radiograph of the knee in a 45-year-old woman shows a large lytic lesion in the lateral femoral condyle *(arrows)*. The radiographic findings and patient's age and gender are unusual for the diagnosis of gout. However, when one sees a very large lytic lesion adjacent to subchondral bone, an articular process should be considered. **B,** CT confirms the mass. Aspiration of the joint effusion showed urate crystals that confirmed the diagnosis. This case, as well as the cases in Figure 21-3 and 21-4, illustrate the old adage that gout can look like anything.

compartments. The hand and wrist may show involvement in the distal interphalangeal (DIP) joints, proximal interphalangeal (PIP) joints, and intercarpal joints, with the metacarpophalangeal (MCP) joints less frequently involved. Gout is a relatively easy diagnosis to make when it follows all of the preceding rules, including being oligoarticular with tophi and discrete, nonmarginal erosions with overhanging edges. However, it may also present as a polyarticular disease, without obvious tophi but with multiple well-marginated erosions. This appearance in an older man should always arouse suspicion for gout, but is often misdiagnosed as rheumatoid arthritis (see Fig. 21-3). Psoriatic arthritis may produce findings suggestive of gout, and serum urate may be elevated in patients with psoriasis. Finally, a younger patient with a gouty tophus may be clinically misdiagnosed with neoplasm. If magnetic resonance imaging (MRI) is done on these patients with atypical clinical and radiographic presentation (see Fig. 21-4), the tophus demonstrates low signal intensity on T1 but variably low to high signal intensity on T2, depending on the amount of calcification present in the tophus. It may even appear inhomogeneous and infiltrative. A gouty tophus usually enhances. It is worthwhile to remember that gout can have a variety of appearances and is relatively common, so should always be kept in mind as a potential diagnosis. Septic arthritis in particular can have a clinical and imaging appearance that is identical to an acute gout attack. Definitive diagnosis is made by inspection of the synovial fluid. Both crystal analysis and microbiological evaluation may be appropriate.

CALCIUM PYROPHOSPHATE DIHYDRATE CRYSTAL DEPOSITION DISEASE (PYROPHOSPHATE ARTHROPATHY)

Calcium pyrophosphate dihydrate (CPPD) crystal deposition disease is common. It is a disorder that results in intra-articular and para-articular CPPD crystal deposition, which leads to an associated arthropathy with radiographically distinctive features. The correct terminology for the arthropathy is *pyrophosphate arthropathy*. However, the clinical presentation of pyrophosphate arthropathy often resembles the intermittent acute attacks of gout, and is more loosely termed "pseudogout." It is important to note that "pseudogout," "chondrocalcinosis," and "pyrophosphate arthropathy" are not synonymous terms. "Pseudogout" can be used correctly only to describe a type of clinical presentation. "Chondrocalcinosis" is the radiographic finding of calcified cartilage, and itself does not imply an arthritis. "Pyrophosphate arthropathy" is the form of arthritis resulting from pyrophosphate crystal deposition, and may or may not have either chondrocalcinosis or a gout-like clinical presentation.

Pyrophosphate arthropathy generally occurs among middle-aged patients, without sex predilection. It may clinically present as pseudogout (acute self-limited attacks simulating gout or infection), pseudo-RA (more continuous acute attacks simulating RA in joint distribution), pseudo-degenerative joint disease (chronic progressive arthropathy but with acute exacerbations), pseudo-degenerative joint disease without acute exacerbations, pseudoneuropathic arthropathy (rapidly destructive form), or even as an asymptomatic arthropathy. The diagnosis is proven by joint aspiration demonstrating CPPD crystals. Most cases have no associated serum biochemical abnormality, but CPPD crystal deposition disease can occur in association with numerous metabolic conditions, including hemochromatosis (see following discussion), gout, hypothyroidism, and hyperparathyroidism. Incidental chondrocalcinosis is common in the elderly. Although most associated disorders may be coincidental, CPPD crystal deposition is definitely associated with hemochromatosis and hyperparathyroidism.

Key Concepts	Calcium Pyrophosphate Dihydrate (CPPD) Terminology

These conditions sometimes occur together but are not synonymous:
Pseudogout: Acute crystal-induced joint inflammation, clinically similar to gout
Chondrocalcinosis: CPPD crystal deposition in cartilage; asymptomatic
Pyrophosphate arthropathy: Distinctive arthropathy of CPPD

Both the radiographic appearance and the location of the arthropathy are quite distinctive. Chondrocalcinosis is generally present, although not invariably. Chondrocalcinosis may be in hyaline cartilage, fibrocartilage, synovium, or the joint capsule (Figs. 21-6–21-8). The most common locations for chondrocalcinosis include the triangular fibrocartilage complex of the wrist, lunatotriquetral ligament of the wrist, menisci of the knee, symphysis pubis, and acetabular labrum. In patients with pyrophosphate arthropathy, bone density is usually normal. Because CPPD deposition disease is a systemic disorder, there is uniform crystal deposition in joint cartilage, and thus there is uniform cartilage destruction, much like that seen in inflammatory arthropathies. Although early disease shows erosive change, more advanced disease appears primarily productive with sclerosis, osteochondral fragments, and osteophytes. This appearance resembles osteoarthritis (OA), but the location of abnormalities is distinctly different from OA, being bilaterally symmetric much like the distribution of rheumatoid arthritis. Subchondral cysts are a very distinctive feature because they are both common and large, occasionally simulating a neoplasm.

<table>
<tr><td>**Key Concepts**</td><td>**Pyrophosphate Arthropathy**</td></tr>
</table>

Shares many features with osteoarthritis (OA), but appears as "OA with a funny distribution"
Chondrocalcinosis usually (although not invariably) present, most frequent in wrist, knee, and symphysis pubis
Large subchondral cysts, occasionally simulate a lytic neoplasm
Knee: Patellofemoral
Wrist: Radiocarpal. Can progress to scapholunate advanced collapse (SLAC) wrist
Hand: Especially second and third MCP joints

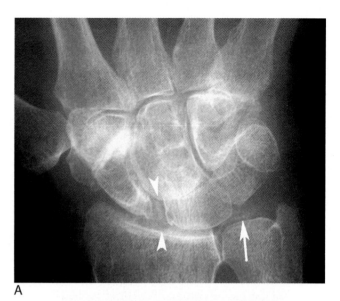

The most frequently involved joints are the knee, wrist, and second and third MCP joints of the hand. The knee generally demonstrates chondrocalcinosis in the menisci, but deposition is also frequently seen in the hyaline cartilage, synovium, and capsule. The arthritic process may be present in all three compartments but is usually seen earliest and most severely in the patellofemoral compartment, as opposed to the medial and lateral compartments (see Fig. 21-7).

Pyrophosphate arthropathy involving the hand and wrist shows a unique distribution. First, the chondrocalcinosis is usually located in the triangular fibrocartilage complex (see Fig. 21-6). However, close observation also may show chondrocalcinosis in the lunotriquetral ligament and the hyaline cartilage of the wrist. In addition, the arthropathy itself has a very specific distribution. Degenerative changes are specifically found in the radiocarpal joint, and late in the disease may be associated with scapholunate dissociation and scaphoid erosion into the distal radial articular surface. Proximal migration of the capitate between the dissociated scaphoid and lunate may result in a scapholunate advanced collapse (SLAC) wrist pattern (see Fig. 21-6; see also Chapter 7). A SLAC wrist may occur with rheumatoid arthritis and after trauma as well as with CPPD. Clues to a diagnosis of CPPD

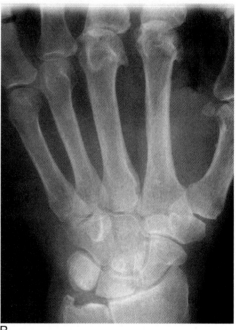

Figure 21-6   Pyrophosphate arthropathy, hand and wrist. **A,** PA radiograph of the wrist in an 81-year-old woman with pyrophosphate arthropathy. Note the chondrocalcinosis seen both in the triangular fibrocartilage (arrow) and between the scaphoid and lunate (arrowheads). There is mild scapholunate disassociation (note the distance measures 3.5 mm at the scapholunate joint). There is mild radiocarpal cartilage loss and prominent cyst formation in the scaphoid, capitate, and hamate. These findings are typical of pyrophosphate arthropathy. **B,** A different patient with pyrophosphate arthropathy. Note the triangular fibrocartilage chondrocalcinosis, early scapholunate advance collapse (SLAC wrist), and prominent osteophytes at the second and third MCP joints. Although SLAC wrist can be seen with other processes, the prominent productive change seen at the third MCP is so typical for pyrophosphate arthropathy that the diagnosis can be made even without the presence of chondrocalcinosis.

(Continued)

include distribution in the radiocarpal and second and third MCP joints (see Fig. 21-6). The IP joints tend to be spared in CPPD, in contrast with OA. This peculiar appearance and distribution is so typical that pyrophosphate arthropathy can often be diagnosed radiographically with a high degree of certainty, even in the absence of chondrocalcinosis in the involved joints.

Hip involvement is less frequent than knee and wrist, but if large subchondral cysts are seen with what otherwise appears to be OA, one should consider pyrophosphate arthropathy as the diagnosis and search for chondrocalcinosis in the joint and elsewhere (Fig. 21-8). Similarly, OA is uncommon in the shoulder

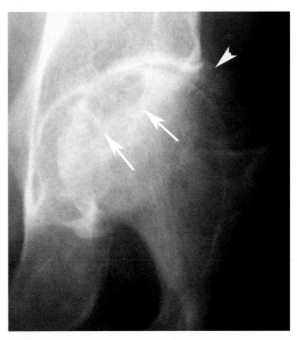

Figure 21-8   Pyrophosphate arthropathy, hip. AP radiograph shows a large subchondral cyst in the femoral head *(arrows)* and chondrocalcinosis in the labrum *(arrowhead)*. This combination of findings establishes the diagnosis of pyrophosphate arthropathy of the hip.

Figure 21-6—(Cont'd)   **C,** Similar pattern in a different patient, who had extensive chondrocalcinosis.

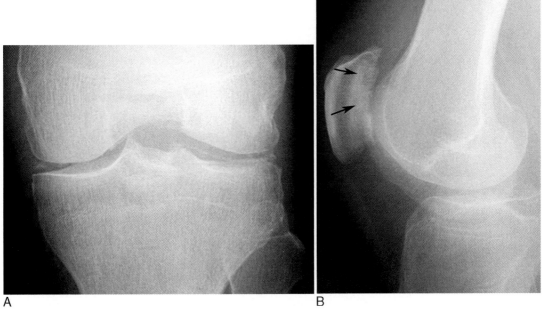

Figure 21-7   Pyrophosphate arthropathy, knee. **A,** AP radiograph of the knee in a 40-year-old woman shows chondrocalcinosis. **B,** Lateral radiographic view shows patellar subchondral cysts. Patellofemoral disease predominates in pyrophosphate arthropathy of the knee.

and elbow in the absence of trauma or occupational injury, and a degenerative joint pattern combined with chondrocalcinosis at these sites often indicates pyrophosphate arthropathy.

HEMOCHROMATOSIS ARTHROPATHY

Hemochromatosis arthropathy develops in up to 50% of patients who have hemochromatosis, thought to be due to accumulation of iron or CPPD crystals in the joints. Hemochromatosis itself may be either primary, owing to increased gastrointestinal absorption of iron, or secondary, owing to blood transfusions, alcoholism, or excess iron ingestion. Onset is usually in the middle-age range and males are more frequently affected than females. The clinical triad of bronze skin, cirrhosis, and diabetes may be present.

The radiographic features of the arthropathy are essentially identical to those of pyrophosphate arthropathy. Thus, chondrocalcinosis is common in hemochromatosis. The disease is primarily productive, with large beak-like osteophytes typical at the MCP joints. However, some erosions may be seen (Fig. 21-9). Subchondral cysts are quite prominent, similar to those found with pyrophosphate arthropathy. The joints most commonly affected are identical to those with pyrophosphate arthropathy, including the radiocarpal joint, second and third MCP joints, and the knee (with the patellofemoral compartment predominating).

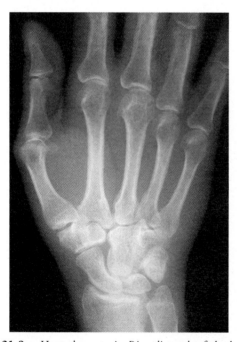

Figure 21-9 Hemochromatosis. PA radiograph of the hand and wrist demonstrates cartilage loss and large osteophytes at the second and third MCP joints in a young man. This distribution is typical of hemochromatosis or pyrophosphate arthropathy. In a younger male, as seen here, hemochromatosis is more probable.

WILSON'S DISEASE

Wilson's disease (hepatolenticular degeneration) is an autosomal recessive process associated with abnormal accumulation of copper in multiple organ systems. Degeneration of the basal ganglia, hepatic cirrhosis, and characteristic brownish-green Kayser-Fleischer rings around the cornea develop between childhood and middle-age. Wilson's disease occurs slightly more frequently in males than females.

The rare associated arthropathy develops later in life. Radiographically, chondrocalcinosis may be present. The bones are osteopenic. Cartilage destruction occurs and the subchondral bone appears indistinct and irregular, with several small fragments or ossicles. This may give the appearance of osteochondritis. The joints most frequently affected are the wrist and hand, particularly the MCPs, followed by the foot, hip, shoulder, elbow, and knee.

CALCIUM HYDROXYAPATITE DEPOSITION DISEASE

Calcium hydroxyapatite deposition disease (HADD) results in periarticular calcifications, is most often monoarticular, and results in an inflammatory reaction that is usually without structural joint abnormality. The cause is unknown but may relate to repeated minor trauma and calcium hydroxyapatite deposition in necrotic tissue. Hydroxyapatite deposition is seen in middle-age and older individuals and affects men and women equally. The key radiographic finding is a homogenous, cloud-like calcification occurring in periarticular locations (tendon, ligament, capsule, or bursa). Occasionally the deposition is intra-articular, producing chondrocalcinosis. The calcification may change over time, showing enlargement or even disappearance.

Key Concepts	Hydroxyapatite Deposition Disease (HADD)
Amorphous, dense soft tissue calcification Calcific tendinitis	

The shoulder is the most frequently involved site, with calcification located in tendons and at the sites of tendon insertion, specifically the rotator cuff, biceps tendons and the subacromial-subdeltoid bursa (Figs. 2-12, 5-5, 21-10). The hand may show periarticular deposits around the MCP and IP joints. The wrist may show hydroxyapatite deposition in any tendon insertion, but this is especially frequent at the flexor carpi ulnaris insertion adjacent to the pisiform. HADD

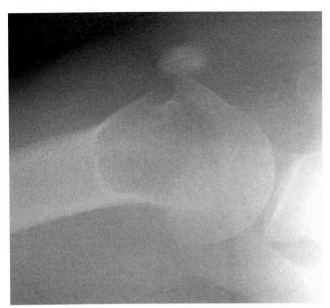

Figure 21-10 Calcium hydroxyapatite deposition disease (HADD). Axillary shoulder radiograph shows amorphous, uniform calcification anterior to the lesser tuberosity of the humerus. This is the typical appearance of HADD in a tendon (calcific tendinitis), in this case in the biceps long head tendon.

at the insertion of the gluteus maximus can be confused with calcification in a soft tissue neoplasm. HADD may be painless, or exquisitely painful. Painful hydroxyapatite deposits may be treated by aspiration under fluoroscopic control or ultrasound guidance, followed by injection of steroids.

ALCAPTONURIA (OCHRONOSIS)

Ochronosis is a hereditary metabolic abnormality arising from the absence of homogentisic acid oxidase and consequent accumulation of homogentisic acid in various organs, including connective tissues. It affects males and females equally, and the arthropathy generally occurs later in life. The radiographic findings are of dystrophic (hydroxyapatite crystal) calcification mostly involving the disks of the spine, but calcification is also occasionally seen in cartilage, tendons, and ligaments. The most specific radiographic appearance is in the spine, which appears osteoporotic with dense disk calcification. Other joints may be involved and show changes of mild degenerative joint disease, but this is a much less specific appearance.

AMYLOIDOSIS

Amyloidosis is a systemic deposition disease that may be either primary or secondary. The secondary form may be associated with multiple myeloma, long-term hemodialysis, RA, familial Mediterranean fever, chronic infection, spondyloarthropathy,

and connective tissue disorders (e.g., systemic lupus erythematosus, scleroderma, and dermatomyositis). Amyloid deposition can result in renal failure, organomegaly, pericardial and myocardial disease, pulmonary septal infiltration, and gastrointestinal tract involvement with submucosal thickening and decreased peristalsis. Between 5% and 13% of patients with amyloidosis have bone or joint involvement, consisting of deposition in bone, synovium, and surrounding soft tissues. The soft tissue deposition results in the formation of bulky nodules, seen particularly about the wrists, elbows, and shoulders. The "shoulder pad" sign has been attributed to amyloidosis, where bulky nodules are superimposed on atrophic shoulder musculature. Magnetic resonance imaging of the nodules shows signal intensity intermediate between fibrocartilage and muscle on all sequences. The MRI findings may help to distinguish amyloid deposits from cellular or free water-containing processes such as inflammation or synovitis (Fig. 21-11). Large periarticular fluid collections can result from chronic joint effusion.

Key Concepts	**Amyloidosis**

Systemic deposition disease
Primary or secondary
Secondary: Multiple causes, notably multiple myeloma, long-term hemodialysis, rheumatoid arthritis (RA), chronic infection
Bulky soft tissue nodules
Arthropathy: Joint space widening
Erosions and subchondral cysts: Sharply marginated
Wrists, elbow, shoulder most frequent
Spine: May resemble discitis or neuropathic disorder

Intra-articular amyloid deposits result in joint space widening due to infiltration, and later narrowing due to cartilage destruction. Erosions and subchondral cysts tend to be sharply marginated (Figs. 21-11, 21-12, 21-13). The joints most commonly involved are the wrists, elbow, and shoulder. Knees and hips are less commonly involved. In patients undergoing long-term hemodialysis, the spine, wrist, and hands are most commonly affected. Also in these patients, spondyloarthropathy often occurs with the appearance of disk space narrowing and end plate irregularity that can mimic discitis, destructive tumor, or neuropathic spondyloarthropathy (Fig. 21-14).

Amyloidosis is most frequently confused with RA because of the nodularity of the soft tissues and the erosive change, particularly of the hands and wrist. The conditions may coexist. The presence of well-defined erosions and frequent preservation of joint space width in amyloidosis may help to differentiate the two. In addition, if the patient is known to have a predisposing factor such as multiple myeloma, the correct diagnosis is more frequently attained.

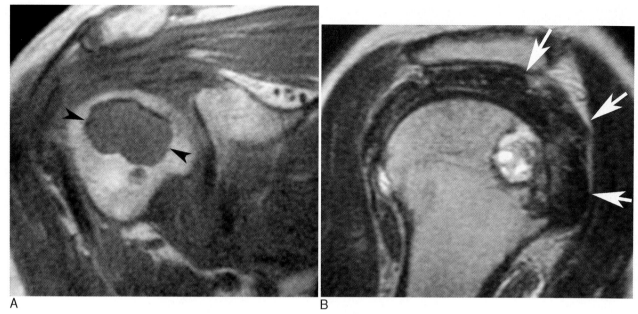

Figure 21-11   Amyloid. **A,** Coronal T1-weighted MR image shows an amyloid deposit within the right humeral head (between *arrows*). Its signal intensity is similar to that of muscle. **B,** T2-weighted sagittal MR image shows the deposit to have heterogeneous signal intensity, with areas of low signal intensity. In addition, note the thickened low-signal supraspinatus and subscapularis tendons, which also contain amyloid deposits *(arrows).*

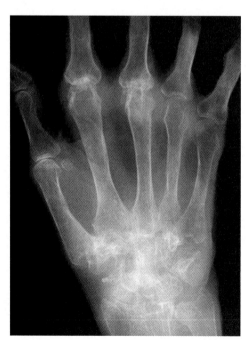

Figure 21-12   Amyloid. PA radiograph of the hand and wrist shows soft tissue swelling of the MCP joints and very prominent, large, well-defined erosions in the carpal bones. When bones are involved with amyloid, the erosions tend to be well defined. This patient had multiple myeloma, with secondary amyloidosis.

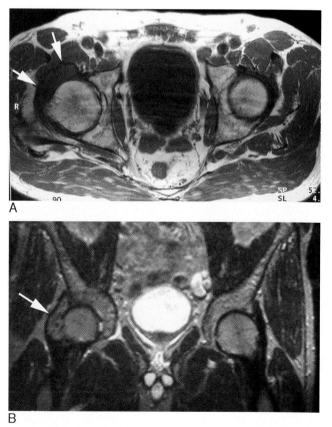

Figure 21-13   Amyloid. Axial T1-weighted (A) and coronal inversion recovery (B) MR images show mass-like capsular thickening of the right hip capsule *(arrows)* with intermediate to low signal intensity on both images. Biopsy showed amyloid.

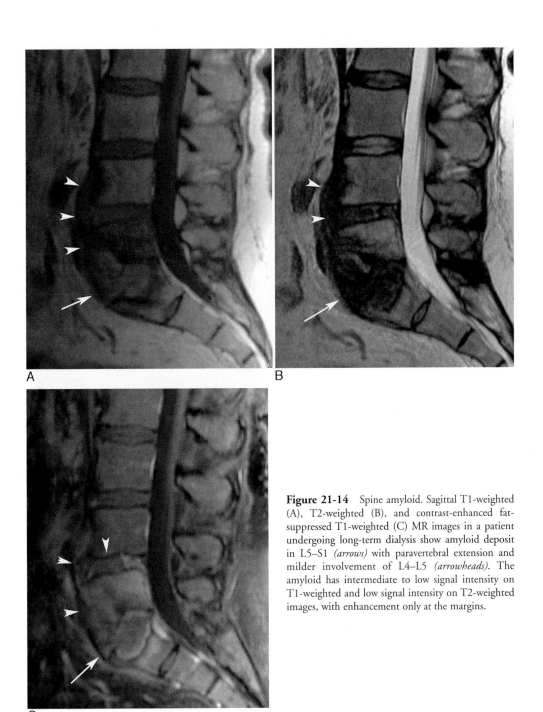

Figure 21-14 Spine amyloid. Sagittal T1-weighted (A), T2-weighted (B), and contrast-enhanced fat-suppressed T1-weighted (C) MR images in a patient undergoing long-term dialysis show amyloid deposit in L5–S1 *(arrows)* with paravertebral extension and milder involvement of L4–L5 *(arrowheads)*. The amyloid has intermediate to low signal intensity on T1-weighted and low signal intensity on T2-weighted images, with enhancement only at the margins.

Avascular Necrosis

ETIOLOGY AND DEMOGRAPHICS
IMAGING
TREATMENT OF ADULT AVN
LEGG-CALVÉ-PERTHES DISEASE
AVN MIMICS

ETIOLOGY AND DEMOGRAPHICS

Avascular necrosis (AVN) of bone, also termed *ischemic necrosis* or *osteonecrosis,* is a poorly understood phenomenon that may be related to traumatic or compressive interruption of arterial inflow, increased marrow pressure with impeded venous drainage, or intraluminal vascular obstruction. The outcome is necrosis of the cellular elements of bone. There are numerous recognized causes of AVN, although many cases are idiopathic. The most common causes of AVN in North America include trauma, steroid use, alcoholism, and sickle cell disease. Many cases are idiopathic. A more complete list of causes is included in the mnemonic "ASEPTIC," for sickle cell anemia, steroids, ethanol abuse, pancreatitis, trauma, idiopathic or infection, and caisson disease. Gaucher's disease and radiation can be added to this list. Avascular necrosis is more common in patients with renal transplants, perhaps only because of steroid use.

It can be useful to search for these conditions when AVN is recognized on a radiograph. An example of the traumatic cause is found particularly in the hip, where delayed reduction of a dislocation or subcapital fracture can result in AVN. Steroid-related AVN may be due to either exogenous or endogenous (Cushing's disease) sources. It is thought that the mechanism of AVN with steroid use is an increase in the size of the fat cells and resultant increased marrow pressure, particularly in the femoral head, with resulting extrinsic compression of intraosseous blood vessels. One may observe a transplanted kidney in the iliac fossa on a pelvis film taken to demonstrate AVN (Fig. 22-1). Alcoholic patients may develop avascular necrosis due to fat emboli and increased marrow pressure. Pancreatic calcification could suggest the diagnosis in this case. Patients with sickle cell disease develop AVN because of microvascular occlusion from the abnormal red blood cells. Abdominal and pelvic radiographs might also demonstrate diffuse patchy sclerosis, vertebral body changes, an absent spleen shadow, or calcified gallstones, all of which suggest sickle cell disease. Sickle cell disease is discussed further in Chapter 41.

Key Concepts	Avascular Necrosis

Radiographs: Sclerosis, followed by subchondral lucency, fracture, collapse and flattening, and secondary osteoarthritis
MRI: Marrow edema followed by double-line sign
Cartilage remains normal until secondary degenerative disease
Causes are numerous. Mnemonic: ASEPTIC: sickle cell anemia, steroids, ethanol abuse, pancreatitis, trauma, idiopathic or infection, and caisson disease ("dysbaric avascular necrosis"); also remember Gaucher's disease and radiation; most common: trauma, steroids, alcoholism, sickle cell disease; many cases idiopathic
Most common sites are femoral head, lunate, proximal pole of the scaphoid, humeral head, vertebral body

The less common causes of AVN also may be evident on plain radiographs. With Gaucher's disease, the sinusoids are packed with Gaucher's cells, increasing marrow pressure. Radiographs show hepatosplenomegaly and bone expansion of the metaphyses of long bones. Gaucher's disease is discussed further in Chapter 39. Radiation has a direct toxic effect on vascular supply to the bone; abnormalities suggesting radiation necrosis, including bone sclerosis and soft tissue edema on magnetic resonance imaging (MRI) (seen in a port-like configuration) may lead to this diagnosis (Fig. 22-2). In patients with systemic lupus erythematosus

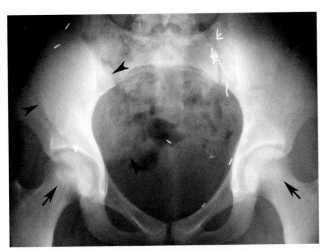

Figure 22-1   Avascular necrosis (AVN), renal transplant. AP radiograph of the pelvis in this 27-year-old woman demonstrates central sclerotic areas within both femoral heads *(arrows),* the earliest radiographic finding of AVN. The cause of AVN is apparent, with the soft tissue mass of the renal transplant seen in the right iliac fossa *(arrowheads).*

(SLE), vasculitis may be additive to these patients' steroid therapy in causing AVN. Avascular necrosis located in unusual sites, such as the talus or humerus, might suggest SLE as a cause. Chapter 20 discusses SLE in more detail.

Caisson disease is nitrogen embolization following rapid decompression after breathing pressurized air. Rapid decompression causes nitrogen dissolved in the blood to form microbubbles that occlude small vessels. This condition was common during construction of New York City's Brooklyn Bridge. The footings for the bridge were dug out by hand under waterproof caissons that contained pressurized air. The workers were decompressed rapidly at the end of each shift. Today, it is divers who most

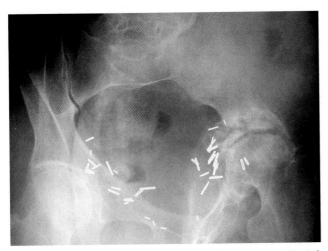

Figure 22-2   Avascular necrosis (AVN), radiation injury. The left femoral head and acetabulum show the mixed sclerosis and lucency of radiation osteonecrosis, with collapse of the femoral head and fragmentation of the acetabular roof in this 64-year-old man who underwent radiation for prostate cancer. The pelvic clips indicate a lymph node dissection.

frequently have this condition. Before the epidemic of caisson disease in New York, most cases of hip osteonecrosis were caused by infection, especially tuberculosis, hence the term "aseptic necrosis" for today's most frequent causes.

Bone cell death depends on the duration of ischemia. Marrow elements are the most vulnerable to prolonged anoxia, and die after about 6 to 12 hours. Osteocytes, osteoblasts, and osteoclasts die after 12 to 48 hours, and marrow fat cells die after 2 to 5 days. Thus, pathologic findings depend on the duration of anoxia. After bone necrosis, revascularization and granulation ingrowth occur along a *reactive interface,* advancing into the bone infarct, replacing dead bone with weaker reparative tissue. Thus, the healing process weakens the bone. Later, the reparative tissue is converted to normal bone. The process is termed *creeping substitution* (of dead bone by new bone).

IMAGING

Avascular necrosis of the hip is discussed here as the prototypical example of the radiographic features of AVN. Initially, the articular cartilage is unaffected by AVN because it is nourished by synovial fluid. The first radiographic sign in hip AVN occurs weeks or months after the bone infarct. This is radiographically apparent as sclerosis, generally in the center of the femoral head (see Fig. 22-1). Initially, the sclerosis is relative in nature, as the vascularized bone surrounding the necrotic bone becomes osteopenic due to hyperemia. Later in the process, the reactive interface develops, with bone formation and repair causing a zone of increased density. The new bone is relatively sclerotic. The classic linear subchondral fracture, also termed a "crescent sign," typically develops subsequently during bone healing due to hyperemia-induced osteoporosis and bone weakening. In the hip, this is best seen on a frog-leg lateral view, but is often discerned on an anteroposterior (AP) view as well (Figs. 22-3, 22-4). The subchondral fracture often leads to progressive subchondral fragmentation, flattening, and deformity. Secondary osteoarthritis may occur much later, and relates to deformity of the articular surface from subchondral fracture.

Radionuclide bone scanning may depict AVN before it is visible on radiographs, seen initially as a photopenic region, followed by increased activity with revascularization and repair, and secondary OA.

Magnetic resonance imaging is the most sensitive imaging tool for detection of avascular necrosis. When the typical features are present, MRI may be highly specific as well. However, at some stages the MRI appearance may be nonspecific. The earliest finding is diffuse marrow edema, which may also be seen in early infection or transient osteoporosis (see discussion later in this chapter and in Chapter 27). However, as the condition evolves, the specific, classic double-line sign develops,

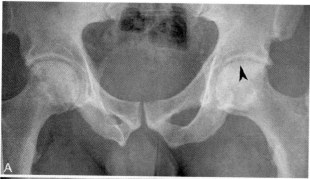

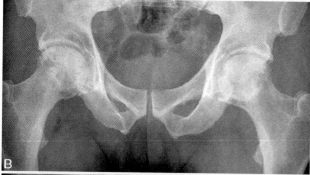

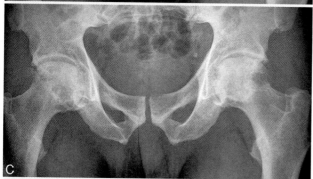

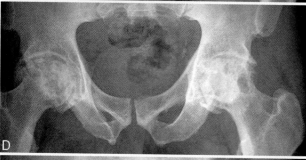

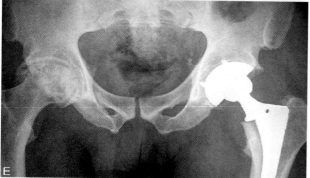

which is seen as a serpiginous (undulating) low-signal-intensity line of uniform width on both T1 and T2 sequences, with an adjacent rim of increased signal intensity on T2 (Fig. 22-5). The double-line sign can occasionally overlap in appearance with a subchondral fracture. Subchondral fractures are usually straight or gently, uniformly curved. Thus, a serpiginous double-line sign is virtually pathognomic for AVN.

An AVN classification system based on the MRI findings has been developed and is used by some authors. In class A, the central femoral head marrow signal is isointense to fat. In class B, the central signal is isointense to hemorrhage. In class C, the central signal is isointense to fluid. Class D shows a central signal isointense to fibrous tissue or bone. These classes are roughly equivalent to the radiographic stages I to IV (I is normal, II shows trabecular changes without collapse, III shows collapse, and IV is AVN with secondary osteoarthritis [OA]); Figs. 22-3, 22-6). It should be remembered that MRI has 98% specificity in differentiating normal from abnormal bone, but only 85% specificity in differentiating AVN from non-AVN disease.

The superb sensitivity of MRI in detection of AVN has lead to an interesting observation that AVN may be clinically occult. Moreover, the marrow changes in some cases of asymptomatic AVN resolve spontaneously. Therefore, the value of screening at-risk but asymptomatic patients has not been established.

Survey radiographs of hip AVN include AP and frog-leg pelvis (see Fig. 22-4). Screening with MRI includes T1 coronal, T2 coronal, and either T1 or T2 sagittal. Fat suppression of the T2-weighted sequences or inversion recovery is needed for optimal sensitivity. The evaluation

---

WHAT THE CLINICIAN WANTS TO KNOW:
AVASCULAR NECROSIS

Extent of disease in coronal and sagittal planes (face of clock analogy)
Femoral head flattening/collapse, and its extent
Contralateral side involvement (may be clinically silent)
Development of secondary osteoarthritis (OA)
Any progression over time

Figure 22-3   Hip avascular necrosis (AVN). Radiographic progression over time in a 45-year-old man with bilateral AVN. **A,** Initial radiograph shows sclerosis in both femoral heads and a left femoral head subchondral crescent with early collapse *(arrowhead)*. **B,** Three months later, the left crescent is no longer visible because of further collapse. Note the flattening of the right femoral head. **C,** One year after the image in part B, bilateral femoral head collapse is progressing and secondary osteoarthritis (OA) is developing, with subchondral sclerosis and osteophyte formation. **D,** Twenty months after the image in part C, collapse and secondary OA are more prominent. **E,** Five months later, a left total arthroplasty has been placed. The right will be replaced soon.

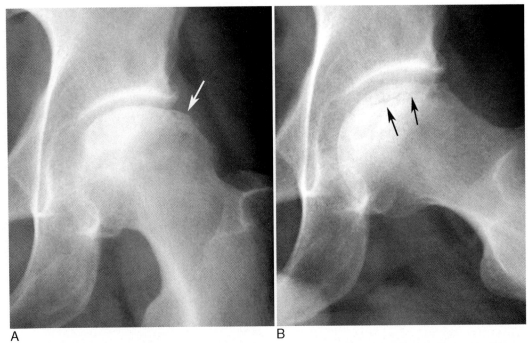

A   B

Figure 22-4   Avascular necrosis (AVN) radiographic evaluation, value of frog-leg lateral view. **A,** AP radiograph of the left hip in this 37-year-old man with AVN due to steroids demonstrates mild femoral head flattening due to mild subchondral collapse. This has created a lateral femoral head ridge that suggests an osteophyte *(arrow).* **B,** The frog-leg lateral radiograph shows a subchondral fracture *(arrows),* making the diagnosis of AVN easy. (Reprinted with permission of the American College of Radiology learning file.)

should be done to determine not only the diagnosis but also to assess for femoral head flattening and secondary OA. It is also important to indicate the extent and location of AVN in the coronal and sagittal planes, referring to locations with a clock-face description. The extent of AVN roughly corresponds to the amount of femoral head at risk for collapse. This helps the surgeon determine whether the patient can be best treated by core decompression (Fig. 22-7), osteotomy with realignment to a noncollapsed weight-bearing portion, or prosthesis placement (see Fig. 22-3).

The most common sites of occurrence of AVN depend on the underlying cause. Sickle cell disease and SLE are common causes of AVN of the humeral head and talus. Bones that are extensively covered with articular cartilage are especially vulnerable to AVN after fracture. These include the femoral head, proximal pole of the scaphoid, humeral anatomic head, and talar body and dome (see Fig. 1-30). Lunate AVN, also termed "lunate malacia" and "Kienböck's disease," is believed to be due most frequently to trauma. It has been questionably associated with ulnar minus variance (Fig. 22-8; see also Chapter 7). Freiberg's disease is subchondral collapse, likely due to AVN of a metatarsal head, most commonly the second and third metatarsal

heads (Fig. 22-9). Freiberg's disease tends to be seen in teenage females and may be related to the trauma of bearing weight in high-heeled shoes.

Imaging of avascular necrosis of the spine may be nonspecific, with increased density of the vertebral body and collapse. However, if gas is seen within the partially collapsed vertebral body, this is virtually pathognomonic for AVN and is a useful sign with which to exclude an underlying tumor. This benign radiographic finding is known as Kümmell's disease. This is thought to be due to a vacuum phenomenon, similar to gas in a healthy joint. The gas-containing space is dark on all MRI sequences but may rapidly fill with fluid or granulation (Fig. 22-10). Sickle cell and Gaucher's disease produce an "H-shaped" vertebra in which the midportion of the superior and inferior endplates of osteonecrotic vertebrae are impacted.

TREATMENT OF ADULT AVN

Treatment of AVN depends on the site. Avascular necrosis of the lunate due to ulnar minus variance may be treated with ulnar lengthening. Scaphoid AVN is managed conservatively. Associated nonunion may require screw fixation and bone grafting. The treatment of AVN of the hip is con-

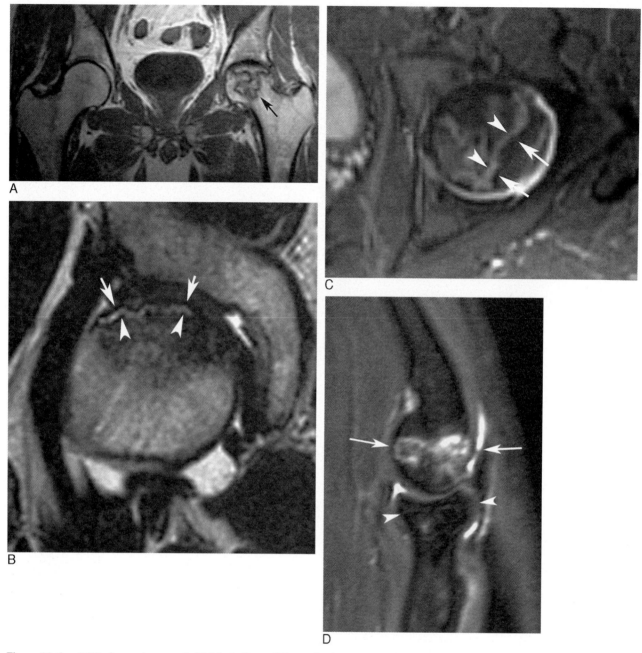

Figure 22-5 MRI of avascular necrosis (AVN). **A,** Coronal T1-weighted MR image of the hips shows classic serpiginous lines *(arrow)* in the left femoral head. Also note mild flattening of the superior aspect of the left femoral head. **B,** Sagittal T2-weighted MR image in a different patient shows the double-line sign of serpiginous low *(arrows)* and high *(arrowheads)* signal intensity. **C,** Axial fat-suppressed T2-weighted MR image in the same left hip as shown in part A also shows the bright *(arrowheads)* and dark *(arrows)* lines, although the latter is less conspicuous with fat suppression. **D,** Humeral capitellum AVN after trauma. Sagittal fat-suppressed T2-weighted MR image in a patient with ongoing pain after successful reduction of a radial head dislocation several months previously shows AVN of the capitellum *(arrows)*. The normal radial head is marked by *arrowheads*.

troversial. There is no medical therapy. Surgical intervention is considered optimal if initiated at the earliest stages, often before the imaging or clinical findings are definite for AVN. Surgical intervention consists of core decompression,

seen radiographically as a cylindrical lucency extending from the femoral neck into the head. A vascularized fibular graft may be placed at this site to stimulate healing and revascularization (see Fig. 22-7).

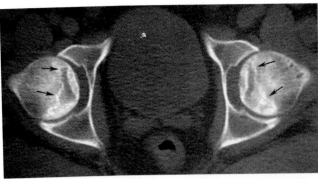

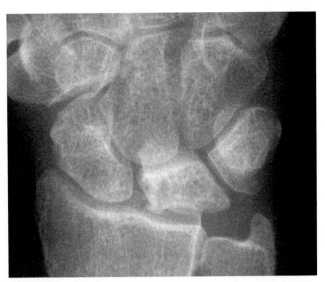

Figure 22-6   CT of bilateral hip avascular necrosis (AVN). The serpiginous lines of AVN on MRI are seen on CT as thin sclerotic lines *(arrows)*.

Figure 22-8   Kienböck's disease (lunate AVN). PA radiograph of the wrist shows a dense lunate with proximal collapse, representing AVN.

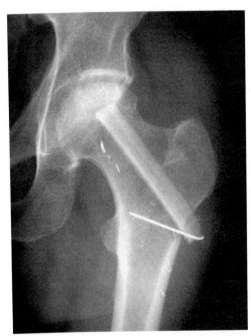

Figure 22-7   Vascularized fibular graft. The AP radiograph of the hip demonstrates the packing of the femoral head with bone graft following decompression, as well as the placement of the vascularized fibular graft within the neck.

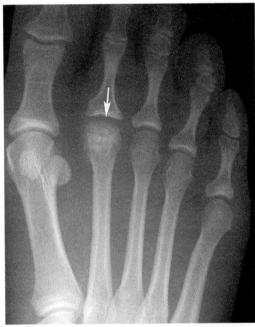

Figure 22-9   Freiberg's necrosis. AP radiograph of the foot in a 26-year-old woman demonstrates slight flattening and fragmentation of the head of the second metatarsal bone *(arrow)*. The location and sex are typical of this condition.

LEGG-CALVÉ-PERTHES DISEASE

Legg-Calvé-Perthes disease (LCP; Figs. 22-11, 22-12) is AVN of the pediatric hip, seen most frequently from age 4 to 8 years, when the vascular supply to the femoral head is most at risk. It is seen more frequently in boys than girls and may be bilateral in 10% of cases, although the presentation in such cases is usually asymmetric. The first radiographic sign may be

effusion, and the clinical presentation may mimic infection. Later, the involved capital femoral epiphysis ossification center may appear smaller than the contralateral normal side. Later still, mechanical forces combined with weakening of the capital femoral epiphysis by the necrosis and healing process result in fragmentation and flattening of the femoral head. Metaphyseal

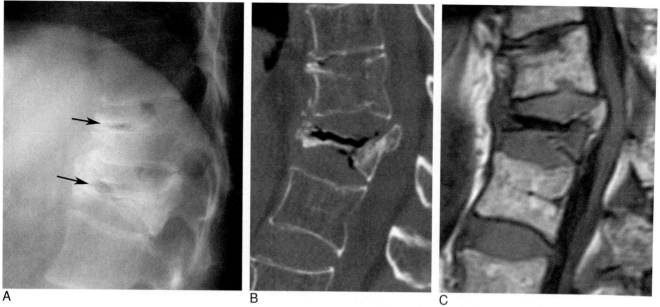

Figure 22-10   Avascular necrosis: spine. **A,** Lateral radiograph of the spine in a man taking steroids for an organ transplant demonstrates gas in the collapsed T12 and L1 bodies *(arrows).* The presence of gas in a collapsed vertebral body is known as Kümmell's disease and is considered pathognomonic for benign collapse rather than neoplasm. **B and C,** Sagittal CT reformat (B) and T1-weighted MR image (C) in a different patient with collapse of T12 show similar findings. Note the signal void of the gas in part C. Another possible cause of a fairly linear signal void in a vertebral body is methyl methacrylate from a vertebroplasty.

irregularity and lucent metaphyseal "cysts" adjacent to the physis (Fig. 22-11B) are manifestations of growth abnormality that results in a short, wide femoral neck. The latter was emphasized in an old term for LCP, *coxa magna.* Femoral head deformity induces secondary deformity in the acetabulum, with flattening

and irregularity. Intra-articular bodies may occur. The outcome varies. Some cases have a normal or near-normal outcome. However, most children have some lasting decrease in range of motion, and early OA is common. The acetabular labrum may become deformed or torn, resulting in the painful "lateral rim

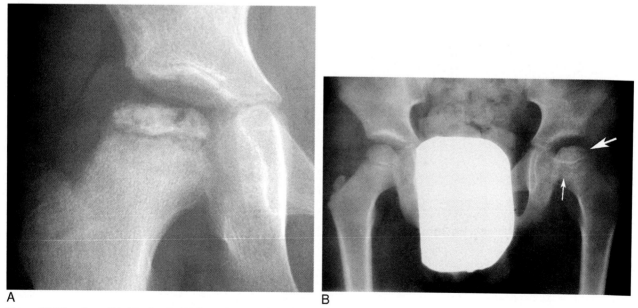

Figure 22-11   Legg-Calvé-Perthes (LCP) disease. **A,** AP radiograph of the hip in a 7-year-old girl shows fragmented and flattened femoral capital epiphysis. **B,** Early LCP. Note subtle irregularity of the capital femoral epiphysis *(large arrow)* and subtle "metaphyseal cyst" *(small arrow-head)* adjacent to the physis.

Pediatric hip avascular necrosis (AVN)

Presentation: Age 4 to 8 years, more frequently in males than females

Present with pain, effusion; can simulate infection

Femoral head fragmentation and flattening

10% bilateral

Early osteoarthritis (OA)

Younger patients and boys tend to have better outcomes

Cases with >50% femoral head involvement tend to have worse outcome

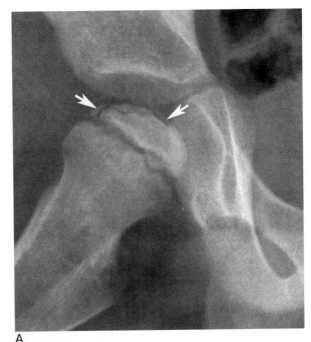

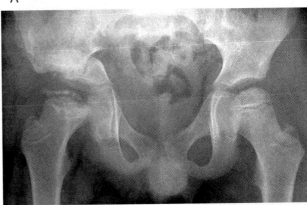

syndrome" (see discussion of femoroacetabular impingement in Chapter 11).

Prognostic factors in LCP are the age of the child at the time of diagnosis and the amount of the femoral head involvement. Older children at the time of diagnosis and females (who are generally more skeletally mature than males of the same age) have a poorer prognosis because they have less remaining growth, and thus less time for the hip to remodel back to a more normal configuration. Involvement of greater than 50% of the femoral head also indicates a worse prognosis. Incomplete coverage of the femoral head ossification center by the acetabular roof also indicates a greater risk for early OA.

Multiplanar MRI can be used to assess the extent of femoral head osteonecrosis as well as femoral head coverage by the acetabulum (see Fig. 22-12). It can also help diagnose bony bridging across the physis, which could result in growth arrest or deformity. Despite these benefits, MRI is not frequently used in managing LCP because most management is conservative, with salvage procedures such as femoral or acetabular osteotomy performed only after a clinical problem has developed.

AVN MIMICS

Meyer's dysplasia is delayed and irregular ossification of the capital femoral epiphysis ossification centers that can simulate LCP. Radiographic findings are usually seen in a younger age group (2 to 4 years). Hypothyroidism, sickle cell disease, Gaucher's disease, and epiphyseal dysplasias can cause fragmentation of the capital femoral epiphyses, which is usually bilateral (in contrast with LCP).

In the past, some authors attempted to unify the osteochondroses with AVN on the basis of the theory that any condition associated with subchondral bone irregularity or collapse was initiated by AVN. Current understanding is that osteochondritis dissecans, Panner's disease (fragmentation of the capitellum), Sever's disease (calcaneus apophysis), Köhler's disease (tarsal navicular), Scheuermann's disease of the spine, and many other radiographically similar conditions are not AVN-related. These conditions are discussed in the Chapter 23.

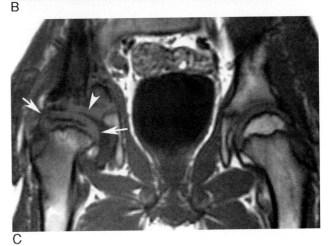

Figure 22-12 Legg-Calvé-Perthes disease. **A,** Frog-leg lateral radiograph shows subchondral lucencies *(arrows)* in the right capital femoral epiphysis. **B,** AP radiograph over one year later shows typical progression, with broad, fragmented capital femoral epiphysis, wide femoral neck, and irregular acetabulum. **C,** Coronal T1-weighted MR image shows similar findings. Note the greater thickness of the intermediate-signal-intensity cartilage of the right femoral head *(arrows)* and acetabulum *(arrowhead)* compared with the normal left.

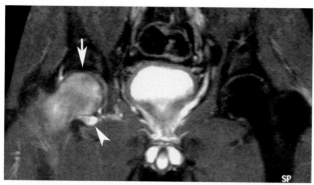

Figure 22-13 Transient osteoporosis of the hip. Coronal inversion recovery MR image shows intense edema in the femoral head *(arrow)* and neck, and an effusion *(arrowhead).* Early avascular necrosis could have this appearance. However, this patient recovered without complication. See also Figure 27-4.

A stress-related insufficiency fracture of the subchondral femoral head may simulate AVN clinically and on imaging studies. The overlying fragment may impact, stimulating AVN with collapse. A similar condition occurs in the subchondral femoral condyle, which was originally thought to represent spontaneous osteonecrosis and therefore named SONK ("spontaneous osteonecrosis of the knee," a term that is falling out of favor, see Chapter 13). In either site, one must carefully look for the subtle low signal line of the subchondral fracture roughly parallel subchondral cortex. With or without collapse, a subchondral insufficiency fracture line usually has a relatively smooth contour, as opposed to the serpiginous line or lines seen with true osteonecrosis.

Transient regional osteoporosis (TRO) is painful but self-limited osteoporosis and regional erythema, seen most frequently in middle-aged men (also occurring in pregnant women), most frequently in the hip, although any lower-extremity joint may be involved. Upper-extremity involvement is unusual. Some authors distinguish transient osteoporosis of the hip (TOH) as a separate entity, but these probably are the same condition. Magnetic resonance imaging shows marked marrow edema (Fig. 22-13). Bone scanning shows increased tracer uptake (Fig. 27-4). Radiographic findings of osteopenia and sometimes periosteal reaction are first seen 4 to 8 weeks after the onset of symptoms. Cartilage is preserved. Transient bone loss may be severe, with risk of pathologic fracture. Transient regional osteoporosis is otherwise a benign, self-limited disease, with full recovery usually within 10 to 12 months; the process may recur, however, often at a different joint a few years later. Transient regional osteoporosis may mimic early AVN clinically and on MRI, and for this reason some authors have suggested that TRO is a transient, self-limited variant of osteonecrosis. Because treatment may be different for TRO and AVN, diagnosis is important. It may show edema in the acetabulum, a finding that is not seen in early AVN. If onset has been recent, waiting a few weeks and repeating radiography may show the typical osteoporosis of the TRO. Alternatively, a double-line sign may be present, or the edema may be localized to a subchondral location, suggesting AVN. Transient osteoporosis of the hip and transient regional osteoporosis are discussed further in Chapter 27 (see Fig. 27-4).

SYNOVIAL CHONDROMATOSIS
OSTEOCHONDROSES
HYPERTROPHIC OSTEOARTHROPATHY
LEAD ARTHROPATHY
ACROMEGALY

SYNOVIAL CHONDROMATOSIS

Synovial chondromatosis is a synovial metaplastic disorder in which cartilaginous nodules form within a joint. The cause is unknown. The cartilaginous nodules may grow and become loose or reattach to the synovium. Additionally, the nodules may undergo enchondral ossification *(synovial osteochondromatosis)*. Although synovial chondromatosis is not an inflammatory condition, the bodies can cause cartilage destruction when trapped between articular surfaces. Mechanical erosions and eventually secondary osteoarthritis (OA) may ensue. Synovial chondromatosis is seen more frequently in males than females and generally in the third through fifth decades of life, although it can be seen in children or older adults as well.

Key Concepts	Synovial Chondromatosis

Metaplasia of synovium into multiple small round or multifaceted cartilage intra-articular bodies
Bodies tend to be of uniform size within a joint
May undergo enchondral ossification to synovial osteochondromatosis
Usually monoarticular
Most frequent sites: Knee, hip, elbow, shoulder
Secondary osteoarthritis (OA) due to mechanical damage to joint
Radiography, CT: Often diagnostic if bodies are adequately mineralized; MRI for problem cases

Radiographically, the process is most frequently seen as an effusion with *multiple round bodies of similar size and variable mineralization.* The bodies are round or multifaceted, and occasionally appear lamellated (calcified cartilage variant) or contain trabeculae (osseous bodies). Although the individual body size may range from 1 mm to 2 cm, most are often only a few millimeters and are uniform in size (Fig. 23-1). Synovial chondromatosis occurs most frequently in the knee but is also seen in the hip, shoulder, and elbow. It is usually, although not invariably, monoarticular.

Magnetic resonance imaging (MRI) is usually not required to make the diagnosis. However, on MRI one sees the effusion conforming to a distended joint capsule and multiple round or multifaceted bodies, which follow the signal of bone or cartilage on all sequences (Fig. 23-2). Magnetic resonance imaging is especially helpful in unusual presentations of synovial chondromatosis, especially when synovial chondromatosis is not detected radiographically because of a lack of mineralization of the bodies. An even more confusing picture might be that of erosive change due to synovial chondromatosis with unmineralized bodies. In either of these cases, MRI clarifies the diagnosis.

The main differential diagnostic consideration is primary or secondary OA with intra-articular bodies, osteochondritis dissecans, avascular necrosis (AVN), chronic joint infection by low-virulence organisms such as *Mycobacterium tuberculosis,* and trauma. Cartilaginous and osteochondral fragments sloughed off by these processes are usually of varied sizes, and often few in number, in contrast with the relatively uniform body size in synovial chondromatosis. If the bodies are not calcified, the differential diagnosis becomes broader and includes mass-like synovial conditions such as pigmented villonodular synovitis, amyloid lipoma arborescens (discussed in Chapter 34), and synovial neoplasms (see Chapter 36). Magnetic resonance imaging is helpful in distinguishing these possibilities.

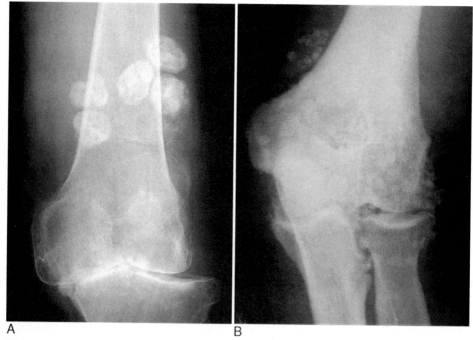

Figure 23-1   Calcified intra-articular bodies. **A,** AP radiograph of the knee in a 66-year-old an shows multiple large round ossified bodies in the suprapatellar bursa. They are all of similar size and density. The bodies in this case are likely related to osteoarthritis. **B,** AP radiograph of the elbow in a 55-year-old man shows many more bodies, all within the joint, and all much smaller. The most common appearance of synovial chondromatosis is multiple cartilage bodies of uniform size (whether large or small).

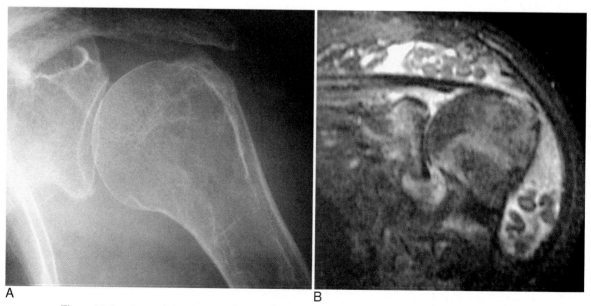

Figure 23-2   Synovial chondromatosis, noncalcified bodies. **A,** AP radiograph of the shoulder in a 54-year-old woman that demonstrates osteopenia but no ossified bodies. The patient had a soft tissue mass. **B,** Oblique coronal T2-weighted MR image shows multiple round intermediate- to low-signal-intensity cartilage bodies located in both the glenohumeral joint and the subacromial-subdeltoid bursa.

OSTEOCHONDROSES

The osteochondroses represent an artificial grouping of benign disease processes, all once believed to be initiated by AVN. Current understanding is that while many are associated with osteonecrosis, most are traumatically induced, and only a few truly are initiated by osteonecrosis. Some are normal variants that are grouped with the pathologic osteochondroses only by tradition and because they carry eponyms that suggest they are pathologic.

The osteochondroses arise in skeletally immature patients or young adults. With the exception of Freiberg's necrosis (discussed in Chapter 22), males are affected more frequently than females. The traumatically induced osteochondroses often show bony fragments within a lucent bed, sometimes with flattening of a convex surface. The overlying cartilage is often intact.

Osgood-Schlatter disease and *Sinding-Larsen-Johansson* disease are painful fragmentation and swelling of the tibial tubercle and lower pole of the patella, respectively. Typical age range is 10 to 15 years. These conditions were discussed in Chapter 12.

Blount disease is considered by some to be an osteochondrosis of the medial aspect of the proximal tibial metaphysis and by others to be a physeal injury with secondary deformity. The first theory seems more likely. Diminished growth or occasionally fragmentation at this site results in a genu varum (bow leg) deformity (Fig. 23-3). This altered anatomy increases the compressive force across the medial knee, exacerbating the growth disturbance in the medial tibial metaphysis and potentially injuring the medial physis as well. Two major forms are recognized. *Infantile tibia vara* is most common, occurs in toddlers, is more common among black children,

and is often bilateral and painless. It evolves when the normal physiologic bowing of the lower extremity worsens with weight bearing, especially in children who walk at an early age. This is not felt to be a true necrosis but a result of persistent microtrauma of weight bearing and abnormal pressure resulting in fragmentation of the medial metaphysis. *Adolescent tibia vara* disease is unilateral and painful, tends to have milder deformity than the infantile form, and relates directly to either trauma or infection causing bony bridging of the medial growth plate.

Scheuermann's disease is painful adolescent kyphosis and may be classified as an osteochondrosis of the spine, specifically the endplate. This condition is discussed in Chapter 43 (see Fig. 43-12).

Several normal variants show fragmented ossification centers in the skeletally immature patient and may simulate osteochondroses. The most frequently seen is that in the femoral condyles, previously discussed in Chapter 12. Another location that may show a dense and fragmented apophysis is the calcaneus. This appearance has been termed *Sever's disease,* but this represents a normal variant, hence the newer term *Sever's phenomenon.* Similarly, the humeral trochlea and lateral epicondyle, as well as the anterior tibial apophysis and tarsal navicular, may ossify in a fragmented fashion. The tarsal navicular should be termed *Köhler's disease* only when fragmentation occurs in a previously seen normal tarsal navicular in a patient who reports pain at that site. Similarly, irregularity can be found at the ischiopubic synchondrosis in the skeletally immature patient, termed *Van Neck's phenomenon.*

Kienböck's disease (lunate) and *Freiberg's disease* (metatarsal heads) are thought to be due to AVN and were discussed in Chapter 22. *Osteochondritis dissecans* (OCD) was discussed in Chapter 3. Briefly, OCD is a subchondral fracture probably

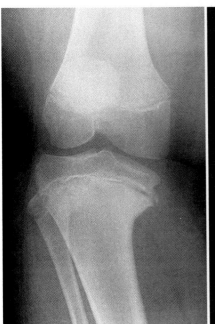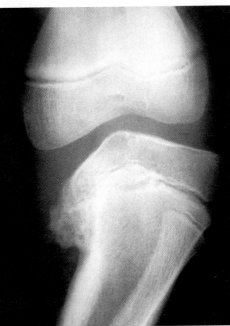

A   B

Figure 23-3   Blount's disease. **A,** Note the depression of the medial tibial metaphysis causing varus alignment, with relative preservation of the physis and epiphysis. **B,** More advanced example in a 14-year-old male shows more severe irregularity of the metaphysis and epiphysis. The physis is narrowed. (Part B reprinted with permission from the American College of Radiology learning file.)

due to chronic shear stress that may become loose in situ or displace into the joint. The knee is the most frequent site, especially the lateral aspect of the medial femoral condyle. *Panner's disease* is fragmentation of the humeral capitellum, and is a type of OCD. This condition was discussed in Chapters 3 and 6.

HYPERTROPHIC OSTEOARTHROPATHY

Hypertrophic osteoarthropathy is a disease process of unknown cause that presents clinically as arthralgia with painful, swollen joints. Radiographically, the joints appear normal, with possible swelling and effusions but no erosive or productive changes. The major abnormality is found on the "corner" of a joint radiograph, where symmetric diaphyseal and metaphyseal periosteal new bone formation is seen. The periosteal new bone may show onion skinning, irregularity, or waviness, and its thickness and extent probably depend on the duration of the disease. (Patterns of periosteal new bone formation are discussed in detail in Chapter 29.)

Hypertrophic osteoarthropathy may be primary or secondary. The primary form is also termed *pachydermoperiostitis,* which is a spectrum of diseases ranging from mere periostitis (periosteal new bone formation) to the complete process of periostitis, clubbed digits, and thickening of the skin, particularly at the forehead and dorsum of the hands (Fig. 23-4).

Primary HOA is often familial and is much more common in males than females. It develops during adolescence, and the process usually spontaneously arrests in young adulthood.

Key Concepts	Hypertrophic Osteoarthropathy (HOA)

Presents clinically as arthralgia
Radiographically normal joints
Bilaterally symmetric thick periosteal metaphyseal and diaphyseal new bone
Primary or secondary
Search for associated condition: lung cancer, chronic chest and gastrointestinal conditions

Secondary HOA is a painful periostitis in the extremities associated with several disease processes, especially bronchogenic carcinoma. It can also occur with other malignant, benign, or chronic suppurative diseases of the lung, cyanotic heart disease, or chronic gastrointestinal processes such as biliary cirrhosis or inflammatory bowel disease. The mechanism of the reaction is unknown. A humoral or neurologic mediator is hypothesized. Interestingly, a thoracotomy may lead to clinical remission almost immediately, with slower radiographic

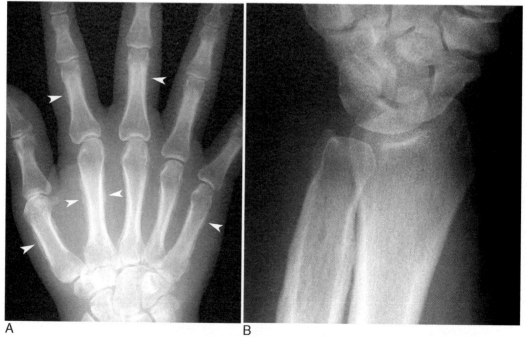

Figure 23-4   Pachydermoperiostosis (primary hypertrophic osteoarthropathy). **A,** PA radiograph of the hand in this 26-year-old man demonstrates thick periosteal reaction along the proximal phalanges as well as metacarpals *(arrowheads).* The radiograph alone does not make the diagnosis of pachydermoperiostosis but is diagnostic when occurring in combination with the thickening of the skin over the hands and forehead seen clinically. **B,** Distal forearm in a different patient also shows thick, solid periosteal new bone.

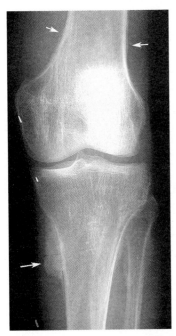

Figure 23-5   Secondary hypertrophic osteoarthropathy. AP radiograph of the knee in this 73-year-old man with bronchogenic carcinoma demonstrates solid, undulating metaphyseal and diaphyseal periosteal new bone in the distal femur and more extensively in the proximal tibia *(arrows).*

ACROMEGALY

Acromegaly results from an excess of growth hormone. In the skeletally immature patient, excess growth hormone produces a proportional increase in size of the bones, leading to gigantism. In the skeletally mature patient, the bones cannot lengthen, but respond to growth hormone by tubular bone widening and acral growth.

In the adult, radiographic abnormalities include soft tissue thickening, especially over the phalanges and in the heel pad. The skull may show an enlarged sella due to the pituitary adenoma. The facial bones and mandible become quite prominent, as does the occipital protuberance. The paranasal sinuses may be enlarged and excessively pneumatized. The spine demonstrates an increased vertebral body and disk height and posterior vertebral body scalloping. There may be an exaggerated thoracic kyphosis.

In the appendicular skeleton, hand and foot changes predominate over those in the more proximal bones. The phalanges and metacarpals may be wide, with spade-like distal phalangeal tufts (Fig. 23-6). Excrescences at the tendon attachments along the phalanges may be prominent. The hyaline cartilage increases in width. Beak-like osteophytes may eventually develop into secondary degenerative joint disease. Throughout the skeleton, there may be bony proliferation at the entheses.

resolution. It is critical to consider secondary HOA when diffuse extremity periostitis is observed, and to seek an underlying disease process, starting with a chest radiograph (Fig. 23-5).

The differential diagnosis of the periostitis seen in HOA includes *thyroid acropachy,* which can occur after surgical resection of the gland for hyperthyroidism. The character of periostitis in thyroid acropachy is said to be more feathery and spiculated and predominately located on the hands and feet. Periosteal reaction in the lower limbs can also be seen in patients with vascular insufficiency.

LEAD ARTHROPATHY

Lead bullets lodged in bursae and joint spaces can result in lead poisoning due to dissolution of the lead by synovial fluid. With progressive degradation, the fragments are spread throughout the joint, lining the synovium and cartilage (see Fig. 13-27B). Synovial inflammation and foreign body mechanical damage to cartilage lead to productive change and secondary OA. Clinical lead poisoning requires sufficient breakdown of fragments to produce a large surface area of lead and is more likely from an inflamed joint or bursa. Lead bullets in extra-articular soft tissues dissolve much more slowly and are not associated with lead intoxication.

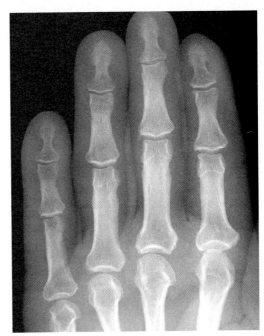

Figure 23-6   Acromegaly. This PA radiograph demonstrates widening of the cartilage spaces, overgrowth of the soft tissues, and overgrowth of the tufts of the distal phalanges, all typical of acromegaly. (Reprinted with permission of the American College of Radiology learning file.)

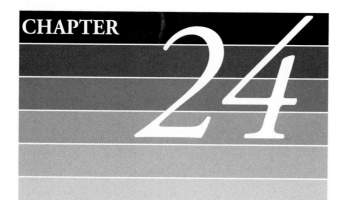

CHAPTER 24

Joint Arthroplasty

Joint arthroplasties are common today, especially in the hip and knee. Imaging analysis of arthroplasties includes evaluation for anatomic placement, fracture and dislocation, loosening of the prosthesis, mechanical wear, granulomatous reaction to worn microscopic particles, and infection. This section will concentrate on total hip arthroplasties for two reasons: First, it is the most frequent arthroplasty encountered, and second, the principles of evaluation of the total hip arthroplasty are generalizable to other protheses.

Key Concepts	Component Loosening: Radiographic Findings

Change in component alignment
>2-mm lucency at cement-bone or prosthesis-bone interface
Scalloped contour of lucency around component
Component, bone, or cement fracture

Total arthroplasty refers to resurfacing both sides of a joint. *Hemiarthroplasty* is replacement of only one side. In the hip, hemiarthroplasty is often performed for treatment of a hip fracture that is at risk for avascular necrosis (AVN) or nonunion. This is a comparatively quick and easy procedure, allowing the patient to return to weight bearing relatively quickly compared with total arthroplasty. Total arthroplasty is used most often for management of osteoarthritis (OA), and the specific indication is refractory pain. Most hip arthroplasties consist of metal alloy femoral and acetabular components lined with polyethylene plastic. The femoral component is composed of a stem that is inserted into the femoral shaft, a neck, and a round head that is smaller than the native femoral head. The components may be fixed with methylmethacrylate, screws, or press fit after careful reaming of the native bone for a tight fit. Press fit ("noncemented") components have a porous surface to allow ingrowth of bone for better biological

fixation, and are often coated with materials that stimulate bony ingrowth. Often, the ingrowth tissue is fibrous rather than bone, but this seems to provide good fixation. In addition to metal-on-polyethylene, metal-on-metal and ceramic protheses are available. These have the advantage of producing fewer microscopic particles as they wear, which reduces the rate of failure due to loosening or particle disease. This is discussed later in the chapter.

Failure of a total hip arthroplasty frequently relates to improper positioning of the components. In the total hip, the acetabular and femoral components should be placed in the expected anatomic site of each. The following parameters should be assessed:

1. The alignment of the acetabular component in the coronal plane is important. The lateral opening of the acetabulum (horizontal version) is measured as the angle of opening relative to the transischial line (a line drawn between the two ischial tuberosities, used throughout this section as a convenient landmark for measurement). The lateral opening angle of the acetabular component normally measures 40 ± 10 degrees (Fig. 24-1). An increased lateral opening angle puts the patient at risk for dislocation. A decreased lateral opening angle limits abduction and may result in anterior dislocation when the hip is placed in forced abduction.

2. The angle of the acetabulum in the axial plane is also important. As seen on a groin lateral film or on an axial computed tomography (CT), the acetabulum should be anteverted (oriented anteriorly) 10 to 15 degrees. Zero-degree anteversion may be acceptable if there is anteversion at the femoral neck-shaft angle, but retroversion of the acetabular component is never acceptable and predisposes to posterior dislocation. It is important to note that on an anteroposterior (AP) radiograph, one can see that the acetabular component is angled, but one cannot determine whether the angulation is anteversion or retroversion without the added information from the groin lateral film (Fig. 24-2) or axial CT.

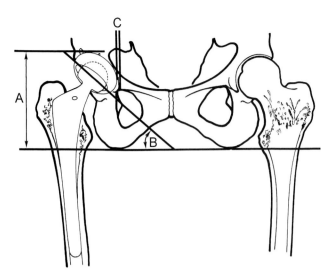

Figure 24-1 Evaluation of total hip arthroplasty. The reference line for most of what should be evaluated in a total hip arthroplasty is the transischial line. The distance labeled A is used to evaluate effective limb length; another way to evaluate this would be to compare the levels of the lesser trochanters with one another. B indicates the opening angle (lateral inclination) of the acetabular cup. The measurements between the lines indicated by C is used to evaluate for either excessive or lack of medialization of the cup.

3. Medial-lateral positioning of the acetabular component is also important. The acetabular component should be placed such that the horizontal center of rotation of the femoral head component is similar to that of the normal femoral head (see Fig. 24-1). If the acetabular component is too medial in position, there may be excessive thinning of the wall and risk of failure. If the acetabular component is placed too far laterally, the iliopsoas tendon will cross medially to the femoral head center of rotation and muscle contraction will tend to force the head from the socket, increasing the probability of dislocation.

4. Equal limb length must be maintained. This can be evaluated by choosing a femoral landmark, such as the greater or lesser trochanter, and comparing it with the opposite side relative to the transischial line (Fig. 24-1, 24-3). Limb length can be affected by placement of the acetabular component, placement of the femoral component, length and size of the femoral neck and head, and thickness of the polyethylene liner. If the hip ends up too short, contracting muscles will be ineffective and the hip subject to dislocation. If the hip is placed such that there is overlengthening of the limb, the

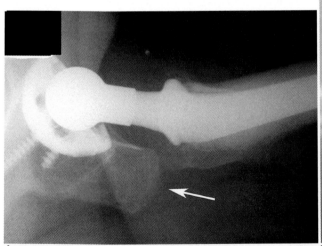

A

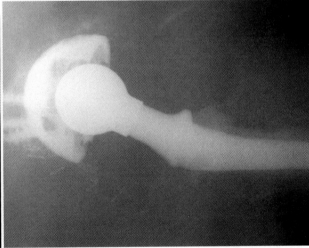

B

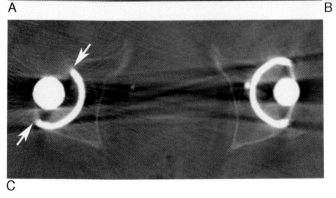

C

Figure 24-2 Anteversion of the acetabular component. **A,** Groin lateral view shows the ischium *(arrow)* that is a posterior structure and therefore showing anteversion (anterior angulation) of both the acetabular component and the femoral neck. **B,** Groin lateral film taken in a patient who chronically dislocates her hip. The reason for the dislocation is shown, with the retroverted acetabular component. **C,** Axial CT image in a different patient shows excessive anteversion of the right acetabular component *(arrows)* and neutral alignment (inadequate anteversion) of the left acetabular component. The white disks in the center of each acetabular component are the prosthetic femoral heads.

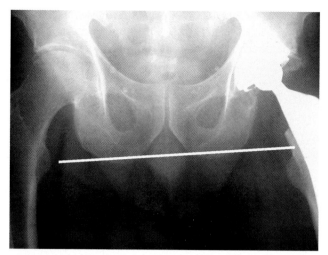

Figure 24-3   Abnormal limb length. The transischial line is used for evaluation of effective limb length. Note that the patient's normal right hip shows the lesser trochanter to be at the level of the transischial line, whereas the total hip replacement results in extension of the lesser trochanter beyond the line. In this case, the total hip results in an effective overlengthening of the left leg.

neurovascular bundle will be stretched and the muscles likely to spasm, again subjecting the hip to dislocation.

5. The femoral component should be placed in a neutral to slight valgus position (with the prosthesis resting against the lateral cortex proximally and against the medial cortex distally). A varus position predisposes the femoral component to loosening.

6. Inappropriate sizing of implant components may result in failure of the arthroplasty. The acetabular cups are sized for complete osseous coverage. Uncemented stems are chosen for optimal proximal fit rather than distal canal fit, with the goal of providing maximal surface contact to promote bone ingrowth and to prevent *subsidence* (inferior movement of the implant into the femoral shaft) of the prosthesis.

In evaluating follow-up films of prostheses, it is crucial to have a comparison film taken at or around the time of placement of the prosthesis. Comparison with this index film may reveal subtle changes in position of a component, which may not be seen with the most recent comparison film (Fig. 24-4). *Loosening* can definitely be diagnosed when there is migration of a component (generally superiorly and medially with an acetabular component, inferiorly with a femoral component), or a change in alignment of a component with the adjacent bone. Therefore, at follow-up, specific evaluation of limb length, lateral opening angle of the acetabulum, and positioning of the components relative to their position at the time of initial placement must be made. If there is no definite change in position or alignment, loosening may still be identified. In a cemented prosthesis, one may expect to see thin (1- to 2-mm) radiolucent zone at portions of the cement-bone interface. This radiolucent zone is considered normal if it is less than 2 mm wide, is not continuous around the component, and does not widen over time. These lucencies are particularly common around the superolateral portion of the acetabular component and tip of the femoral stem. If, however, a portion of the radiolucent zone measures greater than 2 mm, or

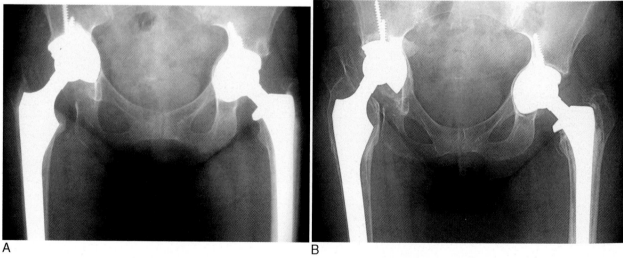

A   B

Figure 24-4   Failed total hip arthroplasty. **A,** Baseline examination shows cementless right total hip arthroplasty and hybrid left total hip arthroplasty, with the components appropriately aligned and showing no evidence of loosening. **B,** Four years later there has been a significant change, with loosening of all the components. The right acetabular component has tilted and is superiorly subsided. The right femoral component shows a lucency surrounding it at the bone component interface with subsidence of the component by approximately 2 cm. The left acetabular component shows a 2-mm lucency surrounding it, with slight tilt, indicating loosening. The left femoral component shows a 2- to 3-mm lucency surrounding the cement-bone interface. This is loose as well. Finally, both acetabular components show superior migration of the femoral heads relative to the acetabular components, indicating polyethylene wear.

shows progressive widening, the component is considered loose. A final finding of loosening of a cemented component is fracture of the cement (Fig. 24-5) or a component (Fig. 24-6).

As with a cemented component, the most convincing sign of loosening in a cementless component is progressive change in position, either subsidence or tilt (Fig. 24-7). However, other signs may be of value. First, it is important to note that prominent calcar resorption is common in cementless prostheses. (Recall that the calcar is the cortex of the medial femoral neck.) This resorption is due to stress shielding of the proximal femur, including the calcar, by the stiff femoral component, which transmits force from the prosthetic femoral head to the distal aspect of the stem. The bone that is not under stress is resorbed. This unfortunate consequence is one reason that *revision arthroplasty*

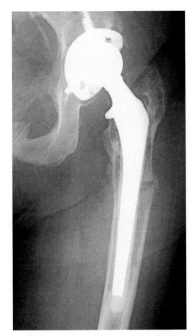

Figure 24-5   Failed cemented femoral component. AP radiograph demonstrates a wide lucency at the cement-bone interface of the femoral component, with fracture in the proximal shaft of the femur. Additionally, there is polyethylene wear, with superior migration of the femoral head within the acetabular component.

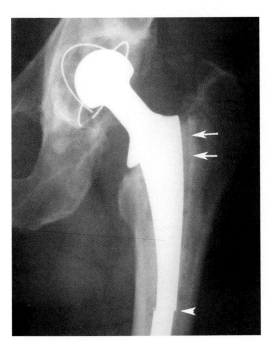

Figure 24-6   Fractured femoral component. Note the separation of the cement from the proximal femoral component *(arrows)* and fracture across the distal prosthesis *(arrowhead).*

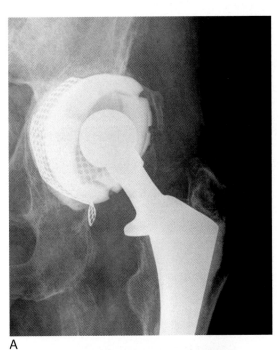

A

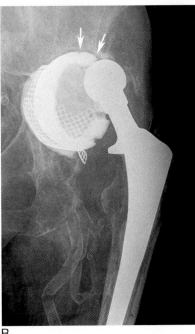

B

Figure 24-7   Failed acetabular component. **A,** Baseline AP radiograph after surgery. **B,** One year later, the acetabular component has rotated and the femoral head is subluxed superiorly. Note the increase in lucency at the superior margin *(arrows).*

(i.e., replacement of an arthroplasty with a new arthroplasty) requires a longer stem for purchase into healthy bone. Femoral components may include a "calcar shelf," which is a medial flange intended to transmit some force to the calcar to reduce bone loss due to stress shielding. However, despite this and many other design modifications, proximal femur bone loss due to stress shielding is common. Cortical thickening and endosteal sclerosis is often present around the distal stem in response to this locally elevated stress as a normal finding. A narrow radiolucent zone between the bone and prosthesis is frequently seen, often with a fine, uniform sclerotic margin. If the radiolucent zone at the bone–prosthesis interface is greater than 2 mm wide, it is likely to represent loosening. Furthermore, excessive cortical hypertrophy and endosteal bone bridging at the tip of the femoral stem, or excessive endosteal scalloping, also probably represent loosening, particularly if progression is shown (Fig. 24-8).

Besides component loosening, failure of the construct itself may constitute a complication. Fracture of the prosthesis itself is uncommon, but when present tends to be of the distal stem (see Fig. 24-6). Separation of the polyethylene insert from its backing may be heralded by the presence of small wedge-shaped metallic fragments (Fig. 24-9). Fractures and displacement of the polyethylene can occasionally be seen. Fracture of the host bone is uncommon and can occur in the pelvis as well as the femoral shaft (Fig. 24-10). In the shaft, a fracture usually begins at the tip of the prosthetic stem and progresses longitudinally and anteriorly. This fracture pattern is seen most frequently in long-stem femoral revisions, where the tip of the revision fractures the femoral cortex at its

anterior bow. These fractures are usually nondisplaced and are easily overlooked.

Polyethylene wear is theoretically a trivial problem, but in practice occurs relatively frequently. Polyethylene wear can be subtle and asymmetric, and is revealed by offset of the femoral

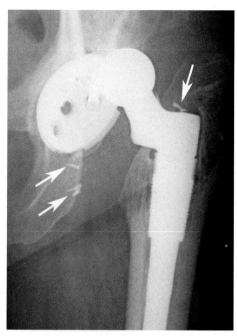

Figure 24-9   Failed total hip arthroplasty. This patient has a dislocated total hip, with multiple wedge-shaped metallic densities *(arrows)*. These spikes are used to hold the polyethylene within the metallic backing of the cup. Their presence indicates failure of the cup.

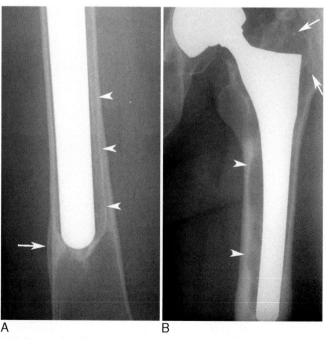

Figure 24-8   Failed cementless femoral component. **A,** AP radiograph shows a wide lucency and sclerotic line surrounding the femoral component *(arrowheads)*. Additionally, there is endosteal and periosteal new bone formation *(arrow)*. **B,** AP radiograph in a different patient shows scalloping of the endosteum *(arrowheads)* as well as bead shedding *(arrows),* indicating failure of this cementless prosthesis. It has also subsided by approximately 1 cm.

head within the acetabular cup, where the wear in the polyethylene occurs superolaterally in the weight-bearing portion (see Figs. 24-4, 24-5). Polyethylene wear itself can cause mechanical symptoms. Also, polyethylene wear is a major source of the small particles that can lead to component loosening. Small particles can initiate an immune-mediated granulomatous reaction that can result in bone lysis, in some cases very extensive (Figs. 24-11, 24-12). This osseous destruction, related to granulomatous disease, has been termed "particle disease" or "massive osteolysis," although the osteolysis is not always massive. It is often localized with scalloped margins. It is important to note that the source of the particles is not important; the particles may be polyethylene, cement, osseous debris, or even metallic microspheres. Rather than the material, the size of the particles seems to elicit the granulomatous reaction. Particles roughly this size of a red blood cell are the problem; larger particles do not initiate the granulomatous reaction.

Infection is a serious complication of total joint arthroplasty. Plain radiographic findings are usually neither helpful nor specific in identifying prosthetic infections. The radiographs may appear normal or may mimic loosening or particle disease. If infection is suspected, aspiration under strict aseptic condition, supplemented if necessary with nonbacteriostatic (preservative-free) saline injection, enables detection of most prosthetic infections. Radionuclide imaging for detection of infection or loosening can be problematic as tracer uptake is a normal postoperative finding and expected for at least 1 year after surgery, with different uptake patterns observed for cemented and noncemented prostheses.

Many of the generalizations discussed previously for total hip arthroplasty also apply to total knee arthroplasties. The tibial component should be placed 90 ± 5 degrees to the long axis of the tibial shaft on the AP radiograph and ranges from 90 degrees to the long axis of the tibia to a slight posterior tilt on the lateral radiograph. The femoral component is placed in 5 ± 5 degrees to the long axis of the femoral shaft on the lateral, with 4 to 7 degrees of valgus angulation as seen on the AP radiograph. Of all the components, the tibial is most likely to loosen. Early loosening is usually followed by tilting of the tibial component into a varus position with subsidence into the medial tibial plateau and collapse of the cancellous bone. Polyethylene wear, fragmentation, and dislocation may follow (Figs. 24-12, 24-13). Patellar complications occur frequently, including subsidence, polyethylene wear, polyethylene dissociation from the metal backing, disintegration of the metal backing with metallosis (metal particles lining the polyethylene and capsule) (Fig. 24-14), and patellar AVN or fracture. An additional abnormality to watch for in follow-up of knee prostheses is a periprosthetic fracture. Patients who are osteoporotic with knee prostheses (e.g., patients with rheumatoid arthritis [RA]) are particularly prone to developing fractures in the metaphyseal region of either the distal femur or proximal tibia. Fracture may be seen as a minor change in contour or a sclerotic line of fracture healing (Fig. 24-15). If a patient has had a previous tibial tubercle transfer, proximal tibial fracture is even more likely following placement of a total knee arthroplasty.

Resurfacing of other joints is less common because of lower frequency of disabling arthritis and difficulty in producing a functional, durable arthroplasty. Shoulder arthroplasty is often achieved by hemiarthroplasty with replacement of the humeral head. The prosthetic head is normally high riding and abuts the glenoid and undersurface of the acromion. Total shoulder arthroplasty seems to come in and out of favor. A major difficulty is successful resurfacing of the small glenoid, but the procedure has the potential to provide better function and pain relief than a hemiarthroplasty

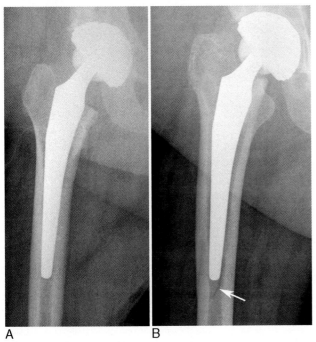

Figure 24-10 Fracture. **A,** Postoperative baseline radiograph. **B,** Several months later, the patient developed acute pain. AP radiograph shows a femur fracture *(arrow)* with subsidence of the femoral component.

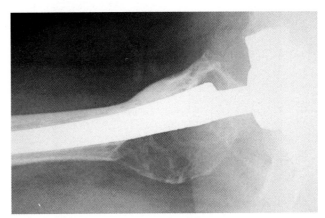

Figure 24-11 Particle disease. Frog-leg lateral radiograph demonstrates an expanded lytic lesion in the proximal femoral metaphysis. This osteolysis most frequently is related to particle disease.

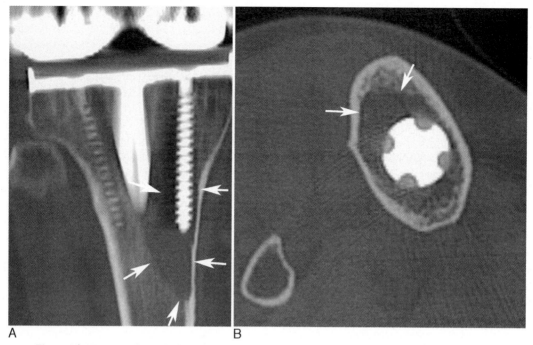

A   B

Figure 24-12   CT of particle disease. **A,** Coronal CT reconstruction of the proximal tibia in a patient with a total knee arthroplasty shows well-circumscribed lysis around a tibial fixation screw. **B,** Axial CT image through the proximal leg in a different patient with a knee arthroplasty shows subtle bone lysis anterior to the cemented tibial stem component *(arrows)*.

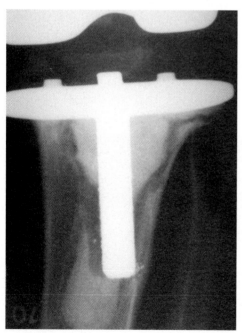

Figure 24-13   Tibial component loosening. AP radiograph demonstrates gross tibial component loosening, with medial tilt of the component, fracture of the cement, and bead shedding.

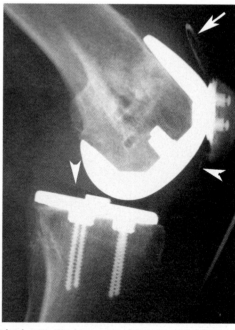

Figure 24-14   Patellar component failure. Lateral radiograph demonstrates superior subsidence of the patellar component. It also shows dissociation of some of the metal backing, with displacement into the suprapatellar bursa *(arrow)*. Finally, the patient is developing metallosis in the joint, with metallic fragments lining the polyethylene and joint capsule *(arrowheads)*.

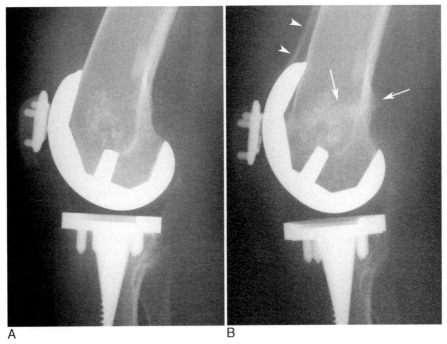

A   B

Figure 24-15   Periprosthetic fracture. **A,** Lateral radiograph of the knee arthroplasty at the time of placement. **B,** The same knee several months later. The patient has developed a fracture in the distal femoral metaphysis *(arrow),* angulation at the fracture site, and healing reaction seen at the anterior femoral cortex *(arrowheads).*

(Fig. 24-16). Ankle arthroplasty also is occasionally performed (Fig. 24-17). The medial or lateral compartment of the knee also may be selectively resurfaced (Fig. 24-18). The same principles of follow-up evaluation as for total knee and hip arthroplasties apply to other joints.

Silastic arthroplasties are radiolucent, flexible silicon rubber implants that are used for replacement of small joints made painful and dysfunctional by long-standing arthritis, usually RA. These implants are most commonly seen at the wrist, MCP, and MTP joints. If the arthroplasty is of the Swanson variety,

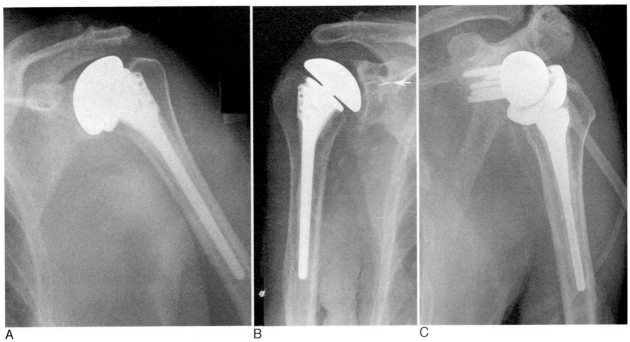

A   B   C

Figure 24-16   Shoulder arthroplasty. **A,** Hemiarthroplasty. **B,** Total arthroplasty. Note the metal marker *(arrow)* in the cemented polyethylene glenoid component. **C,** Total arthroplasty. This system reverses the normal anatomy by placing the ball component in the glenoid and the cup component in the humerus.

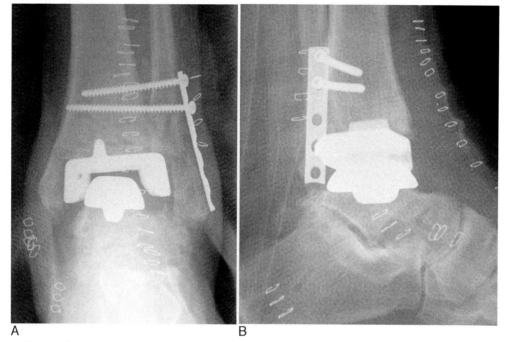

A   B

Figure 24-17   Ankle arthroplasty. **A,** AP radiograph. **B,** Lateral radiograph.

it is most at risk for fracture at the thinnest part, that which acts as the "hinge" at the junction of the flange and the body. In addition, dislocation of the flange may occur, especially in diseases such as RA that have soft tissue imbalance or contractures. Finally, as these prostheses are usually not cemented, repetitive motion results in particle breakdown; in addition,

particle disease with prominent osteolysis can develop (Fig. 24-19). The same process can be seen with silastic carpal implants (Fig. 24-20).

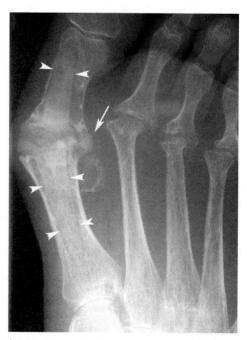

Figure 24-19   Silastic (flexible plastic) prosthesis with particle disease. Silastic implants work best in small joints with low loads, and are most often used in late-stage rheumatoid arthritis. AP radiograph of the great toe demonstrates first metatarsophalangeal Swanson silastic prosthesis *(arrowheads)* in a patient with late-stage rheumatoid arthritis. The prosthesis has failed, with fracture of the lateral body *(arrow)* and osteolysis around the prosthesis.

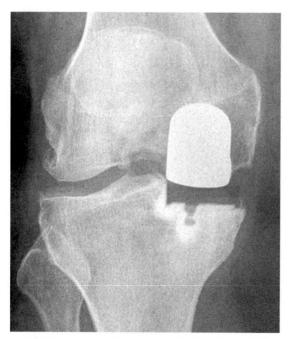

Figure 24-18   Knee partial arthroplasty. Both surfaces of the medial compartment have been replaced.

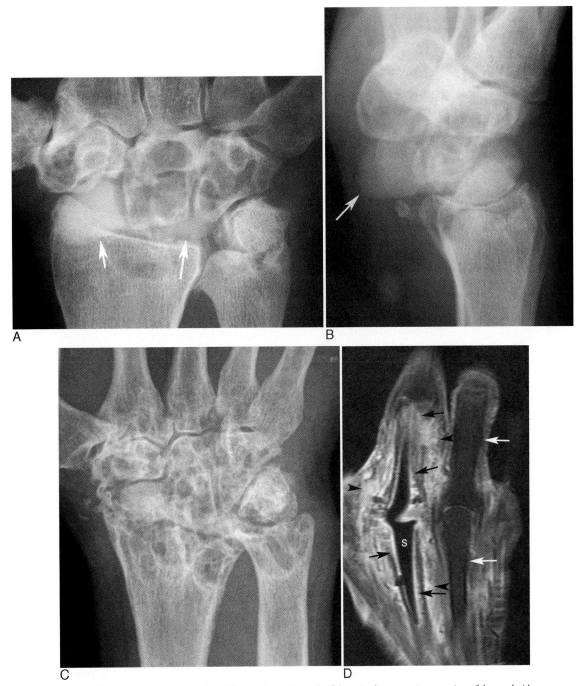

Figure 24-20   Silastic carpal implant failure. **A,** PA radiograph of the wrist demonstrating resection of the scaphoid and lunate and replacement by silastic prostheses *(arrows)*. There is significant particle disease, with large cysts seen in the trapezium, capitate, and hamate. **B,** Lateral view shows palmar dislocation of one of the carpal prostheses *(arrow)*. **C,** PA radiograph in a different patient with a silastic carpal implant shows extensive cyst-like lysis in the carpal bones. **D,** Coronal-contrast-enhanced, fat-suppressed, T1-weighted MR image shows low signal intensity silastic implant(s) in the third finger across the MCP joint, with intense surrounding intraosseous *(back arrows)* and extraosseous *(arrowheads)* enhancement due to granulomatous reaction to the silastic. Contrast with the normal adjacent fourth metacarpal and proximal phalanx *(white arrows)*.

Part IV Sources and Suggested Readings

Basset L, Blocka K, Furst D, et al: Skeletal findings in progressive systemic sclerosis (scleroderma). AJR 136:1121–1126, 1981.

Bjorkengren A, Weisman M, Pathria M, et al: Neuroarthropathy associated with chronic alcoholism. AJR 151:743–745, 1981.

Bock G, Garcia A, Weisman M, et al: Rapidly destructive hip disease: Clinical and imaging abnormalities. Radiology 186:461–466, 1993.

Bollow M, Braun J, Hamm B, et al: Early sacroiliitis in patients with spondyloarthropathy: Evaluation with dynamic gadolinium enhanced MR imaging. Radiology 194:529–536, 1995.

Brower A, Allman R: Pathogenesis of the neurotrophic joint: Neurotraumatic versus neurovascular. Radiology 139:349–354, 1981.

Cobby M, Adler R, Swartz R, Martel W: Dialysis related amyloid arthropathy: MR findings in four patients. AJR 157:1023–1027, 1991.

Glickstein M, Burk D, Schiebler M, et al: Avascular necrosis versus other diseases of the hip: Sensitivity of MR imaging. Radiology 169:213–215, 1988.

Hermann KA, Althoff CE, Schneider U, et al: Spinal changes in patients with spondyloarthritis: Comparison of MR imaging and radiographic appearances. Radiographics 25:559–570, 2005.

Kaplan P, Montesi S, Jardon O, Gregory P: Bone in-growth hip prostheses in asymptomatic patients: Radiographic features. Radiology 169:221–227, 1988.

Kiss E, Keusch G, Zanetti M, et al: Dialysis-related amyloidosis revisited. AJR 185:1460–1467, 2005.

Kopecky K, Braunstein E, Brandt K, et al: Apparent avascular necrosis of the hip: Appearance and spontaneous resolution of MR findings of renal allograft recipients. Radiology 179:523–527, 1991.

Link T, Steinbach L, Ghosh S, et al: Osteoarthritis: MR imaging findings in different stages of disease and correlation with clinical findings. Radiology 226:373–381, 2003.

Manaster B: Total hip arthroplasty: Radiographic evaluation. Radiographics 16:645–660, 1996.

Manaster B: Total knee arthroplasty: Post-operative radiographic findings. AJR 165:899–904, 1995.

Murphey M, Wetzel L, Bramble J, et al: Sacroiliitis: MR imaging findings. Radiology 180:239–244, 1991.

Rafto S, Dalinka M, Scheibler M, et al: Spondyloarthropathy of the cervical spine and long term hemodialysis. Radiology 166:201-204, 1988.

Resnick D (ed): Diagnosis of Bone and Joint Disorders, ed 4. Philadelphia: W.B. Saunders, 2002.

Sommer OJ, Kladosek A, Weiler V, et al: Rheumatoid arthritis: A practical guide to state-of-the-art imaging, image interpretation, and clinical implications. Radiographics 25:381–398, 2005.

Steinbach L, Resnick D: Calcium pyrophosphate dihydrate crystal deposition disease revisited. Radiology 200:1–9, 1996.

Tervonen O, Mueller D, Matteson E, et al: Clinically occult avascular necrosis of the hip: Prevalence in an asymptomatic population at risk. Radiology 182:845–847, 1992.

Wagner S, Schweitzer M, Morrison W, et al: Can imaging findings help differentiate spinal neuropathic arthropathy from disk space infection? Initial experience. Radiology 214:693–699, 2000.

Weissman B, Rappaport A, Sosman J, et al: Radiographic findings in the hands in patients with systemic lupus erythematosus. Radiology 126:313–317, 1978.

Yang B, Sartoris D, Djukic S, et al: Distribution of calcification in the triangular fibrocartilage region in 181 patients with calcium pyrophosphate dihydrate crystal deposition disease. Radiology 196:547–550, 1995.

Yu J, Chung C, Recht M, et al: MR imaging of tophaceous gout. AJR 168:523–527, 1997.

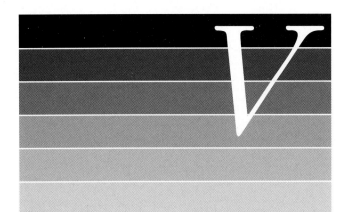

METABOLIC BONE DISEASE

CHAPTER 25

Disorders of Calcium Homeostasis

HYPERPARATHYROIDISM
OSTEOMALACIA
RICKETS
RENAL OSTEODYSTROPHY

Bone is mostly mineral (calcium hydroxyapatite) deposited on a matrix (osteoid) composed primarily of collagen. Both the mineral and collagenous components must be normal and present in normal amounts for normal bone strength. Metabolic, hormonal, or genetic conditions can alter the composition or quantity of the matrix or the calcium hydroxyapatite, resulting in bones that are weak, deformed, or demineralized, often in a characteristic pattern. This chapter and Chapter 26 review metabolic bone diseases. Osteoporosis and Paget's disease have some features in common with metabolic conditions and are discussed in subsequent chapters.

Understanding the means by which the body maintains calcium and phosphate homeostasis is key to understanding the metabolic bone diseases of the musculoskeletal system. Calcium-phosphate balance and sodium-phosphate balance are critical in cellular electrolyte equilibrium and maintenance of numerous energy-dependent cellular transactions, not the least of which is the integrity of adenosine triphosphate (ATP) production. Not only is bone important structurally, but it provides a large reserve for calcium and phosphate. Serum calcium and phosphate levels are constant. Normal levels are maintained by gut absorption of electrolytes, use of mobile bone reserves, and kidney tubular action. The hormones responsible for interacting with these targets are parathyroid hormone, vitamin D, and calcitonin. *Parathyroid hormone* is produced by the four parathyroid glands. Low serum levels of calcium induce the glands to produce the hormone. Parathyroid hormone acts on several sites to increase calcium levels in the serum. For example, in the kidney, the hormone acts on the proximal tubules to enhance phosphate excretion and calcium reabsorption through calcium-phosphate pumps. At the bone surface, parathyroid hormone stimulates osteoclast-mediated bone resorption, which results in hydroxyap-

Key Concepts	Calcium Homeostasis

Parathyroid hormone and vitamin D are the two main regulators of calcium and phosphate homeostasis.
Parathyroid hormone acts on bone and kidney to increase serum calcium while maintaining phosphate levels constant.
Vitamin D depends on dietary intake and normal function in small bowel, liver, and kidney.
Vitamin D acts on bone and gut to calibrate serum calcium and phosphate levels. Phosphate balance is the target.

atite dissolution and thus increases calcium and phosphate levels in the blood. The net effect from action of the hormone in bone and kidney is increased calcium and stable phosphate levels. Finally, parathyroid hormone acts in the kidney as a cofactor to enhance the synthesis of 1,25-hydroxy-vitamin D and in the action of vitamin D in bone and gut, thus indirectly increasing calcium levels through vitamin D action.

The endogenous form of *vitamin D* (vitamin D_3) is derived from cholesterol and is synthesized in the skin after exposure to ultraviolet light. Most vitamin D, however, comes from dietary supplementation as vitamin D_2. Exogenous forms of vitamin D are absorbed through the gut and converted in the liver to 25-hydroxy-vitamin D. However, the active form of the vitamin is produced in the kidney, where it is 1-hydroxylated. The 1,25-hydroxylated form is the active form of the hormone; it acts on bone, gut, kidney, parathyroid glands, and other tissues, including the skin. In bone, the vitamin binds with intranuclear receptors and causes transcription of osteocalcin, osteopontin, and alkaline phosphatase. This action results in mobilization of calcium and phosphorus, and also promotes maturation and mineralization of osteoid matrix. For this activity, vitamin D requires the presence of parathyroid hormone as a cofactor. In the gut, 1,25-hydroxy-vitamin D causes the production of calcium-binding protein and thus increased intestinal calcium transport, with passive absorption of phosphate. This action of vitamin D requires parathyroid hormone as a cofactor. It also acts to increase phosphate resorption in the proximal renal tubules, also requiring the presence of parathyroid hormone. The active form of vitamin D inhibits the release of parathyroid hormone from the parathyroid glands and is a cofactor of action of parathyroid hormone in bone. Thus, vitamin D acts to increase calcium and phosphate levels in the blood. Activation of vitamin D through 1-hyroxylation in the kidney is increased in the setting of hypophosphatemia and hypocalcemia. Vitamin D is self-regulated as well: renal 1-hydroxylation decreases in the setting of increased levels of 1,25-hydroxy-vitamin D.

Calcitonin is a hormone produced primarily by the parafollicular cells of the thyroid gland. While not critically important in humans, it is a physiologic antagonist to parathyroid hormone. The hormone is under the direct control of blood calcium levels such that increased blood levels of calcium results in increased levels of calcitonin. The hormone's action is to inhibit osteoclast-mediated bone resorption and to stimulate renal calcium clearance.

HYPERPARATHYROIDISM

This disease can take three forms: primary, secondary, and tertiary hyperparathyroidism. Primary hyperparathyroidism occurs in the setting of a parathyroid gland adenoma in most cases (60% to 90% of cases), although occasionally parathyroid gland hyperplasia, or, rarely, glandular adenocarcinoma, is a cause. In about 10% of cases, adenomas can be multiple. Familial forms are associated with the multiple endocrine neoplasia (MEN) syndromes, including MEN I in 95% of cases and MEN II in 33% of cases.

In primary hyperparathyroidism, serum levels of calcium are elevated whereas serum levels of phosphate are decreased. Patients usually present clinically with generalized weakness, urolithiasis, peptic ulcer disease, pancreatitis, and bone and joint pain and tenderness.

Key Concepts	**Hyperparathyroidism**

Proportion of mineralized bone to osteoid is normal (versus osteomalacia).

Primary hyperparathyroidism: Most commonly due to adenomas. Associated with the multiple endocrine neoplasias.

Secondary hyperparathyroidism: Due to renal disease that causes physiologic activation of the hormone.

Radiographs:

Demineralization at multiple sites, most classically subperiosteal demineralization radial aspects of second and third middle phalanges

Clues to primary versus secondary:

Calcium pyrophosphate deposition (CPPD), brown tumors favors primary.

Bone sclerosis, periostitis, soft tissue calcification favors secondary.

Secondary hyperparathyroidism implies elevated hormone levels due not to disease of the parathyroid glands themselves but rather to other causes, with resultant physiologic activation of the parathyroid glands to produce increased amounts of hormone. The most common cause of secondary hyperparathyroidism is renal failure. In renal failure, there is tubular dysfunction and diminished capacity to excrete phosphate. Elevated serum phosphate levels result in calcium-phosphate binding and nonmeasurable diminished serum calcium, which in turn promotes parathyroid hormone synthesis. The result is the maintenance of normal serum calcium levels at the expense of elevated parathyroid hormone levels.

Tertiary hyperparathyroidism, which occurs in situations of long-standing secondary hyperparathyroidism, refers to a condition in which the cause for secondary hyperparathyroidism has been corrected but the parathyroid glands function autonomously, producing hormone despite a lack of calcium imbalance to induce hormone synthesis.

The effect of increased parathyroid hormone levels in bone is hydroxyapatite crystal dissolution. As the hormonal effect is generalized, the bone loss is diffuse and most apparent at sites of greatest surface area. Generalized bone demineralization is therefore a uniform feature of this disease (Fig. 25-1). Bone loss in the skull can yield a "salt-and-pepper" appearance (Fig. 25-1B). In addition, bone resorption can be seen in typical sites of high bone surface area, including subperiosteal, intracortical, endosteal, trabecular, subchondral, and subligamentous locations (Figs. 25-1, 25-2). This nonpreferential loss of bone is an important feature of the disease, and can appear extremely aggressive.

Subchondral bone loss can mimic inflammatory arthropathy and is especially seen in the sacroiliac, acromioclavicular, sternoclavicular, and temporomandibular joints, and at the symphysis pubis (see Fig. 25-2). Subligamentous bone resorption is most common at the trochanters, ischial tuberosities, inferior surface of the calcaneus and distal clavicle, and elbow. Intracortical and subperiosteal changes can mimic highly aggressive neoplasia, and endosteal bone resorption can mimic endosteal erosion that is seen in marrow dyscrasias, such as multiple myeloma (Fig. 25-3). Important areas to look for bone resorption that is specific for hyperparathyroidism include the subperiosteal locations of the radial aspects of the second and third middle phalanges (Fig. 25-1C and D). Other sites of subperiosteal bone resorption include the medial aspect of the humerus, femur, and tibia (Fig. 25-1E); the superior and inferior aspects of the ribs; and the lamina dura of the teeth. Hyperparathyroidism can produce tuftal bone resorption similar in appearance to acro-osteolysis (Fig. 25-1C and D). Weakened bone due to osteopenia risks the occurrence of insufficiency fracture.

Other radiographic features of hyperparathyroidism can give clues to its diagnosis. These include soft tissue calcification, periostitis (Fig. 25-4), brown tumors (Fig. 25-5), calcium pyrophosphate dihydrate deposition (CPPD), and bone sclerosis (Fig. 25-6). Soft tissue calcification, periostitis, and osteosclerosis are more frequently seen in secondary hyperparathyroidism.

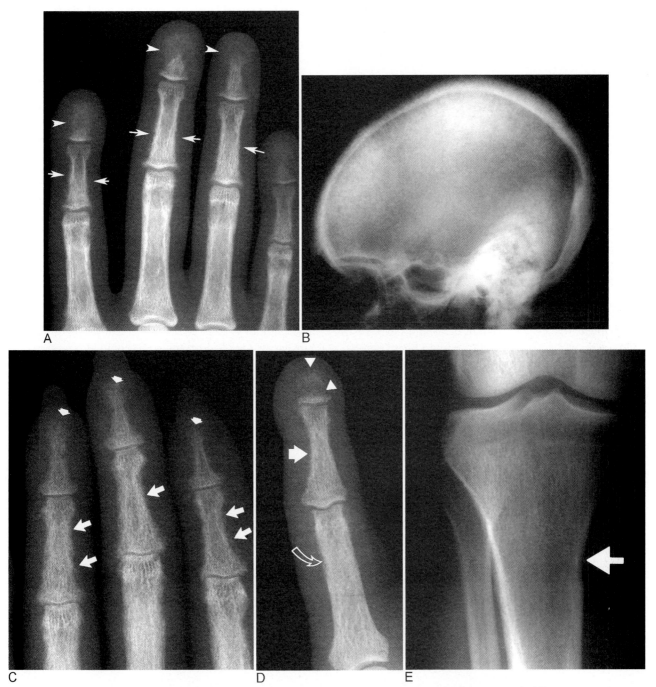

Figure 25-1   Radiographic features of hyperparathyroidism. **A,** PA radiograph of fingers reveals diffuse bone demineralization. The trabecula are fuzzy because of diffuse resorption. Note the presence of localized resorption of bone at the distal phalangeal tufts *(arrowheads)* and along the middle phalanges *(arrows).* **B,** Lateral skull radiograph shows salt-and-pepper appearance. **C,** PA radiograph of fingers demonstrating subperiosteal bone resorption in phalanges *(arrows)* and subcortical tuft resorption *(arrowheads).* **D,** PA radiograph of finger demonstrates subperiosteal bone resorption *(closed arrow)* that is greater on the radial side (left side of the image). Also note intracortical *(open arrow)* and tuftal *(arrowheads)* bone resorption. **E,** AP radiograph of proximal tibia demonstrates subperiosteal bone resorption at the medial aspect of the proximal tibial metaphysis.

(Continued)

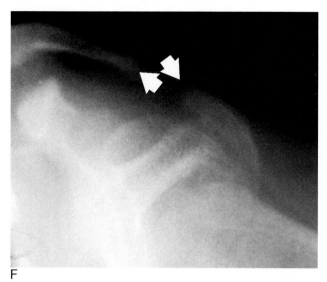

F

Figure 25-1—(Cont'd) **F,** Angled radiograph of the acromioclavicular joint shows subchondral bone resorption *(arrows)* mimicking inflammatory arthropathy.

Both CPPD and brown tumors are more frequent in primary hyperparathyroidism. The former can occur in up to 40% of patients with primary hyperparathyroidism. *Brown tumors,* which are accumulations of osteoclasts and fibrous tissue, can be multiple and tend to heal after treatment of the underlying disorder. They appear as eccentric, occasionally intracortical, lytic, and often expansive lesions that can be confused radiographically with giant cell tumor and fibrous dysplasia. Brown

tumors can also be seen in secondary hyperparathyroidism and, in fact, account for more cases of brown tumors even though their relative incidence is greater in primary hyperparathyroidism. This is because the prevalence of secondary hyperparathyroidism is far greater than that of primary hyperparathyroidism. Finally, patients with hyperparathyroidism are prone to tendon and ligament laxity and rupture (Fig. 25-7).

OSTEOMALACIA

Any pathophysiologic process that interferes with the production of vitamin D will result in osteomalacia. In the absence of vitamin D, bone mineral is not laid down, although osteoid production is normal. Understanding how the hormone is produced allows one to determine a differential of potential causes. These include lack of dietary intake and diminished gut absorption of the vitamin or of calcium, as can occur with malabsorption syndromes such as Crohn's disease or with small bowel resection. Liver (both biliary and hepatocellular) and renal diseases will also interfere with hormone production. Biliary diseases will result in problems with gut absorption of vitamin D, whereas hepatocellular disease will interfere with 25-hydroxylation of vitamin D.

With renal disease, osteomalacia also has two causes. First, renal failure can interfere with 1-hydroxylation of 25-vitamin D. Second, renal tubular disorders (vitamin D resistant rickets), such as X-linked hypophosphatemia and cystinosis, result in abnormally increased clearance of inorganic phosphorus

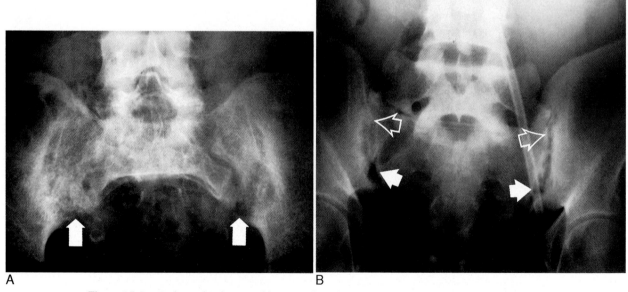

A   **B**

Figure 25-2 Radiographic features of hyperparathyroidism, pelvis. **A,** AP radiograph of sacroiliac joints shows bilateral subarticular bone resorption *(arrows)* mimicking inflammatory arthropathy. **B,** AP radiograph of sacroiliac joints shows subarticular *(closed arrows)* and subligamentous *(open arrows)* bone resorption of both sacroiliac joints. Recall that the true synovial articulation of the sacroiliac joints is located at the inferior two thirds and the anterior third of the sacroiliac interspace. The remainder of the interspace is a syndesmosis.

(Continued)

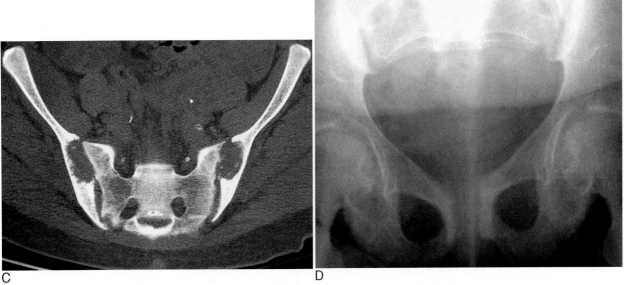

Figure 25-2—(Cont'd)   C, Axial CT in a different patient with hyperparathyroidism due to chronic renal failure shows extensive iliac subarticular resorption. **D,** AP radiograph of the pelvis shows subarticular bone resorption of the symphysis pubis and, to a lesser extent, the sacroiliac joints.

(hypophosphatemia) and thus diminished ability to mineralize osteoid. In these disorders, there is also an intrinsic defect in osteoblast hydroxylase function—normally, hypophosphatemia stimulates production of 1,25-hydroxy-vitamin D. However, in the X-linked form of disease, there is a failure to stimulate the hydroxylase; thus, vitamin D levels are abnormally low for the level of phosphate depletion.

Another cause for osteomalacia is rare receptor resistance to vitamin D action, which can also interfere with mineralization of osteoid. Certain drugs, such as Dilantin and phenobarbital, can interfere with vitamin D hydroxylation and thus function.

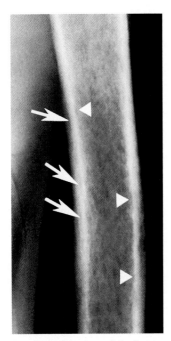

Figure 25-3   AP radiographic view of the humerus in patient with secondary hyperparathyroidism shows numerous intracortical lucencies *(arrows)* and endosteal bone resorption *(arrowheads)* mimicking aggressive neoplasia.

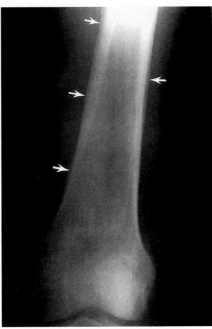

Figure 25-4   AP radiograph of distal femur in patient with secondary hyperparathyroidism shows solid periosteal new bone formation *(arrows).*

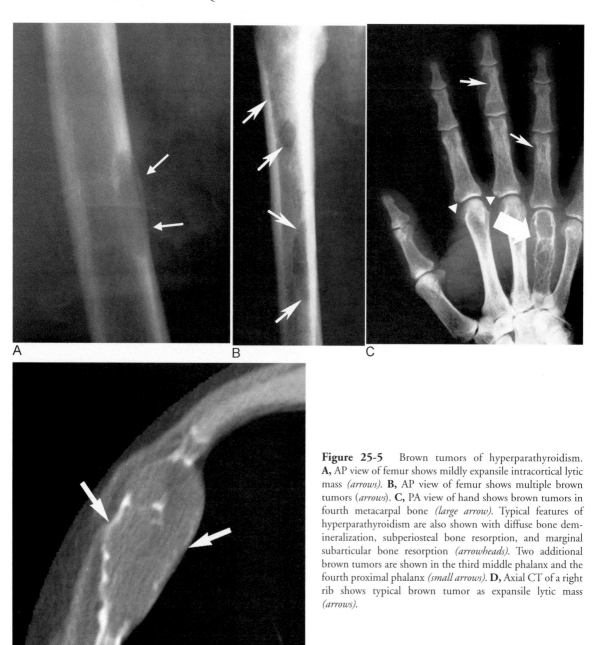

Figure 25-5 Brown tumors of hyperparathyroidism. **A,** AP view of femur shows mildly expansile intracortical lytic mass *(arrows)*. **B,** AP view of femur shows multiple brown tumors *(arrows)*. **C,** PA view of hand shows brown tumors in fourth metacarpal bone *(large arrow)*. Typical features of hyperparathyroidism are also shown with diffuse bone demineralization, subperiosteal bone resorption, and marginal subarticular bone resorption *(arrowheads)*. Two additional brown tumors are shown in the third middle phalanx and the fourth proximal phalanx *(small arrows)*. **D,** Axial CT of a right rib shows typical brown tumor as expansile lytic mass *(arrows)*.

Finally, a rare oncogenic form of osteomalacia due to hormone production by tumors interferes with tubular resorption of phosphate. Often, these tumors are very small, benign, and asymptomatic, and curiously are found in bone. Such lesions include hemangioma, nonossifying fibroma, and giant cell tumor of bone. In this setting, the osteomalacia is cured by resection of the lesion. Diagnosis is helped by laboratory analysis, which is similar to that found with renal tubular disorders, with high levels of urine phosphate.

Generalized bone demineralization is a major feature of osteomalacia, as it is in hyperparathyroidism. However, unlike the proportionate loss of mineral and cartilaginous osteoid matrix that is seen histologically in hyperparathyroidism, there

is disproportionately decreased mineral relative to osteoid matrix found in osteomalacia. This occurs in osteomalacia because of the loss of osteoblastic capacity to deposit hydroxyapatite crystals on the cartilaginous matrix. Thus, osteomalacia is a pathologically distinct disease.

Radiographic findings in osteomalacia reflect the underlying histologic characteristics: osteomalacic bone appears lucent, coarsened, and smudgy (Fig. 25-8), which is probably due to a mixture of decreased bone density and possibly radiographic density contributed by nonmineralized osteoid. A highly specific feature of osteomalacia is the appearance of *Looser's zones,* or pseudofractures, which are linear foci of undermineralized osteoid at sites of mechanical loading (Fig. 25-9). Often bilateral

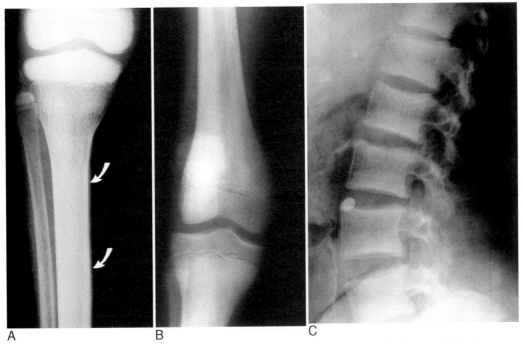

Figure 25-6   Secondary hyperparathyroidism and bone sclerosis. **A,** AP radiograph of proximal tibia shows epiphyseal bone sclerosis and tibial diaphyseal solid periosteal new bone *(arrows).* **B,** AP radiograph of knee shows generalized increased bone density. Note increased thickness of cortical bone. **C,** Lateral radiograph of lumbar spine shows typical features of rugger jersey spine with alternating bands of density and lucency. The denser bone is located in the subendplate regions.

and symmetric, these appear as linear lucencies perpendicularly oriented to the cortex of the bone, with incomplete penetration of the bony width. They usually occur along the concave (compressive) margins of the curvature of the bone, unlike the fatigue fractures of Paget's disease (sometimes termed "pseudofractures") that typically occur along the convex (tensile) margins of curves. Characteristic locations of Looser's zones include the medial aspects of the proximal femurs, the pubic bones, the dorsal aspect of the proximal ulnae, the distal parts of the scapulae, and the ribs.

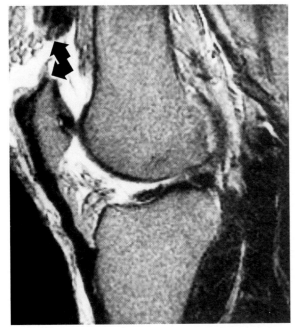

Figure 25-7   Tendon rupture in hyperparathyroidism. Sagittal T2-weighted MR image of knee in a patient with primary hyperparathyroidism shows acute rupture of quadriceps tendon at patellar insertion *(arrows).*

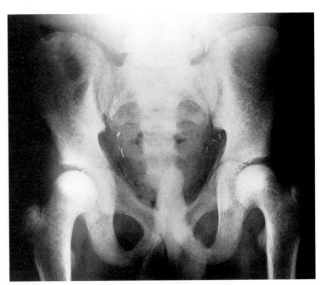

Figure 25-8   AP radiograph of the pelvis in patient with osteomalacia shows diffuse bone demineralization and coarsened appearance of bone typical for osteomalacia.

RICKETS

Rickets is osteomalacia in the immature skeleton. Features include undermineralization of osteoid at metabolically active sites, namely the metaphyseal zones of provisional calcification. The disease is especially well demonstrated at sites of rapid bone growth, such as the proximal and distal femur, the proximal tibia, the proximal humerus, and the distal radius.

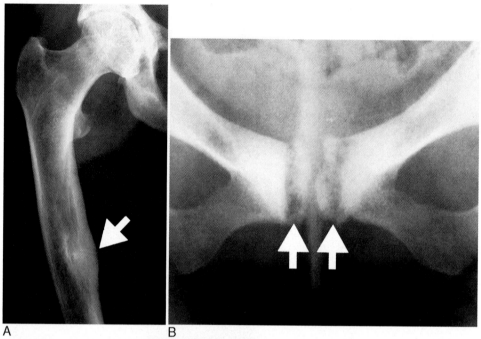

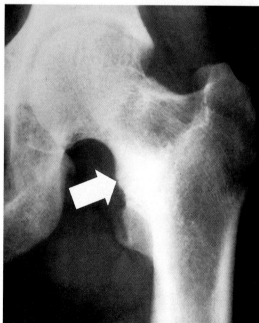

Figure 25-9   Pseudofractures (Looser's zones). **A,** AP radiograph of femur shows typical appearance of pseudofracture as incomplete linear lucency along concave, or weight-bearing, aspect of the femur *(arrow)*. **B,** AP radiograph of pelvis shows bilateral symmetric linear lucencies in os pubis *(arrows)* consistent with pseudofractures. **C,** AP radiograph of the left femur shows ill-defined linear lucency at weight-bearing, medial margin of the basicervical femoral neck with surrounding sclerosis *(arrow)*.

(Continued)

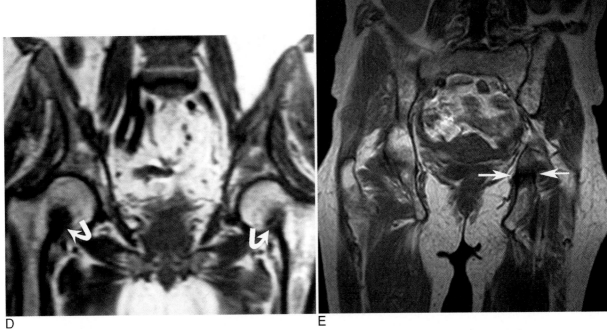

Figure 25-9—(Cont'd)   **D,** Coronal T1-weighted MR image of hips in same patient as in part C shows bilateral, symmetric pseudofractures in the femoral necks. The broad zones of diminished signal *(arrows)* correlate with sclerosis on the radiographs. **E,** Coronal T1-weighted MR image of the pelvis in a different patient shows Looser's zone in the left ischium (between *arrows*).

The appearance is that of widened and irregularly shaped physeal lucencies, often with flaring of the metaphyses (Fig. 25-10A). In the ribs, a rachitic rosary will appear (Fig. 25-10B) because of the same physeal pathophysiology at multiple costochondral junctions. The bones are soft, sometimes resulting in bizarre deformities after the onset of weight bearing, which results from repeated insufficiency fractures (Fig. 25-10C). Severe cases may have short, squat bones. Children with rickets are also at substantial risk of displaced Salter-Harris I fractures (slipped epiphyses), which occur most commonly bilaterally at the hips. Correcting the metabolic deficiency will reverse the findings at the growth plates, although bone deformities will persist (Fig. 25-11).

There are two important differential diagnoses to consider for rickets. The first is metaphyseal dysplasia (Schmid type) that looks similar to osteomalacia, with growth plate widening, but this disease is due to an inborn error in enchondral ossification. Laboratory values and bone mineralization are normal. The other is hypophosphatasia, in which bone is severely osteopenic, growth plates are wide, and multiple fractures are seen. However, in this disease serum alkaline phosphatase level is low, unlike other causes of rickets in which the enzyme level is elevated.

RENAL OSTEODYSTROPHY

Renal osteodystrophy represents the clinical, pathologic, and radiologic manifestations of osteomalacia combined with secondary hyperparathyroidism that occur in chronic renal failure. Renal failure results in hyperphosphatemia and thus increased synthesis of parathyroid hormone. In addition, renal failure results in decreased 1,25-vitamin D production in the kidney. Furthermore, diminished gut calcium absorption as a result of diminished vitamin D production activates parathyroid hormone synthesis. Thus, these patients will manifest features of both metabolic disorders (Fig. 25-12). In truth, the mechanisms of action are quite complicated; for example, there is skeletal resistance to parathyroid hormone action because vitamin D is a cofactor of parathyroid hormone action in bone. In addition, patients with renal failure are often undergoing dialysis, and aluminum in the dialysate, which is present to bind phosphate,

Key Concepts	Rickets

Rickets = osteomalacia in children.
Wide physes (unmineralized zone of provisional calcification).
Metaphyseal irregularity, fraying. Metaphyses may become dense with treatment.
Leg bone bowing (other causes: congenital, Blount's disease, neurofibromatosis type 1 [NF1], osteogenesis imperfecta, achondroplasia).
Large rib ends (rachitic rosary).
Salter-Harris I fractures, slipped capital femoral epiphysis.

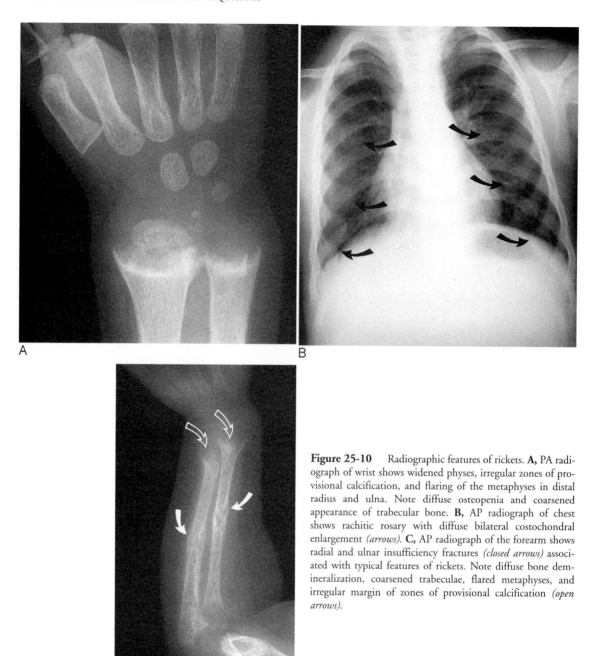

Figure 25-10 Radiographic features of rickets. **A,** PA radiograph of wrist shows widened physes, irregular zones of provisional calcification, and flaring of the metaphyses in distal radius and ulna. Note diffuse osteopenia and coarsened appearance of trabecular bone. **B,** AP radiograph of chest shows rachitic rosary with diffuse bilateral costochondral enlargement *(arrows).* **C,** AP radiograph of the forearm shows radial and ulnar insufficiency fractures *(closed arrows)* associated with typical features of rickets. Note diffuse bone demineralization, coarsened trabeculae, flared metaphyses, and irregular margin of zones of provisional calcification *(open arrows).*

can lead to bone toxicity that mimics osteomalacia. Amyloidosis also can be seen in patients undergoing dialysis, leading to findings in joints and spinal disk spaces that can appear similar to infection (see Fig. 21-14). Further compounding these patients' skeletal findings are the risk for osteomyelitis and septic arthritis because of chronic immune suppression, the risk for avascular necrosis due to long-term steroid therapy, and traumatic subchondral bone collapse in osteopenic bone.

Key Concepts	Renal Osteodystrophy

Long-standing renal failure.
Combined features of hyperparathyroidism and osteomalacia are seen; one or the other may dominate.
Tumoral calcinosis, aluminum toxicity.
Amyloidosis.

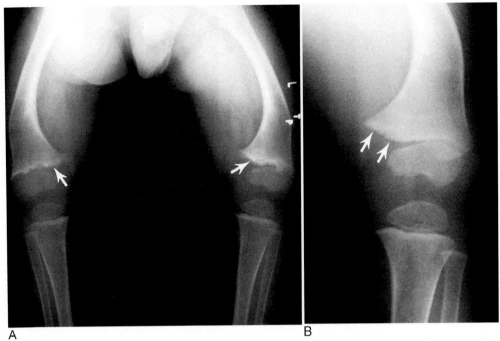

Figure 25-11 Rickets before and after treatment. **A,** AP radiograph of knees shows irregular contour of femoral metaphyseal zones of provisional calcification *(arrows),* metaphyseal flaring, and varus deformity of distal femurs. **B,** After treatment, AP radiograph of left knee shows narrowing of physes, restored smooth contour of distal femoral metaphyseal zones of provisional calcification *(arrows),* and diminished metaphyseal flaring. Femoral varus deformity persists.

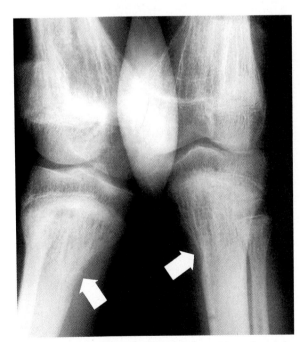

Figure 25-12 AP radiograph of knees in boy with renal osteodystrophy shows combined features of osteomalacia and hyperparathyroidism. Note coarsened trabecular appearance typical of osteomalacia, and subperiosteal bone resorption in the concave cortex of the proximal tibias *(arrows)* typical of hyperparathyroidism. Genu valgum, as shown in this case, is often found in children with hyperparathyroidism.

Patients with renal osteodystrophy can show areas of decreased bone density and osteosclerosis, with sclerosis often predominating at the endplate regions of the spine, known as the "rugger jersey spine." ("Rugger" is British for rugby.) Rugby players traditionally wear jerseys with horizontal stripes. Occasionally diffuse osteosclerosis can be found (see Fig. 25-6). In addition, profuse soft tissue calcifications can be seen, including vascular calcifications and para-articular accumulations of calcium-phosphate precipitates, which can occasionally take on a liquid form as milk of calcium; these accumulations can be massive and are referred to as *tumoral calcinosis* (Fig. 25-13). Insufficiency fractures and Looser's zones can be found in addition to the classic features of hyperparathyroidism (Fig. 25-14).

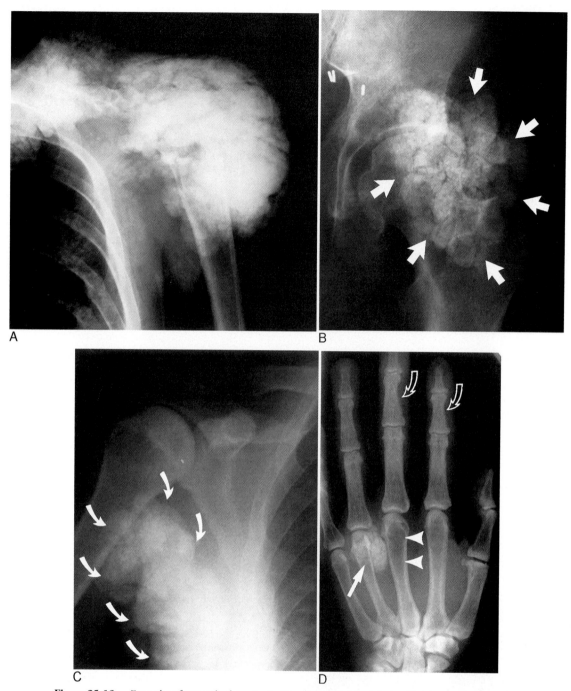

Figure 25-13   Examples of tumoral calcinosis. **A,** AP radiograph of the left shoulder demonstrates massive para-articular soft tissue calcification due to tumoral calcinosis. Note the diffuse demineralization of bone and multiple left rib fractures. **B,** AP radiograph of left hip shows multiple para-articular calcifications *(arrows)* due to tumoral calcinosis. **C,** AP radiograph of the right shoulder shows massive tumoral calcinosis *(arrows)*. **D,** PA radiograph of the right hand shows soft tissue deposit of tumoral calcinosis *(closed arrow)* as well as features of hyperparathyroidism with diffuse demineralization of bone, subperiosteal bone resorption *(open arrows)*, and third metacarpal brown tumor *(arrowheads)*.

(Continued)

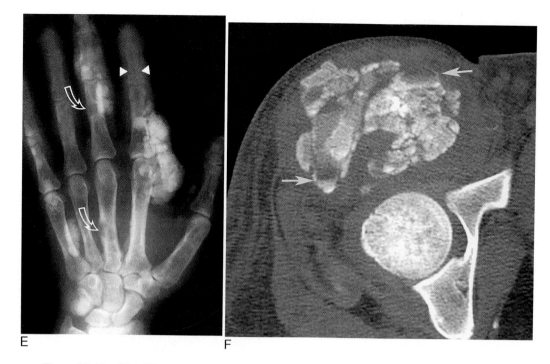

E   F

Figure 25-13—(Cont'd)   E, PA radiograph of the right hand shows multiple deposits of tumoral calcinosis, diffuse bone demineralization, third metacarpal and phalangeal brown tumors *(open arrows)*, and Looser's zone in second middle phalanx *(arrowheads)*. **F,** Patient undergoing long-term dialysis who has tumoral calcinosis anterior to the right hip. Note the subtle layering within some of the calcium-filled cysts *(arrows)*. This is the same patient as shown in Fig. 25-2C.

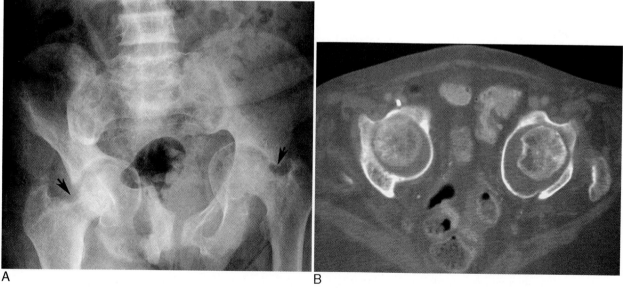

A   B

Figure 25-14   Renal osteodystrophy. **A and B,** AP pelvis radiograph (A) and axial CT image (B) show severe findings of renal osteodystrophy, including protrusio acetabuli, sacroiliac and symphysis pubis subchondral bone resorption, bilateral femoral neck subperiosteal bone resorption (*arrows* in part A), rugger jersey spine, right pubic insufficiency fractures, diffuse coarsening of trabeculae, and mixed pattern of increased and decreased bone density.

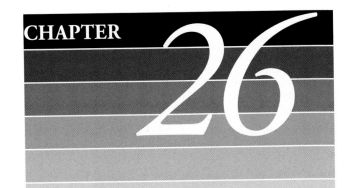

Miscellaneous Metabolic Bone Diseases

FLUOROSIS, HYPERVITAMINOSIS A, AND
 HYPERVITAMINOSIS D
HEAVY METAL POISONING
SCURVY
HYPOTHYROIDISM
HYPOPARATHYROIDISM AND RELATED CONDITIONS

This chapter reviews additional metabolic conditions that need to be discussed, although this discussion is far from exhaustive.

FLUOROSIS, HYPERVITAMINOSIS A, AND HYPERVITAMINOSIS D

Fluorosis (fluoride toxicity), vitamin A toxicity (hypervitaminosis A), and vitamin D toxicity (hypervitaminosis D) are due to overingestion. Each tends to cause increased bone density (Fig 26-1, Table 26-1) and periostitis due to metastatic deposition of calcium salts. Fluorosis and hypervitaminosis A can cause flowing ossification of the anterior longitudinal ligament of the spine that is so pronounced it can mimic diffuse idiopathic skeletal hyperostosis and seronegative spondyloarthropathy. Retinoic acid derivatives, which are related to vitamin A and are used for treating acne, may also cause this finding (Fig. 26-2). The teeth of children with fluorosis are mottled in appearance and highly resistant to caries.

Children with hypervitaminosis A may develop hydrocephalus. Periosteal new bone formation can be prominent (Fig. 26-3), and may be so extensive as to mimic Caffey's disease (infantile cortical hyperostosis; see Chapter 46), but the mandible is usually spared in hypervitaminosis A. Patients of any age may become jaundiced because of hepatic toxicity.

Hypervitaminosis D causes hypercalcemia, hypercalciuria, phosphaturia, soft tissue calcification, and cortical and trabecular thickening. The skull may become dense. In children, the provisional zone of calcification widens.

Thyroid acropachy, which is seen, rarely, after treatment for thyrotoxicosis, can also manifest as prominent, fluffy, solid periosteal new bone deposition, particularly in the

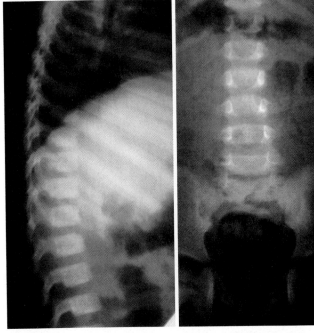

Figure 26-1 Fluorosis. This 4-year-old African child lives in an area with elevated fluoride in drinking water. Note the diffusely increased bone density, best appreciated on the lateral radiographic view.

Table 26-1	Differential Diagnosis of Diffuse Increased Bone Density (3MsPROF)
Myelofibrosis	
Mastocytosis	
Metastatic disease, rarely myeloma	
Sickle cell anemia	
Paget's disease, pyknodysostosis	
Renal osteodystrophy	
Osteopetrosis	
Fluorosis	

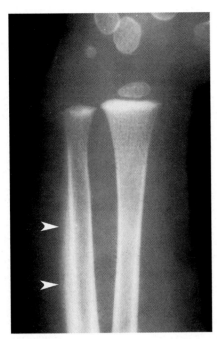

Figure 26-2   Hypervitaminosis A. Note the solid periosteal new bone formation on the distal ulna *(arrows)*, which is a nonspecific finding. This child had been given excessive oral vitamin A.

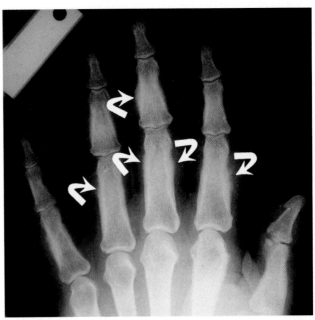

Figure 26-4   PA radiograph of hand in woman with thyroid acropachy shows exuberant fluffy periosteal new bone formation *(arrows)* in the proximal and middle phalanges and generalized swelling of the fingers.

metacarpals/tarsals and phalanges in the hands and feet (Fig. 26-4). Clubbing can be seen in this disease, and soft tissue swelling is found, such as in the orbits (exophthalmos) and lower extremities (myxedema).

HEAVY METAL POISONING

Several heavy metals, most notably lead, are osteoclast poisons that result in increased bone density and undertubulation in the metaphyses due to unopposed osteoblast action. Dense metaphyseal bands can also be seen physiologically in growing children, although their presence in the proximal fibula and distal ulna strongly suggest lead poisoning (Fig. 26-5). Healing rickets can also cause dense metaphyseal bands. The clinical

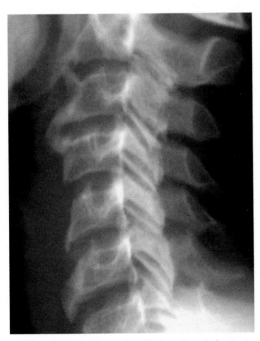

Figure 26-3   Retinoid arthropathy. The lateral cervical spine in this 22-year-old man demonstrates prominent anterior osteophyte formation in the cervical spine, an incongruent finding in a patient of this age. He was using retinoids, which are vitamin A analogs, for a skin condition. (Reprinted with permission of the American College of Radiology learning file.)

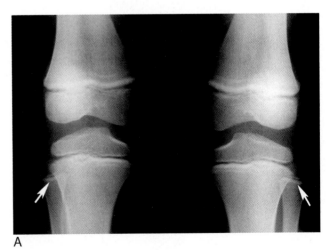

A

Figure 26-5   Two patients with lead poisoning. **A,** AP radiograph of knees shows multiple dense metaphyseal bands bilaterally in the femur, tibia, and fibula *(arrows)*. The presence of the increased density in the fibular metaphyses strongly suggests heavy metal poisoning. Note mild metaphyseal undertubulation.

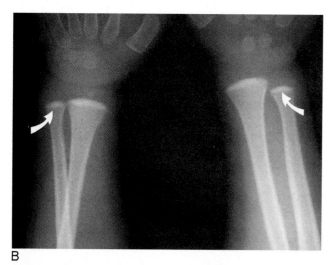

B

Figure 26-5—(Cont'd) **B,** AP radiograph of wrists shows dense metaphyseal bands in distal radius and ulna *(arrows)* bilaterally. The presence of the increased density in the distal ulnar metaphyses is highly suggestive of lead poisoning.

Key Concepts	Differential Diagnosis of Dense Metaphyseal Bands
Normal variant Heavy metal (lead) poisoning Hypervitaminosis D Metaphyseal stress lines Rickets (after treatment) Scurvy (rare)	

history, as well as other findings of rickets (e.g., metaphyseal widening), may help to make the correct diagnosis. Rarer causes of dense metaphyseal bands include hypervitaminosis D, treated hypothyroidism, and, very rarely, scurvy.

SCURVY

Scurvy, a disease caused by low dietary intake of vitamin C, is rarely encountered today. Vitamin C is required for collagen formation and therefore is needed for bone matrix, cartilage, tendon, and ligament synthesis. Without the vitamin, production of collagen and thus bone production is diminished with diffuse bone demineralization, and there is increased tendency toward insufficiency fracture. In children, bleeding risk can result in extensive pronounced subperiosteal hemorrhage and subsequent periosteal ossification. Other signs found in the immature skeleton are named and include *Wimberger's sign,* which is a sclerotic epiphyseal rim related to disorganized bone production at the epiphyseal center of ossification, *Frenkel's line,* which is a dense metaphyseal line of similar pathophysiology, and *Pelkin's fracture,* which is a metaphyseal corner fracture.

HYPOTHYROIDISM

Hypothyroidism manifests with mild osteoporosis, soft tissue edema, and myopathy. The juvenile form manifests with severe delay in skeletal maturity, in which skeletal age lags markedly behind clinical age (Fig. 26-6A). Dental development is also severely delayed. Other characteristic findings in juvenile

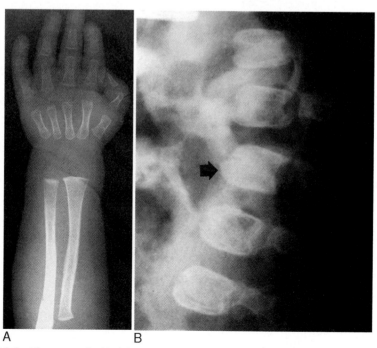

A   B

Figure 26-6 Eleven-month-old girl with congenital hypothyroidism. **A,** PA radiograph of hand and forearm shows severe delay in skeletal maturity, with complete absence of ossification of the carpal bones and epiphyses. **B,** Lateral radiograph of thoracolumbar junction shows bullet-shaped vertebra *(arrow).*

hypothyroidism include wormian bones, a bullet-shaped vertebra at the thoracolumbar junction (Fig. 26-6B), and epiphyseal fragmentation (which, in the proximal femur, can mimic Legg-Calvé-Perthes disease).

HYPOPARATHYROIDISM AND RELATED CONDITIONS

Key Concepts	Hypoparathyroidism

Radiographs: Metastatic deposition of calcium phosphate salts, often in subcutaneous locations
Osteosclerosis, localized or generalized
Osteoporosis (rare)

Hypoparathyroidism is associated with incapacity of the parathyroid glands to produce sufficient hormone for calcium homeostasis. This occurs most commonly after parathyroid gland resection for hyperparathyroidism and results in hypocalcemia and hyperphosphatemia. Clinical manifestations predominate with irritability, seizures, and tetany. Radiographically, metastatic deposition of calcium phosphate salts can occur, often in subcutaneous locations or the basal ganglia of the brain, and osteosclerosis can be localized or generalized. Rarely osteoporo-

Key Concepts	Pseudohypoparathyroidism and Pseudo-Pseudohypoparathyroidism

Shares clinical features with hypoparathyroidism
Added clinical features: Short stature, obesity, brachydactyly
Radiographs: Small osteochondromas, short metacarpals/tarsals

sis is seen. *Pseudohypoparathyroidism* has similar clinical manifestations but represents target cell resistance to parathyroid hormone in which the patients are clinically hypocalcemic but have high serum levels of parathyroid hormone. These patients have a characteristic body type: they are short and obese, with short metacarpals and metatarsals, especially in the first, fourth, and fifth metatarsals (Fig. 26-7). Short stature and short metacarpals are due to accelerated, early growth plate closure. Thick calvaria and intracranial and soft tissue calcifications can be seen. Also seen are unusual small osteochondromas, projecting at right angles to the shafts of the bones (Fig. 26-7D). Radiographic features are otherwise similar to those seen with hypoparathyroidism. *Pseudo-pseudohypoparathyroidism* is clinically and radiologically the same as pseudohypoparathyroidism but serum hormone levels of parathyroid hormone and calcium are normal.

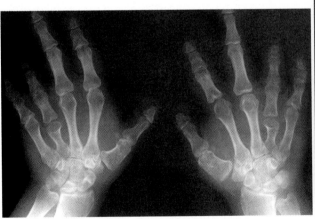
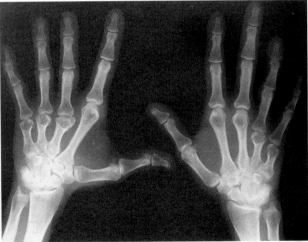

A   B

Figure 26-7   Characteristic features of pseudohypoparathyroidism. **A,** PA radiograph of hands shows characteristic shortening and mild widening of multiple small tubular bones, particularly the first and fourth metacarpals in this patient. **B,** PA radiograph of hands in another patient shows pronounced shortening of the right third through fifth and the left fourth and fifth metacarpal bones.

(Continued)

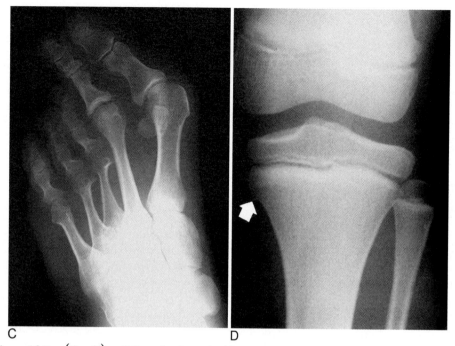

C

D

Figure 26-7—(Cont'd)   **C,** Frontal radiograph of foot shows third through fifth metatarsal shortening. **D,** AP radiograph of knee shows tiny osteochondroma *(arrow)* arising at a right angle from medial aspect of proximal tibial metaphysis.

CHAPTER 27

Osteoporosis

GENERALIZED OSTEOPOROSIS
REGIONAL OSTEOPOROSIS

Osteopenia is a general term for diminished radiographic bone density due to decreased bone mineral density (BMD). *Osteoporosis* is a more specific term for decreased bone mass *with qualitatively normal bone.* (Both terms are also used in a somewhat different and very specific way in interpreting dual x-ray absorptiometry (DEXA) bone density scans, as discussed later in this chapter). Osteoporosis is the most common cause of decreased BMD, but keep in mind that there are other causes such as osteomalacia (unmineralized osteoid) that are not associated with qualitatively normal bone.

GENERALIZED OSTEOPOROSIS

Osteoporosis is a disease of diminished bone quantity. The ratio of osteoid matrix to hydroxyapatite mineral is normal. Histologically, the bone is normal, but there is less of it, with cortical thinning and diminished quantity and thickness of trabecular bone. Laboratory values that are markers for accelerated bone turnover are normal. Although the exact cause for most cases of osteoporosis is not known, it is clear that there is an imbalance in the normal bone turnover process, with bone loss exceeding bone production. Over time, this leads to grossly diminished bone mass.

Senile osteoporosis is associated with advancing age. *Postmenopausal osteoporosis* is associated with the diminished estrogen levels of postmenopausal women. Thus, amenorrhea is a risk factor for osteoporosis. Other contributing factors include low body weight in women, low levels of weight-bearing exercise, and a family history of osteoporosis. Among women, the incidence of osteoporosis is greater among white and Asian persons than it is among black persons. Bone loss typically begins in the fourth decade in women and the fifth or sixth decades in men. In fact, 30% to 50% of women older than age 60 years show evidence of significant bone loss.

Key Concepts	Generalized Osteoporosis

Major worldwide health problem
Major complication is fracture: Spine, hip, forearm most frequent.
Diagnosis: Dual x-ray absorptiometry (DEXA)
  T-score: Relative to normal young adults
    World Health Organization criteria: −1 to −2.5 indicates osteopenia; lower than −2.5 indicates osteoporosis
  Z-score: Relative to age-matched reference group; less useful
Diagnosis: Other quantitative tests: quantitative CT, US, for calcaneus
Radiography is insensitive
Radiographic findings
  Semiquantitative: Cortical tunnels, cortical thinning
  Qualitative: Decreased bone density, accentuated trabecular bone contrast, and increased contrast between cortical and medullary bone
Common causes of generalized osteoporosis:
  Advanced age
  Alcoholism
  Poor nutrition
  Smoking
  Diffuse marrow replacement (metastatic disease, myeloma, Gaucher's disease)
  Endocrine: Hypogonadism, hyperthyroidism, hyperparathyroidism, Cushing's disease
  Drugs: Heparin, Dilantin, corticosteroids
  Multiple myeloma (osteoclast activation)
  Congenital diseases (e.g., osteogenesis imperfecta)
  Inborn errors of metabolism (e.g., homocystinuria)

Besides senile and postmenopausal osteoporosis, which are together termed *primary osteoporosis,* secondary causes of osteoporosis include hypercorticism (steroid therapy or Cushing's disease); effects of other drugs, especially heparin (Table 27-1); alcoholism; smoking; congenital diseases such as osteogenesis

Table 27-1	Drug-Induced Changes in Bone

Heparin: Osteoporosis (dose-related)
Dilantin and phenobarbital: Osteomalacia
Corticosteroids: Osteoporosis, avascular necrosis
Warfarin: Embryopathy with stippled epiphyses
Lead and other heavy metals (e.g., bismuth): Osteoclast poison, dense metaphyseal bands, and undertubulation of metaphyses
Vitamin A: Painful periostitis
Vitamin D: Increased bone density, periostitis, soft tissue calcifications
Fluorosis: Increased bone density, periostitis, ligament ossification, stress fractures
Alcohol: Fetal alcohol syndrome, osteoporosis, avascular necrosis
Prostaglandins: Periostitis in infants

Key Concepts	Osteoporosis in Children

Causes: Idiopathic, corticosteroid use, immunocompromise, neuromuscular conditions (disuse), methotrexate therapy, osteogenesis imperfecta, prematurity
Easily overestimated on radiographs

imperfecta; and inborn errors of metabolism such as homocystinuria and ochronosis. Other less common causes of generalized osteoporosis include amyloidosis, hyperthyroidism, mastocytosis, and rare idiopathic juvenile forms of osteoporosis. Bone loss in myeloma can be extensive but histologically is typically shown to be due to plasma cell infiltration of the marrow space or plasmacytomas, and is not generally considered osteoporosis.

The major complication of osteoporosis is fracture; the most common locations are the spine, the hip, the proximal humerus, and the distal forearm. It is this fracture risk that makes osteoporosis a major health issue throughout the world because of its high prevalence in elderly women and enormous impact on morbidity, mortality, and societal cost.

Effective treatments for osteoporosis include calcium supplementation, estrogen therapy, and bisphosphonate drugs such as etidronate. The bisphosphonate drugs are so effective that bone loss can be reversed. Although the optimal time to intervene with drug therapy in patients with or at risk for osteoporosis is still unclear, most women regardless of bone mass are advised to undergo dietary supplementation with calcium and to undertake exercise programs.

The radiologist's role is to detect osteoporosis and to monitor progression of disease after the initiation of treatment. Both DEXA and quantitative computed tomographic (CT) densitometry provide quantitative, reasonably accurate, and reproducible measurements of bone density. Specialized ultrasonographic (US) equipment can measure the density of the calcaneus, but this technique is less widely used. The World Health Organization has established guidelines for diagnosis of osteoporosis, with emphasis on fracture risk, using DEXA. With DEXA, BMD is reported at several sites in absolute value (g/mL), relative to normal young adults (standard deviation is the T-score), and relative to age- and sex-matched reference populations (standard deviation is the Z-score). T-scores between −1 and −2.5 (that is, bone density between 1 and 2.5 standard deviations below the average of normal young adults of the same sex) are defined as *osteopenic*. T-scores below −2.5 are defined as *osteoporotic*. Be aware that these definitions of osteopenia and osteoporosis are specific to reporting on DEXA scans.

In evaluating DEXA scans, the radiologist's role is to assure proper placement of regions of interest for BMD measurement and to assure absence of radiographic abnormalities that might interfere with measurement. Such confounders include osteophytes in the spine, compression fractures, and soft tissue calcification (e.g., diffuse idiopathic skeletal hyperostosis or aortic calcification), any of which can erroneously increase a BMD value on DEXA. Usually, measurements at four lumbar levels are averaged and a measure of the proximal femur and occasionally the wrist are obtained. Measurements at each site of risk are more predictive of fracture risk at that site than is a measurement from a remote site. Thus, the risk for hip fracture is best determined from a BMD measurement of the hip. Measurements at two or three sites are routine in patients undergoing DEXA.

Quantitative CT densitometry is more sensitive than DEXA because the cross-sectional nature of data acquisition allows evaluation limited to trabecular bone where generalized osteoporosis is most greatly manifested. Computed tomographic densitometry may be more accurate for assessing bone density than DEXA in patients with diffuse idiopathic skeletal hyperostosis, aortic calcification, spine fracture, and excessive degenerative osteophyte formation. Computed tomographic densitometry is less popular because of higher cost and radiation dose.

Radiography provides less quantitative evaluation of bone density. Approximately 30% to 50% of bone mineral must be lost for grossly diminished bone density to be subjectively apparent on radiographs. The least subjective radiographic finding of osteoporosis in long bones is cortical bone loss. A specific location to look for cortical thinning is in the second and third metacarpal shafts, where middiaphyseal cortical width should account for at least 50% of bone width in individuals with normal bone density (Fig. 27-1). The relatively rapid bone loss associated with hyperparathyroidism, hyperthyroidism, disuse, regional hyperemia, and reflex sympathetic dystrophy can cause small, discrete areas of endosteal or subperiosteal cortical bone loss, as well as fine linear radiolucencies within the diaphyseal cortex termed *cortical tunnels* or *intracortical lucencies,* which are difficult to see without magnification radiographs (Fig. 27-2). Cortical tunnels are part of the normal bone turnover process, as aggregates of osteoclasts create these cylindrical defects in lamellar bone that are normally promptly repaired by osteoblasts. The development of radiographically visible cortical tunnels reflects the delayed and diminished osteoblastic activity in osteoporosis. These subtle defects are less than 0.5 mm in diameter, several millimeters in length, and parallel to the long axis of the bone.

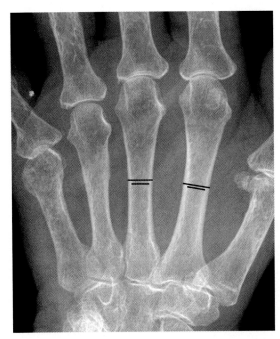

Figure 27-1 Cortical thickness in the metacarpals and metatarsals can serve as a rough guide to the presence or absence of generalized osteoporosis in adults. In this elderly woman with osteoporosis, the transverse width of the medullary spaces (illustrated by *short lines* across metacarpals 2 and 3) excede one half the transverse width of the shafts *(long lines)*, due to cortical bone loss. This generalization does not apply to children.

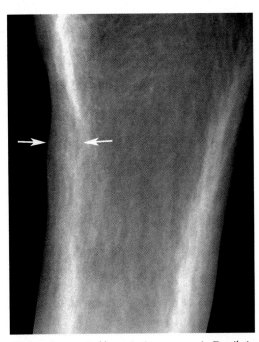

Figure 27-2 Intracortical lucencies in osteoporosis. Detail view of the femur in a 65-year-old man immobilized for a fracture shows subtle radiolucent lines parallel to the cortex (e.g., between *arrows*).

Additional findings of osteoporosis in long bones include accentuation of stress- or load-bearing trabeculae (because these are the last to be resorbed), insufficiency fractures, and transverse trabeculae in the diaphysis or metaphysis, termed *bone bars* or

reinforcement lines. Progressive loss of trabeculae in the proximal femur reflects the least important trabecular lines of force, starting with the secondary tensile trabeculae, followed by the primary tensile trabeculae, then the secondary compressive followed by the primary compressive trabeculae (Fig. 27-3).

There are numerous radiographic findings in osteoporosis in the spine. Vertebral endplates may appear thinned, with exaggerated contrast between vertebral body endplate and central density (see Fig. 27-3). Compression fractures might be seen, taking the shape of anterior wedging, biconcavity of endplates, or generalized loss of height. In addition, osteoporosis can be manifested with increased conspicuity of vertically oriented trabecular bone in the spine due to generalized dropout of horizontally oriented trabeculae.

Bone scans in patients with primary osteoporosis are normal, unless arthritis or a stress fracture with healing response is present. Magnetic resonance imaging (MRI) is highly sensitive for detection of insufficiency fractures and is more sensitive than bone scanning, especially within the first few days after the fracture. Vertebral body marrow often has a mottled appearance on T1-weighted MR images in patients with osteoporosis, but this appearance is neither sensitive nor specific.

REGIONAL OSTEOPOROSIS

There are regional forms of osteopenia that are of unclear cause. The best known are transient osteoporosis of the hip (TOH, introduced previously in Chapter 22), and regional migratory osteoporosis. It is unclear whether these diagnoses are unique or related, and whether they are related to transient forms of avascular necrosis (AVN) or occult stress fracture.

Key Concepts	Regional Osteoporosis

Local osteopenia, often symptomatic, may appear radiographically aggressive
Regional migratory osteoporosis
Transient osteoporosis of the hip. Might be forme fruste of avascular necrosis (AVN)
Reflex sympathetic dystrophy
Local hyperemia: Healing fracture, hypervascular tumor, infection, synovitis
Diminished loading, disuse

Transient osteoporosis of the hip is seen most commonly among middle-aged men (either hip) and pregnant women (usually the left hip), and often occur in patients with no history of significant trauma or known risk factors for AVN. Patients present with sudden onset of severe hip pain. Asymmetric diminished bone density is seen radiographically in the affected hip. Magnetic resonance imaging shows marrow

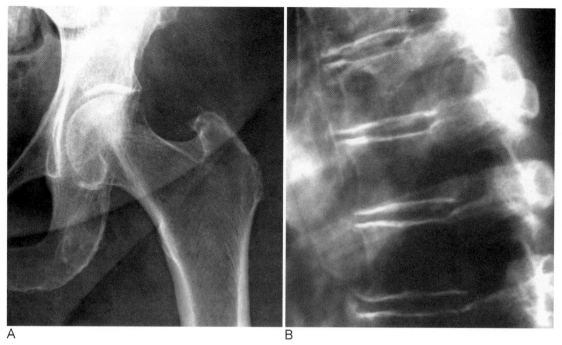

Figure 27-3   Osteoporosis. **A,** AP view of hip shows exaggerated trabecular pattern in primary compressive lines of force. The tensile lines of force are largely absent, indicating advanced osteoporosis. **B,** Lateral radiograph of spine shows exaggerated contrast between the endplates and the medullary bone.

edema with diminished signal on T1-weighted images (Fig. 27-4), increased signal on fat-suppressed T2-weighted or inversion recovery MR images (see Fig. 22-13), and contrast enhancement throughout the femoral head and neck, often associated with a joint effusion. This marrow edema is in marked contrast with generalized osteoporosis, which does not show marrow edema except if a fracture or other focal pathologic process is present. As implied by its name, TOH is self-limited, usually reversing after several months. No treatment other than conservative therapy is needed. As noted in Chapter 22, TOH may be a specific manifestation of transient regional osteoporosis (TRO), also termed regional migratory osteoporosis. Unlike TOH, however, multiple consecutive joints in TRO become affected with bone marrow edema, usually in the lower extremities at and distal to the knee. Treatment and natural history are otherwise the same as with TOH.

Reflex sympathetic dystrophy is thought to be mediated by dysfunction of the sympathetic nervous system. Its cause is unknown

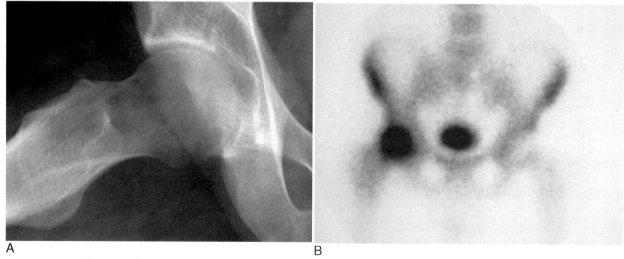

Figure 27-4   Transient regional osteoporosis. **A,** AP radiograph of the right hip in this 45-year-old man shows subtle demineralization. **B,** Radionuclide bone scan shows increased uptake in the right femoral head.

(Continued)

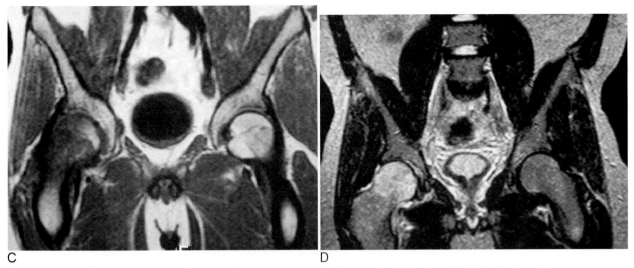

C   D

Figure 27-4—(Cont'd)   **C and D,** T1-weighted (C) and T2-weighted (D) spin-echo MR images show diffuse low signal and high signal intensity, respectively, due to marrow edema (see also Fig. 22-13).

but the condition is associated with traumatic, neurologic, or vascular events. It is associated not only with severely diminished bone density but with soft tissue trophic changes (Fig. 27-5), including swelling and hyperesthesia followed by atrophy and contracture of an entire extremity at and distal to the affected site.

Localized bone demineralization is also to be expected in the setting of hyperemia because hyperemia induces osteoclast activation and thus bone resorption. Thus, inflammatory arthropathy, hypervascular tumors, reflex sympathetic dystro-

phy, and healing fractures are associated with regional osteoporosis. Disuse of a limb is also associated with localized diminished bone density because bone mass is directly proportional to the forces acting across the bone. Casting of a fracture combines disuse and hyperemia related to the injury. Localized forms of osteoporosis can appear aggressive owing to active remodeling of bone, with evidence of intracortical lucencies, metaphyseal band-like lucencies, and subcortical/subchondral resorption of bone (Figs. 27-1, 27-5, 27-6, 27-7).

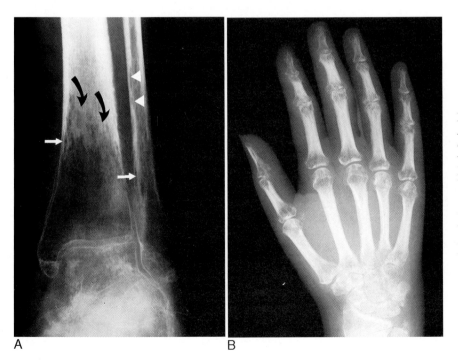

A   B

Figure 27-5   Reflex sympathetic dystrophy. **A,** AP view of the ankle shows pronounced bone demineralization in the distal leg and hindfoot with aggressive features, including intracortical lucency *(straight arrows)*, endosteal resorption of bone *(arrowheads)*, and broad zone of transition *(curved arrows)* to more normal appearing proximal tibial and fibular diaphyses. **B,** PA radiograph of the hand of another patient shows pronounced periarticular osteopenia and diffuse soft tissue swelling in the wrist and hand.

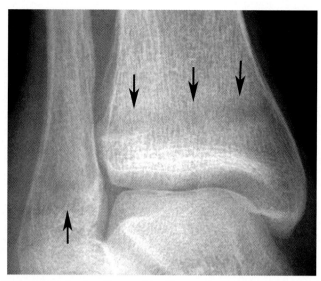

Figure 27-6 Osteoporosis related to disuse and local hyperemia. Disproportionate focal demineralization of the metaphysis after casting. This radiograph was obtained during a cast change for a fifth metatarsal fracture. Note the transverse band of demineralization *(arrows)* in the distal tibia and fibula, proximal to the former position of the physes. The metaphysis of children has a rich blood supply that can persist into adulthood, resulting in focally greater bone loss during immobilization.

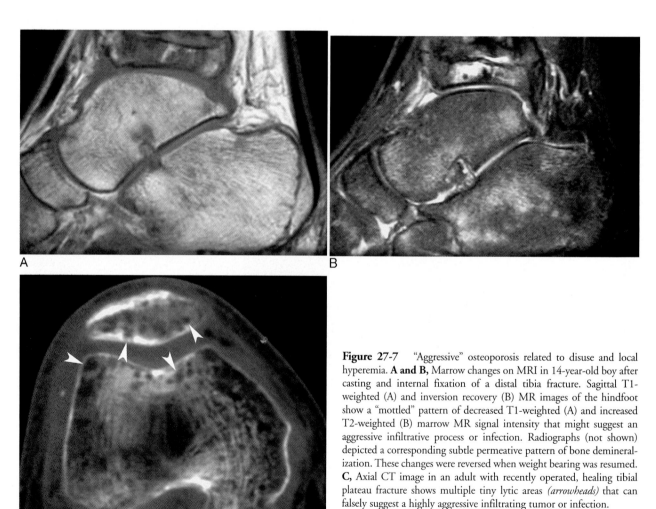

Figure 27-7 "Aggressive" osteoporosis related to disuse and local hyperemia. **A and B,** Marrow changes on MRI in 14-year-old boy after casting and internal fixation of a distal tibia fracture. Sagittal T1-weighted (A) and inversion recovery (B) MR images of the hindfoot show a "mottled" pattern of decreased T1-weighted (A) and increased T2-weighted (B) marrow MR signal intensity that might suggest an aggressive infiltrative process or infection. Radiographs (not shown) depicted a corresponding subtle permeative pattern of bone demineralization. These changes were reversed when weight bearing was resumed. **C,** Axial CT image in an adult with recently operated, healing tibial plateau fracture shows multiple tiny lytic areas *(arrowheads)* that can falsely suggest a highly aggressive infiltrating tumor or infection.

CHAPTER 28

Paget's Disease

Paget's disease is not a metabolic disease per se but has in common with many metabolic bone diseases a disturbance of osteoblast and osteoclast equilibrium. Paget's disease was first described as "osteitis deformans" by Sir James Paget in 1877. It is a chronic progressive skeletal disorder expressed initially as bone resorption that is localized to one or more bones. It is a disease that can cross joints. Most frequent sites of bone involvement are the skull, spine, pelvis, and femur. The cause is not known with certainty, but the osteoclast is considered to be the problem cell. Electron microscopy shows paramyxovirus inclusion bodies within osteoclasts, suggesting paramyxovirus infection as the cause. Adding to suspicion of an infectious cause, Paget's disease is more frequent in extreme north and south latitudes and has low incidence in Asia and Africa. Among those who migrate from low-incidence to high-incidence areas, disease prevalence becomes the same as the prevalence in the new area. In the United States, Paget's disease is rare before age 40 years, occurs in 3% of people older than 40 years old, and occurs in 10% of people older than 80 years old, with a 2:1 male:female occurrence. The incidence of Paget's disease is decreasing for unknown reasons.

Three sequential, although often coexistent, stages are described for Paget's disease. Stage I is the osteolytic phase, also termed the "hot" phase. Stage II is the mixed lytic and blastic phase, and corresponds to the onset of osteoblastic activation in response to osteoclastic bone resorption. Stage III is the sclerotic phase.

Paget's disease is a disease of osteoclasts. Osteoclasts are activated with resultant osteolysis, followed by an osteoblastic response until a new equilibrium is established between bone production and bone lysis. The rapid, disordered bone resorption and production results in an abnormal, mosaic-like histologic appearance of osteoid. Serum phosphorus and calcium levels are normal, but serum alkaline phosphatase and hydroxy proline are elevated, reflecting increase bone production and resorption, respectively.

In long bones, the disease usually begins at the ends of bones and extends roughly 1 cm per year toward the diaphysis. (In the tibia, Paget's disease occasionally begins in the diaphysis.) The

Key Concepts	Paget's Disease

Mechanism: Activated osteoclasts

Three sequential phases: Lytic, mixed lytic and sclerotic, and sclerotic

Radiographs:

Hallmarks: Bone expansion, cortical and trabecular bone thickening

Leading edge of lytic phase: "Blade of grass" = "flame-shaped" margin; equivalent finding in skull: Osteoporosis circumscripta

Later phases: spine: picture frame vertebrae; skull: "Cotton wool" diploe

Complications

Osteoarthritis

Bone deformity ("bone softening"): Basilar skull invagination, insufficiency fractures, protrusio acetabuli, insufficiency fracture, and proximal femoral varus

Cranial nerve palsies

Osteomyelitis

Malignant transformation (new-onset pain); look for new lytic lesion; poor prognosis

Giant cell tumors

leading edge represents the osteolytic phase, and usually has a sharply defined wedge-shaped margin between the normal and involved bone, a feature highly uncharacteristic of neoplasia (Fig. 28-1). The long bone lysis is often described as having a "flame-shaped" or "blade of grass" appearance (Fig. 28-2). The equivalent finding in the skull is termed "osteoporosis circumscripta," which describes acutely marginated bone demineralization during the lytic phase of disease (Fig. 28-3).

Behind the lytic leading edge, mixed lytic and sclerotic phase disease develops in a frequently disorganized pattern. Resulting findings are often pathognomonic for Paget's disease. "Picture frame vertebra" is a term that describes the mixed lytic and sclerotic phase in the spine (Fig. 28-4); "cotton wool" describes

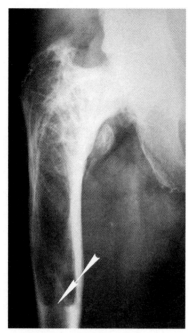

Figure 28-1   Paget's disease. AP radiograph shows sharp linear transition between pagetic and normal bone *(arrow)*. This finding is highly uncharacteristic of neoplasm. Moderate bone expansion, increased cortical thickness, and trabecular bone thickening assures the diagnosis of Paget's disease.

the mixed lytic and sclerotic phase in the skull (Fig. 28-5). The pathognomonic triad of findings in the mixed lytic and sclerotic phase of Paget's disease is bone expansion, cortical bone thickening, and trabecular bone thickening (Fig. 28-6). These findings reflect the pathophysiology of the disease and indicate

accelerated bone turnover, including bone deposition and bone expansion. An often-quoted classic clinical presentation involves the story of a man who is asked by his doctor whether his hat size has increased, and the man says, with hand to ear, "Eh?" The cause for deafness can be from otosclerosis related to enlargement and diminished function of the middle ear ossicles or expansion of surrounding bone in the inner ear.

Several complications occur in the setting of Paget's disease. First are those related to disorganized and fragile bone production. Pagetic bone is "soft" and prone to fracture and deformity (Fig. 28-7). Weakened subchondral bone leads to osteoarthritis, which occurs in 50% to 96% of patients with Paget's disease (Fig. 28-6A). Basilar skull impression is common, occurring in one third of patients. Neurologic complications related to osseous expansion include sensorineural and conductive hearing loss and spinal stenosis. Neoplastic transformation, most commonly osteosarcoma, occurs in 1% of patients with Paget's disease (Fig. 28-8), although in the skull, giant cell tumor is the most common form of neoplastic transformation. New-onset pain in a patient with Paget's disease should alert the clinician to the possibility of sarcomatous transformation, which has a 1% survival at 2 years as the sarcomas resulting from Paget's disease are highly aggressive. Osteomyelitis is more common in patients with Paget's disease, and is thought to relate to the hypervascularity and subsequent increased risk that organisms such as *Staphylococcus aureus* would seed affected bones. Crystal deposition diseases, including monosodium urate and calcium pyrophosphate dihydrate, occur, possibly because of increased calcium mobilization in patients with Paget's disease. High-output cardiac failure is a rare complication of the disease, due to the high vascularity of

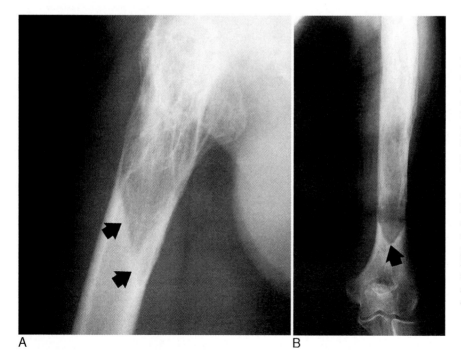

A   B

Figure 28-2   Paget's disease, long bones: blade of grass. **A,** Frog-leg lateral radiographic view of the right proximal femur shows the mixed lytic and sclerotic phase in the proximal aspect of pagetic bone and the lytic phase in the distal portion of pagetic bone. This indicates that the advancing front of Paget's disease is in the distal aspect of pagetic bone. The sharp, blade-like appearance of the margin between pagetic and normal bone *(arrows)* is shown, a feature that would be highly uncharacteristic for neoplasm. **B,** AP view of humerus in a different patient shows a flame-shaped distal margin of Paget's disease with abrupt transition to normal bone *(arrow)*. Note the mixed phase of Paget's disease in the more proximal humerus, where bone expansion, cortical bone thickening, and trabecular bone thickening are shown. At the flame-shaped margin, the appearance of Paget's disease is purely lytic.

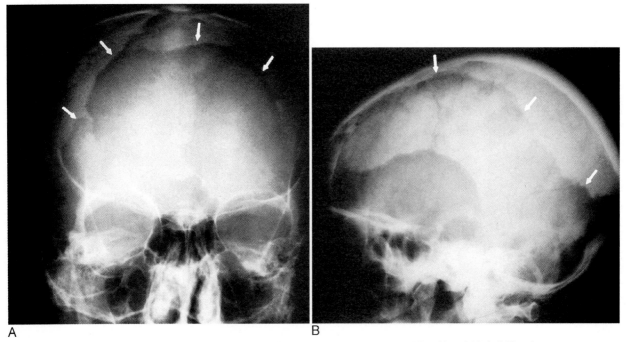

A   B

Figure 28-3   Paget's disease, lytic phase, skull: osteoporosis circumscripta. AP (A) and lateral (B) skull films show broad calvarial lytic region with sharp margins *(arrows)* between pagetic and normal bone in the acute, lytic phase of disease.

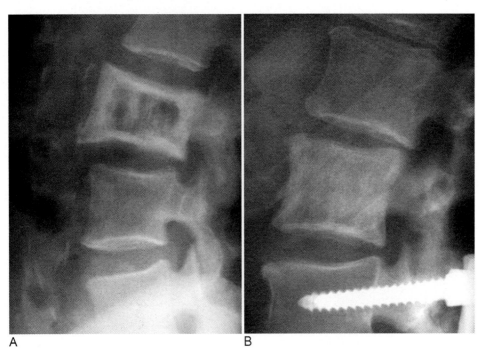

A   B

Figure 28-4   Paget's disease, mixed and sclerotic phase, spine. **A,** Lateral radiograph of lumbar spine shows picture frame appearance of L3 vertebral body. Note the increased density of the vertebral body, with greater density at the margins, trabecular bone thickening, and overall bone expansion. **B,** Subtler example of the same findings in a different patient. (Part A reprinted with permission from the American College of Radiology learning file.)

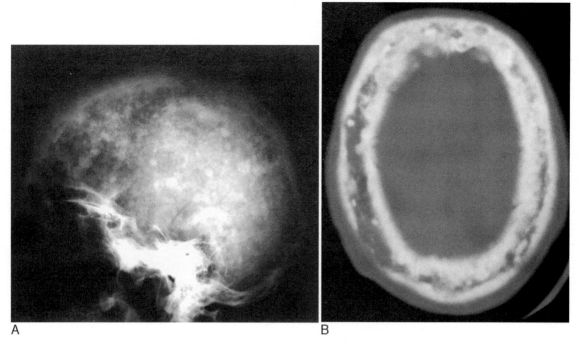

Figure 28-5 Paget's disease, mixed lytic and sclerotic phase, "cotton wool" skull. **A,** Lateral radiograph of the skull shows a cotton wool appearance due to the mixed lytic and sclerotic phase of Paget's disease. **B,** Axial CT in a different patient shows the patchy sclerosis, with thickening of the tables of the skull.

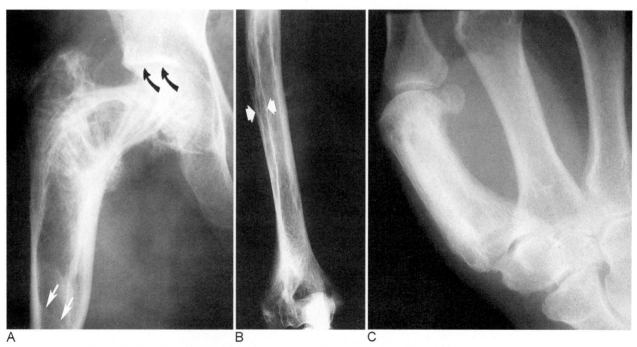

Figure 28-6 The essential features of Paget's disease are bone expansion, cortical bone thickening, and trabecular bone thickening. **A,** AP radiograph of the right hip shows bone expansion, cortical bone thickening, and trabecular bone thickening. Note also the abrupt transition to normal bone *(straight arrows)*. In addition, there is moderate osteoarthritis of the hip *(curved arrows)*, a common complication of Paget's disease adjacent to a joint. **B,** AP radiograph of humerus shows bone expansion, cortical bone thickening *(arrows)*, and trabecular bone thickening. **C,** Thumb metacarpal Paget's disease. Any bone can be involved with Paget's disease, although fibular involvement for some reason is extremely rare.

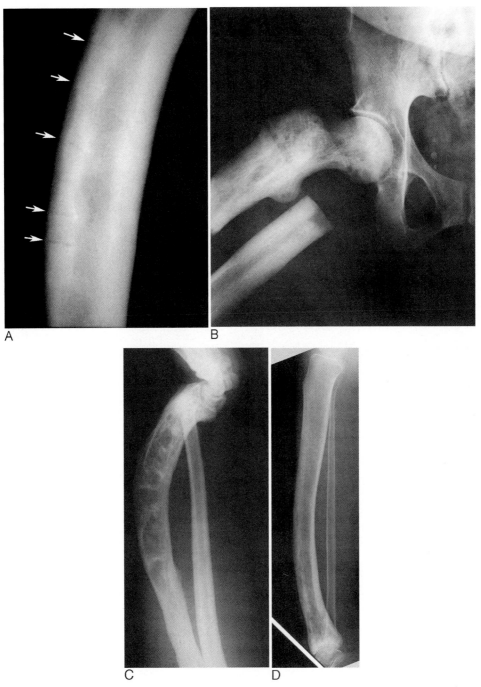

Figure 28-7   Complications of Paget's disease. **A,** Detail of a femur radiograph shows "banana fractures" *(arrows),* which are distraction insufficiency fractures on the convex side of a long bone curved by Paget's disease. **B,** Frog-leg lateral radiograph of the right hip shows insufficiency fracture of subtrochanteric femur and features of Paget's disease at and proximal to fracture site. **C,** Lateral radiograph of the left forearm shows substantial bone expansion in radius associated with cortical and trabecular bone thickening associated with angular deformity of radius due to multiple healed insufficiency fractures. **D,** Lateral radiograph of the leg shows Paget's disease of the distal tibia with anterior bowing. Note that the leading edge is well defined, but is subtler than the examples in Fig. 28-2. Also note the varus of the proximal femur in Fig. 28-6A, termed "shephard's crook deformity," which is a common complication.

pagetic bone. Anemia can occur because of the increase in plasma volume associated with high output failure. Occasional occurrence of metastasis in pagetic bone may relate to

increased vascularity as well. Another occasional complication of increased bone turnover in these patients is the possibility of rapid osteolysis that may occur when equilibrium between

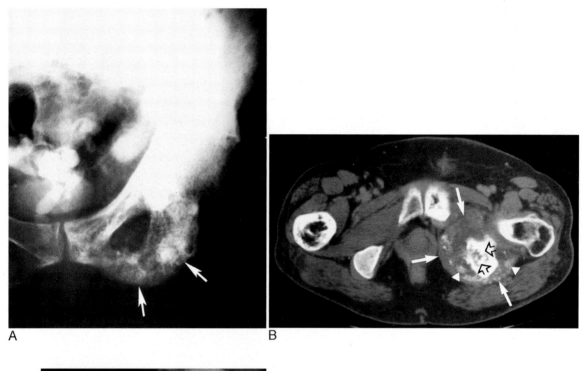

A

B

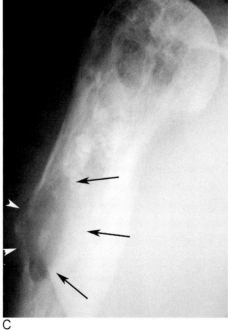

C

Figure 28-8   Paget sarcoma. **A,** AP radiograph of left pelvis shows bone expansion, cortical bone thickening, and trabecular bone thickening in pubic bone diagnostic for Paget's disease. In the ischium, however, there is an ill-defined mix of lysis and sclerosis *(arrows)* suspicious for sarcomatous transformation. **B,** Axial CT shows pagetic left ischium with cortical bone thickening and slight bone expansion. However, the ischium is surrounded by a large soft tissue mass *(closed arrows)* with associated fluffy matrix calcifications *(arrowheads)*. Similar calcifications are shown centrally in the ischium *(open arrows)*. The diagnosis at surgery was osteosarcoma with background of Paget's disease. **C,** Sarcomatous transformation in a different patient. Proximal humerus radiograph shows Paget's disease and a lytic lesion *(arrows)* with lateral cortical destruction *(arrowheads)* that was a new finding. This was a high-grade osteosarcoma.

bone production and lysis is disrupted in situations in which patients become non–weight-bearing (Fig. 28-9).

Treatment with bisphosphonates that inhibit osteoclast-mediated bone resorption can be helpful in patients with severe manifestations of Paget's disease. Calcitonin is occasionally used for treatment.

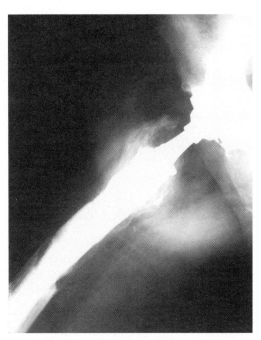

Figure 28-9   Frog-leg lateral radiograph of right proximal femur in patient with Paget's disease obtained 1 month after total hip replacement. In the interval, there has been rapid osteolysis of the pagetic bone due to non–weight-bearing in the perioperative period.

Part V Sources and Suggested Readings

Holick MF, Krane SM, Potts JT: Calcium, phosphorus, and bone metabolism: Calcium regulating hormones. In Fauci AS, Braunwald E, Isselbacher KJ, et al. (eds): Harrison's Principles of Internal Medicine, ed. 14. New York, McGraw-Hill, 1998.

Knockel JP: Disorders of phosphorus metabolism. In Fauci AS, Braunwald E, Isselbacher KJ, et al. (eds): Harrison's Principles of Internal Medicine, ed 14. New York, McGraw-Hill, 1998.

Krane SM, Holick MF: Metabolic bone disease. In Fauci AS, Braunwald E, Isselbacher KJ, et al. (eds): Harrison's Principles of Internal Medicine, ed 14. New York, McGraw-Hill, 1998.

Lenchik L, Sartoris DJ: Current concepts in osteoporosis. AJR 168:905–911, 1997.

Olsen KM, Chew FS: Tumoral Calcinosis: Pearls, polemics, and alternative possibilities. Radiographics 26:871–885, 2006.

Potts JT: Diseases of the parathyroid gland and other hyper- and hypocalcemic disorders. In Fauci AS, Braunwald E, Isselbacher KJ, et al. (eds): Harrison's Principles of Internal Medicine, ed 14. New York, McGraw-Hill, 1998.

Resnick D (ed): Diagnosis of Bone and Joint Disorders, ed 4. Philadelphia, W.B. Saunders, 2002.

Swischuk LE, Hayden CK, Jr: Rickets: A roentgenographic scheme for diagnosis. Pediatr Radiol 8:203–208, 1979.

VI

TUMORS

DISCRIMINATORS
IMAGING TECHNIQUES
   Radionuclide Studies
   Computed Tomography
   Magnetic Resonance Imaging
   Ultrasonography

This chapter provides an introduction to some of the descriptive terminology of tumor imaging, with emphasis on applying this terminology to a concise description of radiographic findings and a narrow differential diagnosis. The equally important topics of tumor staging, tumor biopsy, and assessment of tumor response to therapy are discussed in subsequent chapters, and are reviewed in Chapter 38.

Bone and soft tissue tumors can be categorized as benign or malignant. Malignant tumors can be primary, secondary (that is, due to malignant transformation of a preexisting lesion), or metastatic in origin. Tumor mimics (i.e., musculoskeletal mass lesions that are not true neoplasms) can be considered as another category, but are often lumped with benign tumors. The distinction between benign and malignant can be difficult for many musculoskeletal neoplasms, both for the pathologist and the radiologist. The pathologist often relies heavily on findings made by the radiologist and orthopedic oncologist to make a diagnosis. In many cases, the imaging features are best described in terms of the aggressiveness of the lesion. The terms *aggressive* or *nonaggressive* refer to the local behavior of the tumor. Always keep in mind that many aggressive tumors are not malignant. Examples of benign, radiographically aggressive lesions include Langerhans cell histiocytosis, infection, aneurysmal bone cyst, and giant cell tumor. Also, one should note that many malignant tumors do not have aggressive features on imaging studies. Finally, one must always keep in mind the possibility of metastatic disease.

Tumor imaging may include magnetic resonance imaging (MRI), computed tomography (CT), bone scanning, positron emission tomography (PET), angiography, and ultrasonography (US) but should always include radiography. The radi-ograph is usually the single best imaging test with which to diagnose many tumors, especially primary bone tumors. In fact, in most cases, the radiograph is the only test needed to make a diagnosis and guide patient management. The other tests are mostly used for staging purposes. The remainder of this introductory chapter therefore emphasizes radiographic findings.

DISCRIMINATORS

Some tumors can be diagnosed with simple pattern recognition, but in general an organized approach is needed, analogous to arthritis imaging (Table 29-1). Always consider the following discriminators.

1. *Tumor margin/pattern of bone destruction.* These closely related terms refer to the appearance of the margin between the tumor and the host bone. This extremely important discriminator applies primarily to lytic (radiolucent) bone lesions. Description of the tumor margin/pattern of bone destruction includes analysis of 1) the width of the margin between normal bone and clearly abnormal bone, also known as the *zone of transition,* and 2) the presence or absence of sclerosis at the tumor margin. Lytic bone tumor margins can be divided into five types: types 1A to C (geographic), 2 ("moth-eaten"), and 3 (permeative) (Tables 29-2, 29-3).

Type 1 lesions have a well-defined zone of transition between the abnormal and normal bone. These are also termed

Table 29-1	Key Criteria for Categorizing a Solitary Osseous Lesion on Plain Radiographs

Margin (especially for lytic lesions)
Tumor matrix
Location
Periosteal reaction
Age of patient

Table 29-2	Tumor Margin/Pattern of Bone Destruction

Applies to lytic lesions
Type 1 (Geographic):
    1A: Narrow zone of transition, sclerotic margin; nonaggressive
    1B: Narrow zone of transition, nonsclerotic margin; usually nonaggressive
    1C: Wide zone of transition, nonsclerotic margin; aggressive
Type 2 (moth eaten): Multiple lytic areas; aggressive
Type 3 (permeative): Aggressive

Table 29-3	Tumor Margin Differential Diagnosis

Type 1A margin
Nonaggressive, benign
Numerous benign lesions, including bone cyst,* nonossifying fibroma, fibrous dysplasia, osteoid osteoma, chondroblastoma chronic osteomyelitis,* low grade chondrosarcoma,* Langerhans cell histiocytosis*
Type 1B margin
Nonaggressive
Bone cyst*
Enchondroma
Chondromyxoid fibroma
Giant cell tumor*
Type 1C margin
Aggressive
Giant cell tumor*
Osteosarcoma*
Malignant fibrous histiocytoma
Chondrosarcoma
Osteomyelitis*
Brown tumor
Langerhans cell histiocytosis*
Metastasis*
Type 2 (moth-eaten)
Aggressive
Malignant neoplasms, primary and metastatic*
Osteomyelitis
Langerhans cell histiocytosis
Type 3 (permeated = resorption of bone in Haversian systems)
Aggressive
Neoplastic: Round cell tumors, osteosarcoma,* metastasis*
Metabolic: Hyperparathyroidism
Mechanical: Fracture, aggressive osteoporosis
Osteomyelitis*

*Note that several lesions may have a variety of appearances.

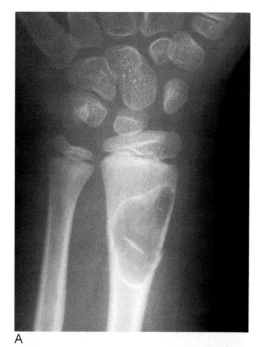

A

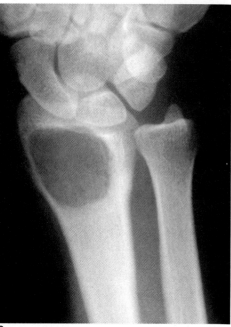

B

Figure 29-1   Nonaggressive tumor margins. **A,** Geographic lesion (mass is easily outlined) with sharp, sclerotic (1A) margins. Note the "fallen fragment sign" of a cortical fracture fragment that has fallen into this solitary bone cyst (*arrow;* see Chapter 37 for further discussion of this sign). **B,** Geographic lesion with sharp but not sclerotic (1B) margins in this giant cell tumor of the distal radius.

*geographic lesion*s because the tumor margins are clearly seen and are reminiscent of a national border on a map. Type 1 lesions are divided according to the width of the zone of transition. Type 1A and 1B lesions have very sharply defined margins (i.e., the zone of transition is very narrow, as if drawn with a sharp pencil) (Fig. 29-1). The difference between type 1A and 1B lesions is the presence or absence of host bone sclerosis at the margin. Type 1A lesions have a sclerotic rim. Type 1B tumors do not have a sclerotic rim. Type 1A lesions are the

least aggressive bone tumors, and are almost always benign (see Table 29-3). Think of the process as so slow growing that the host bone has walled it off with a sclerotic wall. Type 1B lesions usually are nonaggressive. Type 1C lesions have a nonsclerotic margin with a broad zone of transition (Fig. 29-2). Type 1C lesions are aggressive.

Type 2 lesions have a moth-eaten pattern of regional multifocal bone destruction, manifested as multiple discrete holes

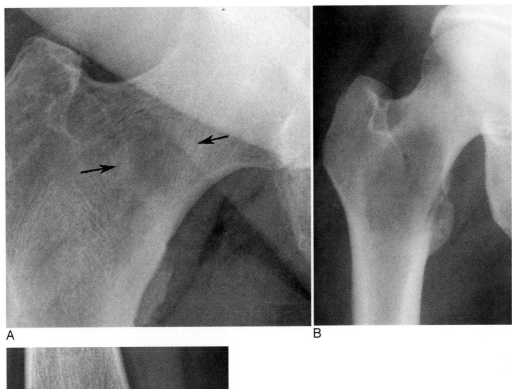

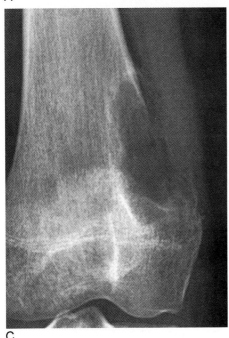

Figure 29-2   Aggressive tumor margins: well-defined margins with broad zone of transition (1C margins). **A,** Subtle femoral neck geographic lesion with "fuzzy" margins (wide zone of transition, 1C), a lung adenocarcinoma metastasis. **B,** Another 1C lesion, with a wider zone of transition and cortical breakthrough. This is a plasmacytoma. **C,** Another lesion with a well-defined but wide zone of transition. This also was a lung cancer metastasis.

(Fig. 29-3). Type 3 lesions have a permeative pattern of bone destruction that represents tumor infiltration and enlargement of the Haversian systems. In both patterns, the zone of transition between clearly normal and clearly abnormal bone is broad, and it is difficult to draw the lesion margins. Distinguishing type 2 from type 3 margins can be difficult but is not always necessary because both indicate a highly aggressive process.

Some authors simplify this system by grouping 1C, 2, and 3 lesions together as "permeative" or "aggressive." Type 1A and 1B lesions are "geographic," either with or without a sclerotic margin. This highly practical approach is used in some of the major musculoskeletal radiology textbooks.

If a lesion has a mixture of findings (e.g., mostly a 1A margin but a small section with a 1B margin), the lesion is considered to be 1B. In other words, always judge a lesion by its most aggressive margin (Fig. 29-4).

The reader should remain aware that some lesions are notorious for causing a variety of bone destruction patterns. Examples of lesions with highly variable radiographic presentation are metastases, osteomyelitis, Langerhans cell histiocytosis, and chondrosarcoma.

Another descriptor of bone destruction is *endosteal scalloping,* which refers to sharply marginated destruction of the inner margin of cortical bone by a medullary tumor. Endosteal

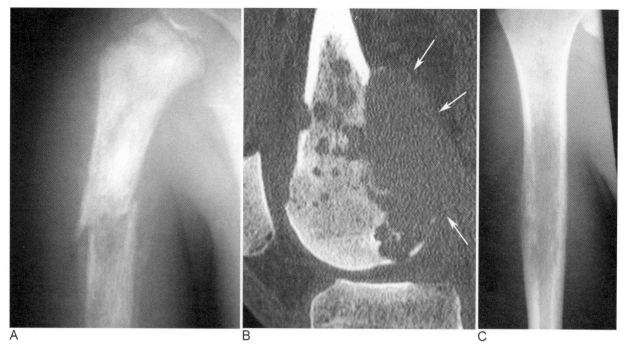

Figure 29-3   Aggressive tumor margins: permeative and moth-eaten lesions (type 2 and 3 margins). **A,** An example of permeative (type 3) bone destruction, with the tumor infiltrating among trabeculae, destroying some but leaving others. This metadiaphyseal lesion is an osteosarcoma arising in an 8-year-old boy. (Reprinted with permission from the American College of Radiology learning file.) **B,** Sagittal CT reconstruction shows moth-eaten pattern (type 2 margin) in the distal femur due to metastatic lung cancer. Note soft tissue mass *(arrows)*. **C,** Lesion with permeative and moth-eaten features (type 2 and 3 margins) due to Ewing's sarcoma in a 14-year-old. Note the subtle lucent areas in the proximal metaphysis. The distinction between type 2 and 3 margins is usually not significant; either indicates a highly aggressive lesion.

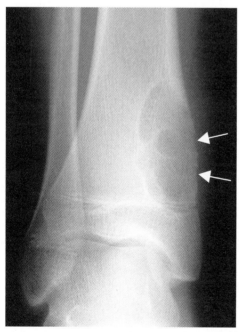

Figure 29-4   Aggressive tumor margins: mixture of aggressive and nonaggressive margins in a 17-year-old male. Most of the margins are sharp and sclerotic (1A, nonaggressive), suggesting a nonaggressive lesion. However, there is cortical breakthrough medially *(arrow)*, an aggressive finding. Despite the nonaggressive appearance of most of the lesion margin, the cortical destruction must be considered a red flag and the lesion must be worked up as an aggressive lesion. At biopsy, this was an osteosarcoma.

bone destruction may progress to cortical breakthrough if the lesion is highly aggressive, or may progress to bone expansion if the periosteum can maintain an intact layer of overlying bone in less aggressive lesions, or may be limited to endosteal scalloping if the lesion is still less aggressive. This latter pattern is frequently seen with enchondromas, low-grade chondrosarcomas, nonossifying fibroma, and adamantinoma

2. *Lesion density/tumor matrix.* Is the lesion purely lytic (radiolucent), purely blastic (radiodense), or mixed lytic and blastic? Note that, when present, bone lysis is due to hormonal and mechanical factors, not direct bone destruction by the tumor. Fifty percent of trabecular bone must be destroyed before a lytic medullary lesion becomes visible on radiographs.

Table 29-4   Tumor Matrix
Chondroid
Arcs and rings
Cartilage-forming tumors: Enchondroma, chondrosarcoma,   chondroblastoma
Osteoid
Cloud-like, amorphous
Bone-forming tumors: Osteosarcoma, osteoid osteoma, osteoblastoma;   also the ground-glass density in fibrous dysplasia
Also can be seen in early fracture healing and early myositis ossificans

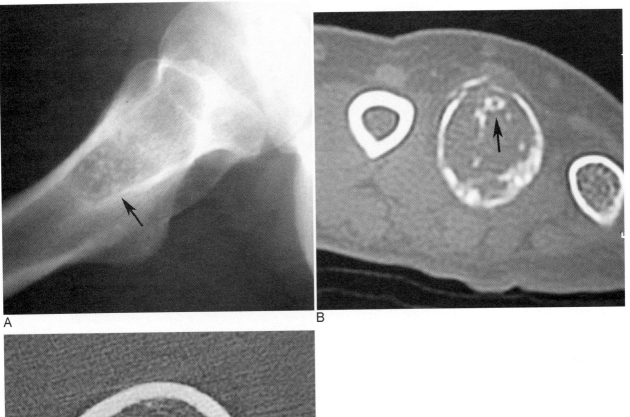

Figure 29-5   Chondroid matrix. **A,** Lateral radiograph of the proximal femur shows the dense "rings and arcs" or "Cs and Js" calcification of chondroid matrix in a grade 1 chondrosarcoma *(arrow).* **B,** Axial CT of a metacarpal enchondroma with associated cortical expansion and fracture. Another description of chondroid matrix is "circles or pieces of circles with a radius of 1 to 2 mm." Note the centimeter markers at the right side of the image and the chondroid matrix, including one complete ring *(arrow).* **C,** Axial CT of an enchondroma in the distal femoral metaphysis shows similar pattern of calcification.

If the lesion is partially calcified, is the calcification in a specific pattern of tumor matrix (Table 29-4)? Chondroid tumors and osteosarcomas often produce a histologically and radiographically distinct tumor matrix (Fig. 29-5). *Chondroid matrix* is endochondral ossification of chondroid nodules. Radiographically, it appears as circles or pieces of circles with a radius of 1 to 2 mm. Other descriptions of chondroid matrix are "arcs and rings," "punctate," "popcorn," or "C- and J-shaped" calcifications. The calcification of chondroid matrix tends to be dense for its size, especially in comparison with osteoid matrix.

Osteoid matrix, which is produced by osteosarcoma, osteoid osteoma, and osteoblastoma, may calcify in an amorphous pattern, sometimes described as "cloud-like," "fluffy," or "cotton wool" (Fig. 29-6). Also, the ground-glass opacification often seen in fibrous dysplasia is due to calcification of osteoid. In contrast, *ossification* (such as normal bone or mature myositis ossificans) is quite different because it has well-defined trabeculae and cortex. Periosteal reaction often coexists with tumor matrix in aggressive osteosarcomas. Calcification of osteoid in early fracture healing and early myositis ossificans can have an identical appearance to tumor osteoid and is therefore a potential diagnostic pitfall, as a benign process can appear as an aggressive process both radiographically and at histology.

If the radiographic findings are indeterminate for presence or type of tumor matrix, CT can be an excellent problem solver because it usually clearly identifies the pattern of calcification.

3. *Location of lesion.* There are three aspects of lesion location, any of which may be important in determining the probable histologic features of the lesion. First, the particular bone in which the lesion is found may be important. For example,

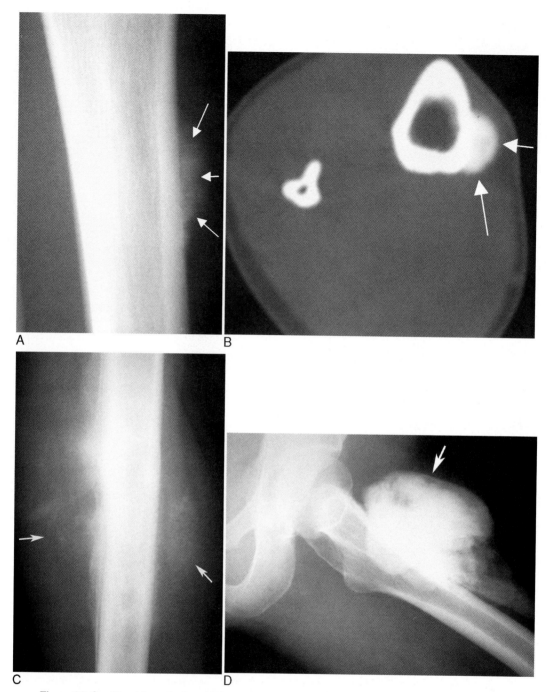

Figure 29-6 Osteoid matrix. **A and B,** AP radiograph (A) and axial CT image (B) of a surface osteosarcoma in the tibia of an 18-year-old man. The lesion arises from the surface of bone, forming amorphous osteoid matrix in the adjacent soft tissues *(arrows).* **C,** Subtle amorphous calcification in the soft tissues of an osteosarcoma *(arrows).* The matrix is less dense than bone and shows no evidence of organized bone formation. **D,** Mixed pattern of dense osteoid matrix and regions of bone formation with trabecula and cortex *(arrow)* in a 22-year-old woman. This is a parosteal osteosarcoma.

certain tumors occur most commonly in specific bones. Localization may refer to a specific bone such as the tibia (a frequent location of adamantinoma, ossifying fibroma, and chondromyxoid fibroma—all rare lesions), or a category of bones such as flat versus tubular, or appendicular versus axial. The second aspect of lesion location is location along the length of a tubular bone (Table 29-5). Although many lesions are meta-

physeal, some lesions are characteristically found in the region of the epiphysis (chondroblastoma) and others are more frequently found in a diaphyseal location (Ewing sarcoma). The third aspect related to location of lesion is location in the transverse plane of a long bone. Many lesions are centrally located ("concentric"), whereas others are eccentrically located or even cortically based or surface lesions (Fig. 29-7, Table 29-6).

Table 29-5   Typical Locations for Solitary Bone Lesions: Longitudinal Location

Epiphysis: Chondroblastoma, subchondral cyst, giant cell tumor (growth plate closed)

Metaphysis: Osteosarcoma, chondrosarcoma, enchondroma, osteochondroma, giant cell tumor (growth plate open)

Diaphysis: Round cell tumors (lymphoma, myeloma, Ewing's sarcoma)

4. *Periosteal reaction.* Periosteal reaction represents new bone formation arising from the periosteum, frequently but not always elevated away from the bone surface (Tables 29-7, 29-8). The terms "periostitis," "periosteal reaction," and "periosteal new bone formation" are often used as synonyms. Periosteal reaction occurs with many processes, most commonly healing fracture, osteomyelitis, and tumor. Mechanical and local hormonal factors promote activation of periosteal new bone formation. The periosteal reaction is not the underlying process, but rather is a response to the process.

As with lesion margins, the pattern of periosteal reaction is an indicator of underlying lesion aggression. Periosteal reaction can be described as uninterrupted (solid) versus interrupted. Descriptors of interrupted periosteal reaction include lamellated, hair-on-end, sunburst, and absent.

Uninterrupted periosteal reaction is uniform cortical thickening (Fig. 29-8). "Solid" or "mature" are synonyms. In general, solid periosteal reaction reflects a slow-growing, nonaggressive lesion,

or a lesion that has healed either spontaneously or following successful treatment. Tumor mimics and other nonneoplastic processes, such as healing fractures, healing or chronic osteomyelitis, or hypertrophic osteoarthropathy, typically follow this pattern of periosteal reaction. Osteoid osteoma and, to a lesser degree, osteoblastoma elicit an intense solid periosteal reaction that can be very painful. Although clinically quite obnoxious, these are not aggressive lesions in terms of bone destruction or malignant potential.

If the tumor has slowly "expanded" the bone, the original cortex has been resorbed and the periosteum has produced a new cortex. This is a type of uninterrupted periosteal reaction. The expanded bone may have only an eggshell-thin new cortex, but if intact, it usually indicates a nonaggressive lesion.

Interrupted periosteal reaction indicates a more aggressive lesion (Fig. 29-9). Types of interrupted periosteal reaction include *lamellated (onionskin), hair-on-end,* and sunburst. Lamellated periosteal reaction is layers of solid periosteal new bone formation parallel to the adjacent cortex separated by thin radiolucent layers of unossified matrix or tumor. Hair-on-end and sunburst periosteal reaction indicate rapidly growing, highly aggressive lesions (Fig. 29-6). A *Codman's triangle* is a triangular area of periosteal calcification that has formed at the margins of an aggressive lesion, with the periosteum not seen elsewhere because it is destroyed or is elevated so rapidly by the tumor that it cannot form visible new bone.

Cortical breakthrough of a bone lesion is created by soft tissue extension of a lesion through the cortex and periosteum

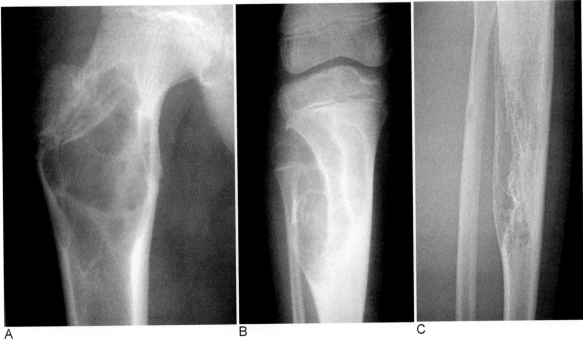

Figure 29-7   Transverse locations of tumors in long bones. **A,** AP radiograph showing a central lesion in the proximal femur, a solitary bone cyst in an 11-year-old boy. **B,** AP radiograph demonstrating an eccentric location of a metaphyseal lesion, in this case a chondromyxoid fibroma in an 18-year-old woman. **C,** A cortically based lesion in the mid-shaft of the tibia in a 14-year-old girl. Although from the radiograph alone one may not be able to determine that the lesion is completely cortically based, CT in part D confirms this.

(Continued)

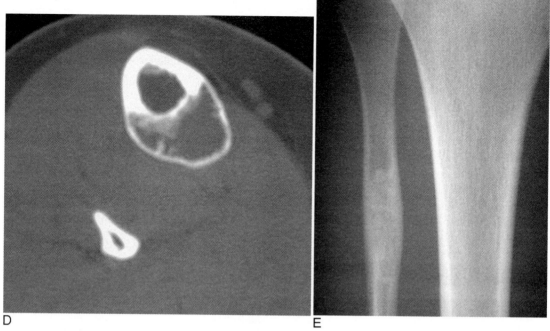

Figure 29-7—(Cont'd) **D,** In this case, the lesion is an unusual manifestation of fibrous dysplasia, which can occasionally be cortically based. **E,** AP radiograph demonstrating a nonossifying fibroma that is healing with sclerosis. Nonossifying fibroma is usually a cortically based lesion; however, when it occurs in very small bones such as the fibula, it fills the entire marrow space and gives the appearance of being a central lesion. For examples of a juxtacortical lesions, see Fig. 29-3.

Table 29-6   Cortical and Juxtacortical Tumor

Cortical
   Osteoid osteoma
   Fibrous lesions: Nonossifying fibroma ("fibrous cortical defect"),
     osteofibrous dysplasia (ossifying fibroma)
   Adamantinoma
Juxtacortical
   Osteochondroma
   Parosteal or periosteal osteosarcoma
   Juxtacortical chondroma
   Ganglion
   Any soft tissue tumor near the bone

Table 29-7   Periosteal Reaction

Solid: Nonaggressive process
Expanded shell: Nonaggressive
Interrupted: Aggressive
   Lamellated ("onionskin")
   Hair-on-end
   Sunburst
   Codman's triangle

Table 29-8   Periosteal New Bone Formation in Children

Infection/inflammation
Healing fracture
Metabolic (scurvy, hypervitaminosis A and D, Gaucher's disease, others)
Physiologic (during rapid growth)
Solid tumors (often aggressive periosteal reaction)
Leukemia
Premature birth (prostaglandin E, physiologic, metabolic disease of
   prematurity)
Melorheostosis

---

and indicates an aggressive lesion. Infection can mimic an aggressive osseous tumor in its pattern of bone destruction as it can extend into the soft tissue as well. The appearance of the soft tissue fascial planes may help to distinguish infection from tumor, as tumor tends to displace fascial planes whereas infection tends to obliterate them.

5. *Age of patient.* This parameter is essential for diagnosis, as some lesions are typically found among certain age groups (Table 29-9). For example, a patient older than age 50 with a solitary lesion lytic lesion should be considered most likely to have metastasis or a plasmacytoma rather than primary bone tumor. Similarly, between 30 and 60 years of age, chondrosarcoma, primary lymphoma, and malignant fibrous histiocy-

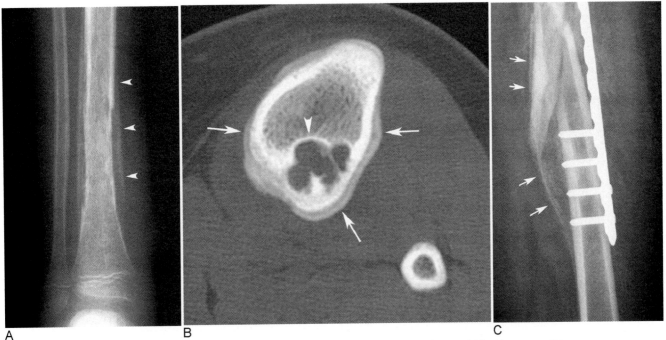

Figure 29-8   Nonaggressive periosteal reaction. **A,** Distal tibia radiograph in a child with osteomyelitis shows uninterrupted periosteal reaction *(arrowheads)*. Note the aggressive bone destruction. The comparatively nonaggressive solid periosteal reaction was an important clue to the correct diagnosis. **B,** CT of a nonossifying fibroma *(arrowhead)* in the distal tibia in a child with an associated pathologic fracture (not shown). In this case, the periosteal elevation *(arrows)* was not caused by the tumor but rather by healing response to a pathologic fracture through the tumor. Note the well-defined, sclerotic (1A) tumor margin. **C,** Detail view of an internally fixed femur shaft shows solid, continuous new bone *(arrows)* formed by periosteum elevated by hematoma. This will remodel into mature bone.

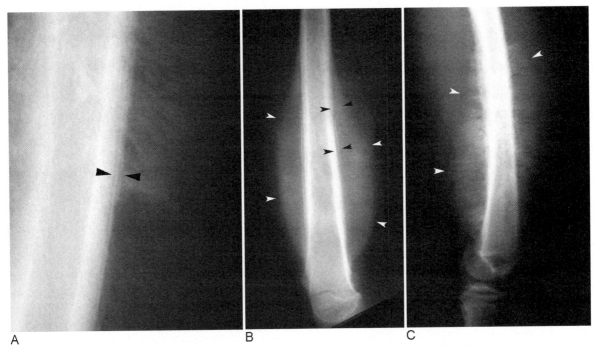

Figure 29-9   Aggressive periosteal reaction. **A,** Detail of a femur radiograph of a child with osteosarcoma shows subtle lamellated (between *arrowheads*) and hair-on-end periosteal reaction. **B,** Lateral femur radiograph in a child with Ewing's sarcoma shows interrupted *(black arrowheads)* and hair-on-end *(white arrowheads)* periosteal reaction. **C,** Older child with an osteosarcoma. Note florid periosteal reaction *(white arrowheads)*.

(Continued)

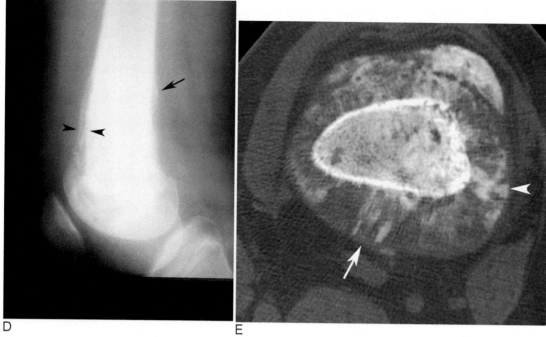

Figure 29-9—(Cont'd)   **D,** Another older child with an osteosarcoma. Note lamellated periosteal reaction (between *black arrowheads*) and Codman's triangle *(arrow)*. **E,** Axial CT image of a teenager with distal femur osteosarcoma shows a mixture of hair-on-end periosteal reaction *(arrow)* and osteoid tumor matrix *(arrowhead)*.

Table 29-9   Age as a Criterion for Osseous Tumor

Age (y)	Lesion
1	Metastatic neuroblastoma
1–10	Ewing's sarcoma
10–30	Osteosarcoma more frequent than Ewing's sarcoma
	Epiphysis, skeletally immature: Chondroblastoma, eosinophilic granuloma, osteomyelitis
	Epiphysis, skeletally mature: Giant cell tumor
30–60	Chondrosarcoma, primary lymphoma, malignant fibrous histiocytoma, fibrosarcoma
50–80	Metastasis, multiple myeloma

toma should be strongly considered. An aggressive lesion in a tubular (long) bone in a child younger than age 10 is more likely to be Ewing's sarcoma than osteosarcoma, but between the ages of 10 and 20 years osteosarcoma is more likely.

Estimates of relative tumor prevalence and distribution by age are limited for many musculoskeletal neoplasms because of their rarity. Investigators from the Armed Forces Institute of Pathology (AFIP) reported the distribution of musculoskeletal tumors by age from their very large registry in 1995 (see Kransdorf, 1995). Some musculoskeletal radiologists use this data to help to guide their differential diagnoses. However, this list is subject to selection bias, as only cases sent to the AFIP are included.

Other features can assist in evaluating a bone tumor. For example, if the lesion is polyostotic it will fall into either the benign polyostotic category (fibrous dysplasia, Paget's disease, histiocytosis, multiple exostosis, multiple enchondromatosis) or the malignant category (metastases, multiple myeloma, primary bone tumors with bony metastases [e.g., Ewing's sarcoma, osteosarcoma, and malignant fibrous histiocytoma], or polyostotic primary neoplasms [e.g., hemangioendothelioma and angiosarcoma]).

The following is a sample template of a radiographic description of a solitary bone tumor:

"There is a ____ cm (central, eccentric, surface, exophytic) (lytic, blastic, mixed density) lesion in the (specific bone and location within the bone-diaphysis, etc.). The tumor margin/pattern of bone destruction (if applicable) is (1A, 1B, 1C, 2 or 3/'geographic with a sclerotic margin,' etc.). The tumor contains (chondroid, osteoid, no) tumor matrix. There is (no, solid, interrupted, lamellated, hair-on-end, etc.) periosteal reaction. There is/is no (bone expansion, cortical breakthrough, extraosseous soft tissue mass). Overall, the lesion has (nonaggressive, aggressive, highly aggressive radiographic features)."

A complete report will also include diagnostic possibilities and recommendations for additional imaging, biopsy, and/or laboratory and clinical evaluation if appropriate. For example, some lesions are "don't touch" lesions (i.e., benign with malignant features at histology, such as myositis ossificans and healing fracture).

IMAGING TECHNIQUES

As noted previously, radiographs are essential for diagnostic work-up of bone tumors and are sometimes helpful in evaluating soft tissue tumors. Other imaging studies are used for staging, and sometimes as diagnostic problem solvers.

Radionuclide Studies

Bone scanning with technetium(99m)Tc methylene diphosphonate is used for staging purposes, to evaluate whether more than one bone lesion is present (i.e., to search for metastatic disease or "skip lesions" of multifocal osteosarcoma). Bone scanning also is used if it is desirable to determine whether an osseous lesion is monostotic or polyostotic. It's also useful for evaluating a blastic lesion because a blastic lesion that is not "hot" on bone scanning is highly likely to be inactive.

Positron emission tomography using 18F fluorodeoxyglucose may be used to evaluate tumor metabolic activity, based on glucose uptake and retention. This is a promising method for tumor characterization and possibly even grading, and for detecting recurrent or residual tumor after therapy.

Computed Tomography

Generally, MRI is preferred for local staging both in osseous and soft tissue tumors. However, CT is often used to evaluate extraosseous extension, and is often preferred for evaluating chest wall masses because respiratory motion is easier to control with CT than with MRI. Computed tomography is excellent for diagnostic purposes for demonstrating matrix calcification, assessing for degree and pattern of bone destruction, and detecting a thin rim of calcification over an expansile tumor.

Magnetic Resonance Imaging

Because of its superb soft tissue contrast and multiplanar capability, MRI is often the best test for local staging. However, it is not perfect. First, a high-quality examination is needed, and the entire lesion must be included (Table 29-10). The relationship of the tumor and reactive tissue to critical adjacent structures such as growth plates, neurovascular bundles, and joints must be demonstrated. T1- and T2-weighted images, the latter preferably with fat suppression, are needed for a complete examination. Intravenous gadolinium is occasionally helpful to, for example, distinguish a solid from cystic lesion or guide biopsy to viable (enhancing) tissue rather than necrotic tumor, which does not enhance. Many centers use dynamic gadolinium enhancement to assist in differentiating malignant tumor from reactive tissue, or benign from malignant, as malignant tumors tend to enhance more rapidly. This technique is not widely used in the United States.

Table 29-10   MRI of Musculoskeletal Tumors: Technical Requirements

1. Surface coils must be used if possible.
2. Axial images are required for evaluation of compartments as well as neurovascular bundles.
3. The entire extent of the lesion must be imaged with axial sequences. One longitudinal scan is also included for evaluation of skip metastases.
4. Inclusion of an externally palpable landmark is highly desirable, allowing measurement of distance to the lesion to be accurately translated from the scan to the surgical site.
5. T1-weighted imaging must be included because it shows high tumor-to-fat contrast.
6. T2-weighted sequences are generally included, showing high tumor-to-muscle contrast.
7. Evaluation of joint involvement often requires coronal or sagittal imaging.
8. Inversion recovery or gadolinium-enhanced imaging may subjectively enhance lesion conspicuity.
9. Gadolinium-enhanced imaging may assist in guiding biopsy of necrotic lesions.

Second, MRI may exaggerate or underestimate tumor size because peritumoral edema signal cannot reliably be differentiated from adjacent tumor. Also, tumor microinvasion into adjacent tissues may not be demonstrated by MRI.

Third, MRI is generally not reliable for diagnosis, or in predicting tumor grade. However, MRI may provide clues to the diagnosis (Tables 29-11–29-13). For example, the lobules of cartilage in chondroid tumors may be detected on T2-weighted sequences (see Chapter 32). Fat signal intensity in a soft tissue mass, confirmed with chemical fat suppression, indicates a lipoma or liposarcoma (Chapter 34). The presence of fluid-fluid levels can narrow the diagnosis (see Table 29-13). In addition, MRI may reveal flow voids in arteriovenous malformation. Highly cellular lesions such as lymphoma tend to have relatively low signal intensity compared with other uncalcified malignancies.

Table 29-11   Differential Diagnosis for Musculoskeletal Mass with Short T1 (High Signal Intensity on T1-Weighted Images)

Common:
   Fat (suppresses with chemical fat suppression): Lion poma, liposarcoma, hemangioma, dystrophic fat
   Methemoglobin: Hematoma, hemorrhage within a tumor
   Gadolinium enhancement
Uncommon:
   Proteinaceous material
   Melanin (high signal within melanoma metastases more likely to be due to methemoglobin)

Table 29-12	Differential Diagnosis for Musculoskeletal Mass with Predominantly Low Signal Intensity on T2-Weighted Images

Hypocellular fibrous tissue
   Tumor (e.g., plantar fibroma)
   Scar tissue
Dense mineralization
Melanin
Blood
   Acute hematoma
   Hemosiderin: Old hematoma, pigmented villonodular synovitis, giant cell tumor of the tendon sheath, synovium in patients with hemophilia
Vascular flow void
Gas
Foreign body
Gouty tophus
Amyloidosis
Methacrylate

Highly cellular tumors such as lymphoma often have intermediate-low signal intensity.

Table 29-13	Musculoskeletal Masses with Fluid-Fluid Levels

Giant cell tumor
Aneurysmal bone cyst
Telangiectatic osteosarcoma
Solitary bone cyst
Tumor necrosis
Hematoma, hemorrhage within a tumor
Chondroblastoma
Hemangioma if large low-flow channels are present
Cystic degeneration within fibrous dysplasia

Fourth, hemorrhage, hematoma, and inflammatory change may produce abnormal signal intensity patterns that can be confused with tumor. Infection (see Fig. 1-4) can involve several compartments, appear highly invasive, and incite prominent tissue reaction. Infections may have nonspecific signal intensity on MRI unless there is an encapsulated abscess (which can be demonstrated with injection of contrast medium). Similarly, hematoma, especially in a chronic stage, may be misdiagnosed as a neoplasm by MRI. Chronic hematomas often incite tremendous adjacent tissue reaction and appear to involve many compartments with a highly inhomogeneous mass (see Fig. 1-4). Hematoma can mask an underlying tumor. If there is a question of whether a lesion thought to be hematoma is truly that lesion, biopsy or close follow-up MRI to complete resolution is recommended.

Ultrasonography

Ultrasonography can depict, localize, and partially characterize relatively superficial soft tissue masses. Tumor vascularity can be assessed. This test can be used to guide percutaneous biopsy or to guide placement of a mammographic hook wire into a tumor to guide surgical resection.

CHAPTER 30

Bone-Forming Tumors: Benign

OSTEOMA
ENOSTOSIS (BONE ISLAND)
OSTEOID OSTEOMA
OSTEOBLASTOMA
OSSIFYING FIBROMA (OSTEOFIBROUS DYSPLASIA)

OSTEOMA

An osteoma is actually a hamartoma, an abnormal proliferation of compact bone without stromal cellular proliferation. Osteomas usually are found within membranous bones, either in the calvaria (usually arising from the external table) or the paranasal sinuses (Fig. 30-1). The entire lesion is densely sclerotic with well-defined margins. The lesion does not behave aggressively, although it can occasionally cause expansion of adjacent bone. Osteomas may be multifocal, especially as part of Gardner's syndrome, a disease of autosomal dominant inheritance that is associated with multiple colonic adenomatous polyps. Diagnosis is made by radiographic characteristics, and no treatment is necessary. If an osteoma is incidentally noted on magnetic resonance imaging (MRI), it will appear with low signal on all sequences because of its dense mineralization.

Differential diagnosis of an osteoma includes blastic metastasis and calvarial hyperostosis adjacent to a meningioma.

ENOSTOSIS (BONE ISLAND)

A bone island is a region of compact bone within the medullary space, surrounded by trabecular bone. Close inspection demonstrates spicules at the margin of the lesion that blend into the normal surrounding trabeculae (Fig. 30-2). This characteristic appearance is pathognomonic. The shape of a bone island is related to the general orientation of adjacent trabecular bone. In the shafts of long bones and at other sites where the trabeculae are mostly oriented longitudinally, the bone island is ovoid, with its long axis parallel to the long axis

of the bone. Bone islands in regions of more random trabecular orientation such as a metaphysis are more spherical. There is no host response to a bone island. There are two theories regarding the origin of bone islands. They may be hamartoma-

Key Concepts	Bone Island

Small round or oval focus of dense bone within medullary space.
Blends into surrounding trabeculae.
Occasionally enlarge slowly or present with large size; may therefore need to be differentiated from slow-growing low-grade osteosarcoma. Negative bone scan excludes osteosarcoma.

tous proliferations, like the osteoma, or they may represent areas of failure of osteoclast activity during bone remodeling. The lesion is very common, and is usually noted incidentally. Its size varies widely, but lesions larger than 1 cm are unusual except in the pelvis, where lesions up to 2.5 cm ("giant bone

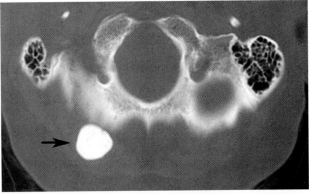

Figure 30-1 Osteoma. Axial CT of the head shows a very dense homogenous round suboccipital mass *(arrow)*, typical for an osteoma.

island") may occur. Lesions larger than these sizes, or lesions increasing in size, can be evaluated with bone scanning to assist in excluding blastic metastases or osteosarcoma (Fig. 30-3). A normal bone scan excludes the possibility of osteosarcoma. Note that a large bone island may show tracer uptake. Correlation with prostate-specific antigen (PSA) also can be helpful in men because it is often, although not always, elevated when metastatic prostate cancer to bone is present. If a bone island is noted on MRI, it will appear with low signal intensity on all sequences, identical to normal cortical bone. *Osteopoikilosis* is multiple bone islands clustered around joints. This condition is discussed further in Chapter 46.

In addition to blastic metastasis and osteosarcoma, the differential diagnosis of a large or atypically shaped bone island includes a dense osteoid osteoma that obscures its nidus and osteoblastoma. Bone islands occasionally increase in size over time, also potentially confusing the diagnosis.

OSTEOID OSTEOMA

Osteoid osteoma is a small lytic lesion (the *nidus*) surrounded by dense reactive bone formation. The nidus is composed of highly vascular fibrous tissue, osteoid, and immature bone. The nidus is the central lucent area on radiography or computed tomography (CT), although it may mineralize partially or nearly completely, potentially obscuring the lesion. Almost all present between the ages of 5 and 25 years. The male-to-female ratio is 2:1.

Osteoid osteomas have a typical clinical presentation of aching pain lasting weeks, months, or years. The pain is often worse at night and is relieved with aspirin. This presentation is not unique but suggests the diagnosis. These symptoms are dramatically relieved by complete excision of the lesion. Although painful, osteoid osteoma is a benign lesion and will spontaneously involute after about 3 years. However, the symptoms are usually so severe that most lesions are treated.

The appearance of an osteoid osteoma varies according to its location. The most common location of osteoid osteoma is the cortex of tubular bones. The local sclerotic reaction may be so dense that the nidus may be masked on plain film (Fig. 30-4). If the nidus is not seen, these lesions could be confused with prominent healing bone formation about a stress fracture or possibly reactive bone formation about a small chronic cortically based abscess (Fig. 30-5). Computed tomography, MRI, or bone scanning can show the cortical nidus when it is not seen on radiography. Cortical osteoid osteoma in children has similar features. Growth deformity can result from hypervascularity of the lesion.

Osteoid osteoma also may occur within a joint capsule, especially along the femoral neck. These lesions can be within cancellous bone rather than the cortex, and can be difficult to diagnose. Unlike the extra-articular cortical osteoid osteomas, these intracapsular lesions elicit little marginal sclerosis or

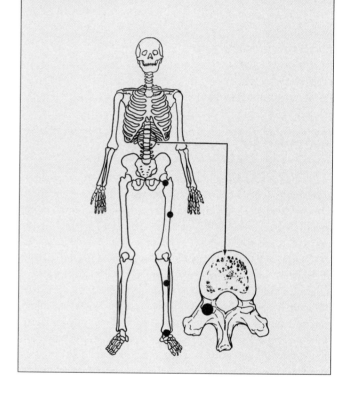

Small round or ovoid lytic lesion (the nidus), <1.5 cm. Nidus may contain sclerotic focus.

Painful, worse at night, relieved with nonsteroidal anti-inflammatory drugs.

Intense reactive sclerosis in long bone diaphyseal lesions. This may obscure nidus on radiographs. CT or MRI may be needed.

Reactive bone formation may occur at some distance from nidus if lesion is intracapsular.

Most common locations: Femoral diaphysis, tibial diaphysis, femoral neck, posterior elements of spine.

Treatment: Resection or ablation, surgically or with CT guidance.

periosteal bone formation because there is no periosteum inside the joint. However, new bone formation is often found at a considerable distance from the nidus, more distally along the cortex, much like the remote periosteal reaction found in chondroblastoma (Fig. 30-6). In addition, host reaction in the form of chronic synovitis can be intense with joint effusion and, over a long period, cartilage loss and osteoarthritis (see Fig. 30-6). If chronic synovitis and lateral subluxation of the femoral head occur in a child with an intracapsular osteoid osteoma, irreversible limb-length discrepancy and a valgus configuration of the femoral neck can result (Fig. 30-7). Because the sclerotic bone reaction is found at some distance from the nidus and the articular reaction can be extreme, the actual culprit in this variety of osteoid osteoma, the nidus, can

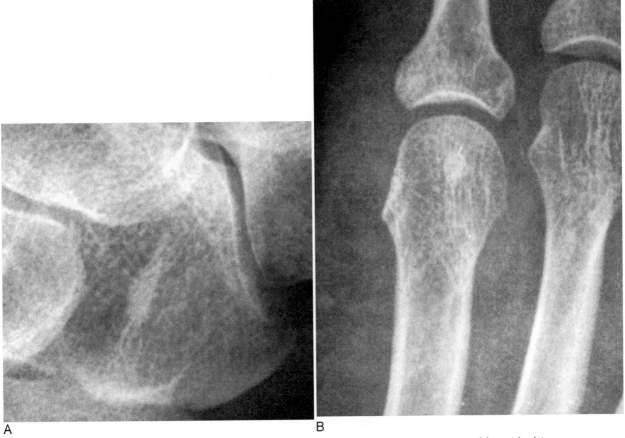

Figure 30-2   Bone island. **A,** Lateral radiograph of the cuboid, demonstrating a typical bone island in which dense bone formation is seen to be homogenous except at its peripheral edges, where it blends into the adjacent normal trabeculae. The lesion is elongate. **B,** AP radiograph shows a bone island in the fifth metatarsal head.

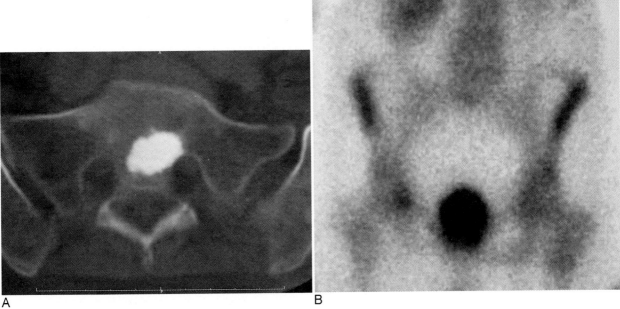

Figure 30-3   Bone scanning as problem solver for giant bone island. **A,** Detail from abdominal CT in a patient with breast cancer shows large sclerotic lesion in the sacrum. **B,** Diphosphonate bone scanning shows no significant tracer uptake by the lesion, excluding an active blastic metastasis or osteosarcoma.

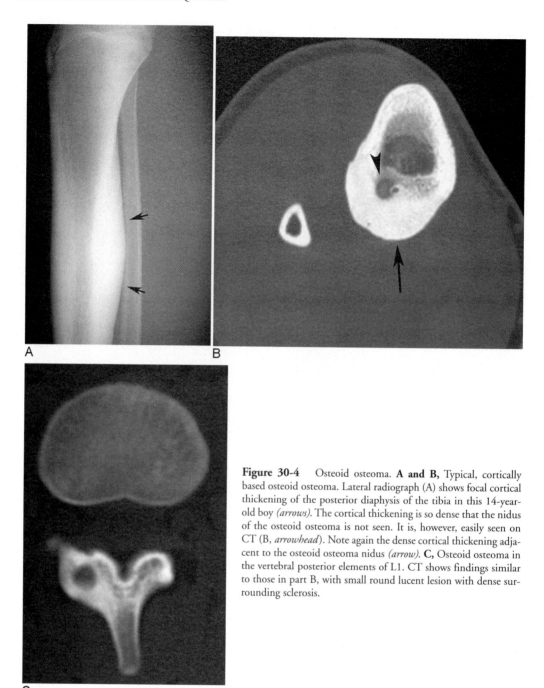

Figure 30-4   Osteoid osteoma. **A and B,** Typical, cortically based osteoid osteoma. Lateral radiograph (A) shows focal cortical thickening of the posterior diaphysis of the tibia in this 14-year-old boy *(arrows)*. The cortical thickening is so dense that the nidus of the osteoid osteoma is not seen. It is, however, easily seen on CT (B, *arrowhead*). Note again the dense cortical thickening adjacent to the osteoid osteoma nidus *(arrow)*. **C,** Osteoid osteoma in the vertebral posterior elements of L1. CT shows findings similar to those in part B, with small round lucent lesion with dense surrounding sclerosis.

be easily missed. Magnetic resonance imaging is the best "problem solver" test when an intra-articular osteoid osteoma is suspected.

The least common variety of osteoid osteoma is found in a subperiosteal location. These are manifest as a round, soft tissue mass located immediately adjacent to bone with underlying scalloping, irregular bone resorption, and little reactive change. The talus is the most common site of this rare variety of osteoid osteoma.

Osteoid osteomas also occur in the spine, especially the posterior elements (see Fig. 30-4C). The patient can develop painful scoliosis, with the lesion being formed at the concave margin of the apex of the curve. This scoliosis has no rotatory component. Because of the sclerotic reaction to the underlying nidus, an osteoid osteoma in the posterior elements of the spine can be mistaken for a blastic metastasis or sclerosis related to abnormal stress, particularly in a patient with contralateral spondylolysis.

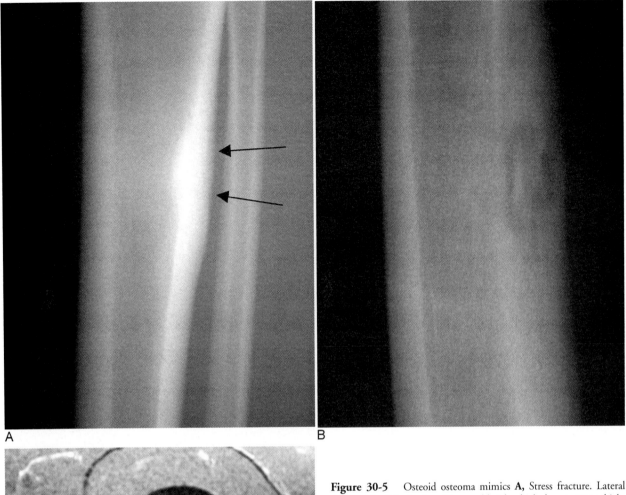

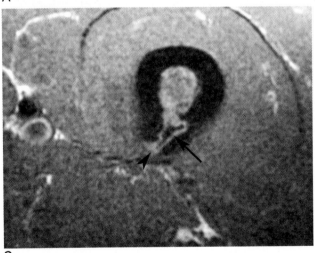

Figure 30-5   Osteoid osteoma mimics **A,** Stress fracture. Lateral radiograph of the leg in a 16-year-old girl, which demonstrates thickening of the cortex of the tibia in the posterior medial position in its proximal third *(arrows)*. This is a typical location for a stress fracture, which it proved to be. However, the radiographic appearance is not always distinguishable from an osteoid osteoma with the nidus obscured. **B and C,** Intracortical abscess with sequestrum. **B,** Lateral radiograph of the middiaphysis of the femur in a 15-year-old boy demonstrates thickening of the cortex, this time with an irregularly shaped lytic lesion and central density *(arrowheads)*. Although this could represent an osteoid osteoma with central calcified nidus, the fat-suppressed, contrast enhanced, T1-weighted MR image (C) demonstrates irregularly shaped, low-signal-intensity sequestrum *(arrow)* with surrounding enhancement, and interruption of the cortex *(arrowhead)*.

By definition, the nidus of an osteoid osteoma is less than 2 cm in size, and most are only a few millimeters in size. A lesion with a nidus larger than 2 cm is considered to be an osteoblastoma, which is histologically identical but has different clinical features. Osteoid osteoma may not be truly neoplastic because it has limited growth potential and does not metastasize. In contrast, the larger osteoblastoma has unlimited growth potential and may undergo malignant transformation, although some authors dispute the latter.

Magnetic resonance imaging to localize the nidus of an osteoid osteoma requires high-resolution imaging with a small field of view, surface coils, and thin sections. The nidus often but not always has high T2 signal, and almost always enhances intensely after gadolinium administration (Fig. 30-8). The adjacent marrow may show either edema or sclerosis, with the attendant expected signal intensities. If the nidus is not noted, the appearance in the region of host reaction may mislead one toward a diagnosis of a larger, more aggressive lesion.

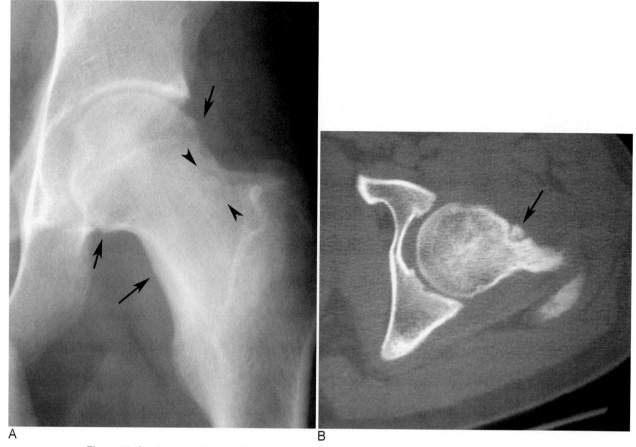

A   B

Figure 30-6   Intracapsular osteoid osteoma. **A and B,** 17-year-old boy. AP hip radiograph (A) shows reactive change in the form of femoral head osteophytes and calcar buttressing (thickening of the medial femoral neck cortex, *short arrows*). The nidus of the osteoid osteoma is in the anterior femoral neck cortex *(arrowheads),* better seen with CT (B, *arrow*).

Bone scanning in extra-articular osteoid osteoma shows intense tracer uptake in the nidus as well as in the reactive bone. Classically, the nidus uptake is greater, resulting in the "double-density sign" of punctate intense activity at the nidus surrounded by a larger region of less intensely increased activity.

The differential diagnosis of a cortical osteoid osteoma includes osteoblastoma, chronic osteomyelitis, and stress fracture (see Fig. 30-5). Chronic infection may have a percutaneous draining sinus. Computed tomography may show a small channel between the nidus of infection and the adjacent soft tissues termed a *cloaca* (sewer) that is not present in osteoid osteoma. The temporal pattern of pain associated with a stress fracture is different from that associated with an osteoid osteoma because pain with the former improves at night and with rest.

The differential diagnosis of an intra-articular osteoid osteoma includes any cause of monoarticular synovitis such as infection and inflammatory arthritis. In children, early Legg-Calvé-Perthes disease may have similar clinical features.

The radiologist often plays a key role in the treatment of these lesions. Computed tomography–guided resection with a

drill, or radiofrequency ablation or thermoablation under general anesthesia, is effective and generally causes less morbidity than surgical resection because less bone is removed. If preoperative localization for surgical resection is requested, a drop of methylene blue can be injected into the periosteum overlying the lesion using CT guidance (Fig. 30-9). Alternatively, a needle can be left in place over the lesion. Such localization allows the surgeon to minimize the amount of cortical bone destroyed in the resection, decreasing the risk of postoperative fracture.

OSTEOBLASTOMA

Osteoblastoma is a rare benign bone-forming tumor that may be difficult to differentiate from osteoid osteoma histologically but is quite distinct radiographically. Osteoblastoma may be characterized by its common location in the posterior elements of the spine (42%). The remainder occur mostly in long bones. Osteoblastomas are usually type 1A geographic lesions with a narrow zone of transition and sclerotic margin, with expansion of the underlying bone. Although these are

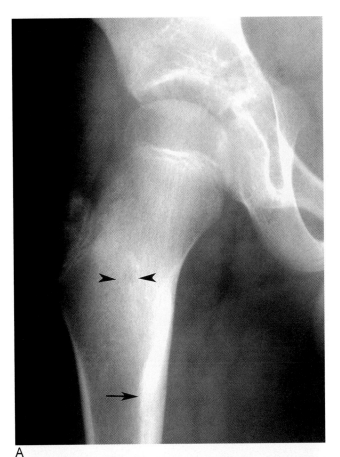

A

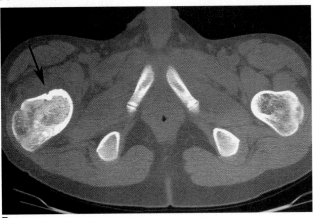

B

Figure 30-7   Osteoid osteoma with resultant growth deformities in a 10-year-old boy. **A,** AP radiograph of the hip shows dense and remote cortical reactive bone formation *(arrows),* a wide and valgus femoral neck, and the faintly seen lucent nidus of the osteoid osteoma *(arrowheads).* **B,** The intracapsular nidus is localized with CT *(arrow).* Growth disturbance can also occur with extracapsular lesions but is less frequent and tends to be less severe. (Reprinted with permission from the American College of Radiology learning file.)

bone-forming tumors, they have a wide range of density on radiography and CT, from lucent to a mixed pattern to a completely blastic appearance (Fig. 30-10). Because of this range of mineralization, the signal intensities seen on both T1- and T2-weighted MR imaging can vary widely. Generally, the lesions

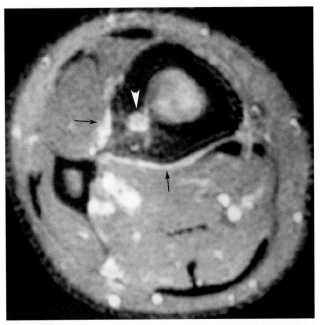

Figure 30-8   MRI of osteoid osteoma. Axial fat-suppressed T1-weighted image with intravenous gadolinium shows intensely enhancing nidus *(arrowhead)* in the posterolateral tibial cortex and intense periosteal enhancement *(small arrows)* overlying the thickened cortex adjacent to the nidus.

appear nonaggressive, with only occasional cortical breakthrough. Treatment is with curettage or marginal excision, and recurrence is rare. Differential diagnosis includes osteoid osteoma, osteomyelitis, and aneurysmal bone cyst in the spine; in addition, because of the occasional finding of osteoid matrix, these lesions can be mistaken for osteosarcoma. Unlike osteoid osteomas, they may rarely undergo malignant transformation (Fig. 30-10B).

Key Concepts	Osteoblastoma

Expansile and usually nonaggressive.
Most common location: Posterior elements of the spine.
Variable osteoid formation. Ranges from lytic (most common) to densely sclerotic.
Histologically identical to osteoid osteoma, but has unlimited growth potential and small risk of malignant transformation to osteosarcoma.

OSSIFYING FIBROMA (OSTEOFIBROUS DYSPLASIA)

Ossifying fibroma (also called osteofibrous dysplasia) is an extremely rare, benign osseous dysplasia found almost exclusively in the anterior proximal tibia. It most often appears in

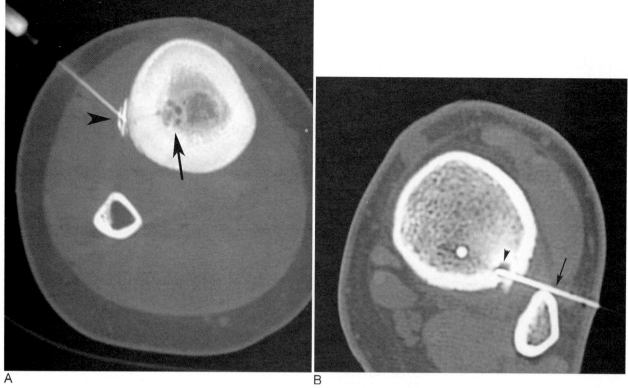

A   B

Figure 30-9 Radiologist participation in osteoid osteoma management. **A,** Subperiosteal contrast and methylene blue injection for localization for open surgical resection. Note the subcortical tibial osteoid osteoma *(arrow)* with circumferential cortical reactive bone formation in the middiaphysis of the tibia of this 14-year-old boy. **B,** Radiofrequency ablation. CT shows radiofrequency ablation electrode *(arrow)* placed percutaneously into a distal tibial osteoid osteoma *(arrowhead).* Biopsy was performed before ablation.

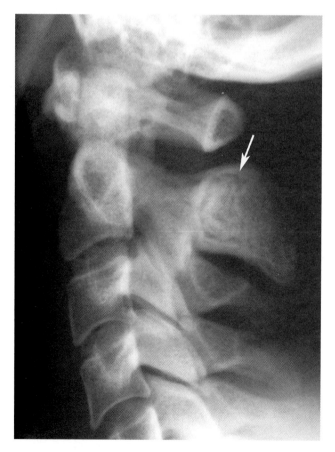

Figure 30-10 Osteoblastoma. Lateral radiograph shows mixed lytic and blastic lesion expanding the spinous process of C2 *(arrow);* typical appearance of osteoblastoma in this 36-year-old woman.

the first through third decades of life and appears as a cortically based geographic, oval lesion. It is associated with cortical bowing and generally causes local expansion of bone. It has a sclerotic rim and may be entirely lucent or may contain osteoid matrix. This is an interesting lesion because it can be histologically and radiographically similar to cortically based fibrous dysplasia or adamantinoma. It is differentiated from fibrous dysplasia by the presence of osteoblastic rimming around bony trabeculae, which is not found in fibrous dysplasia. It is differ-

entiated from adamantinoma by the lack of epithelial cells, which are found in adamantinoma. These three lesions are believed by some authors to represent a spectrum of lesions, although there are subtle histologic differentiating characteristics. Therefore, as there are no other radiographic distinguishing features, the radiologist should consider ossifying fibroma as well as cortically based fibrous dysplasia and adamantinoma in the differential diagnosis with this location and appearance (Fig. 30-11).

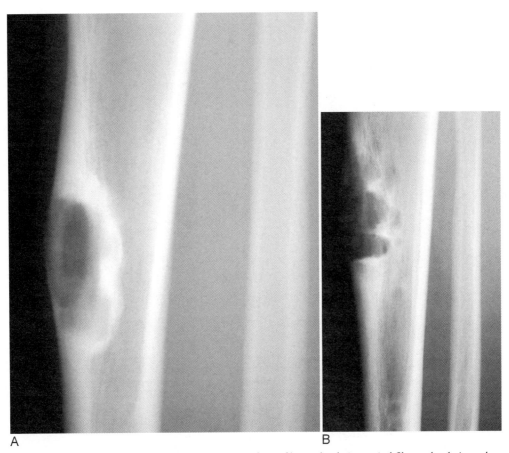

A   B

Figure 30-11   Similarity of imaging appearance of osteofibrous dysplasia, cortical fibrous dysplasia, and adamantinoma. **A,** AP radiograph of a cortically based lytic lesion in the proximal tibia of a 12-year-old girl. This is typical of osteofibrous dysplasia (also known as ossifying fibroma). However, it is not always radiographically distinguishable from a cortically based fibrous dysplasia or adamantinoma. **B,** Cortically based lytic lesion in the anterior tibia of a 12-year-old girl. This lesion has adjacent daughter lesions and at biopsy was found to be fibrous dysplasia.

(Continued)

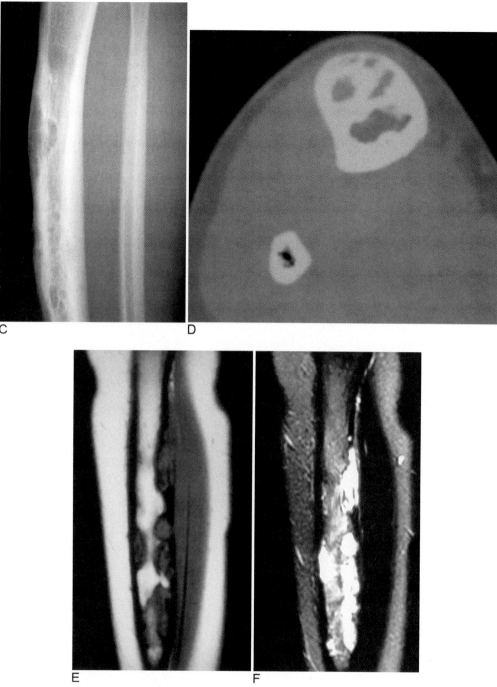

Figure 30-11—(Cont'd) **C,** Cortically based lytic lesions in the anterior tibia, this time in a 10-year-old boy, which proved to be adamantinoma. **D,** CT confirms the cortical nature of this lesion. Note that there are no radiographically distinguishing features among these three lesions. **E and F,** Oblique sagittal T1-weighted (E) and T2-weighted (B) MR images of the tibia in a different patient with osteofibrous dysplasia show the lucent areas on radiographs to have intermediate T1 and high T2 signal. The radiograph in this patient (not shown) resembles findings in part C. The MR imaging findings, like the radiographic findings, are not specific for osteofibrous dysplasia rather than adamantinoma or cortically based fibrous dysplasia.

Bone-Forming Tumors: Malignant (Osteosarcoma)

HIGH-GRADE INTRAMEDULLARY (CONVENTIONAL)
  OSTEOSARCOMA
TELANGIECTATIC OSTEOSARCOMA
PAROSTEAL OSTEOSARCOMA
PERIOSTEAL OSTEOSARCOMA
HIGH-GRADE SURFACE OSTEOSARCOMA
LOW-GRADE INTRAOSSEOUS OSTEOSARCOMA
SOFT TISSUE OSTEOSARCOMA
OSTEOSARCOMATOSIS (MULTICENTRIC OSTEOSARCOMA)
OSTEOSARCOMA IN THE OLDER AGE GROUP

Osteosarcoma is the most common primary malignant bone tumor in adolescents. Among all ages, it is second only to myeloma in frequency of primary bone malignancy (15% to 20%). Several types of osteosarcoma are described and, because of their varying prognosis, treatment, and imaging features, we consider them individually.

HIGH-GRADE INTRAMEDULLARY (CONVENTIONAL) OSTEOSARCOMA

Conventional osteosarcoma makes up 75% of all osteosarcomas (Figs. 31-1–31-5; see also examples in Chapter 29). Most arise in children between 10 and 25 years of age. Most conventional osteosarcomas (90%) are metaphyseal in origin, but they can be diaphyseal. Despite the metaphyseal origin, the tumor frequently crosses the physeal plate to involve the epiphysis. Such epiphyseal involvement is found in 75% of cases and, although infrequently detected by radiography, can be easily seen on magnetic resonance imaging (MRI). Epiphyseal spread of tumor must be sought because there are significant therapeutic implications (the preferred allograft cannot be used; rather, osteoarticular graft or a prosthesis must be placed).

Conventional osteosarcoma occurs most frequently at the sites of most rapid growth: the distal femur is the most common site, followed by the proximal tibia and the proximal humerus. Although flat bones are less frequently involved than long bones, osteosarcoma of the iliac wing deserves mention.

Key Concepts	Conventional Osteosarcoma

Most common primary bone sarcoma in the adolescent age group.
Frequently located about the knee, originating centrally in the metaphysis and often extending across the physeal plate to the epiphysis.
Highly aggressive, rapid growth.
Permeative margins, cortical breakthrough, and soft tissue mass.
Most show osteoid matrix, but occasionally presents as a purely lytic lesion.
Aggressive periosteal reaction: Hair-on-end, sunburst, or Codman's triangle. May be absent.
Spread: Direct invasion, local lymphatic; hematogenous metastasis to bone, lung.

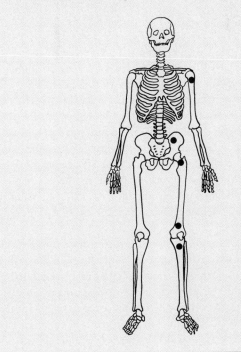

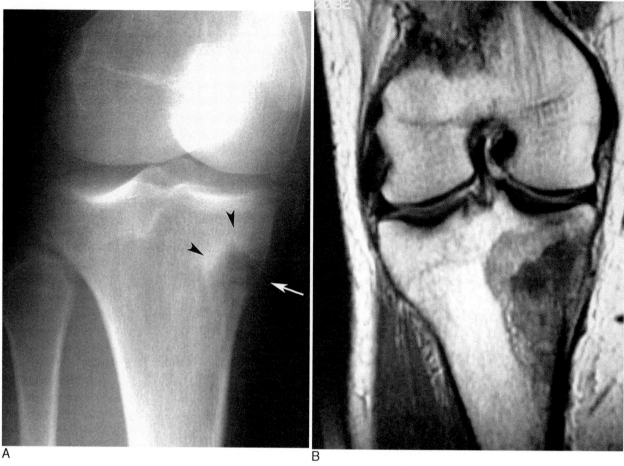

Figure 31-1   Central osteosarcoma. **A,** Oblique radiograph shows an aggressive predominately lytic lesion in the proximal tibia metaphysis. Note cortical breakthrough *(arrow)* and wide zone of transition. A very small region of sclerosis within the bone *(arrowheads)* could represent either tumor matrix or reactive bone formation. **B,** Coronal proton density MRI shows that the lesion is larger than suggested by radiography.

Conventional osteosarcomas have a very rapid doubling rate and frequently are large when first noticed. They are highly aggressive in appearance, with a permeative pattern and wide zone of transition. Cortical breakthrough is usually seen, often with a large soft tissue mass. Periosteal reaction is usually present and often appears aggressive, with a hair-on-end, sunburst, or Codman's triangle pattern. The MRI signal intensity is never high on T1-weighted images unless there is hemorrhage or gadolinium has been administered. T2 signal intensity varies. Densely calcified tumors can have low signal intensity on all sequences.

As with all sarcomas, pathologists classify a tumor as an osteosarcoma not according to its point of origin but rather the presence of histologic features, in this case bone, notably the production of osteoid. Most osteosarcomas produce osteoid matrix that is visible on radiography or computed tomography (CT). The amount of matrix and the degree of matrix calcification vary widely, so the radiographic appearance

may range from densely blastic to nearly completely lytic. The matrix most often appears amorphous or cloud-like because it is less dense than normal bone and lacks an organized trabecular pattern. Osteosarcomas can be histologically quite heterogeneous, and pathologists further classify these tumors on the basis of predominant features: 50% produce enough osteoid to be termed "osteoblastic," whereas 25% produce predominately cartilage (chondroblastic) and 25% produce predominately spindle cells (fibroblastic). The radiographic appearance often corresponds to these histologic findings, with the matrix calcification in the cartilage and spindle cell variety being more subtle relative to that of the osteoblastic variety. It should also be noted that the matrix usually appears denser in the intraosseous portion of an osteosarcoma than in the extraosseous portion. This is an artifact, as the matrix within the soft tissue mass is not superimposed over adjacent remaining bone.

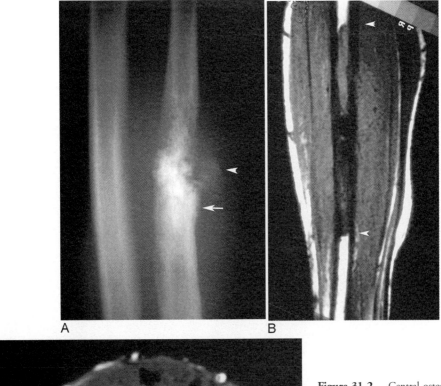

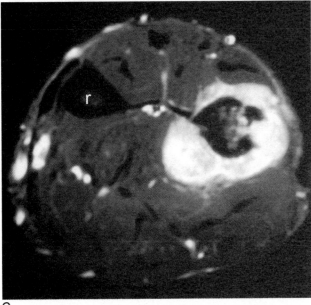

Figure 31-2 Central osteosarcoma in the ulna of a 20-year-old man. **A,** Detail view of frontal radiograph shows permeative lesion in the ulnar midshaft. Note cloud-like osteoid matrix *(arrowhead)* and small area of lamellated periosteal reaction *(arrow)* adjacent to areas of completely absent periosteal reaction, indicating a highly aggressive lesion. **B,** Sagittal T1-weighted MR image shows the true intraosseous extent of the tumor (between *arrowheads*). Complete imaging requires evaluation of the entire involved bone for skip lesions (not shown). **C,** Axial fat-suppressed T1-weighted MR image with intravenous gadolinium shows intensely enhancing intra- and extraosseous tumor. r, radius.

Because so many of these lesions occur around the knee, coronal or sagittal imaging is useful to evaluate for joint involvement. In addition, careful attention must be paid to imaging the remainder of the involved bone to detect "skip" lesions (i.e., metastatic lesions to the same bone), which occur in 1% to 10% of cases.

Radiographs are pathognomonic if the lesion shows osteoid matrix in the soft tissue mass and is typical in location. The differential diagnosis for osteosarcoma can include Ewing's sarcoma. Although Ewing's sarcoma tends to be diaphyseal in location, it can be metadiaphyseal. Furthermore, Ewing's sarcoma can elicit an extensive reactive bone formation that can mimic osteoid matrix. However, the reactive bone formation is restricted to the involved bone and does not extend into the soft tissue mass in a Ewing's sarcoma. This usually helps differentiate the two.

Any lesion that produces immature bone can be confused with osteosarcoma, including healing fractures, early myositis ossificans (see Chapter 2), and the so-called cortical desmoid of the posteromedial distal femur (Chapter 13). It is important

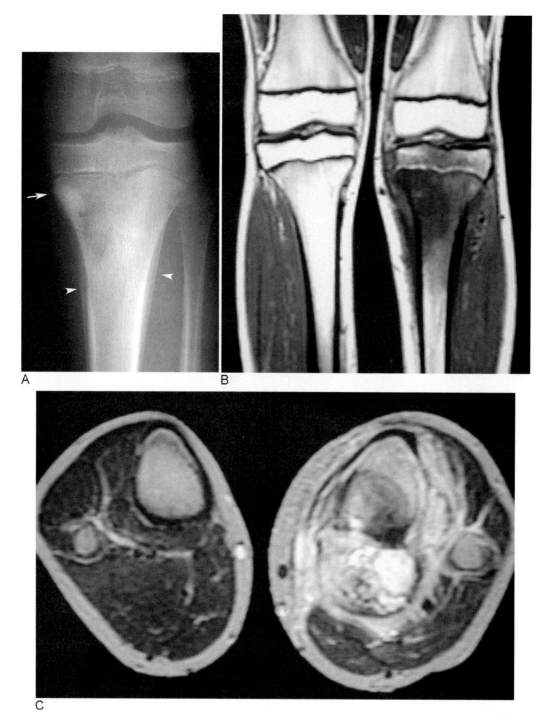

Figure 31-3   Central osteosarcoma. **A,** AP radiograph demonstrates a mixed lytic and sclerotic geographic lesion with a wide zone of transition in the metadiaphysis of the tibia in this 14-year-old boy. The lesion is highly aggressive, with abundant periosteal reaction *(arrowheads)* that is interrupted medially and lamellated laterally. Tumor matrix *(arrow)* causes the increased density in the medial metaphysis. By radiographic criteria, this is the classic appearance of osteosarcoma. Also, by radiographic criteria, the epiphysis appears spared. **B and C,** However, MRI better demonstrates the true tumor size. The T1-weighted coronal MR image (B) shows abnormal signal in the epiphysis and more extensively in the metaphysis and diaphysis due to tumor extension. The axial T2-weighted MR image (C) demonstrates the large soft tissue mass involving both the anterior and posterior compartments as well as the popliteal neurovascular bundle.

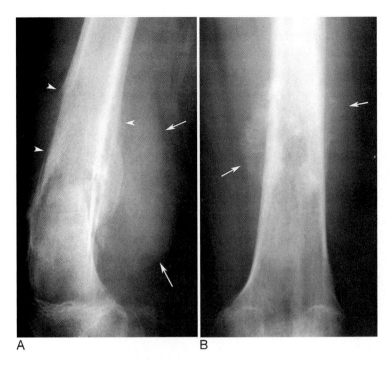

Figure 31-4   Central osteosarcomas. **A,** Lateral radiograph of a highly aggressive lesion involving the distal metaphysis of the femur in a 12-year-old girl. Note interrupted periosteal reaction *(arrowheads)*. A large soft tissue mass extends well beyond the periosteal reaction *(arrows)*, which contains very subtle amorphous tumor matrix. **B,** AP radiograph of an osteosarcoma in a different patient that shows much more obvious osteoid matrix formation in the soft tissue mass *(arrows)*. The range of density of osteoid can be wide, and periosteal reaction also contributes to tumor density on radiographs.

A   B

to recognize these lesions to avoid biopsy, as tissue obtained during the active repair phase may be difficult to distinguish histologically from osteosarcoma. Careful evaluation, including patient history and radiographic analysis, may mitigate a potentially confusing biopsy.

WHAT THE CLINICIAN WANTS TO KNOW: OSTEOSARCOMA

Tumor margins: MRI often better shows medullary involvement than other modalities
Epiphyseal spread
Muscles, joints involved
Neurovascular bundle involvement
Skip lesions within the same bone
Metastases: Lung (CT), bones (bone scanning)

The metastatic potential of conventional osteosarcoma is high, with hematogenous spread to lungs and bones and lymphatic spread locally. As noted previously, metastasis to the same bone is termed a skip lesion. Metastases are found in 10% to 20% of patients at clinical presentation. As with most sarcomas, pulmonary metastases tend to be small, so chest CT is required for staging. Eighty percent of tumor relapses occur in the lung, and 20% occur in bone. Both local recurrence and systemic disease usually occur within 2 years after initial diagnosis.

The radiologic work-up begins with radiography, which usually establishes the diagnosis. Bone scanning is used to ensure that the lesion is monostotic, chest CT is done to exclude metastatic disease to the lung, and MRI is performed

to evaluate the local extent of the lesion. Magnetic resonance imaging is used to plan the biopsy and definitive therapy. The field of view should be extended on one or two sequences to include the entire involved bone in order to search for skip lesions. Treatment begins with induction chemotherapy, which helps to control the development of micrometastases and to allow easier excision. Following chemotherapy, the tumor is restaged with MRI and biopsy. A 90% histologic tumor cell death is considered a good response and predicts a better outcome. Note that a good response is not necessarily associated with significant tumor shrinkage on imaging studies. This is especially common with osteosarcoma. For example, the tumor cells may mature in response to chemotherapy, and increased areas of ossification may be seen. A pathologic fracture may develop during therapy, with associated hemorrhage complicating the MRI appearance.

Regardless of the success of chemotherapy (or radiation, if that is chosen), wide surgical excision is required to prevent local recurrence. Limb salvage is preferred if possible because it improves the quality of life without significantly affecting longevity. The patient concludes therapy with adjuvant multidrug chemotherapy. As with most sarcomas, follow-up imaging is performed more frequently during the first 2–5 years after treatment because most recurrences occur during this time.

TELANGIECTATIC OSTEOSARCOMA

Telangiectatic osteosarcoma is a rare osteosarcoma variant that occurs in the same age range and location as conventional osteosarcoma. Telangiectatic osteosarcoma is expansile and lytic, and frequently has type 1C margins and cortical breakthrough

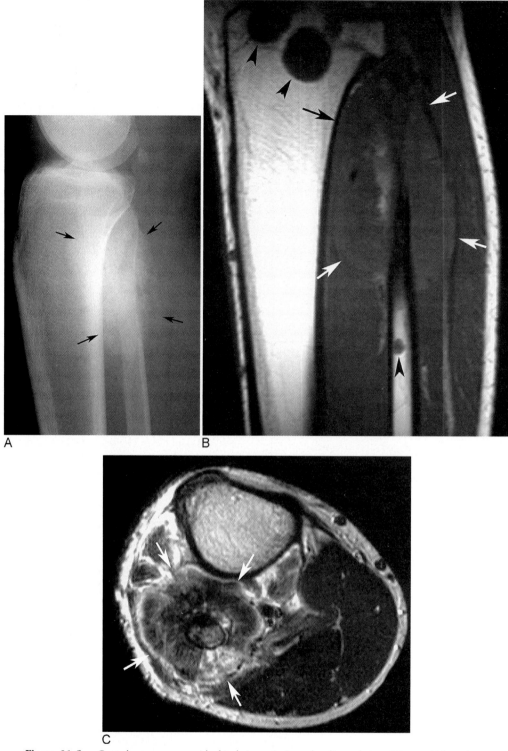

Figure 31-5 Central osteosarcoma with skip lesions. **A,** Lateral radiograph in a 17-year-old boy shows cloud-like osteoid matrix surrounding the proximal fibula. **B and C,** Sagittal T1-weighted (B) and axial T2-weighted (C) MR images show the tumor mass *(arrows)* and also show marrow metastases in the proximal tibia and fibula *(arrowheads* in part B).

(Fig. 31-6). This geographic pattern can mislead the unwary into underdiagnosis; it is essential to identify the broad zone of transition that distinguishes this as an aggressive lesion. Telangiectatic osteosarcoma is highly vascular and contains necrotic tissue and large pools of blood, with tumor located only at the periphery and along septations. Thus, fluid-fluid levels and findings of hemorrhage on MRI are frequent. With careful observation, the peripheral tumor can be seen to appear nodular in some areas, and irregular in others. Careful observation is required to avoid misdiagnosing telangiectatic osteosarcoma as the less aggressive aneurysmal bone cyst or even giant cell tumor, both lesions that can contain fluid-fluid levels. Aneurysmal bone cysts usually do not have tumor nodules along the periphery. In these lesions, the zone of transition on radiographs is not as broad as for an osteosarcoma.

The metastatic potential, work-up, prognosis, and therapy are identical to those for conventional osteosarcoma.

PAROSTEAL OSTEOSARCOMA

Parosteal osteosarcoma is a surface lesion that represents the second most common variety of osteosarcoma (Figs. 31-7–31-10). Although there is a wide age range, including adolescence, more than 80% of cases occur between the ages of 20 and 50 years.

Thus, the median age is older than is found with conventional osteosarcoma. This is one of the few sarcomas that is not more common in males (male-to-female ratio, 2:3). The lesion also tends to be of low grade and is better differentiated than conventional and telangiectatic osteosarcoma, resulting in a substantially better prognosis.

This surface osteosarcoma is found most frequently at the posterior distal femoral metaphysis; other common locations are the proximal tibia and proximal humerus. The site of origin is the bone surface, but the tumor is otherwise located nearly entirely in the soft tissues, usually with lobulated margins. This results in a cleavage plane between much of the lesion and the underlying bone. There is local invasion of the underlying bone in approximately 50% of cases. This is usually not seen on radiography but is confirmed on MRI.

Parosteal osteosarcoma is often large by the time of discovery. The tumor matrix is usually densely sclerotic centrally, while peripherally the matrix may be less mature or even nonossified. This zoning pattern is the reverse of myositis ossificans, in which more mature bone is found peripherally. Computed tomography can demonstrate this zoning phenomenon, as may MRI. The MRI appearance varies depending on the degree of matrix ossification. If it is not cellular and contains little cartilage, there will be low signal on all sequences. However, more cellularity is often present, as well

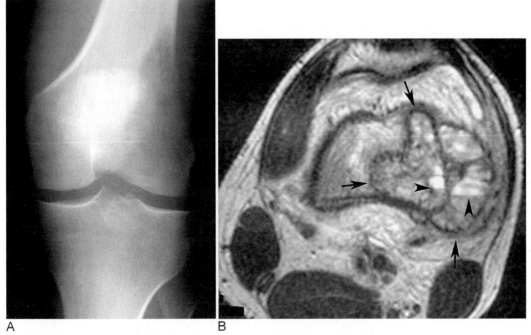

A   B

Figure 31-6   Telangiectatic osteosarcoma. **A,** AP radiograph demonstrates a geographic lytic lesion with a wide zone of transition (type 1C margin) in the distal femoral metaphysis extending to the subchondral region. This aggressive pattern of bone destruction is sometimes erroneously interpreted as nonaggressive, particularly when compared with the highly aggressive osteosarcomas seen in Figs. 31-1–31-4. Telangiectatic osteosarcomas are often misjudged as being nonaggressive lesions. **B,** Axial T2-weighted MR image demonstrates the large extraosseous soft tissue mass *(arrows)* that contains fluid levels *(arrowheads)*. This is the classic MR appearance of telangiectatic osteosarcoma, but this appearance may be seen in other lesions, notably aneurysmal bone cysts and giant cell tumors. Combined with the aggressive radiographic appearance, telangiectatic osteosarcoma is a likely preoperative diagnosis.

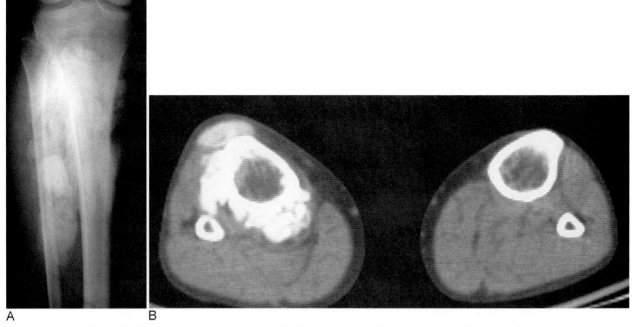

Figure 31-7 Parosteal osteosarcoma. **A and B,** Extensive lesion with dense matrix. **A,** AP radiograph shows a dense, well-defined osteoid matrix forming this tumor, which appears to "wrap around" the proximal tibial metadiaphysis in this 41-year-old man. **B,** The appearance of the tumor as a surface lesion wrapping around the underlying bone is confirmed on CT. This is a large parosteal osteosarcoma in a typical location with characteristic dense osteoid formation.

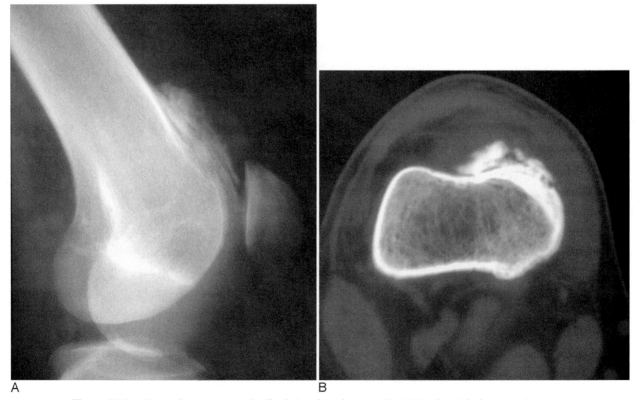

Figure 31-8 Parosteal osteosarcoma. Smaller lesion than shown in Fig. 31-7, also with dense matrix. **A,** Lateral radiograph shows dense calcification anterior to the distal femoral cortex. **B,** Axial CT better demonstrates the location and position of the surface lesion.

(Continued)

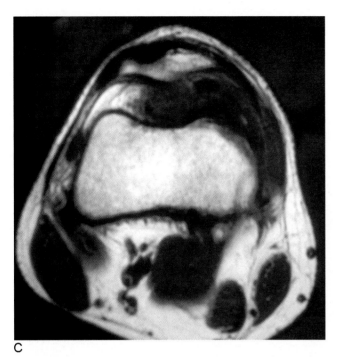

C

Figure 31-8—(Cont'd)   C, Axial T1-weighted MR image shows low signal in the tumor, reflecting the dense calcification, with minimal marrow invasion *(arrows).*

as cartilaginous regions and soft tissue mass, which gives an heterogeneous appearance. The extent of marrow involvement should be carefully assessed, along with regions that are more cellular; these might suggest a higher grade or dedifferentiation.

Parosteal osteosarcomas tend to be slow growing and low grade, but with inadequate excision may recur locally in a more aggressive form. With multiple recurrences they may dedifferentiate into a high-grade sarcoma. These lesions can be ideal for limb salvage techniques with wide resection. Because of the low-grade nature of the lesion, chemotherapy is generally not necessary. Metastases to the lung in parosteal osteosarcoma occur both later and with considerably less frequency compared with metastases in conventional osteosarcoma.

Parosteal osteosarcoma is generally not a difficult diagnosis to make radiographically. In its earliest stages, it could be mistaken for myositis ossificans, although the zoning of the mature bone differentiates the two both radiographically and histologically. Parosteal osteosarcoma is easily distinguished from an osteochondroma as the latter should show cortical and marrow continuity with the underlying bone.

PERIOSTEAL OSTEOSARCOMA

Periosteal osteosarcoma is a rare surface osteosarcoma. It has a distinct radiographic appearance compared with parosteal or conventional osteosarcomas. Because it is a surface lesion, it usually causes scalloping of the underlying cortex, although occasionally cortical thickening is seen (Fig. 31-11).

Periosteal osteosarcomas are usually located in a more diaphyseal position than either conventional or parosteal osteosarcomas. The femur and the tibia are the most common locations for periosteal osteosarcoma. They tend to wrap around the circumference of the bone. At the knee, periosteal osteosarcoma may be suggested rather than parosteal osteosarcoma by medial rather than posterior location. The soft tissue mass extends from the surface of the lesion, usually with spicules of bone emanating in a sunburst pattern. Periosteal reaction is common, often in the form of Codman's triangles.

Key Concepts	Osteosarcoma

High grade intramedullary (conventional, central) (75%)
Telangiectatic: Expansile with fluid-fluid levels. High grade.
Surface types:
    Parosteal > periosteal > high grade surface
    Parosteal:
        Low grade
        Posterior distal femur
        Surface mass
        May calcify densely (especially centrally)
    Periosteal:
        Intermediate grade
        Medial distal femur, tends to wrap around the bone
        Cortical scalloping, bone spicules radiate from cortex
        Intraosseous involvement is rare
    Parosteal and Periosteal: Older mean age and better
        prognosis than conventional osteosarcoma
Extraosseous: Rare. Soft tissue mass, may calcify. High grade.
    Poor prognosis.
Secondary: Poor prognosis. Common: Paget's, radiation.
    Rare: Fibrous dysplasia, preexisting bone infarct.

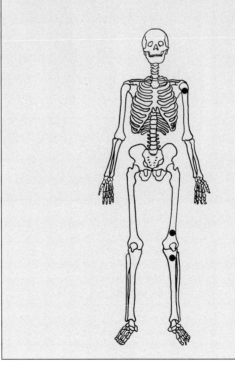

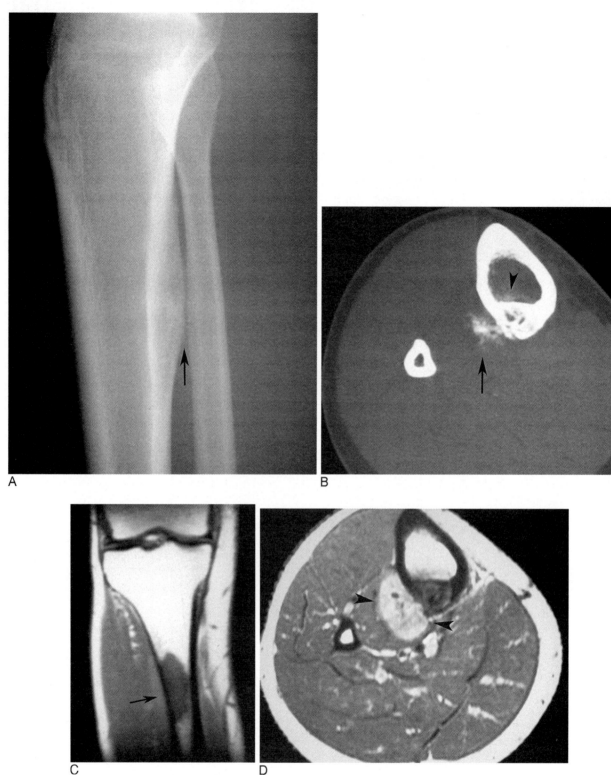

Figure 31-9 Parosteal osteosarcoma, with only minimal visible tumor calcification. **A,** Lateral radiograph shows prominent focal cortical bone formation in the posterior tibial metadiaphysis, a location that is typical for a stress fracture in this active 28-year-old man. There is extremely subtle osteoid matrix posterior to the thickened cortex *(arrow)*. **B,** CT demonstrates the matrix in the soft tissues *(arrow)* as well as subtle new bone formation within the medullary canal *(arrowhead)*. The dense cortical new bone formation is also demonstrated. CT confirms the diagnosis of an early parosteal osteosarcoma. **C,** Coronal T1-weighted MR image confirms that the surface parosteal osteosarcoma has invaded the marrow cavity *(arrow)*. Fifty percent of parosteal osteosarcomas show focal marrow invasion. **D,** Axial T2-weighted MR image shows the soft tissue mass *(arrowheads)*. Because this sequence was performed without fat suppression, the marrow extension is difficult to distinguish from normal marrow fat.

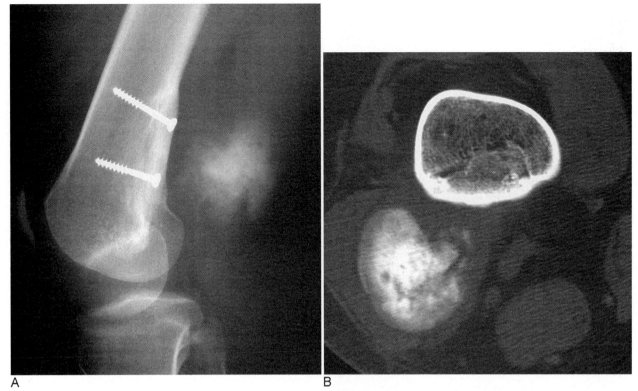

Figure 31-10   Recurrent parosteal osteosarcoma. **A,** Lateral radiograph demonstrating a previously resected parosteal osteosarcoma with bone graft secured with screws at the posterior cortex, now incorporated. The recurrent tumor is in the soft tissues and demonstrates the zoning phenomenon typical of parosteal osteosarcoma; the more mature bone formation is located centrally in the mass and the periphery shows less mature osteoid formation. **B,** The zoning phenomenon is emphasized on CT, where the dense center *(long arrow)* is surrounded by less mature peripheral osteoid formation *(short arrows).*

Magnetic resonance imaging demonstrates the extent of the soft tissue mass and usually shows no intramedullary extension of the lesion, although the rare intramedullary extension of lesion should be sought because this will affect limb salvage plans. The MRI signal is nonspecific: low intensity on T1-weighted images and high intensity on T2-weighted images. The perpendicular reactive bone formation may be seen as low-signal linear rays on all sequences.

Periosteal osteosarcomas generally arise in the second or third decade of life, similar to or slightly later than conventional osteosarcomas. They frequently show some chondroid differentiation at histology, and are usually of intermediate grade. Treatment is by wide excision. Their prognosis is better than that of conventional osteosarcomas, although not as good as that of parosteal osteosarcomas. The major differential diagnosis is juxtacortical chondroma, another surface lesion that can have a very similar appearance (see Fig. 32-14). The rare high-grade surface osteosarcoma can be difficult to differentiate as well.

HIGH-GRADE SURFACE OSTEOSARCOMA

High-grade surface osteosarcoma is rare. Like periosteal osteosarcomas, these lesions tend to involve the diaphysis of long bones. They are similar in appearance to periosteal osteosarcomas, although intramedullary involvement is more frequent in the high-grade surface lesions. High-grade surface osteosarcomas have a prognosis identical to that of conventional osteosarcoma.

LOW-GRADE INTRAOSSEOUS OSTEOSARCOMA

Low-grade intraosseous osteosarcoma is a rare variant that is entirely intraosseous. Its appearance ranges from being well circumscribed and very nonaggressive to a more permeative pattern. The lesion is diaphyseal or metadiaphyseal in the long bones. It can range from being entirely lytic to quite sclerotic. The median age is slightly older than for conventional osteosarcoma.

If the lesion is not highly aggressive in appearance, it may be mistaken for fibrous dysplasia, bone island, or a cartilage lesion. If it is more aggressive in appearance, it may be mistaken for Ewing's sarcoma, lymphoma, or malignant fibrous histiocytoma. Occasionally, an enlarging bone island can suggest a densely sclerotic osteosarcoma. As noted in Chapter 30, bone scanning of these lesions does not show the intense tracer uptake that would be expected in a sclerotic osteosarcoma.

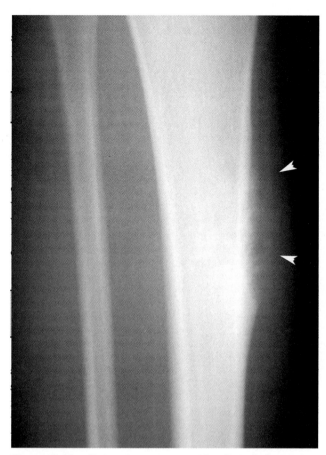

Figure 31-11   Periosteal osteosarcoma. AP radiograph demonstrates the surface periosteal osteosarcoma in a 12-year-old girl, with the typical tumor osteoid arising from the surface of the lesion and a faint scalloping of the cortex *(arrows)*. For another example of periosteal osteosarcoma, see Fig. 29-6.

If the lesion is recognized initially and completely resected, survival is excellent. With recurrence, a higher-grade lesion may be found.

SOFT TISSUE OSTEOSARCOMA

This is a rare extraosseous osteosarcoma, generally occurring later in life (40 to 70 years). It is found most frequently in the thigh, with less frequent occurrence in the upper extremity and retroperitoneum. The soft tissue mass has variable amounts of mineralized osteoid. Treatment is with wide resection and adjuvant chemotherapy or radiation therapy; prognosis is poor, worse than that for conventional osteosarcoma.

OSTEOSARCOMATOSIS (MULTICENTRIC OSTEOSARCOMA)

Osteosarcomatosis is a rare process, with the synchronous appearance of osteosarcoma at multiple sites, often bilaterally symmetric. The lesions are nearly always osteoblastic and are

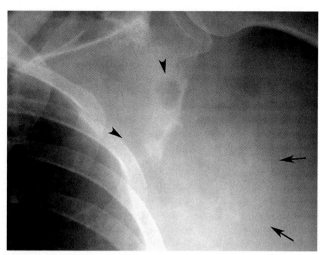

Figure 31-12   Secondary osteosarcoma. AP radiograph of the shoulder demonstrates destruction of the scapula *(arrowheads)*, along with a large soft tissue mass in the axilla containing subtle osteoid matrix *(arrows)*. This 66-year-old woman had axillary radiation for breast carcinoma and 12 years later developed a radiation-induced osteosarcoma.

rapidly progressive. Although this was originally considered a truly synchronous development of multicentric osteosarcomas, this condition more likely represents rapidly progressive metastatic disease. The current theory is supported by the fact that in many cases there are a dominant bone lesion and pulmonary metastases at the time of diagnosis. Although the origin of osteosarcomatosis may be controversial, the results unfortunately are not—all these patients have an extremely poor prognosis.

OSTEOSARCOMA IN THE OLDER AGE GROUP

Osteosarcomas arising in patients older than age 60 years often do not have the classic appearance of conventional osteosarcoma. Their location tends to be different (one fourth in the axial skeleton, often in the cranial/facial bones, and with greater frequency in the soft tissues). Eighty percent of the bone lesions present as purely lytic with aggressive margins. Although some are primary osteosarcomas, about half arise in pre-existing lesions. Common pre-existing lesions for secondary osteosarcoma include Paget's disease, previously radiated bone, and dedifferentiated chondrosarcoma. It is likely that no more than 1% of patients with Paget's disease are at risk for developing osteosarcoma; when osteosarcoma does occur in such patients, there is generally long-standing and severe Paget's disease. Postradiation osteosarcomas (Fig. 31-12) have locations that parallel that of commonly irradiated areas (shoulder girdle for breast carcinoma, pelvis for genitourinary tumors). Osteosarcoma is the most frequent malignancy to arise from radiated bone, with the interval between radiation and diagnosis ranging from 3 to 40 years (average, 14 years). Other sarcomas that occur in radiated bone include malignant fibrous histiocytoma, chondrosarcoma, and undifferentiated sarcoma.

Up to 10% of well-differentiated chondrosarcomas can dedifferentiate into osteosarcoma or other high-grade sarcoma. Radiographically, there is often a sharp transition between the well-differentiated chondrosarcoma and the highly aggressive dedifferentiated tumor. This tumor may contain elements of fibrosarcoma, malignant fibrous histiocytoma, and high-grade chondrosarcoma, as well as osteosarcoma. Osteosarcoma may also rarely arise from benign conditions, including osteochondroma, osteoblastoma, bone infarct, and fibrous dysplasia.

Treatment of secondary osteosarcoma is with radical excision and chemotherapy. However, survival is poor, averaging 37% at 5 years in older patients with primary osteosarcomas and 7.5% in patients with osteosarcoma arising in a preexisting lesion.

ENCHONDROMA
MULTIPLE ENCHONDROMATOSIS (OLLIER'S DISEASE AND
    MAFFUCCI'S SYNDROME)
EXOSTOSIS (OSTEOCHONDROMA, OSTEOCHONDRAL
    EXOSTOSIS)
MULTIPLE HEREDITARY OSTEOCHONDROMAS
DYSPLASIA EPIPHYSEALIS HEMIMELICA (TREVOR
    DISEASE)
JUXTACORTICAL (PERIOSTEAL) CHONDROMA
CHONDROBLASTOMA
CHONDROMYXOID FIBROMA
CENTRAL CHONDROSARCOMA
CLEAR CELL CHONDROSARCOMA
DEDIFFERENTIATED CHONDROSARCOMA
MESENCHYMAL CHONDROSARCOMA

Cartilage-forming tumors are common. Many have chondroid matrix (Fig. 29-5) or other features discussed later that allow easy diagnosis. However, the distinction between benign cartilage-forming tumor and chondrosarcoma can be extremely difficult in some situations. Chondrosarcoma is the third most common primary malignant bone tumor following multiple myeloma and osteosarcoma; it is frequently misdiagnosed. Thus, this chapter emphasizes imaging features that help to distinguish benign from malignant chondroid tumors.

ENCHONDROMA

Enchondromas (occasionally termed chondromas) are common benign cartilaginous neoplasms, which are thought to arise in the medullary canal owing to continued growth of residual benign cartilaginous rests that are displaced from the growth plate. Enchondromas are most frequently discovered incidentally because they are usually asymptomatic in the absence of pathologic fracture or malignant transformation.

Key Concepts	Enchondroma

Common, usually incidental benign cartilage-forming neoplasm.

Central, metaphyseal location.

Chondroid matrix, but may be entirely lytic (especially in the hand or foot).

Geographic, although often without a sclerotic margin.

MRI shows lobulated bright signal on T2-weighted images, with low-signal-intensity calcifications.

Fifty percent of cases occur in tubular bones of hands and feet. May present with bone expansion, pathologic fracture.

Small risk of malignant transformation in axial skeleton and proximal extremity enchondromas.

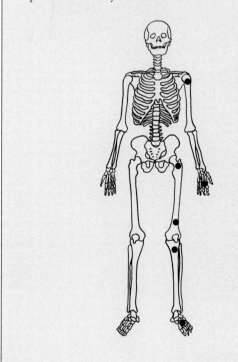

Enchondromas are especially common in the tubular bones of the hands or feet, and up to 50% of all enchondromas occur in one of those locations (Fig. 32-1). They are also commonly distributed among metaphyseal regions of the long tubular bones, especially the humerus, femur, and tibia, but occur only rarely in the axial skeleton.

The most common appearance of an enchondroma is that of a discrete geographic lesion, often with lobulated margins (see Figs. 29-5, 32-1). The lesion may mildly expand bony margins, with cortical thinning. Sclerotic margins are most common in the hands and feet, but lesions in the small tubular bone may expand and present with a pathologic fracture. Often, no sclerotic margin is seen in the metaphyseal lesions of the larger tubular bones. Enchondromas usually contain cartilaginous matrix, which may appear as stippled and curvilinear (arcs and rings) calcification, generally appearing denser than normal bone. However, enchondromas can also appear lytic

and be discovered only incidentally by magnetic resonance imaging (MRI) or inferred radiographically by cortical thinning or endosteal erosion (Fig. 32-1C). There should be no cortical breakthrough, soft tissue mass, or host response in the absence of pathologic fracture; these findings suggest chondrosarcoma.

Enchondromas are usually monostotic. They may, however, be multiple when found in the hands or feet (see Fig. 32-1). Patients with multiple enchondromatosis (Ollier's disease; see later discussion) have more than one enchondroma in locations other than the hands or feet.

With MRI, an enchondroma appears as a mass with lobules of intermediate (as seen with muscle) signal intensity on T1-weighted images and very high signal intensity on T2-weighted images (Fig. 32-2). The very high T2 signal intensity is due to the high water content of the mucopolysaccharide extracellular matrix of the tumor. The stroma between the chondroid nodules

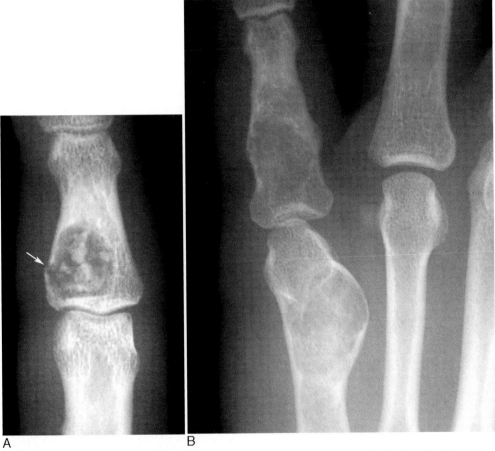

A   B

Figure 32-1 Enchondroma in the hand. Fifty percent of enchondromas arise in the hands or feet. Note the wide variety of appearance of cartilaginous matrix in these cases. Similar-appearing lesions located proximal to the hands or feet would be concerning for chondrosarcoma. See also Fig. 29-5B. **A,** AP radiograph of the middle phalanx of a finger in a 35-year-old man. In this case there is a geographic lesion with a narrow zone of transition, dense calcifications, and pathologic fracture *(arrow)*. This is a pathognomonic appearance of an enchondroma. **B,** AP radiograph of the fourth and fifth fingers in a different patient, a 23-year-old man. In this case the matrix is much less dense and the lesions are expansile. These also are typical for enchondroma. A patient can have more than one enchondroma in the hands or feet without a suggestion of multiple enchondromatosis.

(Continued)

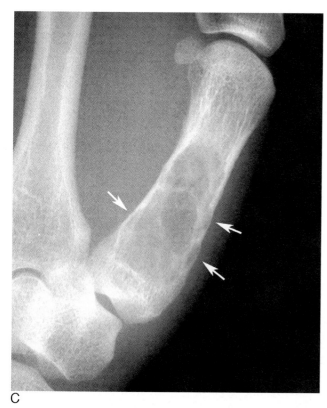

C

Figure 32-1—(Cont'd)   C, AP radiograph of the thumb in a third patient shows a lytic central lesion, without matrix, with endosteal scalloping and minimal expansion *(arrows)*. Because there is no matrix, a complete differential diagnosis for this lesion includes solitary bone cyst, giant cell tumor, aneurysmal bone cyst, or fibrous dysplasia, but the location in the hand makes enchondroma by far the most likely diagnosis.

Key Concepts	Enchondroma Versus Chondrosarcoma

Strongly favors enchondroma:
   Location in hands or feet
Favors enchondroma:
   Small lesion, stable over time
   No endosteal cortical scalloping
   Asymptomatic
Favors chondrosarcoma:
   Proximal location
   Large size
   Enlarging
   Pain without mechanical cause
   Destruction of previously present matrix
   Endosteal cortical scalloping greater than two thirds of
     cortical thickness
   Cortical breakthrough

The major diagnostic consideration at sites other than the hands and feet is low-grade chondrosarcoma. There is considerable histologic and radiographic overlap between enchondroma and low-grade chondrosarcoma. Chondrosarcoma can develop de novo or occur as malignant transformation within an enchondroma or other cartilaginous tumor. The difficulty in distinguishing low-grade chondrosarcoma from enchondroma lies in the fact that these benign and malignant lesions may be indistinguishable radiographically. Even with serial radiography, bone scanning, computed tomography (CT), and MRI, no

may enhance with gadolinium. Occasional internal septations, and punctate signal voids representing matrix calcifications, are also seen. However, this appearance is not specific for enchondroma, as a low-grade chondrosarcoma can be indistinguishable from enchondroma on all imaging studies.

The differential diagnosis of an enchondroma in the hands or feet is different from that of an enchondroma in the more proximal tubular bones. Chondrosarcoma is rare in the hands or feet, regardless of the radiographic appearance. If the lesion shows no matrix calcification, one might also consider a diagnosis of giant cell tumor, epidermoid inclusion cyst, aneurysmal bone cyst, solitary bone cyst, and fibrous dysplasia. Statistically, giant cell tumor is the second most common neoplasm in the small tubular bones. Symptomatic enchondromas of the hands and feet are generally treated with curettage and bone grafting. Lesions that present with pathologic fracture are usually allowed to heal before curettage.

In sites other than the hands or feet, enchondroma may occasionally be confused with bone infarct, although the serpiginous pattern of calcification found in a bone infarct usually allows clear differentiation. If a well-circumscribed lytic lesion of the proximal tibia lacks chondroid matrix and has a sclerotic margin, chondromyxoid fibroma also could be considered, but this is an exceedingly rare tumor.

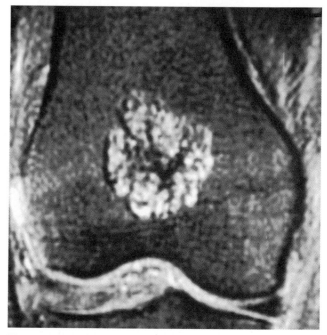

Figure 32-2   Coronal T2-weighted image of the distal femur shows typical MR appearance of a chondroid tumor with multiple lobules of high T2 signal.

interval change may be shown with low-grade chondrosarcomas. Chondrosarcomas may be histologically heterogeneous, so biopsy is not reliable. Thus, the surgeon and the pathologist may rely heavily on clinical and radiographic features in forming a diagnosis. Local pain in the absence of fracture or joint-related pathology is a highly suspicious clinical finding for chondrosarcoma. Radiologists may be asked to perform an intra-articular injection of lidocaine to distinguish joint-related pain from tumor pain (tumor pain will not resolve, whereas joint pain will resolve). Important radiographic clues that favor chondrosarcoma over enchondroma include endosteal scalloping of greater than two thirds of the cortical thickness, cortical breakthrough, increasing tumor size, and development of lucency within previously ossified chondroid matrix (Fig. 32-3).

MULTIPLE ENCHONDROMATOSIS (OLLIER'S DISEASE AND MAFFUCCI'S SYNDROME)

Multiple enchondromatosis is a rare developmental abnormality characterized by the presence of enchondromas in the metaphyses and diaphyses of multiple bones. The disease appears in early childhood and is neither hereditary nor familial. It tends to be unilateral and localized to one extremity. The lesions may look like typical enchondromas or may be much larger and may appear grotesque, especially in the fingers. The lesions in the metaphases of the long bones frequently do not have a typical appearance of enchondroma, but rather appear striated, with vertical lucencies and densities. Most have some chondroid matrix (Fig. 32-4). The involved limb usually is short and demonstrates epiphyseal deformities. The risk of malignant transformation (usually chondrosarcoma) ranges from 10% to 25%. The disease probably results from the ectopic deposition of cartilage rests from the physis, which continue to grow, causing the bony deformities.

Maffucci's syndrome falls in the spectrum of multiple enchondromatosis, in which enchondromatosis is found in combination with soft tissue and visceral hemangiomas. Phleboliths may be present, which, in addition to the features of enchondromatosis, make the radiographic diagnosis (Fig. 32-5). Maffucci's syndrome is believed to have a much higher malignant potential than enchondromatosis alone.

EXOSTOSIS (OSTEOCHONDROMA, OSTEOCHONDRAL EXOSTOSIS)

Exostoses are one of the most common benign tumors, seen in approximately 3% of the population. Exostoses are the result of displaced growth plate cartilage, which causes lateral bone growth from the metaphyseal region. The displaced physeal cartilage produces new bone, creating an excrescence from the underlying metaphyseal bone. This results in the essential feature of an exostosis: continuity of the normal marrow, cortex, and periosteum between the exostosis and the host bone. The exostosis is covered by a cartilaginous cap, which is its source of growth. Chondroid matrix may be seen within the cartilaginous cap, but otherwise the appearance is that of deformed but otherwise normal bone. The size may range from small to very large, and soft tissues are displaced by the bony mass.

An exostosis can be *pedunculated* (cauliflower-like, Fig. 32-6) or *sessile* (broad-based, Fig. 32-7). The most common locations are the distal femur, proximal humerus, tibia, and fibula, all

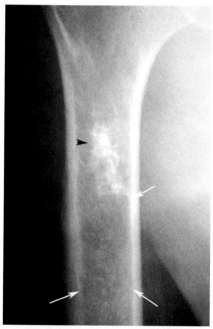

Figure 32-3 Enchondroma with malignant transformation. AP radiograph of the proximal humerus in a 58-year-old man. Note the chondroid matrix in the proximal portion of the lesion *(arrowhead),* which represents a benign enchondroma. However, lytic change distal to the matrix *(arrows)* represents destruction of bone and the distal portion of the parent enchondroma by chondrosarcoma. This more distal portion of the enchondroma has transformed to a chondrosarcoma.

Key Concepts	Exostosis (Osteochondroma)

Metaphyseal: Exostosis usually points away from adjacent joint.
Around knee most common location, but can occur anywhere.
Ninety-five percent of cases found in extremities; most are solitary.
Distinct appearance, with normal marrow, cortex, and periosteum extending from the underlying bone into the exostosis, and a cartilage cap, which may or may not show chondroid matrix.
Growth ceases at skeletal maturity.
Mechanical complications are common.
Pain or continued growth after skeletal maturity warrants exclusion of sarcomatous transformation.

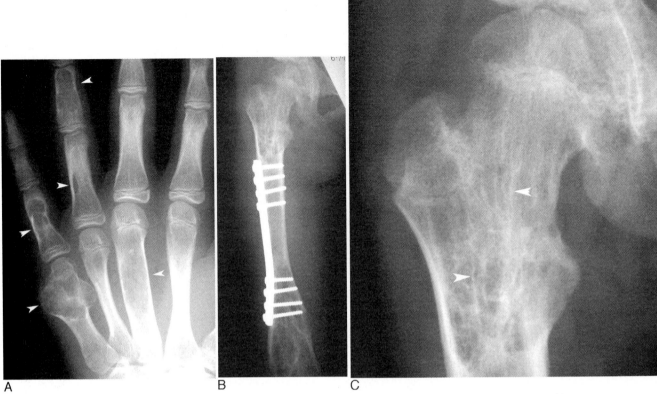

Figure 32-4   Multiple enchondromatosis (Ollier's disease). **A,** AP radiograph of the hand in a 13-year-old boy shows several enchondromas *(arrowheads)*. Several of these show chondroid matrix typical of enchondromas. Bone expansion by enchondromas in Ollier's disease can be much greater than in this example, to the point of being grotesque. **B,** AP radiograph of the femur in a 9-year-old patient with Ollier's disease. Note that the dysplasia involves the metaphyses and epiphyses but not the diaphyses. In this case, the patient has undergone limb lengthening, which is the reason for the lateral plating. **C,** Detail of the proximal femur from part B. The vertical striations that can be seen in multiple enchondromatosis are shown *(arrowheads)*. Notice that the appearance of the dysplasia in multiple enchondromatosis can be very different from that of a routine enchondroma (e.g., Fig. 32-1). Chondroid matrix need not be seen in multiple enchondromatosis. (Parts B and C reproduced with permission from the American College of Radiology learning file.)

regions of rapid growth. Pedunculated exostosis usually grows away from the adjacent joint. Ninety-five percent of cases occur in the extremities and 36% are found around the knee. Ninety percent are solitary. Growth of an exostosis normally ceases at skeletal maturity.

The MRI appearance of an exostosis is characteristic, with continuity of normal-appearing host bone marrow and cortex extending into the lesion. The overlying hyaline cartilage cap is high signal on T2-weighted MR images, typical of cartilage, and is uniform in thickness, generally less than 1 cm thick (see Figs. 32-6, 32-8).

The imaging appearance of an exostosis usually is pathognomonic. The pedunculated or cauliflower variety of exostosis should be differentiated from a parosteal osteosarcoma by the type of matrix and the lack of continuity of the cortex and marrow with host bone seen in the osteosarcoma. Occasionally, myositis ossificans that is adjacent to the cortex may be confused with an exostosis, but careful examination demonstrates

no cortical or marrow continuity with myositis ossificans. Computed tomography may be helpful when differentiation is difficult. The broad-based sessile type of exostosis may be confused with old postfracture deformity, a metaphyseal dysplasia, or the occasional cortically based fibrous dysplasia.

Complications of a solitary exostosis include formation of an overlying bursa that may become inflamed (Fig. 32-9A); mechanical complications such as limitation of motion and compression of adjacent nerves, muscles, or blood vessels; fracture of the neck of a pedunculated lesion (Fig. 32-9B); and, very rarely, malignant transformation. Bursa formation can be painful and cause an apparent enlargement. Nerve impingement and pseudoaneurysm formation can occasionally occur, especially in the region of the popliteal fossa. Scapular blade lesions that protrude anteriorly can cause pain and palpable vibration with motion as they slide over the ribs (see Fig. 32-6D). All these findings are demonstrated with MRI and can help differentiate these benign painful lesions from malignant transformation to chondrosarcoma.

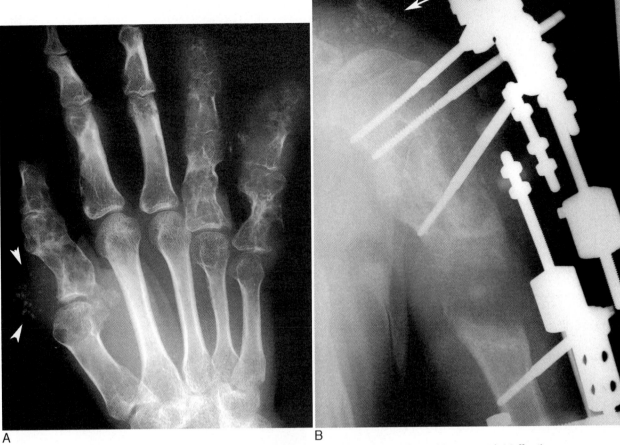

A   B

Figure 32-5   Maffucci's syndrome. **A,** AP radiograph of the hand in a 31-year-old patient with Maffucci's syndrome. Note the multiple, fairly typical-appearing enchondromas. There also are soft tissue hemangiomas, the most prominent seen at the proximal phalanx of the thumb, where phleboliths are seen in the soft tissue mass *(arrowheads)*. **B,** AP radiograph of the proximal humerus in an 11-year-old girl with Maffucci's syndrome. Note the dysplastic appearance of the proximal humerus, which would be typical of either Ollier's disease or Maffucci's disease. However, the soft tissue hemangioma in the shoulder (note the phleboliths, *arrow*) leads to the diagnosis of Maffucci's syndrome. The external fixation hardware is related to limb lengthening to compensate for severely shortened limbs in Maffucci's syndrome that is due to diversion of growth plate cartilage to the enchondromas.

Few (probably far fewer than 1%) solitary exostoses undergo malignant transformation of the cartilage cap to chondrosarcoma. Specific findings include destruction of exostosis bone, destruction of previously present matrix in the cartilage cap, a thick (>1 cm) or irregular cartilage cap, or growth of the cartilage cap after skeletal maturity (Fig. 32-10). More frequently, there is no early radiographic change but the patient reports pain or growth of the exostosis after skeletal maturity. In the absence of mechanical reasons for pain or the formation of a bursa simulating the growth of the exostosis, such clinical symptoms indicate malignant transformation until proven otherwise. If malignant degeneration is suspected, a chondrosarcoma work-up is done, which includes MRI. Bone scanning usually shows mildly increased uptake in exostoses and variable uptake in chondrosarcomas. Although serial scans may be helpful in distinguishing an exostosis from malig-

nant transformation to chondrosarcoma, a single bone scan may not be specific for diagnosis.

Symptomatic osteochondromas are treated with resection. The entire cartilage cap must be removed to prevent recurrence.

MULTIPLE HEREDITARY OSTEOCHONDROMAS

This is an uncommon autosomal dominant disorder that also may arise sporadically. Patients present with multiple exostoses and short stature, the latter caused by diversion of physeal cartilage to the osteochondromas with consequent diminished longitudinal bone growth. Although some of the osteochondromas are cauliflower-like, most are broad-based sessile lesions. These

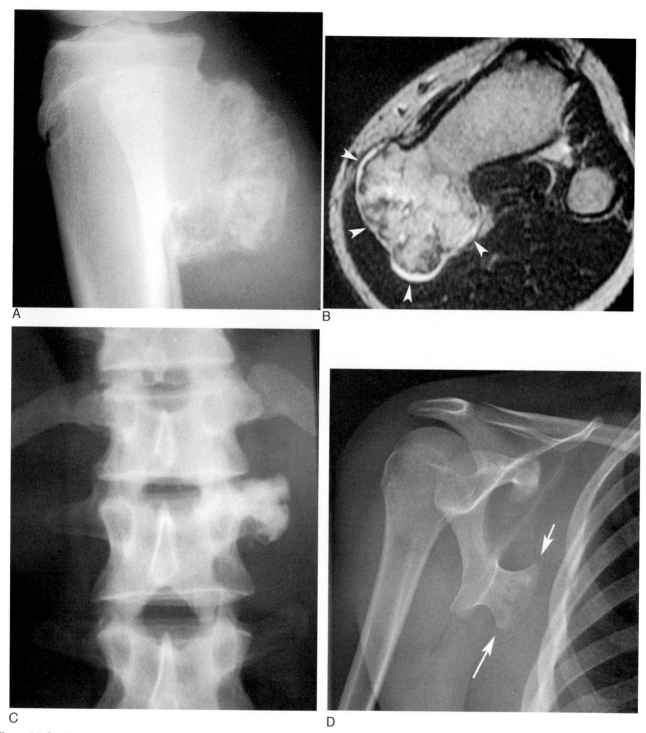

Figure 32-6 Exostosis (osteochondroma). **A,** Lateral radiograph of a typical pedunculated exostosis seen in a 15-year-old boy. The lesion arises from the metaphysis, with continuity of the cortex and the marrow extending from the underlying bone into the exostosis. **B,** This continuity is demonstrated well on the axial T2-weighted MR image. The marrow and cortex extend into the exostosis *(arrows)*. The cartilaginous cap (high signal, *arrowheads*) is uniform and thin. **C,** Pedunculated spine exostosis. **D,** Scapular exostosis (between *arrows*).

sessile osteochondromas result in a greater circumference of the metaphases (Figs. 32-11, 32-12), and the radiographic appearance may simulate a bone dysplasia. A smooth but undulating contour of the cortex in long bone metaphyses and pelvis is common. Coxa valga and Madelung deformity may also be seen. The elbow and wrist joints are often deformed. The lesions first appear in childhood as lumps adjacent to joints.

There is a higher incidence of sarcomatous transformation than in individuals with isolated osteochondromas, especially in the more proximal lesions, reported to be as high as 10% overall. The true risk is likely much lower, about 2% to 5%, and for any particular lesion the risk remains very small.

Treatment of multiple exostoses depends on circumstances, with local resections as necessary for mechanical problems.

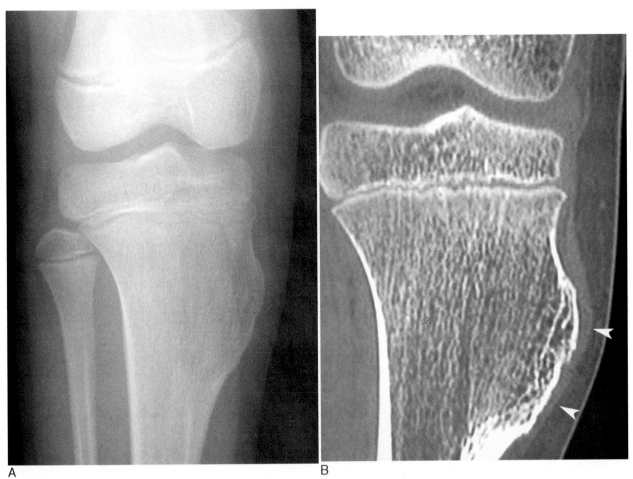

A

B

Figure 32-7 Sessile exostosis **A and B**, AP radiograph (A) and coronal CT reformat (B) show typical bulge-like sessile exostosis at the medial proximal medial metaphysis. Note thin cartilage cap (*arrowheads* in part B).

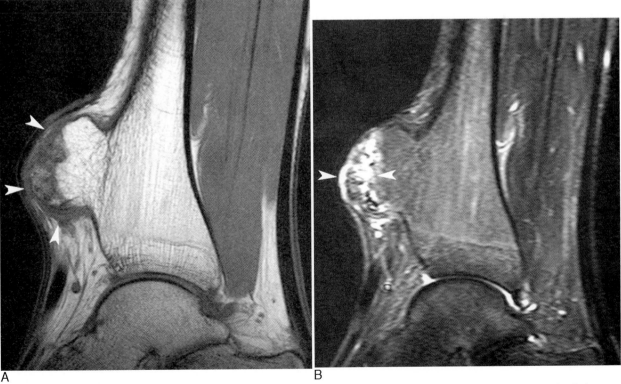

A

B

Figure 32-8 Exostosis: MRI. **A and B**, Sagittal T1-weighted (A) and fat-suppressed T2-weighted (B) MR images of an anterior distal tibia exostosis. Features are similar to those shown in Fig. 32-6B, but the cartilage cap is thicker (*arrowheads*).

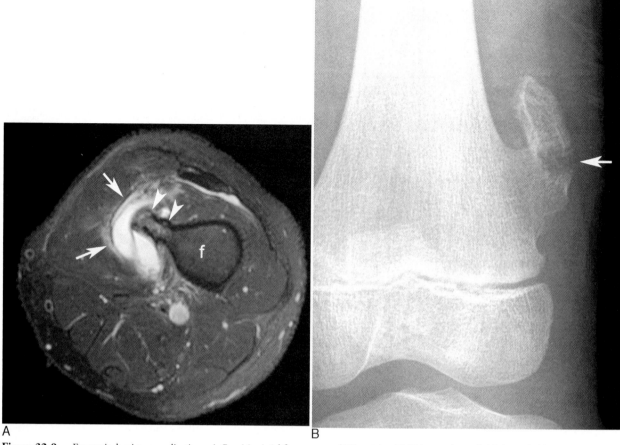

Figure 32-9 Exostosis: benign complications. **A,** Bursitis. Axial fat-suppressed T2-weighted MR image shows fluid-distended bursa *(arrows)* that has formed over a pedunculated medial distal femoral exostosis *(arrowheads).* **B,** Fracture through the base of a pedunculate osteochondroma *(arrow).* f, femur.

The patients are observed for sarcomatous transformation (Fig 32-10) because prophylactic resection is not a realistic option.

DYSPLASIA EPIPHYSEALIS HEMIMELICA (TREVOR DISEASE)

Dysplasia epiphysealis hemimelica, also known as Trevor disease or Trevor-Fairbank disease, is multiple intra-articular epiphyseal osteochondromas (Fig. 32-13). The lesions may occur in single or multiple joints, although generally they occur only in one extremity. The knee and ankle are the most common sites of occurrence. Histologically, the lesions are identical to osteochondromas. Radiographically, they give the appearance of a lobulated mass arising from the epiphysis, which is usually well mineralized. Magnetic resonance imaging can help define the extent of the lesion and its relationship to the joint surfaces. Not surprisingly, Trevor disease causes joint deformity, pain, and limited range of motion. Management is surgical, with resection of the bony excrescences.

JUXTACORTICAL (PERIOSTEAL) CHONDROMA

Juxtacortical chondroma is a benign cartilaginous lesion originating at the periosteal surface (Fig. 32-14). The lesion produces a soft tissue mass and cortical pressure erosion that can be difficult to differentiate from that seen in periosteal osteosarcoma. Furthermore, calcification is produced in the soft tissue mass in about 50% of juxtacortical chondromas, thus making differentiation from periosteal osteosarcoma somewhat problematic.

Juxtacortical chondromas occur in a wide age range and are seen in both large and small tubular bones. Periosteal reaction can be striking, falsely leading one to believe the lesion to be aggressive. The MRI appearance is nonspecific; however, the soft tissue mass adjacent to the bone destruction may make the lesion appear more aggressive by MRI than by radiograph. The clinical behavior, however, is benign. The lesion is treated with wide excision, whenever possible, to preclude recurrence.

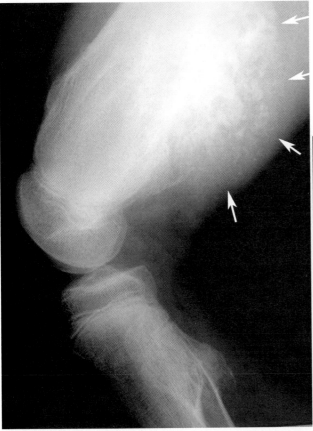

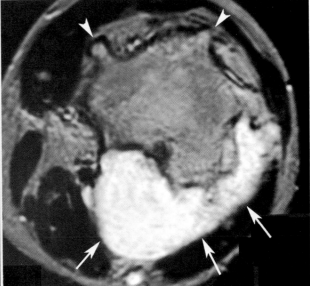

A

B

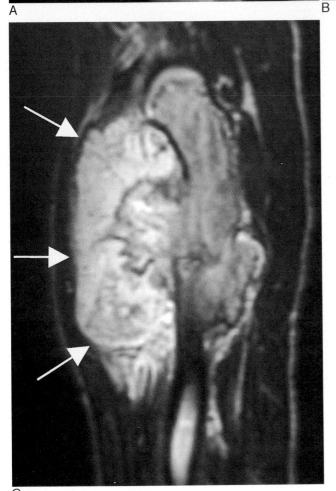

C

Figure 32-10 Malignant transformation of an exostosis. **A,** Lateral radiograph of the knee in a 13-year-old boy who has multiple hereditary exostoses. The posterior lesion in the distal femur shows a large soft tissue mass and abundant chondroid matrix *(arrows),* which was due to transformation of an exostosis to a chondrosarcoma. Radiographs do not always demonstrate a secondary chondrosarcoma. Axial T2-weighted MR image (B) in the same patient shows the multiple small exostoses *(arrowheads)* and the large posterior exostosis and its thick and irregular cartilage cap (high signal intensity, *arrows*). A rule of thumb is that the cartilage cap should not be thicker than 1 cm. The imaging findings in malignant transformation may be much more subtle (e.g., seen as an area of destruction of previously present matrix, or focal enlargement of a portion of the mass). **C,** Malignant transformation in a different patient, with multiple hereditary exostoses. Coronal T2-weighted MR image shows very thick cartilage cap *(arrows)* on a medial femur exostosis in a patient.

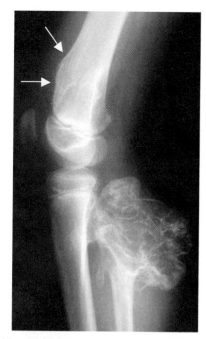

Figure 32-11   Multiple exostoses. Lateral radiograph of the knee in a 7-year-old girl demonstrates the large cauliflower-like exostosis of the proximal fibula and a sessile lesion of the distal femur *(arrows)*. These sessile exostoses occasionally are mistaken for a metaphyseal dysplasia, leading to a missed diagnosis of multiple hereditary exostoses.

The major differential diagnosis, as noted previously, is periosteal osteosarcoma. Giant cell tumor of the tendon sheath can cause cortical "saucerization" (i.e., scalloping of the external bone surface), with a soft tissue mass that appears to be a surface lesion.

CHONDROBLASTOMA

Chondroblastoma (Codman's tumor) is a rare benign cartilaginous tumor found almost exclusively in the epiphysis in skeletally immature patients. This is one of the few neoplasms found in the epiphysis. The lesion typically has geographic and sclerotic margins. Margins are often lobulated, best appreciated with MRI or CT, typical of cartilaginous lesions. The tumor is predominately lytic, although 50% show some amount of chondroid matrix. This may be very subtle, seen only by CT. Even though the lesion is nonaggressive in appearance, most chondroblastomas elicit a thick periosteal reaction along the metaphysis, a location remote from the lesion (Fig. 32-15). The cause for this finding is uncertain, but the reaction may be mediated by hormone-like factors released by the tumor. Chondroblastoma tends to be eccentrically located within the epiphysis. If there is partial physeal closure, the lesion may extend into the metaphysis. The most

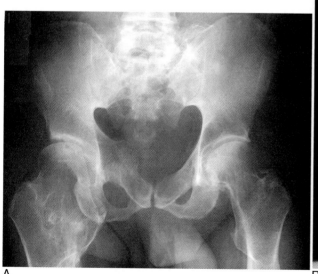

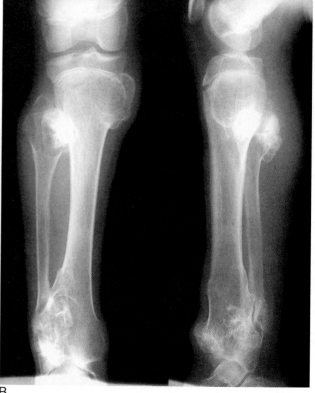

A

B

Figure 32-12   Multiple hereditary exostoses. **A and B,** Radiographs of the pelvis (A) and right tibia and fibula (B) in an older child show multiple osteochondromas. Leg bone shortening is evident because of diversion of growth plate cartilage to the exostoses, creating a radiographic appearance that might be mistaken for dwarfism or metaphyseal dysplasia.

common site of involvement is the proximal humerus, followed by the proximal femur, distal femur, and proximal tibia. The bones of the hindfoot may also be involved.

Magnetic resonance imaging shows signal intensity isointense with muscle on T1-weighted images and intermediate heterogeneous to high signal intensity on T2-weighted images, often in a lobulated pattern. A joint effusion may be present. Magnetic resonance shows not only the prominent periosteal reaction in the metaphyseal region but also intense bone marrow and adjacent soft tissue edema. It therefore suggests a more aggressive lesion than is demonstrated by radiography. However, as was noted in Chapter 29, the radiographic features are more reliable in assessing the aggressiveness of a tumor.

Patients present with localized pain. Diagnosis is made by radiography, and CT can be helpful in confirming matrix calcification. Magnetic resonance imaging generally does not contribute to diagnosis but can help establish the relationship of the chondroblastoma to the adjacent joint and physis. Treatment is by curettage and bone graft. Recurrence rate is 15%, but metastatic potential is almost negligible, with only isolated case reports of malignant chondroblastoma. The major differential diagnoses in the adolescent or young adult include giant cell tumor crossing into the epiphysis, articular lesions with large cysts (e.g., pigmented villonodular synovitis), and clear cell chondrosarcoma. In children, the differential diagnosis includes eosinophilic granuloma and epiphyseal osteomyelitis.

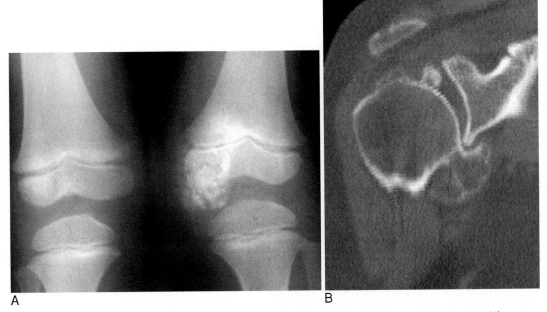

A   B

Figure 32-13 Trevor-Fairbank disease. **A,** AP radiograph of the knees of a 9-year-old boy is typical for Trevor-Fairbank disease, demonstrating exostosis-like lesions arising from the epiphysis. This intra-articular process is usually unilateral. **B,** Coronal CT reconstruction of the proximal right humerus in a different patient shows similar findings. (Part A reproduced with permission from the American College of Radiology learning file.)

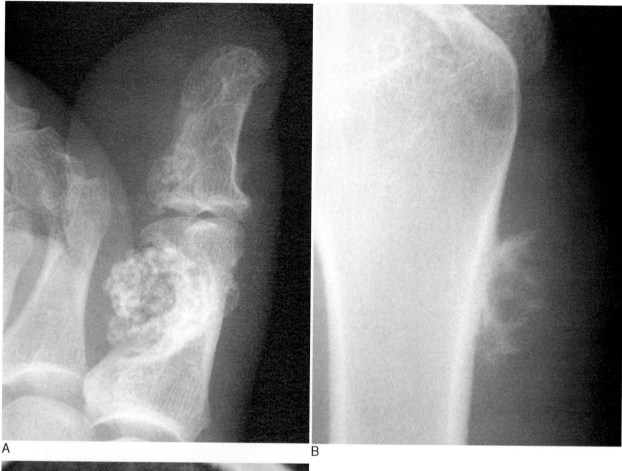

A   B

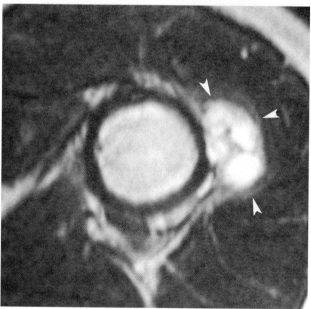

C

Figure 32-14   Juxtacortical chondromas. **A,** Lateral radiograph of the great toe in a 50-year-old woman. Note the lesions in both the proximal and distal phalanx, with each showing scalloping of the underlying bone and a densely calcified chondroid matrix. These findings are of a surface lesion, and each is a typical example of a juxtacortical chondroma. It is unusual to see two adjacent lesions. **B,** Another example, with a somewhat different appearance, is seen in an AP radiograph of the proximal humerus in an 18-year-old woman. Again, a surface lesion is demonstrated, this time without scalloping and with prominent matrix extending into the soft tissues. **C,** Axial T2-weighted MR image shows a juxtacortical mass with high-signal-intensity lobules *(arrowheads),* which is suggestive of cartilage but is not specific. Although this proved at biopsy to be a juxtacortical chondroma, an imaging diagnosis of parosteal osteosarcoma would be reasonable on the basis of the imaging characteristics.

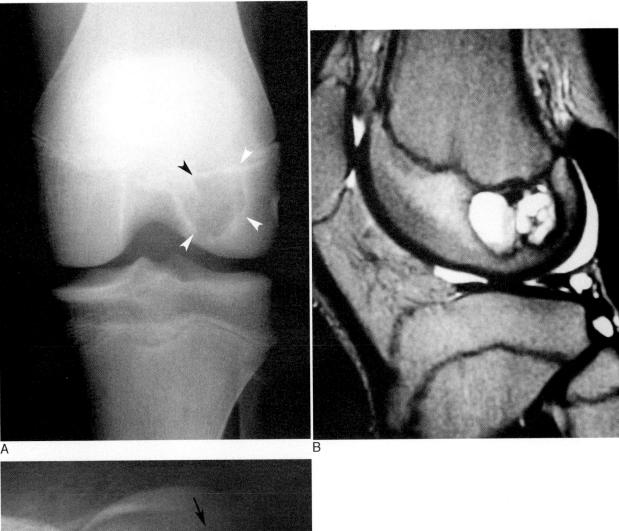

Figure 32-15 Chondroblastoma. **A**, AP radiograph of the knee in a 14-year-old boy shows a geographic lytic lesion in the epiphysis with a narrow zone of transition and sclerotic (type 1A) margin *(arrowheads)*, a typical appearance of chondroblastoma with the open physis. **B**, T2-weighted sagittal MR image demonstrates the epiphyseal location, as well as the largely homogenous high signal appearance that can be typical of cartilage lesions. Also note surrounding bone marrow edema and joint effusion. **C**, AP radiograph of a chondroblastoma in a different patient, an 18-year-old man. In this case, the lytic lesion is again located predominately in the epiphysis and has a partially nonsclerotic margin *(arrows)*. Note the very dense, mature periosteal reaction in the metaphysis *(arrowhead)*, remote from the tumor. Both the location of the lesion in the proximal humerus epiphysis and the dense periosteal reaction away from the tumor are typical of chondroblastoma.

CHONDROMYXOID FIBROMA

Chondromyxoid fibroma is a very rare benign cartilaginous lesion, which also contains fibrous and myxoid tissue. This lesion is so rare that it should very rarely be offered as a likely differential diagnostic possibility. Although the age range is wide, it is most frequently seen in the second and third decades. Patients present with local pain and swelling. Lesion margins are geographic and sclerotic, often lobulated. The tumor is usually occurs eccentrically in the metaphysis.

Chondromyxoid fibroma usually has a thick sclerotic margin and may cause mild cortical expansion (see Fig. 29-7B). Although this is a cartilaginous lesion, it is rare to find calcified tumor matrix within it. The MRI appearance is nonspecific, with low signal intensity on T1 and high signal intensity on T2, which is often inhomogeneous. One third of the lesions are found in the proximal tibia, with the others distributed in the proximal and distal femur, flat bones, tarsal bones, and other small bones of the hand or foot. The lesion follows a benign course and undergoes malignant transformation only rarely. Treatment is with curettage and bone grafting. The recurrence rate is high (approximately 25%) following curettage, perhaps because of incomplete removal of this lobulated lesion.

CENTRAL CHONDROSARCOMA

Central chondrosarcoma may be either primary or secondary (i.e., arising de novo or from malignant transformation from a pre-existing benign lesion, most often an enchondroma) (see Figs. 32-3, 32-16). In general, proximal chondrosarcomas tend to be primary, and peripheral chondrosarcomas tend to arise from pre-existing lesions. These lesions are usually central and metaphyseal in location, and are particularly common in the proximal long bones, the pelvis, and the shoulder girdle. Although enchondroma is common in the hands and feet, these lesions almost never undergo malignant transformation; thus, chondrosarcoma is rare in these locations. Chondrosarcoma occurs most frequently in the fourth through sixth decades of life. Ninety percent of central chondrosarcomas are low grade. Although low-grade chondrosarcomas are generally large (>5 cm) at presentation, they tend to be well defined. Like enchondromas, low-grade chondrosarcomas may show only mild endosteal scalloping. Endosteal scalloping that removes more than two thirds of the cortical thickness favors a chondrosarcoma over an enchondroma. (Please see discussion of distinguishing enchondroma from chondrosarcoma in the endochondroma section of this chapter.) Low-grade chondrosarcomas can have a narrow zone of transition, without sclerotic margins. The amount of chondroid tumor matrix varies, ranging from completely lytic lesions to lytic lesions with only a few

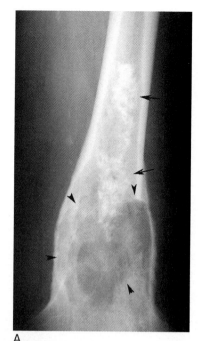

A

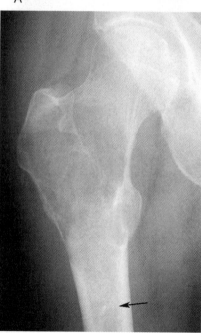

B

Figure 32-16 Intramedullary chondrosarcoma. **A,** AP radiograph of the distal femur in a 79-year-old man. This demonstrates the typical matrix of an enchondroma in its proximal portion *(arrows)*, extending into a highly destructive lesion more distally *(arrowheads)*. This is a chondrosarcoma arising in an enchondroma (see also Fig. 32 1-28B). **B,** AP radiograph of a geographic lytic lesion with a mildly widened zone of transition (type 1C) margin in the proximal femur of a 52-year-old man. There is subtle chondroid matrix in the proximal femoral shaft *(arrow)*. With the aggressive lesion margins, chondroid matrix, proximal location, and patient's age, the diagnosis can only be chondrosarcoma. Note the spectrum of chondroid matrix one might expect to see in chondrosarcoma.

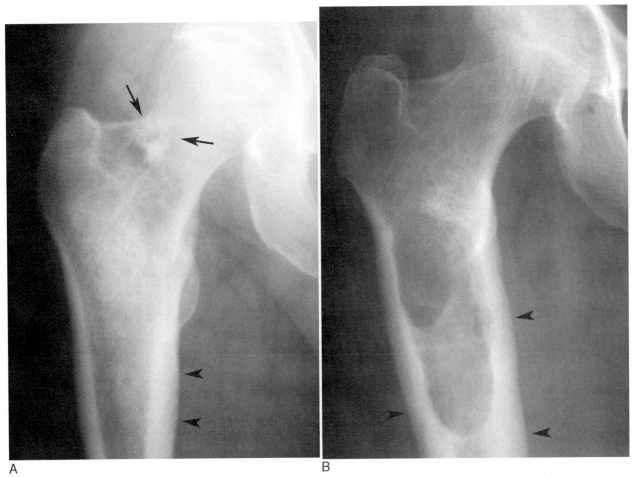

A   B

Figure 32-17   Intramedullary chondrosarcoma. **A,** AP radiograph of the proximal femur in a 38-year-old man. There is chondroid matrix in the proximal portion of the lesion *(arrows),* and the lesion shows a destructive pattern with a wide zone of transition. These features alone make it a chondrosarcoma. Additionally, there is prominent thickening of the cortex *(arrowheads),* also a finding that may be seen in intramedullary chondrosarcoma, although it is not specific. **B,** AP radiograph of the hip in a 51-year-old woman, also an intramedullary chondrosarcoma. In this case, there is no visible chondroid matrix. The zone of transition is narrow but not sclerotic (type 1B margin), and there is cortical thickening with mild expansion related to slow tumor growth *(arrowheads).* The location, age of the patient, and endosteal and periosteal thickening suggest the diagnosis of chondrosarcoma despite the absence of chondroid matrix.

flecks of calcification, to dense aggregates of chondroid matrix (see Fig. 32-16). In general, low-grade tumors contain more myxoid tissue and therefore tend to have less chondroid matrix. There often is no soft tissue mass, although high-grade lesions can be associated with cortical breakthrough with a soft tissue mass. Because there may be no cortical breakthrough, periosteal reaction is variable: there may be none, or the endosteum may be significantly thickened (Fig. 32-17). This latter feature of endosteal thickening, when present, may suggest the diagnosis of chondrosarcoma. It is seen in only a few other aggressive lesions in patients of this age group, including primary lymphoma of bone, Ewing's sarcoma in a younger age group, and osteomyelitis.

It is very important to be aware that chondrosarcomas are common malignant tumors of bone, and most are not aggressive in radiographic appearance. Therefore, if a central lesion in the correct age group appears slightly to moderately aggressive, with a questionable widened zone of transition or endosteal scalloping, the diagnosis of chondrosarcoma should be offered, whether or not definite chondroid matrix is found. Note the variety of appearances central chondrosarcoma can show in Figures 32-16 and 32-17. This lesion is commonly underdiagnosed because it so often appears nonaggressive. Underdiagnosis results in undertreatment, which puts the patient at risk for recurrence or metastatic disease.

A well-differentiated chondrosarcoma may show the lobulated T2-bright features of hyaline cartilage typical of benign

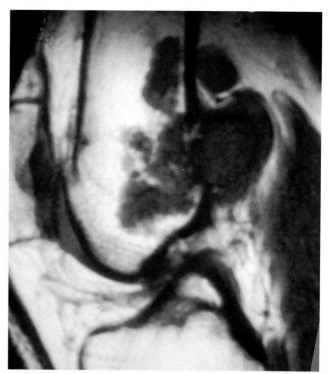

Figure 32-18   Chondrosarcoma. Sagittal T1-weighted image of the distal femur in a 24-year-old woman. The multilobular, low-signal-intensity mass has both intraosseous and extraosseous location, never a normal finding in an enchondroma. Only faint matrix was present on radio-graphs and CT (not shown).

cartilage lesions. The fibrous stroma between the chondroid nodules often enhances intensely, but this is nonspecific because benign enchondromas can have a similar pattern of enhancement. Higher-grade lesions will appear nonspecific and have inhomogeneous high signal intensity on T2-weighted imaging. Mineralized matrix will be seen as low signal intensity on all sequences.

The major differential diagnosis of a central chondrosarcoma is enchondroma. Distinguishing features were discussed previously. If the lesion appears more aggressive and calcification is present, it can be confused with sarcomatous transformation of a bone infarct. If no chondroid matrix is present, the differential diagnosis includes metastasis, plasmacytoma, malignant fibrous histiocytoma, fibrosarcoma, and lymphoma. If the lesion is less aggressive in appearance and without matrix, giant cell tumor might be considered.

Peripheral (exostotic) chondrosarcomas may be either primary or may secondarily arise as malignant transformation of an osteochondroma (exostosis). They are seen most frequently in the third, fourth, and fifth decades of life. They are large extraosseous lesions, arising from the metaphyses of long bones as well as the pelvis, shoulder girdle, sternum, and ribs (see Fig. 32-10). They most frequently show normal-appearing underlying host bone extending into an exostosis but with a large cartilaginous cap (>1 cm thick). Changes over time in the appearance of chondroid calcification in an exostosis may help to diagnose transformation to a chondrosarcoma, but MRI may frequently be necessary to evaluate the cartilaginous cap thickness. Higher-grade lesions may show destruction of the stalk as well as soft tissue mass beyond that of the cartilaginous cap (Fig. 32-18). As described with osteochondromas, transformation to chondrosarcoma may produce no distinct radiographic signs. Therefore, clinical signs of new-onset nonmechanical pain and increased size after growth plate closure should be considered of primary importance in suggesting the diagnosis of peripheral chondrosarcoma.

Ninety percent of chondrosarcomas, either central or peripheral, are low-grade lesions. Therefore, local recurrence is more common than is metastatic disease. Higher grade tumors can be seen with recurrence. Prognosis is worse for proximal and axial lesions than distal lesions. Five-year survival is approximately 75%, and this can be improved by a more prompt radiologic diagnosis and meticulous surgical technique. Chondrosarcoma can be readily implanted in soft tissues because it does not need a blood supply to survive. Therefore, recurrences may be due to tumor spill at the time of biopsy or resection. Wide excision is the therapy of choice. Radiation and chemotherapy do not improve survival or decrease local recurrence rates.

CLEAR CELL CHONDROSARCOMA

Clear cell chondrosarcoma is a very rare lesion that is most often mistaken for a chondroblastoma because it can be identical in imaging appearance and location in the epiphyses, especially of the proximal femur and humerus. These lesions may in fact be related. Clear cell chondrosarcoma occurs in older patients than does chondroblastoma, peaking in the third decade. It is usually geographic in appearance, with a narrow zone of transition and sclerotic margin. Periosteal reaction and cortical breakthrough are rare. Chondroid matrix is usually absent.

If left untreated, clear cell chondrosarcoma may become much more aggressive. Treatment is wide excision; curettage alone can result in an aggressive recurrence.

DEDIFFERENTIATED CHONDROSARCOMA

A portion of a low-grade chondrosarcoma may dedifferentiate into a high-grade, highly aggressive lesion. This dedifferentiation results in a neoplasm that may have several elements, including fibrosarcoma, malignant fibrous histiocytoma, high-grade chondrosarcoma, and osteosarcoma. As many as 10% of chondrosarcomas dedifferentiate.

The radiographic appearance of dedifferentiated chondrosarcoma follows the pathologic findings, and usually shows areas with features of low-grade chondrosarcoma, with other areas with highly aggressive features such as bone lysis. It is important to choose a biopsy site that includes the more aggressive portion of the lesion.

Prognosis of dedifferentiated chondrosarcoma is poor, with a 5-year survival rate of only 20%. Metastases to the lung are common. Treatment is with radical excision and chemotherapy.

MESENCHYMAL CHONDROSARCOMA

This is an exceedingly rare, high-grade chondrosarcoma. The age group for mesenchymal chondrosarcoma is younger than for standard chondrosarcoma (first through fourth decades). The site is unusual, with one third to half arising in the soft tissues. In the skeleton, rib and jaw lesions are common, whereas long bone lesions are typically not seen. Chondroid calcification is usually present, which, combined with a radiographically aggressive lesion in such unusual location and younger age, suggests the diagnosis.

CHAPTER 33

Fibrous Tumors and Tumor-Like Conditions

FIBROUS DYSPLASIA
FIBROMATOSES
NONOSSIFYING FIBROMA/BENIGN FIBROUS CORTICAL
  DEFECT (FIBROXANTHOMA)
BENIGN FIBROUS HISTIOCYTOMA
LIPOSCLEROSING MYXOFIBROUS TUMOR
  (POLYMORPHIC FIBRO-OSSEOUS LESION OF BONE)
MALIGNANT FIBROUS HISTIOCYTOMA/FIBROSARCOMA

FIBROUS DYSPLASIA

Fibrous dysplasia not a neoplasm but rather a hamartomatous fibro-osseous metaplasia or dysplasia consisting of a fibrous stroma with islands of osteoid and woven bone. The lesion is relatively common. Although there is a wide age range of occurrence, it most often is detected in the second and third decades of life. Thirty percent of cases of fibrous dysplasia are polyostotic. Polyostotic fibrous dysplasia has a more aggressive clinical and radiographic appearance and usually presents before the age of 10. Interestingly, in 90% of polyostotic cases, the lesions are hemimelic (i.e., involve a single limb).

Fibrous dysplasia can be found in any bone but is uncommon in the spine. The most common areas of involvement include the tubular bones (in which the lesions are usually central and metadiaphyseal), ribs, pelvis, skull (particularly the base of skull), and facial bones. There is no consistently seen matrix pattern in fibrous dysplasia. The lesions range from being completely lucent, through a uniform mildly radiopaque appearance termed ground-glass density, to densely sclerotic. The density depends on the amount of woven bone present in the fibrous stroma.

Fibrous dysplasia has a range of radiographic appearances, depending on whether it is found in the skull, pelvis, or tubular bones. Lesion density tends to depend on location. In general, lesions in the base of the skull tend to be sclerotic (Fig. 33-1). Calvarial lesions range from lytic to dense and show a nonaggressive expansion of bone. Fibrous dysplasia in the ribs and tubular

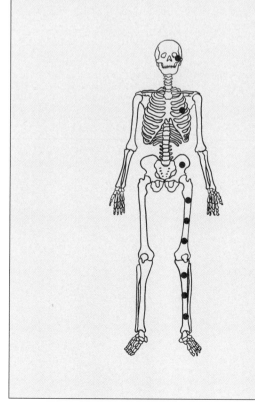

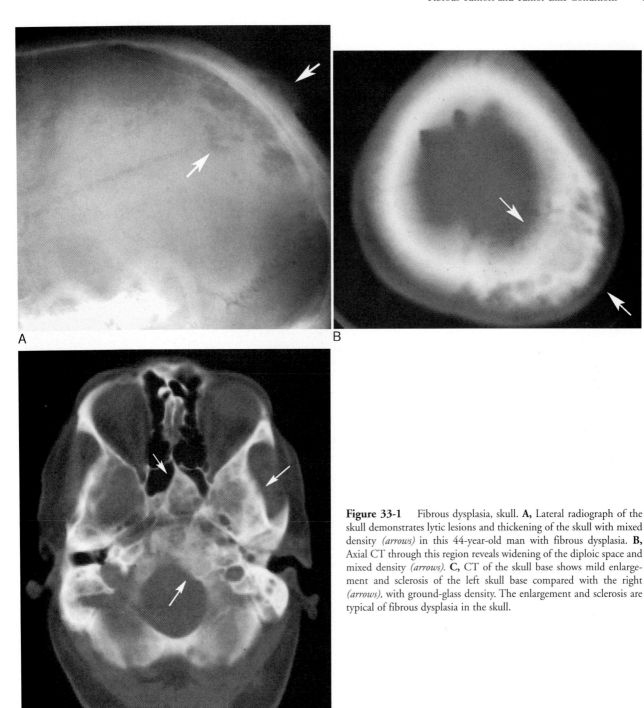

Figure 33-1   Fibrous dysplasia, skull. **A,** Lateral radiograph of the skull demonstrates lytic lesions and thickening of the skull with mixed density *(arrows)* in this 44-year-old man with fibrous dysplasia. **B,** Axial CT through this region reveals widening of the diploic space and mixed density *(arrows)*. **C,** CT of the skull base shows mild enlargement and sclerosis of the left skull base compared with the right *(arrows),* with ground-glass density. The enlargement and sclerosis are typical of fibrous dysplasia in the skull.

bones tend to have ground-glass density (Fig. 33-2). On the other hand, pelvic lesions may be bubbly and expansile (Fig. 33-3).

Bones involved with fibrous dysplasia are frequently expanded, often with cortical thinning (Fig. 33-4). The thin expanded bones are "soft," and long bones may develop bowing and angulation with weight bearing. The term "shepherd's crook" represents severe varus of the femoral neck (Fig. 33-5).

Polyostotic disease with deformed bones, often with a ground-glass density and lacking trabecular definition, makes for a distinct radiographic appearance. Although the lesions in the long bones are usually central, fibrous dysplasia can also be cortically based. When this occurs in the tibia, it can appear identical to osteofibrous dysplasia (ossifying fibroma) and adamantinoma (see Fig. 30-11).

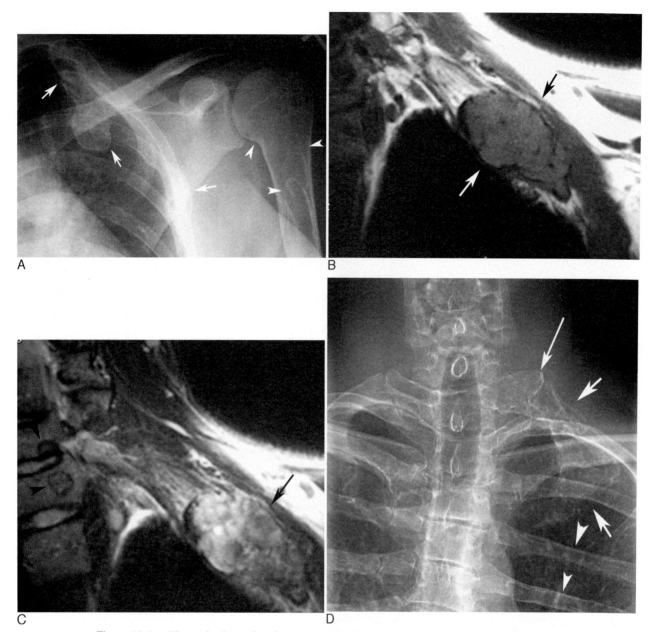

Figure 33-2   Fibrous dysplasia, rib. Ribs are a common location for fibrous dysplasia. This 24-year-old woman had a brachial plexopathy. **A,** AP radiograph demonstrates expanded ribs *(arrows)*, as well as typical lesions in the proximal humerus *(arrowheads)*. **B and C,** Coronal T1-weighted (B) and T2-weighted (C) MR images in the same patient show mass-like enlargement of the first rib *(arrows)*, which is isointense with muscle on T1 and has heterogeneous signal intensity on T2. This mass compresses the brachial plexus. Note additional lesions in the adjacent vertebrae *(arrowheads)*. **D,** AP radiograph in a different patient with fibrous dysplasia shows expanded left first rib *(arrows)*, left T1 transverse process *(long arrow)*, and irregular cortical thinning in the posterior left fourth and fifth ribs *(arrowheads)*.

Craniofacial involvement (leontiasis ossea) is common, especially in patients with polyostotic fibrous dysplasia, with predilection for the sphenoid bones. Frontal, maxillary, and ethmoid involvement is also common. The bone expansion can cause facial deformity, cranial nerve compression, and exophthalmos. The radiographic appearance may suggest Paget's disease, but the cortex is not as thickened, and ground-glass density rather than trabecular thickening is frequently present.

Bone scans of fibrous dysplasia show increased tracer uptake. Magnetic resonance imaging (MRI) is nonspecific, with low to intermediate signal on T1-weighted and variable signal on T2-weighted sequences. The lesions frequently enhance, often uniformly. Cystic degeneration occurs occasionally, which can result in a fluid-fluid level.

Fibrous dysplasia is usually easily diagnosed with radiography. Visualization of skull lesions may benefit from computed tomography (CT). Differential diagnosis may include Paget's disease,

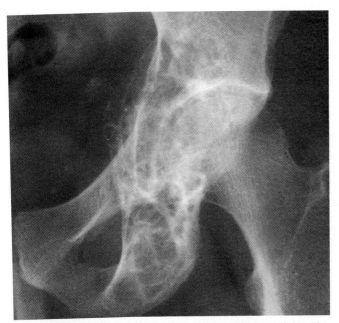

Figure 33-3   Fibrous dysplasia, pelvis. Fibrous dysplasia of the pelvis most frequently appears as a bubbly and expanded lesion, as is seen in this 29-year-old man. Findings suggesting a diagnosis of fibrous dysplasia include the narrow zone of transition, lack of cortical breakthrough, and relatively long length of the lesion compared with the degree of bone expansion.

neurofibromatosis type 1, and, for localized disease, other fibrous lesions.

Most lesions remain quiescent throughout life, neither improving nor resolving. Only 5% continue to enlarge after skeletal maturity. Malignant transformation, usually to fibrosarcoma or osteosarcoma, is rare. In consideration of these observations, treatment is generally reserved for symptomatic lesions only, such as fractures or deformities. Limb-length discrepancy, angular deformity, and pseudoarthrosis seen in the tibia of young children with fibrous dysplasia may require osteotomy, bone grafting, and immobilization. However, resection or curettage of a nonsymptomatic site of fibrous dysplasia is usually both futile and unnecessary.

Fibrous dysplasia (usually the polyostotic form) may be associated with a variety of endocrine disorders, including hyperthyroidism, hyperparathyroidism, acromegaly, diabetes, and Cushing's syndrome. *McCune-Albright syndrome* is polyostotic fibrous dysplasia, endocrine disorder (most often precocious puberty or hyperthyroidism), and café au lait skin lesions with irregular "coast of Maine" margins (as compared with the "coast of California" margins of neurofibromatosis type I). *Cherubism* is a rare, familial, congenital fibrous dysplasia–like enlargement of the mandible with associated abnormal

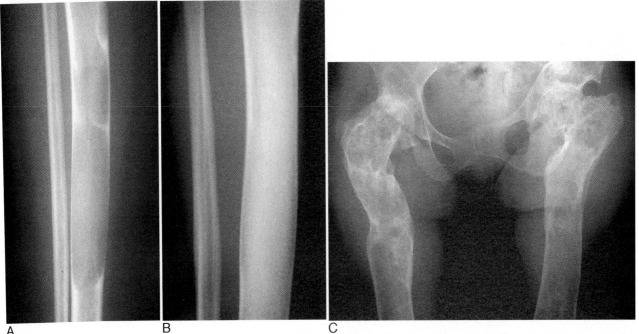

A   B   C

Figure 33-4   Fibrous dysplasia, tubular bones. **A,** AP radiograph of the tibia in a 10-year-old girl demonstrates mild expansion with uniform ground-glass density. This is a typical appearance of fibrous dysplasia in the long bones. **B,** More dense ground-glass appearance, again with mild expansion of the tibia, is seen in a different patient. The juxtaposition of these two cases demonstrates the spectrum of ground-glass density of fibrous dysplasia. Both lesions are relatively long compared with the degree of bone expansion. The zone of transition is narrow and there is no cortical interruption. Remember that although most cases of fibrous dysplasia are central medullary lesions, fibrous dysplasia can occasionally be cortically based. These cortically based lesions can be significantly different in appearance. For examples, please see Fig. 29-7C and D, as well as Fig. 31-11B. **C,** Intermediate density, with unusually marked expansion of the diaphyses. Note the bilateral femoral neck varus configuration which has been termed a "shepherd's crook" deformity and is typical of fibrous dysplasia. Femoral neck varus is also seen with other bone-softening conditions, such as osteomalacia and Paget's disease.

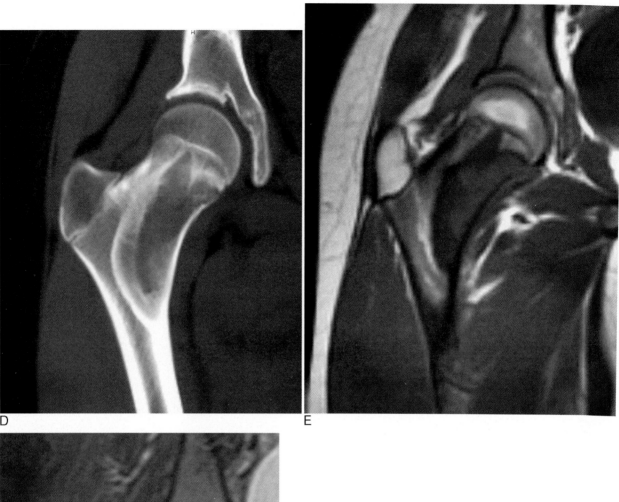

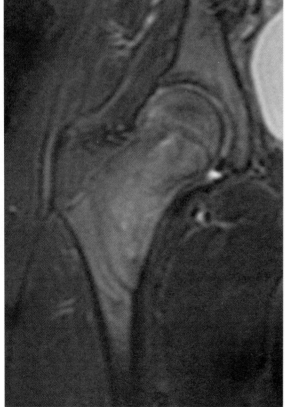

Figure 33-4—(Cont'd) D–F, Fibrous dysplasia of the proximal femur in a 12-year-old girl. Coronal CT reformat (D), coronal T1 (E), and inversion recovery (F) MR images show the typical broad sclerotic margin. This lesion has fairly danse mineralization peripherally, with associated low signal intensity on the MR images. The less densely mineralized central region has MR signal intensity that is commonly seen in fibrous dysplasia and other fibrous lesions, which is intermediate on T1 and only midly increased on fat-suppressed T2 or inversion recovery.

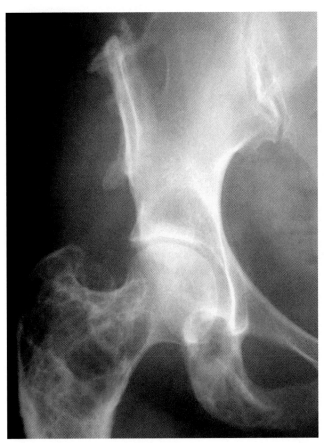

Figure 33-5   Fibrous dysplasia, "bubbly lytic" pattern. AP radiograph shows a geographic expansile "bubbly" lesion in the ischium with a narrow zone of transition, as well as a rather bubbly-appearing expansile lesion in the proximal femur. What is unusual about this case is that this 45-year-old woman has undergone curettage and bone grafting of the femoral neck lesion, with the bone graft obtained from the right iliac wing, which accounts for the iliac wing deformity. Generally, bone grafting and other surgery in the extremities in fibrous dysplasia is reserved for orthopedic complications.

dentition. The jaw usually assumes a more normal morphology by adolescence. The rare *Mazabraud syndrome* is fibrous dysplasia associated with intramuscular myxomas. The myxomas usually occur near the abnormal bones. A *myxoma* is a rare benign mass in the extremities, typically found within skeletal muscle, composed predominantly of myxoid tissue. Myxomas have very high T2 signal, and often enhance only peripherally or along fibrous septae. Their appearance on MRI can resemble an aggressive sarcoma with central necrosis.

FIBROMATOSES

The fibromatoses are a heterogeneous group of tumors that have been described with a variety of terms and classifications, although histologically all the lesions are similar. Fibromatosis histologically is composed of sheets of fibroblasts with herringbone pattern, without evidence for mitoses. Most arise in soft tissue. As a group, soft tissue fibromatoses tend to be large, locally infiltrative, and occasionally multicentric. Tumor often infiltrates through compartmental barriers and has no visible capsule either at surgery or with imaging. This aggressive appearance may lead to a misdiagnosis of a malignant lesion. However, MRI signal characteristics can be helpful in making the correct diagnosis. In up to 80% of cases, the signal intensity is low on both T1 and T2 imaging because of the hypocellularity of the lesion. In the remaining 20% of cases, the nonspecific low signal intensity on T1 and high signal intensity on T2 sequences make the diagnosis more difficult. Enhancement is variable but often intense. The lesions tend to grow along fascial planes, which can be a clue to the diagnosis.

Soft tissue fibromatoses tend to be grouped according to the age and location of occurrence. *Congenital generalized fibromatosis* is a variant that develops in utero, with disseminating lesions involving much of the musculature and viscera. This variant is fulminant and typically fatal within a few months. A second category is *infantile dermal fibromatosis*. In this case, the lesions infiltrate the extensor surfaces of the digits, presenting as firm nodules attached to the skin, tendons, fascia, and periosteum. Bony erosion may occasionally occur. The lesions are usually seen in children 1 to 2 years of age, and recurrence after excision is frequent. Another variant, *juvenile aponeurotic fibroma,* is seen in children and adolescents as a slowly infiltrating lesion arising in the aponeurotic tissue of the hands (usually the volar portion), wrist, and feet (usually the plantar region). This lesion may calcify, especially in the interosseous membrane of the distal forearm (Fig. 33-6). It may be locally aggressive, with recurrence common following resection.

The most common variant of the soft tissue fibromatoses is the *desmoid tumor,* which is also termed *aggressive fibromatosis,* desmoid fibromatosis, or fibrosarcoma grade I desmoid type. (The unrelated and poorly named "cortical desmoid" of the distal femur, which is an avulsive injury and not a tumor, is discussed in Chapter 13.) Aggressive fibromatosis is a fairly common lesion. It presents as a painless infiltrative soft tissue mass, which can originate anywhere, often in the abdominal wall or mesentery. The lesion is often large by the time it is detected, and shows aggressive local infiltration of adjacent muscle, vessels, nerves, and tendons (Fig. 33-7). Rarely, an adjacent bone may be invaded by direct extension of tumor (Fig. 33-7D). When bone is affected by aggressive fibromatosis, it may have a spectacular appearance with huge frond-like excrescences arising from stimulated periosteum, with spicules of bone radiating into the adjacent soft tissue mass. Aggressive fibromatosis often presents in children and young adults and may be indolent for long periods. Although it does not metastasize, it is locally highly aggressive, with a postresection recurrence rate of 65% to 75%. Because the tumor is infiltrative and unencapsulated, the margins can be difficult to assess with imaging studies or by direct palpation at surgery; a wide margin beyond the apparent defined tumor limit should be obtained at surgery.

Two clinical variants of fibromatosis deserve special mention. *Palmar fibromatosis,* also know as *Dupuytren's contracture,*

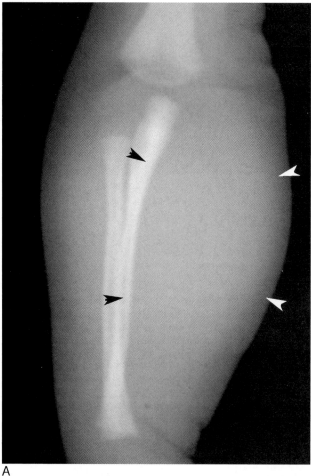

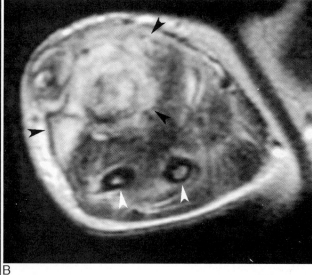

Figure 33-6   Juvenile aponeurotic fibromatosis. **A,** AP radiograph of the forearm in a 6-day-old infant. It demonstrates a large soft tissue mass *(arrowheads)*, along with scalloping and deformity of the forearm bones. **B,** T2-weighted MR image shows the mass *(black arrowheads)* to be volar in location and both heterogeneous and infiltrative. The chronic-appearing bone changes and age of the patient are clues to the diagnosis of congenital form of fibromatosis. The white arrowheads mark the ulna and radius.

is fibromatosis of the palmar hand. Fibrotic bands tether the hand flexor tendons, causing flexion contractures, most frequently of the medial fingers (Fig. 33-8). This is a common condition in elderly patients. *Plantar fibromatosis* presents most often during middle age. This is a benign but potentially locally aggressive lobular tumor-like growth of the plantar fas-

cia. The growths have variable signal intensity and enhancement on all MRI sequences, and are also visible with ultrasonography (US) (Figs. 33-9, 33-10). Diagnosis is usually easy, but this condition can be difficult to treat because of a tendency for local invasion and recurrence. Palmar and plantar fibromatosis often coexist in the same patient.

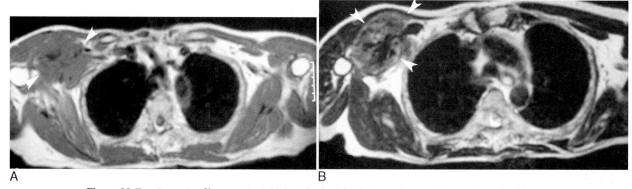

Figure 33-7   Aggressive fibromatosis. **A,** T1-weighted axial MR image shows an intermediate-signal-intensity infiltrative mass involving the anterior chest wall *(arrowheads)* in a 61-year-old man. **B,** T2-weighted MR image shows the mass to remain mostly low signal intensity *(arrows)*. The MR imaging signal characteristics, in combination with the invasiveness of the lesion and location on the chest wall, make the diagnosis of aggressive fibromatosis extremely likely in this case. However, aggressive fibromatosis does not always show low signal characteristics on T2-weighted imaging, as shown in C.

(Continued)

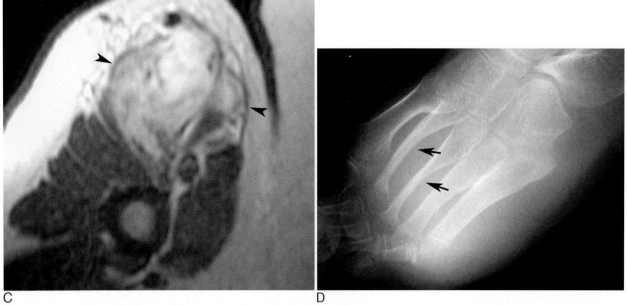

C   D

Figure 33-7—(Cont'd)   **C,** An axial T2-weighted MR image depicting an invasive high-signal-intensity mass lesion *(arrowheads)* in the proximal arm of a 42-year-old man. At biopsy, this proved to also be aggressive fibromatosis. **D,** An oblique radiograph of a foot in a 12-year-old boy showing the osseous deformity *(arrows)* that can occur in cases of aggressive fibromatosis.

Desmoplastic fibroma is the rare form of fibromatosis in bone. Most of these lesions present in the second decade of life and have a geographic pattern with cortical expansion and endosteal erosion. The lesions are located centrally in the metaphysis, most frequently in the long bones but also the pelvis and mandible. The zone of transition varies and can appear aggressive with a wide

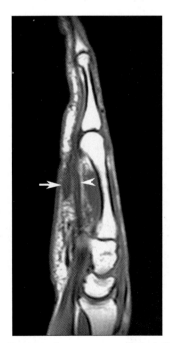

Figure 33-8   Dupuytren's contracture. Sagittal T1-weighted MR image in the hand shows a low-signal-intensity fibrous band *(arrow)* palmar to the flexor tendons *(arrowhead).*

zone of transition. There is no tumor matrix and generally no significant host response. Because these can be radiographically aggressive, they can be difficult to distinguish radiographically as well as histologically from a well-differentiated fibrosarcoma. Their behavior is not malignant, but recurrence is very common.

NONOSSIFYING FIBROMA/BENIGN FIBROUS CORTICAL DEFECT (FIBROXANTHOMA)

Nonossifying fibroma (NOF) and benign fibrous cortical defect are histologically identical, cortically based lesions that in fact are not neoplasms but may arise secondary to physeal defects that migrate away from the physis with growth. The distinction between NOF and fibrous cortical defect is based only on size and propensity for growth; NOF is the larger version. It is estimated that benign fibrous cortical defect occurs in 30% to 40% of children older than age 2. The cause may be related to trauma at muscle attachment sites in the growing skeleton that results in self-limited fibrous proliferation. They are seen infrequently in adults because they convert to normal bone spontaneously after a few years. Most of these lesions are asymptomatic and incidental. Larger lesions may present with pathologic fracture. Hormonal activity resulting in hypophosphatemic vitamin D–resistant rickets has been described, but is very unusual. Multiple NOFs are associated with neurofibromatosis, discussed later in this chapter. Otherwise, these are incidental lesions and are so radiographically specific that they are easily recognizable. Their importance is in their recognition, in that they do not require treatment unless symptomatic.

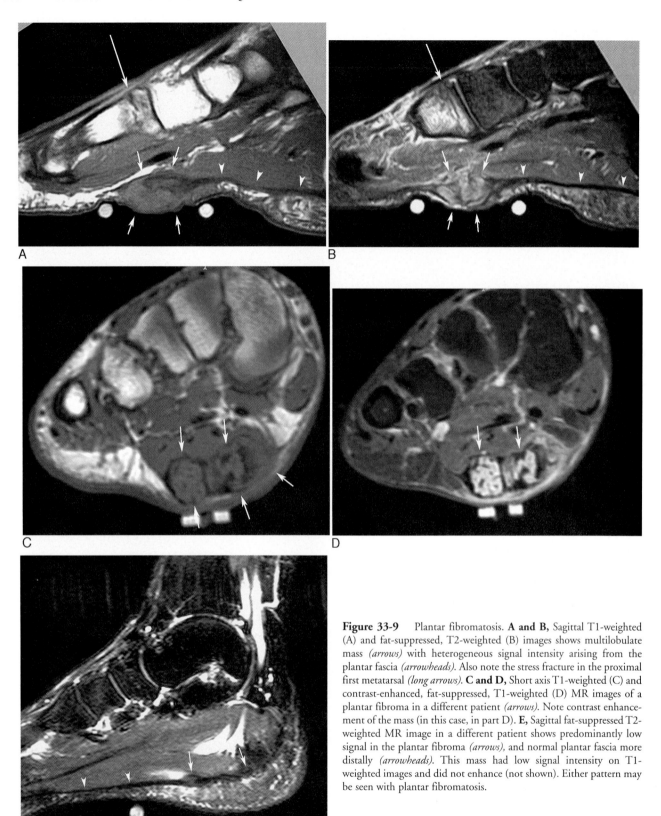

Figure 33-9 Plantar fibromatosis. **A and B,** Sagittal T1-weighted (A) and fat-suppressed, T2-weighted (B) images shows multilobulate mass *(arrows)* with heterogeneous signal intensity arising from the plantar fascia *(arrowheads)*. Also note the stress fracture in the proximal first metatarsal *(long arrows)*. **C and D,** Short axis T1-weighted (C) and contrast-enhanced, fat-suppressed, T1-weighted (D) MR images of a plantar fibroma in a different patient *(arrows)*. Note contrast enhancement of the mass (in this case, in part D). **E,** Sagittal fat-suppressed T2-weighted MR image in a different patient shows predominantly low signal in the plantar fibroma *(arrows),* and normal plantar fascia more distally *(arrowheads)*. This mass had low signal intensity on T1-weighted images and did not enhance (not shown). Either pattern may be seen with plantar fibromatosis.

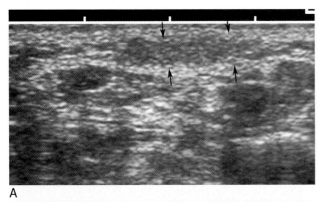

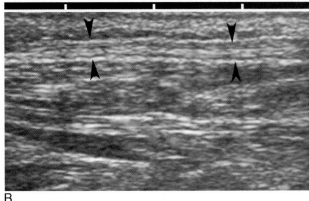

Figure 33-10   US of plantar fibromatosis. Longitudinal images are displayed as they were obtained, with plantar surface of foot at top of image. Note irregularly thickened hypoechoic plantar fascia in (A) *(arrows)*. Contrast with normal thin, uniform, echogenic plantar fascia *(arrowheads)* in (B) at a different site in the same patient.

Key Concepts	Nonossifying Fibroma (NOF), Benign Fibrous Cortical Defect, Fibroxanthoma

Very common, often found incidentally in pediatric radiographs, especially around knee. Does not require further work-up.
Bubbly lytic lesion with sclerotic margins.
Cortical metadiaphyseal lesion.
Larger lesions may present with pathologic fracture.
Most common natural evolution is to be replaced by bone ("heal") over a few years with mild residual sclerosis.

Eighty percent of nonossifying fibromas occur in the diametaphysis of the long bones of the lower extremity. These are eccentric, cortically based lesions. Although they may arise in the cortex, they can enlarge to involve the intramedullary region and even appear central when found in thin bones such as the fibula or ulna (see Fig. 29-7E). These lesions always show a narrow zone of transition, a sclerotic margin, and no matrix calcification (Fig. 33-11). There is no periosteal reaction unless pathologic

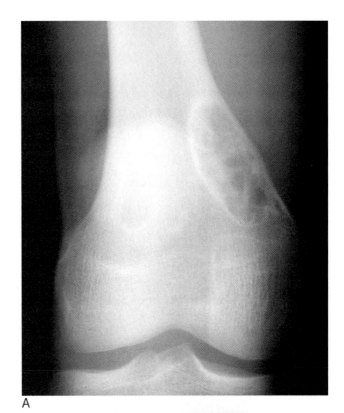

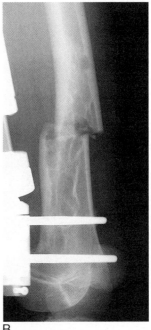

Figure 33-11   Nonossifying fibroma. **A,** AP radiograph shows a cortically based geographic metaphyseal lesion that has a well-defined sclerotic rim in a 19-year-old man. Note that the sclerotic rim is thicker on the medullary margin than the cortical margin, and that the lesion does not extend into the epiphysis. This is a typical nonossifying fibroma, although the patient is a few years older than average. Most nonossifying fibromas have healed by this age, leaving only a faint area of sclerosis. **B,** Pathologic fracture through a large nonossifying fibroma in the distal femur. Note the typical appearance, with sclerotic tumor margins with narrow zone of transition. This fracture, like many pathologic fractures, is transverse. Nonossifying fibromas that extend more than 50% across the transverse diameter of a long bone shaft are at risk for pathologic fracture and may be treated prophylactically if symptomatic.

fracture has occurred. The lesions involute spontaneously, with bone replacing the fibrous tissue. The resulting "healed" NOF may demonstrate homogeneous sclerosis (Figs. 29-7E, 33-12). Not surprisingly, MRI shows low signal intensity on T1-weighted images and variable signal intensity on T2-weighted images, depending on the extent of hypercellular fibrous tissue and hemosiderin versus healing bone that is present (Fig. 33-13).

Many children will have more than one NOF, which is an incidental finding. However, a finding of multiple NOF-like bone lesions (Fig. 33-14) should cause consideration for associated conditions, such as *neurofibromatosis type I* (see Chapter 36) and *Jaffe-Campanacci syndrome*. The latter is multiple nonossifying fibromas with café au lait spots, but without neurofibromatosis. Other associations reported with Jaffe-Campanacci syndrome include mental retardation, precocious puberty, hypogonadism, and cardiovascular and ocular abnormalities.

BENIGN FIBROUS HISTIOCYTOMA

Benign fibrous histiocytoma is a rare osseous lesion that has a histologic appearance very similar to that of nonossifying fibroma but demonstrates different radiographic features: It is geographic and arises centrally in the metaphyseal region of long bones. Both CT and MRI features are nonspecific. Unlike nonossifying fibroma, benign fibrous histiocytoma has a tendency to recur after curettage and may be symptomatic. Benign fibrous histiocytoma may also originate in soft tissue.

LIPOSCLEROSING MYXOFIBROUS TUMOR (POLYMORPHIC FIBRO-OSSEOUS LESION OF BONE)

Liposclerosing myxofibrous tumor (LSMFT) is a benign fibro-osseous bone lesion that usually occurs in the fourth through sixth decades of life, and is most specifically characterized by its location. More than 90% of these lesions occur in the central metadiaphysis of the proximal femur. The lesion usually appears as a lytic or ground-glass geographic lesion with a type 1A margin, often with a markedly sclerotic border (Fig. 33-15). Amorphous mineralization is present in most lesions. The matrix appears globular and irregular. The MRI appearance is nonspecific, with heterogeneous T2 imaging signal. T1-weighted images are more homogeneous, and isointense to muscle. The condition occurs over a wide age range, but most cases are found in adults.

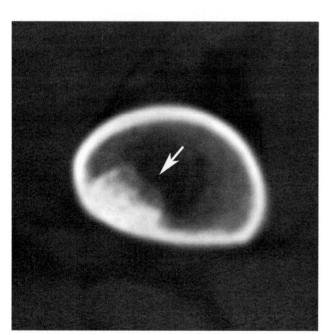

Figure 33-12   Healed nonossifying fibroma. Axial CT through the distal femoral metaphysis in a 21-year-old man shows eccentric uniform sclerosis *(arrow)*. See also Fig. 29-7E.

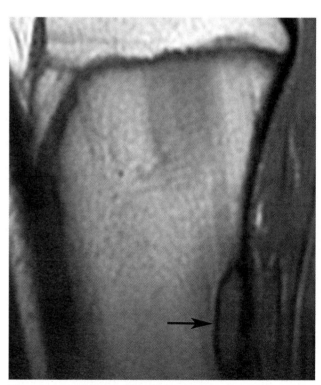

Figure 33-13   Nonossifying fibroma: MRI Sagittal T1-weighted MR image shows small, cortically based intermediate-signal-intensity mass *(arrows)* at the posterior proximal tibial metadiaphysis. The tumor had intermediate signal intensity on T2-weighted images as well.

Histologically, LSMFT is composed of a complex mixture of immature bone and fibrous tissue. Xanthomatous and myxoid elements are frequently present. Ischemic ossification may be found within altered fat. Some feel that LSMFT may be related to fibrous dysplasia or represent an end-stage degeneration of an intraosseous fibrous lesion or lipoma. An important feature of this lesion is its small potential for malignant transformation, despite the initial nonaggressive radiographic appearance. The lesion may present with pain or may be incidental. Because malignant potential has been reported, close clinical and imaging follow-up has been recommended.

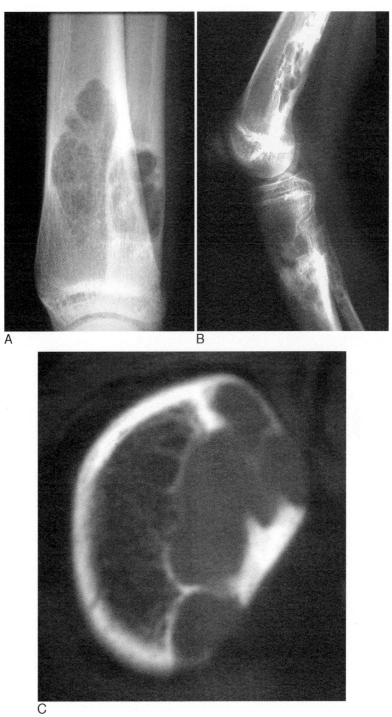

Figure 33-14   Multiple nonossifying fibromas. **A–C,** Lateral ankle (A) and lateral knee (B) radiographs and axial CT through one lesion (C) show multiple bilateral nonossifying fibromas. Note the typical well circumscribed "bubbly lytic" appearance of nonossifying fibroma. These findings should prompt an evaluation for neurofibromatosis type 1.

MALIGNANT FIBROUS HISTIOCYTOMA/FIBROSARCOMA

Malignant fibrous histiocytoma (MFH) is a pleomorphic sarcoma that contains both fibroblastic and histiocytic ele-

ments in varying proportions. Fibrosarcoma is distinguishable histologically, having a more regular appearance of fibroblastic cells. The lesions are not distinguishable radiographically and are discussed together in this section. Both malignant fibrous histiocytoma and fibrosarcoma may originate either in the soft tissues or, less commonly, as osseous lesions.

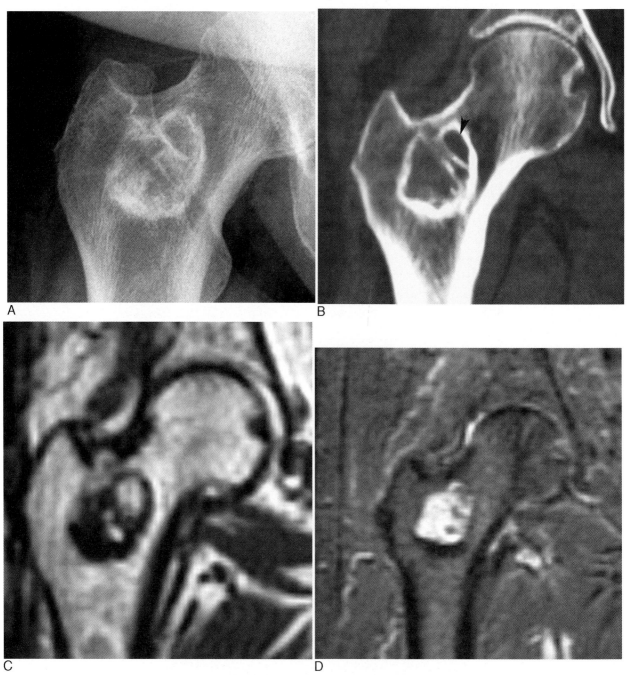

Figure 33-15   Liposclerosing myxofibrous tumor (LSMFT). **A and B,** AP radiograph (A) and coronal CT reconstruction (B) show a geographic mixed density lesion with a fairly broad sclerotic margin in the proximal femur. This is the classic appearance and location of LSMFT. Note that portion of the lesion has fat attenuation (*arrowhead* in part B). **C and D,** Coronal T1-weighted (C) and inversion recovery (D) MR images show the typical mixed signal intensity of LSMFT, including generally high T2 signal intensity.

Key Concepts	Malignant Fibrous Histiocytoma (MFH)

Most common soft tissue sarcoma in adults.

Highly aggressive tumor.

Also relatively common osseous sarcoma, especially in the fourth through seventh decades of life.

Osseous MFH may be primary or secondary.

Lower extremity is the most common site for both soft tissue and osseous MFH.

Dystrophic calcification seen in 15% of cases.

Malignant fibrous histiocytoma is the most frequent soft tissue sarcoma in adults, representing about one fourth of all adult soft tissue tumors (Fig. 33-16). Soft tissue MFH occurs over a wide age range (10 to 90 years of age), with most patients between 30 and 60 years old. Soft tissue MFH is usually located in the extremities; 50% of all cases are found in the lower extremity. Soft tissue MFH is usually not detected by plain radiography, but is worked up with MRI for local staging. The MRI appearance is generally nonspecific: T1-weighted images appear isointense with muscle, and T2-weighted images show inhomogeneous high signal intensity. These lesions may appear to have a reactive pseudocapsule, but must be considered aggressive lesions with tumor cells invariably infiltrating locally at the margins. When the soft tissue mass is adjacent to a long bone, it may cause a smooth cortical pressure erosion. Dystrophic calcification occasionally occurs, usually in the periphery in either a curvilinear or punctate pattern. Internal hemorrhage is common with MFH. A myxoid variety of MFH demonstrates low-signal-intensity central portions on T1-weighted and high signal on T2-weighted images with nodular peripheral enhancement.

Osseous MFH and fibrosarcoma may arise either primarily or secondarily. Malignant fibrous histiocytoma makes up 5% of all primary malignant bone tumors. As with soft tissue MFH, the age range is wide but the peak prevalence is in 30- to 60-year-old patients.

Most osseous MFH lesions occur in the long tubular bones, usually centrally in the metaphysis. Primary MFH usually appears as an aggressive geographic lytic lesion (Fig. 33-17). They generally appear geographic, with a wide zone of transition seen in at least part of the lesion. The lesion is lytic, although dystrophic calcification may be seen in as many as 15% of cases. Magnetic resonance imaging is nonspecific, with low signal intensity on T1- and heterogeneous high signal intensity on T2-weighted images, with occasional low-signal-intensity regions relating to dystrophic calcification.

Although most osseous MFH arises as a primary lesion, up to 20% arise as secondary lesions. Underlying lesions include Paget's disease, previously radiated bone, dedifferentiated chondrosarcoma, nonossifying fibroma, fibrous dysplasia, enchondroma, chronic osteomyelitis, and bone infarct (osteonecrosis). With these secondary forms of MFH, an aggressive lesion will be found in contiguity with the benign lesion from which it arises. For example, MFH arising in bone infarct may demonstrate the nonaggressive serpiginous pattern of calcification commonly seen in bone infarct, immediately contiguous with a highly destructive pattern (Fig. 33-18).

Most MFHs are high-grade tumors, with a 5-year survival rate of 25%. Metastases involve lung, bone, lymph nodes, and liver. Local recurrence after resection is common. Treatment consists of aggressive surgical excision and chemotherapy, often supplemented by radiation therapy.

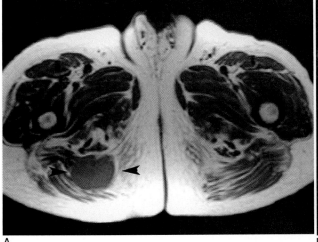
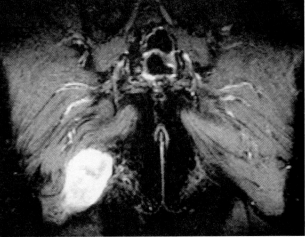

A   B

Figure 33-16   Soft tissue malignant fibrous histiocytoma (MFH). **A,** Axial T1-weighted MR image showing an intramuscular soft tissue mass in the right gluteus maximus that is isointense with muscle *(arrowheads).* **B,** Coronal T2-weighted MR image shows slightly heterogenous but mostly high signal intensity. This is a nonspecific appearance, but a sarcoma must be considered.

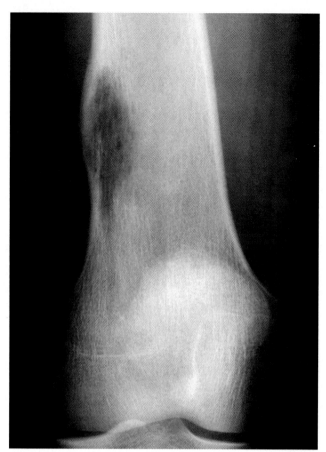

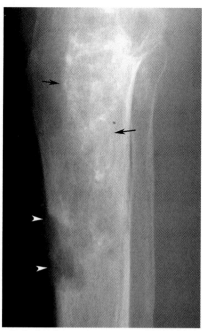

Figure 33-18 Secondary osseous malignant fibrous histiocytoma (MFH). This lateral radiograph of the proximal tibia in a 66-year-old woman demonstrates dystrophic calcific matrix in a serpiginous pattern typical of bone infarct *(arrows)*. However, a more destructive lesion is found in contiguity but slightly distal to the bone infarct *(arrowheads)*. This aggressive lesion arising from a bone infarct represents a secondary osseous MFH. (Reprinted with permission from the American College of Radiology learning file.)

Figure 33-17 Osseous malignant fibrous histiocytoma (MFH). AP radiograph of a moderately aggressive appearing lesion in the distal metadiaphysis of the distal femur in a 22-year-old man. The zone of transition is wide and there is no matrix. This is a nonspecific appearance, but an aggressive lytic lesion in an adult should include MFH as diagnostic consideration.

Fatty and Vascular Tellers

Fatty and Vascular Tumors

FATTY TUMORS
  Lipoma
  Liposarcoma
VASCULAR TUMORS
  Benign
  Intermediate or Indeterminate for Malignancy
  Angiosarcoma

FATTY TUMORS

Lipoma

Lipomas are common tumors consisting of fatty tissue, most often found in soft tissues but rarely arising as an intraosseous lesion. Lipoma and lipoma variants are common benign soft tissue tumors. Eighty percent of lipomas are found in the subcutaneous tissues. Most others are intermuscular or intramuscular. They may extensively infiltrate fascial planes and muscle compartments. Lipomas present as an asymp-tomatic, soft, compressible, mobile mass (Figs. 34-1, 34-2). If they are large enough to be seen on radiographs they may appear as radiolucent (fat tissue density) masses. They show fat attenuation on computed tomography (CT). Magnetic resonance imaging (MRI) is highly characteristic, showing a sharply bordered lesion with high signal intensity matching that of subcutaneous fat on both T1- and T2-weighted imaging, which suppresses with fat saturation. Some lesions can be difficult to differentiate from surrounding fat. Imaging with a marker over a palpable lesion and enlarging the field of view to include both sides to compare symmetry can be helpful for evaluating a small lesion.

Lipomas may contain calcification and ossification, usually representing dystrophic calcification due to prior trauma. Such calcification is usually very dense and often is block-like or in the form of small lines and angles (Figs. 34-3, 34-4). Traumatized subcutaneous fat may show a similar pattern of calcification. Traumatic fat necrosis may have an infiltrative or mass-like appearance on MRI, simulating a neoplasm.

Chondroid tissue is occasionally present within a lipoma, and thus the arcs and whorls pattern of chondroid calcification may rarely be seen as well.

The most frequently encountered difficulty associated with diagnosing lipomas with imaging studies is detecting the rare atypical lipoma or low-grade, well-differentiated liposarcoma. *Atypical lipomas* are histologically well-differentiated lipomas that recur locally but do not metastasize. Magnetic resonance images should be carefully scrutinized to detect any site within a lipoma where typical fat signal is not shown, such as nodules, thickened margins, or areas of irregular or nodular enhancement that may raise concern for low-grade liposarcoma. Lipomas may contain thin enhancing septae, but otherwise do not enhance. Excisional biopsy is required to distinguish these lesions.

Key Concepts	Lipoma Versus Low-Grade Liposarcoma

Lipoma
  Fat density and signal intensity
  May contain thin septations
Low-grade liposarcoma
  Thick, irregular enhancing septations
  Nodules	

Other variants of fat overgrowth are of interest. *Lipomatosis* is a congenital abnormality with multiple lipomas distributed either randomly or symmetrically over the body. Local lipomatosis may occur after local corticosteroid injection. Neural fibrolipoma is discussed in Chapter 36. *Macrodystrophia lipomatosa* is a localized form of gigantism with overgrowth of fat and vascular elements; associated increased blood flow results in overgrowth of the soft tissues and bone, usually in the hand or foot (Fig. 34-5). Other conditions that can cause

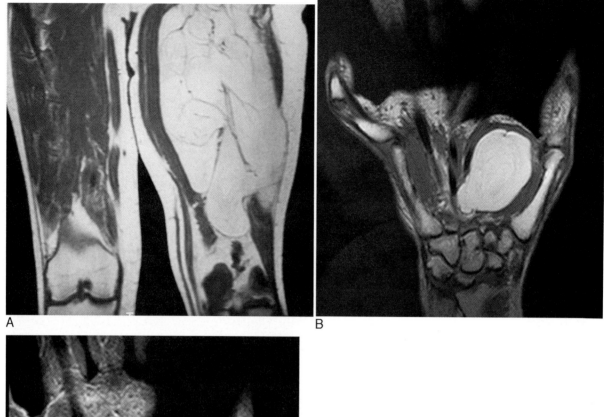

Figure 34-1 Lipoma. **A,** Coronal T1-weighted MR image demonstrates a large mass with uniform high signal and a few thin internal septations infiltrating the left thigh in a 77-year-old man. **B and C,** Coronal T1-weighted (B) and postcontrast fat-suppressed T1-weighted (C) images in a different patient show a lipoma in the palm of the hand. Note that the signal of both tumors is identical to that of the subcutaneous fat. This would hold true on all sequences, including sequences with chemical fat suppression. Also note lack of enhancing nodule or thick septation within the masses, findings that may indicate a liposarcoma.

localized giantism include neurofibromatosis and vascular lesions.

Lipoblastoma is a benign embryonal fatty tumor seen in young children. It simulates liposarcoma histologically. This is a confusing lesion because CT or MRI characteristically show enhancing, nonadipose tissue in the periphery of the lesion. Although recurrence after surgery is common, it is important not to mistake this lesion for liposarcoma. Age at onset is the major factor differentiating lipoblastoma from liposarcoma; the latter occurs almost exclusively in adults, and lipoblastomas are typically found in children younger than 3 years of age.

Other lipomas have characteristic appearances according to their location. *Osseous lipoma* is a rare fatty lesion of bone. This is generally asymptomatic and presents as a lytic lesion with a geographic sclerotic margin and no matrix or host reaction. It usually shows fat density on CT and fat signal intensity on MRI. It may be distinguished by having a central nidus of dystrophic calcification. Osseous lipomas are most often found in the metaphyses of long bones and the calcaneus (Figs. 34-3, 34-6). In the calcaneus, it occurs in the triangular region between the major trabecular arcs (see Fig. 34-3). Occasionally a lipoma is located in a *parosteal* position (Figs. 34-4, 34-7). This

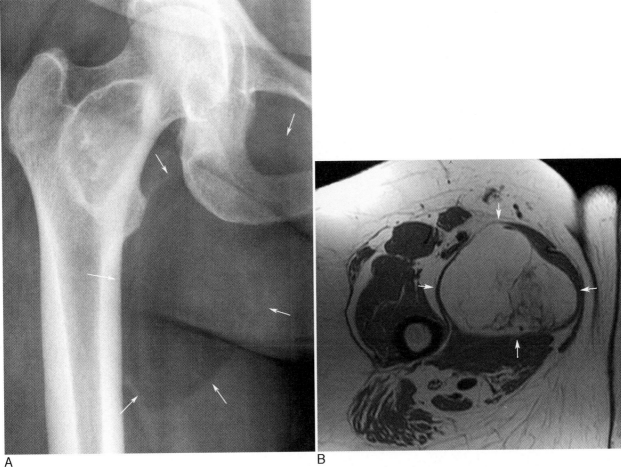

A   B

Figure 34-2   Intramuscular lipoma. **A,** AP radiograph shows low-attenuation mass in the medial thigh *(arrows).* Also note the femoral neck liposclerosing myxofibrous tumor in the proximal femur (compare with Fig. 33-15). **B,** Axial T1-weighted MR image shows the mass *(arrows)* within the adductor musculature. This lipoma contains multiple mildly irregular septations, prompting biopsy, but it is benign.

position may elicit intense periosteal reaction that may take the form of hyperostosis or may produce large bony spicules radiating from the periosteum into the lesion (see Fig. 34-7).

Lipoma arborescens is a rare monoarticular process, usually found in the knee. Features on MRI are characteristic, with hypertrophic synovial villi distended with fat protruding into a large joint effusion. This synovial mass has a signal intensity of fat on all sequences, including those with chemical fat suppression. Although most cases demonstrate a frond-like appearance, it may occasionally appear as mass-like subsynovial fat deposits. Lipoma arborescens can occasionally erode into adjacent bone.

Liposarcoma

Osseous liposarcoma is extremely rare. It is an aggressive neoplasm biologically and at imaging. On the other hand, soft tissue liposarcomas are common and are the second most common malignant soft tissue tumor in adults after malignant fibrous histiocytoma. Soft tissue liposarcoma may range from a well-differentiated to a high-grade lesion. The most common age range is 30 to 60 years, and most cases arise in the buttock, thigh, leg, and retroperitoneum.

Liposarcoma may have a widely variable appearance on imaging studies, depending on the grade and histologic features of the lesion. A low-grade, well-differentiated lesion may show fat density at radiography and CT, and fat signal intensity on MRI. Such well-differentiated liposarcomas can be difficult to differentiate from benign lipomas. Differentiating factors include nonfat nodularity, usually found at the margins of the tumor, or thick and enhancing septa within the fatty tissue. Although benign lipomas can contain septae, these are usually thin, nonenhancing, and few in number. Unlike low-grade liposarcomas, which show fat density or signal, high-grade liposarcomas may be so cellular that no fat is detectable at imaging. Thus, a high-grade liposarcoma may be completely nonspecific at MRI, having low signal intensity at T1-weighted imaging and high inhomogeneous signal intensity at T2-weighted imaging (Fig. 34-8). Other appearances of liposarcoma may relate to the occasional well-differentiated liposarcoma dedifferentiating

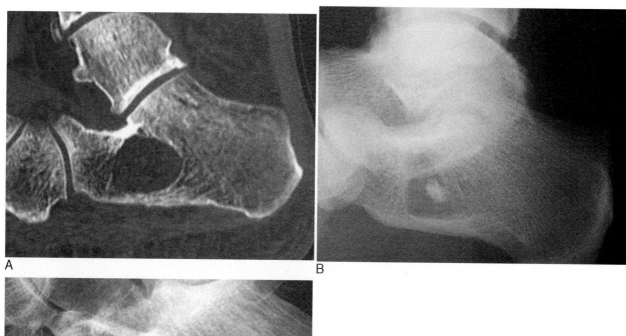

Figure 34-3 Calcaneal lipoma. **A,** Sagittal CT reconstruction shows sharply marginated fat attenuation mass in the central calcaneus. Cysts and numerous other tumors can occur in this location, but the fat attenuation in this case is pathognomonic. **B and C,** Two examples of dystrophic calcification, a classic feature of calcaneal intraosseous lipoma. Common patterns are dense central calcification (B) and a dense ring (C).

into a high-grade sarcoma, giving the appearance of a juxtaposed predominately fatty tumor and more highly cellular tumor. Another variant is myxoid liposarcoma, which can also be potentially confusing in appearance because it contains cyst-like areas of myxoid material, which have intense T2 signal, and may have very little or barely visible fat signal. The uncommon pleomorphic variant is highly undifferentiated and may contain little or no visible fat on imaging studies.

Liposarcoma can metastasize to the lung, liver, and other solid organs and invade locally. High-grade liposarcomas are aggressive and require wide excision and chemotherapy, often combined with radiation therapy.

VASCULAR TUMORS

Benign

The terminology of *vascular malformations* is somewhat varied. *Hemangiomas* are benign proliferations of large (cavernous) or small (capillary) endothelium-lined spaces filled with blood. In current usage, vascular malformations are subdivided into capillary hemangioma, cavernous hemangioma, arteriovenous malformation, and venous angioma or malformation. Vascular malformations may arise anywhere, and may be either osseous or soft tissue in origin. Although the lesions are found most frequently in the fourth and fifth decades of life, the age range is wide. Capillary hemangiomas are primarily dermal lesions in children, and most involute spontaneously during the first decade. Cavernous hemangiomas contain dilated blood-filled spaces. These may present in childhood, do not spontaneously involute, and may enlarge over time. Arteriovenous malformations may be incidental cutaneous lesions. When located in the deep soft tissues, these lesions can be associated with limb overgrowth (due to increased blood flow through the arteriovenous malformation), with large feeding and draining vessels. Venous malformations, when found in the extremities, usually occur within the large muscles of the lower extremity. They may be associated with muscle atrophy, local fatty infiltration, and phleboliths.

Most (75%) osseous vascular malformations are cavernous hemangiomas and are found in the vertebral bodies, skull, and facial bones (Fig. 34-9). In the vertebral bodies, the number of

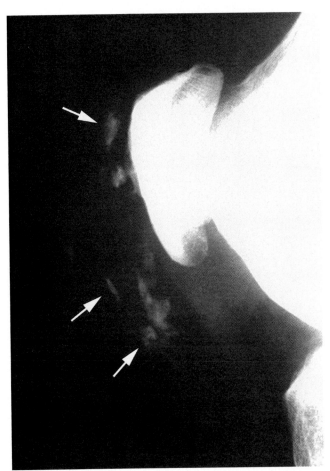

Figure 34-4   Lateral radiograph shows dense, dystrophic calcifications within an anterior patella parosteal lipoma. The location of this tumor resulted in frequent trauma. The calcifications are block-like and linear, which is typical with necrosis.

Key Concepts	Hemangioma
May contain: Fat, feeding or draining vessels, phleboliths	

trabeculae are reduced, leaving only the compressive vertical trabeculae, which are reduced in number but are thickened, usually without collapse. This gives a vertical striated appearance on plain film and a "polka dot" appearance on axial CT. There may be mild expansion and occasionally a soft tissue mass, which may lead to neurologic symptoms due to compression. The expansion is often much more prominent in skull lesions, where the outer table rather than the inner table expands. In the skull lesions, there are also coarsened trabeculae but their pattern is to radiate in a sunburst pattern toward the expanded outer table. This is a pathognomonic appearance. The much less frequent appearance of hemangiomas in other bones generally shows a geographic lytic pattern, sometimes with a radiating or spoke-wheel pattern of ossification. Long bone hemangiomas may have both intraosseus and extraosseous involvement.

The MRI appearance of spinal hemangioma is often characteristic owing to the presence of a variable amount of fatty stroma within the lesion. This fatty stroma leads to an increased signal intensity on both T1- and T2-weighted imaging (see Fig. 34-9). Some hemangiomas do not show increased T1 signal centrally or at all (Figs. 34-10, 34-11). These atypical hemangiomas can be a challenge for the radiologist because they resemble metastatic lesions. However, they often are incidental findings on spine MRI in patients with no history or risk factors for malignancy. Bone scan or repeated MRI after a few months can be an appropriate way to manage these lesions.

Many soft tissue vascular malformations are present as a mass, sometimes containing phleboliths (Fig. 34-12). Feeding or draining blood vessels are more commonly seen with soft tissue lesions. Many soft tissue vascular malformations include numerous tortuous vessels, packed closely together, resulting in a characteristic "can of worms" appearance on CT or MRI (Figs. 34-13, 34-14). Both osseous and soft tissue lesions contain fat in the stroma with high signal intensity on both T1- and T2-weighted images. On MRI, the tortuous vessels are seen either as high signal or flow void, depending on the rate of flow. Soft tissue vascular malformations are usually intramuscular and may scallop or extend into adjacent bone. If a vascular malformation occurs in a skeletally immature patient, it may cause focal bone overgrowth due to chronic hyperemia. The rare *synovial hemangioma* may cause repetitive bleeding into the joint and an appearance similar to hemophilia. The knee and elbow are favored sites for synovial hemangioma; this site preference also makes it difficult to differentiate from the appearance of hemophilia.

Other benign vascular tumors of the extremities are rare, including the extremely uncommon osseous lymphangioma and the somewhat more common soft tissue lymphangioma. Cystic angiomatosis is a rare benign multicentric manifestation of hemangiomatosis or lymphangiomatosis, often with severe visceral involvement. The multiple lytic lesions of bone are nonspecific in appearance unless calcified phleboliths are present in the soft tissues. Another variant is *Gorham's disease,* or massive osteolysis. This is a disease of multicentric angiomatosis with regional dissolution of bone, which is rapid and severely destructive, spreading contiguously across joints.

Vascular Lesions Intermediate or Indeterminate for Malignancy

Hemangiopericytoma and *hemangioendothelioma* fit within this category. Hemangiopericytoma is a malignant vascular tumor that most often originates from the meninges, sinuses, or elsewhere in the head and neck. Peak incidence is in the fourth and fifth decades. Primary hemangiopericytoma of bone is very rare and may have a variety of radiographic appearances that range from a nonaggressive to an aggressive. The axial and proximal appendicular skeletons are the most frequent sites. Discovery of a skeletal hemangiopericytoma should prompt a search for a meningeal or head and neck primary tumor.

Hemangioendothelioma is also a low-grade malignant lesion, which can be difficult to differentiate histologically

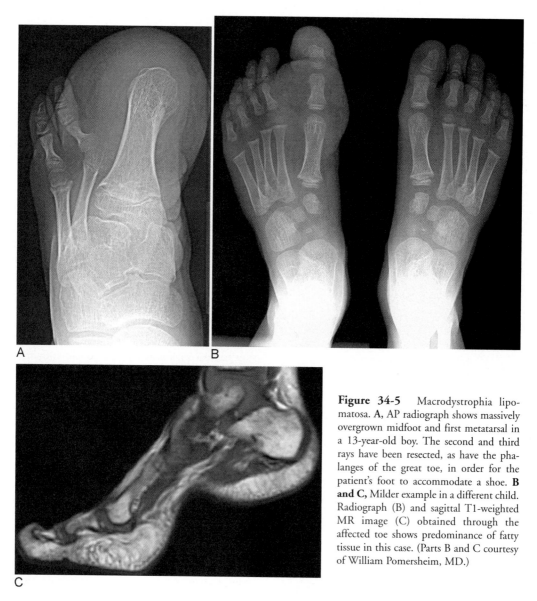

Figure 34-5 Macrodystrophia lipomatosa. **A,** AP radiograph shows massively overgrown midfoot and first metatarsal in a 13-year-old boy. The second and third rays have been resected, as have the phalanges of the great toe, in order for the patient's foot to accommodate a shoe. **B and C,** Milder example in a different child. Radiograph (B) and sagittal T1-weighted MR image (C) obtained through the affected toe shows predominance of fatty tissue in this case. (Parts B and C courtesy of William Pomersheim, MD.)

from angiosarcoma. Patients are typically younger (third and fourth decades). As with hemangiopericytoma, the soft tissue portions of the mass usually are not mineralized. Radiographs of an osseous lesion show osteolysis—sometimes multifocal, sometimes expansile—with variably aggressive tumor margins.

The MRI appearance of these tumors is variable and non-specific, although vascular channels are occasionally seen. There is no underlying fatty stroma as there is in hemangioma. These vascular tumors may be multicentric and can metastasize. Interestingly, when they are multicentric, they tend to involve several bones of a single extremity, often the feet. The lesions that are multicentric tend to have a better prognosis than the solitary lesions.

Angiosarcoma

Angiosarcoma is a rare malignant vascular tumor that may involve bone and soft tissues (Fig. 34-15). Angiosarcoma may

be difficult to differentiate histologically from the less aggressive hemangioendothelioma. Angiosarcoma is seen most frequently in the fourth and fifth decades, but can be seen in younger patients if it is multifocal. Osseous angiosarcomas are extremely rare, permeative, aggressive-appearing lesions without matrix. The most common location is metaphyseal, in the femur, tibia, humerus, and pelvis. Soft tissue angiosarcoma can develop in chronic lymphedema (with exception of congenital lymphedema), such as in the upper extremity after axillary lymph node dissection. Tumors in this setting can resemble nonspecific soft tissue edema without discrete mass.

Thirty-eight percent of angiosarcomas are multifocal. When multifocal, the lesions tend to be regional in distribution. Furthermore, the prognosis is somewhat improved if the lesions are multifocal. Five-year survival is poor for patients who have solitary lesions, with metastases spreading to the lungs or skeleton. Treatment consists of wide resection.

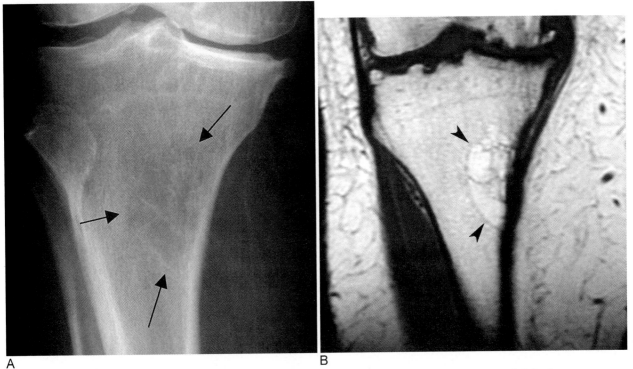

Figure 34-6 Osseous lipoma. **A,** AP radiograph of the proximal tibia in a 60-year-old man. An ill-defined lytic lesion in the tibial metaphysis *(arrows)* does not have an aggressive appearance but is otherwise nonspecific. **B,** MRI allows definitive diagnosis. Coronal T1-weighted MR image shows the lesion *(arrowheads)* to have the same signal intensity as nearby subcutaneous fat.

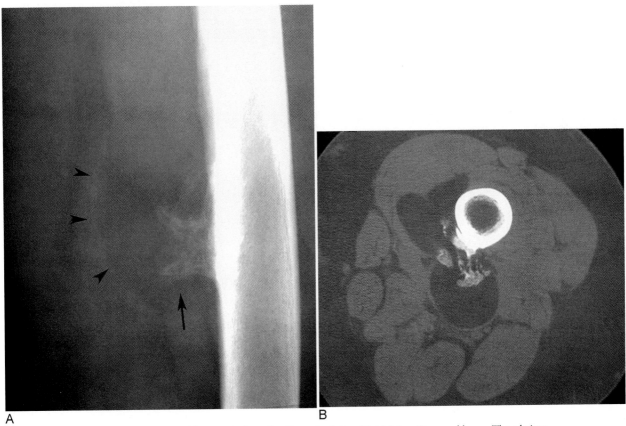

Figure 34-7 Parosteal lipoma. **A,** Lateral radiograph of the mid-thigh in a 63-year-old man. These lesions typically show subtle fat density in the soft tissues *(arrowheads)* and exuberant osseous reaction *(arrow)*. Both this radiograph and the CT image (B), which mirrors the findings of the osseous reaction and lipomatous lesion, make the diagnosis of parosteal lipoma.

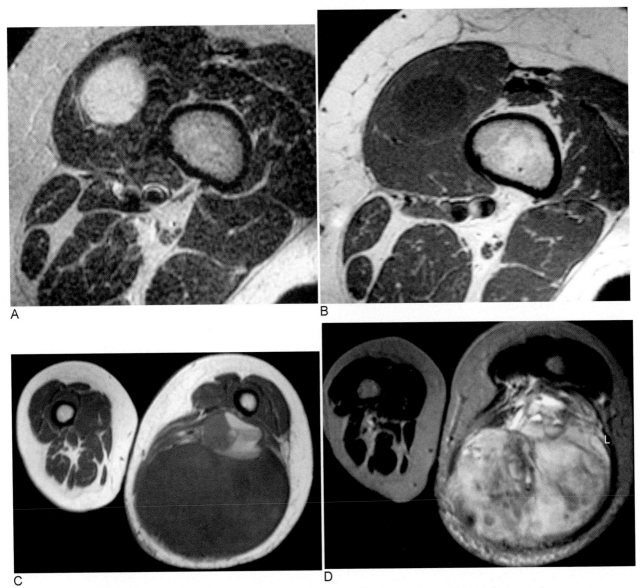

Figure 34-8 Liposarcoma. **A,** T2-weighted axial MR image shows a round mass with signal intensity similar to that of subcutaneous fat in the vastus medialis. **B,** The T1-weighted MR image, however, shows the lesion to be of low signal intensity, different from that of the subcutaneous fat. This was a high-grade liposarcoma. **C,** Very large lesion in the left thigh of a 46-year-old woman. This T1-weighted MR image shows that most of the lesion is low signal intensity but that there is high signal intensity adjacent to the femur. This was misinterpreted as representing a hematoma. **D,** T2-weighted MR image shows most of the lesion to be inhomogeneous and high signal. This is a high-grade liposarcoma. Although the specific variety of sarcoma cannot be diagnosed from the MR image, it is important to remember that large sarcomas can have intratumoral necrosis and bleeding; these must not be mistaken for hematoma.

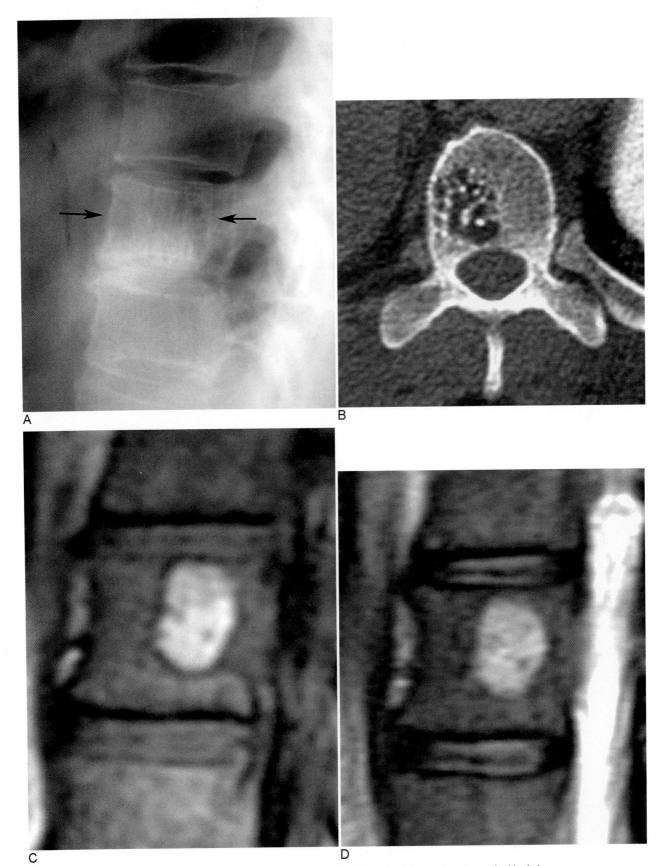

Figure 34-9 Vertebral body hemangioma. **A,** Lateral radiograph of a lower thoracic vertebral body hemangioma *(arrows)* showing the vertical striations that are typical of hemangioma. **B,** Axial CT image shows typical CT appearance, a well-circumscribed lesion with fatty or water density tissue between trabeculae that are thick but few in number. **C and D,** Sagittal T1-weighted (C) and T2-weighted (D) MR images show high signal on both sequences, reflecting the fat and free water within these lesions. (Part A reprinted with permission from the American College of Radiology learning file.)

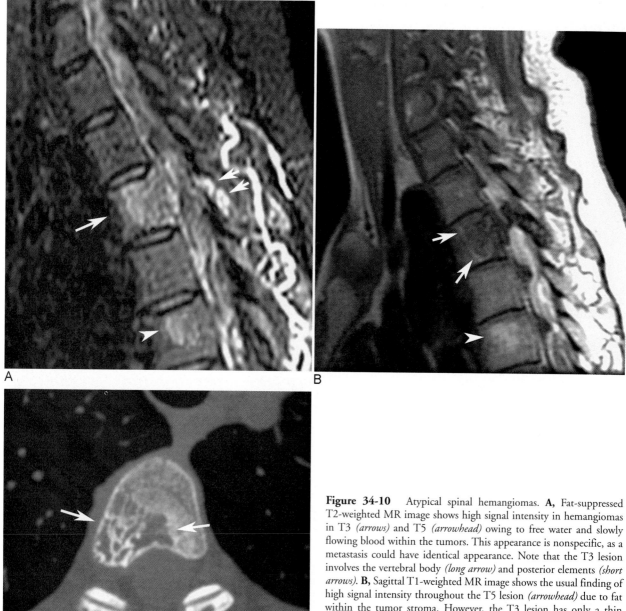

Figure 34-10 Atypical spinal hemangiomas. **A,** Fat-suppressed T2-weighted MR image shows high signal intensity in hemangiomas in T3 *(arrows)* and T5 *(arrowhead)* owing to free water and slowly flowing blood within the tumors. This appearance is nonspecific, as a metastasis could have identical appearance. Note that the T3 lesion involves the vertebral body *(long arrow)* and posterior elements *(short arrows)*. **B,** Sagittal T1-weighted MR image shows the usual finding of high signal intensity throughout the T5 lesion *(arrowhead)* due to fat within the tumor stroma. However, the T3 lesion has only a thin peripheral rim of high signal intensity *(arrows)*. This is enough to make the diagnosis of hemangioma. Some spinal hemangiomas contain no high T1 signal, and can be difficult to diagnose. **C,** CT through T3 lesion shows the typical thickened vertical trabeculae, with extension through the posterior elements *(arrows)*.

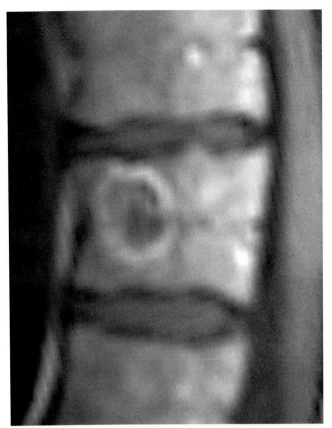

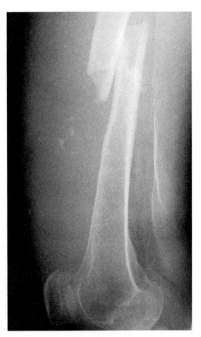

Figure 34-12 Soft tissue vascular malformation. Lateral radiograph shows a large soft tissue mass in the anterior thigh that contains multiple phleboliths. The phleboliths are diagnostic of hemangioma. In this case, the hemangioma caused extrinsic scalloping and thinning of the anterior femoral cortex, which resulted in pathologic fracture.

Figure 34-11 Spine hemangioma: halo sign. Sagittal T1-weighted MR image shows only a high-signal halo around the periphery of this otherwise low-signal hemangioma. This is a benign pattern.

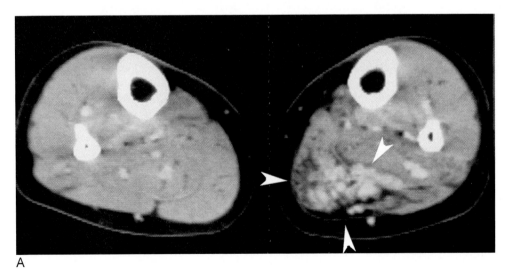

A

Figure 34-13 Soft tissue vascular malformations. **A,** CT performed with administration of contrast medium in a patient with a cavernous hemangioma in the posterior compartment of the leg *(arrowheads)*. Note the enhancing, tortuous vessels within the lesion that have been likened to a "can of worms" and the fatty stroma within the lesion.

(Continued)

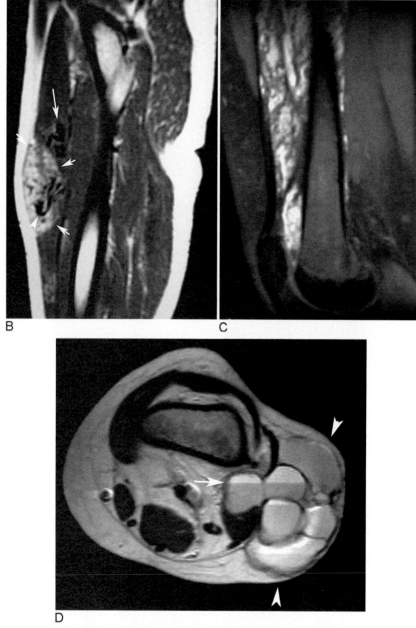

Figure 34-13—(Cont'd) **B,** Lesion with high flow vessels. Intramuscular hemangioma in the anterior thigh a different patient. Sagittal T1-weighted MR image shows high-signal fatty stroma *(short arrows)*, and flow voids within the lesion *(arrowhead)* and a large feeding vessel *(long arrow)*. **C,** Low-flow lesion. Sagittal postcontrast fat-suppressed T1-weighted image in the thigh shows large hemangioma infiltrating the quadriceps muscles and surrounding the femoral shaft. **D,** Low-flow vascular malformation in the distal medial thigh *(arrowheads)*. Axial T2-weighted image shows dilated vascular channels. The channels are enhanced after intravenous contrast administration, excluding a lymphangioma. The flow is so slow that the cellular components are layering, producing fluid-fluid levels *(arrow)*.

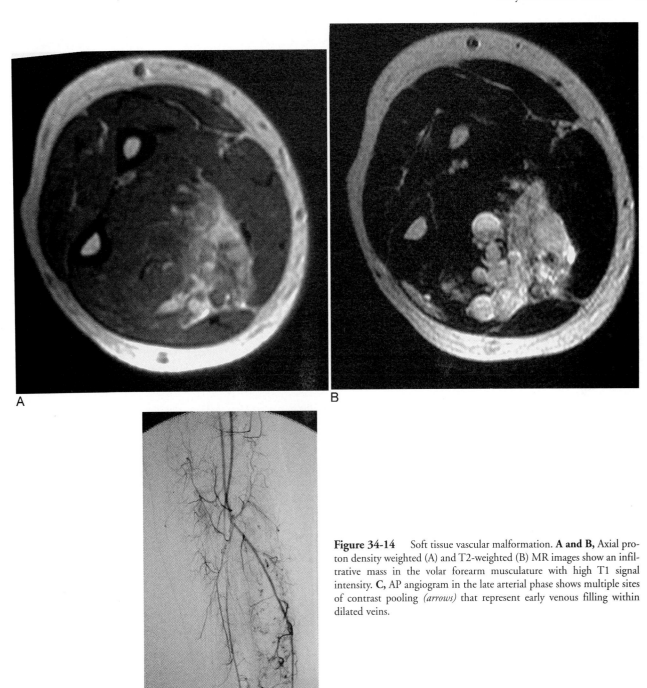

Figure 34-14   Soft tissue vascular malformation. **A and B,** Axial proton density weighted (A) and T2-weighted (B) MR images show an infiltrative mass in the volar forearm musculature with high T1 signal intensity. **C,** AP angiogram in the late arterial phase shows multiple sites of contrast pooling *(arrows)* that represent early venous filling within dilated veins.

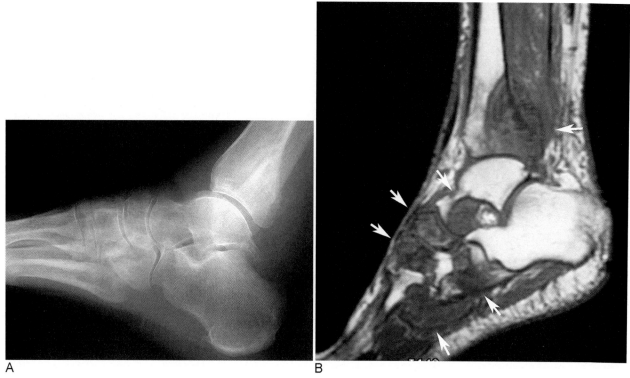

Figure 34-15   Angiosarcoma. **A,** Lateral radiograph of the foot in a 67-year-old man shows an ill-defined destructive lesion involving the posterior aspect of the distal tibia. One might consider that the lucencies seen throughout the bones of the hindfoot and midfoot represent disuse osteopenia. **B,** T1-weighted MR image demonstrates low-signal-intensity lesions involving the multiple bones of the foot and ankle *(arrows).* Multiple tibia involving the lower extremities frequently prove to be vascular tumors. In this case, the diagnosis is angiosarcoma.

CHAPTER 35

Marrow Tumors and Metastatic Disease of Bone

EWING'S SARCOMA
PRIMARY LYMPHOMA OF BONE
HODGKIN'S DISEASE
MULTIPLE MYELOMA
METASTATIC DISEASE OF BONE

EWING'S SARCOMA

Ewing's sarcoma is a highly malignant neoplasm found primarily in children. Along with lymphoma, leukemia, primitive neurectodermal tumor (PNET, with which Ewing's sarcoma shares a specific chromosome 11;22 translocation and is histologically highly similar but not identical), and metastatic neuroblastoma, it is sometimes termed a "small round cell tumor" in reference to a similar histologic appearance. These malignancies, along with osteomyelitis and Langerhans cell histiocytosis, also have a similar radiographic appearance. Ewing's sarcoma is the most common primary malignant bone tumor found in children in the first decade of life. In the second decade, it is second only to osteosarcoma. Ninety-five percent of cases occur between the ages of 4 and 25 years, with the most frequent occurrence between 5 and 14 years. Ewing's sarcoma is a central permeative lesion, most commonly within the diaphysis or metadiaphysis. Seventy-five percent of cases involve the pelvis or long tubular bones. Other sites of involvement include the shoulder girdle, rib, and vertebral body. The expected location relates to the age at presentation; Ewing's sarcoma tends to involve the tubular bones in children younger than age 10 and the axial skeleton, pelvis, and shoulder girdle in patients older than age 10.

Tumor margins are classically permeative, with a large soft tissue mass (Fig. 35-1). No calcified tumor matrix is produced. Most Ewing's sarcomas are completely lytic, but one fourth have minimal reactive bone, and about 15% have marked sclerotic reactive bone (Fig. 35-2). Occasionally, thick reactive endosteal bone formation is seen. The presence of this sclerotic reactive bone might falsely suggest osteosarcoma as the diagnosis. However, the reactive bone in Ewing's sarcoma is found

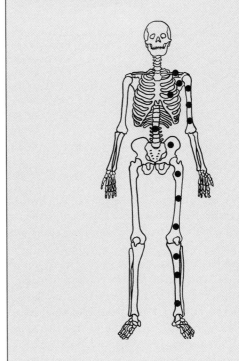

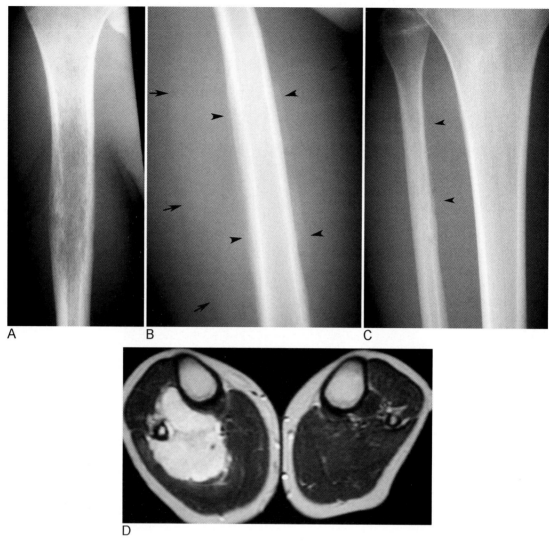

Figure 35-1   Ewing's sarcoma. **A,** Classic appearance of Ewing's sarcoma is a highly permeative lesion in a long bone, as seen in this humerus tumor in a 14-year-old girl. **B,** Sagittal radiograph of the middiaphysis of the femur in a 10-year-old girl. The permeative change in the bone is almost impossible to see, but there is aggressive, interrupted periosteal reaction *(arrowheads)* as well as a large soft tissue mass *(arrows)*. This is also a common radiographic appearance of Ewing's sarcoma. **C and D,** An even more subtle case of Ewing's sarcoma is seen in an AP radiograph (C) of the proximal fibula in a 23-year-old woman. There is subtle permeative change in the medial cortex with equally subtle periosteal reaction *(arrowheads)*. Axial T2-weighted MR image (D) shows the true tumor size, which is larger than suggested by the radiograph.

only within the osseous structures and is not produced within the soft tissue component of the mass. This feature helps to differentiate a sclerotic Ewing's sarcoma from an osteosarcoma, which most frequently shows tumor matrix formation in both the permeative osseous lesion and its soft tissue mass. Aggressive periosteal reaction is a prominent feature of Ewing's sarcoma.

Systemic reaction may be prominent as well, as one third of the patients present with fever, leukocytosis, and elevated erythrocyte sedimentation rate. This clinical presentation simulates infection. Unfortunately, the radiographic appearance as an aggressive permeative lesion with periosteal change also

can be seen in infection. Clinical findings therefore may be misleading. Another interesting clinical feature is that Ewing's sarcoma is rare in black patients.

The magnetic resonance imaging (MRI) appearance of Ewing's sarcoma is nonspecific, with low signal intensity on T1-weighted images and high signal intensity on T2-weighted images. The soft tissue component of the mass is typically large and may contain central necrosis.

Ewing's sarcoma is initially monostotic, but metastases to bone are common so that the lesion may present initially as a polyostotic disease. This can contribute to difficulty in diagnosis.

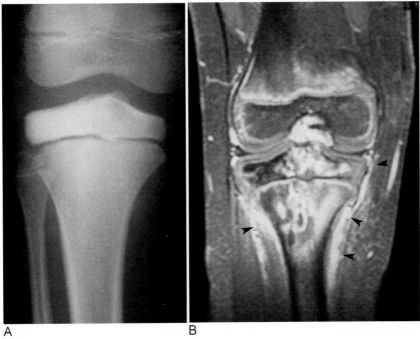

Figure 35-2   Sclerotic Ewing's sarcoma. **A,** AP radiograph of the knee in a 9-year-old boy. The proximal epiphysis of the tibia is sclerotic, but no definite destructive change is seen. Ewing's sarcoma can elicit such dense reactive bone formation that the permeative change can be obscured. **B,** Coronal fat-suppressed, contrast-enhanced, T1-weighted MR image shows that the lesion not only involves the proximal tibial epiphysis but also extends far into the metaphysis. There is an enhancing soft tissue mass *(arrowheads)*, although it is not as large as was seen in Fig. 35-1D).

The differential diagnosis primarily consists of the other "small round cell" lesions (neuroblastoma metastases, lymphoma, PNET, and leukemia), osteomyelitis, and Langerhans cell histiocytosis. Although benign and highly malignant lesions are included in this same differential diagnosis, each of these lesions mentioned previously can have a highly aggressive permeative appearance and require biopsy for diagnosis. The duration of symptoms may be helpful in differentiating among these round cell lesions. Langerhans cell histiocytosis may be one of the most locally aggressive, with the shortest time course of osseous destruction (1 to 2 weeks). Osteomyelitis also has a relatively short course of osseous destruction (2 to 4 weeks). Ewing's sarcoma, although highly aggressive, has a somewhat slower course, with destructive changes seen at 6 to 12 weeks.

The 5-year survival of patients with Ewing's sarcoma has improved to 75%. Central and larger lesions, and lesions with more aggressive histologic features, are associated with a worse prognosis. Fifteen percent to 30% have metastases at the time of diagnosis; these metastases affect lung and bone with equal frequency. Of all the primary bone sarcomas, Ewing's sarcoma most frequently metastasizes to other bones. It should be noted that more

Treatment includes combined radiation and chemotherapy. Amputation and limb salvage surgery with wide resection are secondary options.

PRIMARY LYMPHOMA OF BONE

Primary lymphoma of bone is an uncommon presentation of lymphoma and must be distinguished from secondary osseous involvement by extraosseous primary disease, as the latter requires more aggressive therapy and is associated with a worse prognosis. Although the age range of primary bone lymphoma is wide, the most common range is 30 to 60 years. The lesion is lytic, most frequently moth-eaten or permeative (Fig. 35-3), but it can appear to be of mixed density because of reactive bone formation and prominent endosteal thickening. The lesion tends to arise in appendicular central diaphyseal or metadiaphyseal sites, particularly the femur, tibia, and humerus, but also can occur in the pelvis, scapula, and spine.

This lesion can enlarge rapidly, giving rise to two features seen on radiography, CT, or MRI that can be suggestive of the diagnosis. One of these features is a very large soft tissue mass without extensive cortical destruction. In addition, bone sequestra can be seen. The MRI appearance is nonspecific for diagnosis, but MRI is needed for staging because radiographs do not show the true size and extent of the lesion. The lesions show increased tracer uptake on bone scanning, sometimes before radiographs show any changes.

The major differential diagnosis relates to other aggressive lesions occurring in this age range: in adults, metastases, myeloma, and high-grade sarcomas; in younger patients, osteomyelitis, osteosarcoma, Langerhans cell histiocytosis, and Ewing's sarcoma.

Primary lymphoma of bone can metastasize to lymph nodes and bone. Lung metastases are uncommon, but when present may increase in size and number quickly. Treatment is whole-bone radiation, with chemotherapy reserved for disseminated disease. In contrast, systemic lymphoma with bone involvement is usually treated with chemotherapy. These lesions are often sclerotic, especially when successfully treated.

Metastatic non-Hodgkin's lymphoma to bone indicates an aggressive tumor with relatively poor prognosis (Fig. 35-4).

Key Concepts	Primary Lymphoma of Bone

Permeative. Enormous soft tissue mass with relative preservation of cortex.
Long bones: Usually diaphyseal.
Large tubular bones, pelvis, and scapula.
Sequestra of normal bone surrounded by tumor.
Most common age range: 30 to 60 years.

(Continued)

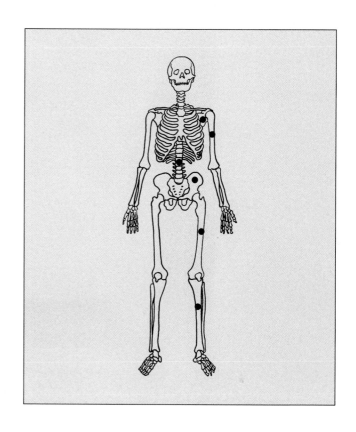

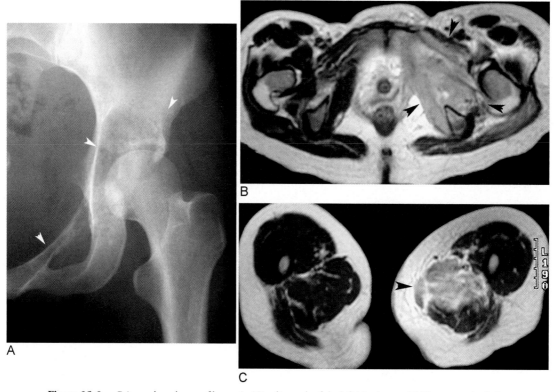

Figure 35-3 Primary lymphoma of bone. **A,** AP radiograph of the left hip shows a highly permeative lesion involving the acetabulum and extending into the superior pubic ramus in a 31-year-old woman. **B and C,** Axial T2-weighted MR images obtained through the low pelvis (B) and thighs (C) demonstrate an unusually extensive soft tissue mass associated with this lesion. In its proximal portion, the soft tissue mass involves both the obturator internus and externus, and the mass extends well down into the proximal half of the thigh, involving the adductor musculature. Such a large, infiltrative soft tissue mass is typical of primary lymphoma.

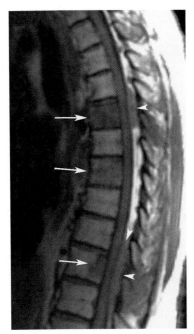

Figure 35-4 Metastatic non-Hodgkin's lymphoma. Sagittal T1-weighted MR image in the thoracic spine of a 50-year-old man shows low signal in vertebral bodies *(arrows)* and epidural tumor *(arrowheads)* with cord compression. Epidural extension is common in lymphoma but is not specific because many tumors may grow within the epidural space. See also Figs. 39-3C and 39-5.

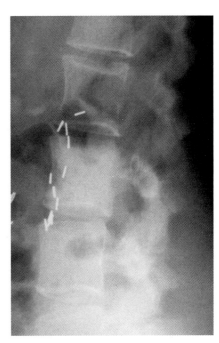

Figure 35-5 Hodgkin's disease. This lateral radiograph of the spine demonstrates an ivory vertebra at L3. Although ivory vertebra can be seen in other disease processes, the periaortic lymph node dissection suggested by the position of the clips helps to make the diagnosis of Hodgkin's disease in this case. (Reprinted with permission from the American College of Radiology learning file.)

HODGKIN'S DISEASE

Hodgkin's disease in bone is almost always metastatic in etiology. Twenty percent of patients with Hodgkin's disease have radiographic evidence of bone involvement, but it is extremely rare as a primary bone tumor. Metastatic Hodgkin's disease can involve bone either by hematogenous dissemination or by contiguous spread from adjacent nodes. The sternum is a common site of contiguous tumor involvement.

Hodgkin's disease of bone is seen most frequently in the second through fourth decades of life. The lesion most frequently is found in the axial skeleton, especially the vertebral bodies. The lesion may be lytic, but most frequently is either blastic or mixed lytic and blastic. The *ivory vertebrae* (Fig. 35-5) is a classic manifestation of Hodgkin's disease, although it is also seen in metastatic disease and Paget's disease. Two thirds of cases are polyostotic. The lesions may be moderately aggressive in appearance and may show a soft tissue mass.

MULTIPLE MYELOMA

Neoplastic proliferation of plasma cells is the most common primary bone tumor. The solitary form of this type of proliferation is called plasmacytoma; the multiple form is much more frequent. Ninety-five percent of patients are older than 40 years of age.

Plasmacytomas are lytic expansile geographic lesions (Fig. 35-6). They have a relatively narrow zone of transition without sclerotic margins. No matrix calcification is present. The most common sites of occurrence for plasmacytoma reflect the distribution of red (hematopoietic) marrow in the skeleton: the vertebral bodies, pelvis, femur, and humerus. The differential diagnosis of plasmacytoma depends on its radiographic appearance. Other lesions that fit the description above include metastasis, high-grade chondrosarcoma, giant cell tumor, and brown tumor of hyperparathyroidism.

Key Concepts	Multiple Myeloma

Most common appearance: Multiple punched-out lytic lesions.
May present as diffuse osteopenia, without focal lytic lesion.
Occasionally presents as a focal lytic expansile lesion (plasmacytoma).
Bone scanning and skeletal radiographic survey are complementary studies, as each misses a large number of myeloma lesions. Whole-body MRI may be used instead.

Seventy percent of patients with plasma cell neoplasia have multiple myeloma, which most often presents with numerous focal, punched-out lytic lesions with a narrow zone of transition.

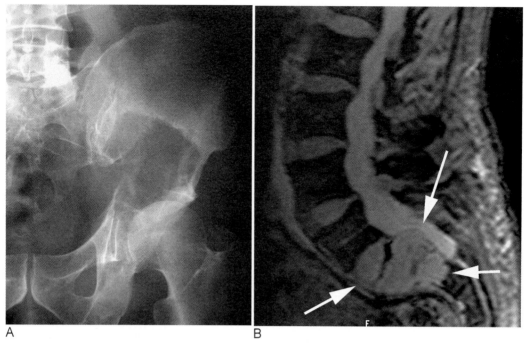

Figure 35-6   Plasmacytoma. **A,** Solitary large lytic lesion of the iliac wing in a 53-year-old man is seen. It is fairly well marginated but shows medial cortical breakthrough. This is a typical appearance of plasmacytoma. **B,** Sacral plasmacytoma in a different patient *(arrows)*. Sagittal T2-weighted MR image. This appearance is not specific, but this is a common presentation of myeloma.

These lesions are generally less than 5 cm in size, often less than 1 cm (Fig. 35-7). Less commonly, multiple myeloma presents as generalized osteopenia (Fig. 35-8), showing no focal lesions. Finding unexplained generalized osteopenia, perhaps with a compression fracture in a middle-aged man, should suggest the diagnosis of multiple myeloma. Whether it presents as focal punched out lesions or as generalized osteopenia, multiple myeloma originates in the red marrow but then progresses to cortex and other areas. Plasmacytoma most frequently involves the skull, vertebral bodies, ribs, and pelvis, followed by the proximal appendicular skeleton. This reflects the distribution of red marrow in the adult. The major differential diagnosis for multiple myeloma is metastatic disease, and the less frequent multiple brown tumors of hyperparathyroidism.

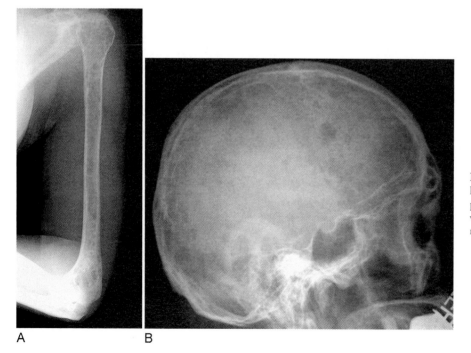

Figure 35-7   Multiple myeloma. The humerus (A) and lateral skull (B) show multiple "punched out" round lytic lesions with very narrow zone of transition typical of myeloma.

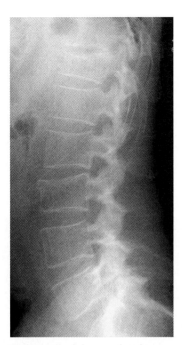

Figure 35-8   Myeloma. A subtle example, where one sees only diffuse osteopenia and compression fractures of the superior endplates of T12 and L3. However, this radiograph of a 32-year-old man who has no known metabolic disease or steroid use. When severe generalized osteopenia is seen in a patient whose age and gender do not suggest senile osteoporosis, multiple myeloma should be strongly considered.

Some manifestations of multiple myeloma are unusual. Ten percent to 15% of cases of multiple myeloma are associated with amyloidosis. When amyloid is deposited in the synovium, the radiographic picture may simulate rheumatoid arthritis. (Amyloidosis is discussed in Chapter 21.) Rarely, multiple myeloma may have a sclerotic pattern, with either a sclerotic margin around lytic lesions or entirely sclerotic round lesions. Such "sclerosing myeloma" (Fig. 35-9) is associated with the *POEMS syndrome.* This acronym stands for the syndrome of polyneuropathy (P), organomegaly (O), endocrinopathy (E), myeloma (M), and skin (S) changes.

The radiologic work-up for multiple myeloma is somewhat controversial because no single study appears to demonstrate all lesions. It seems that skeletal surveys and bone scanning are complementary studies for multiple myeloma: bone scanning detects about one fifth of lesions not seen on skeletal survey, and skeletal survey detects about 40% of lesions not detected on bone scanning. An additional option for determining tumor burden is whole-body MRI, with T1 and inversion recovery sequences. The MRI appearance of both the plasmacytoma and multiple myeloma is nonspecific. T1-weighted imaging demonstrates either a diffuse or mottled decrease in signal intensity or numerous discrete lesions; T2-weighted imaging depicts generalized increased signal intensity.

Most cases of plasmacytoma progress to multifocal or generalized disease within a few years, although a few remain localized. Multiple myeloma is usually a fatal disease with a poor 5-year survival rate, especially in patients who present with more

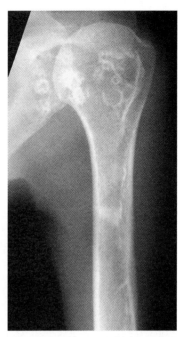

Figure 35-9   Sclerosing myeloma. Multiple myeloma very rarely has lesions that are entirely sclerotic or show a sclerotic rim. Sclerosing myeloma is rare and is part of the POEMS syndrome, discussed in the text.

than one bone lesion and elevated serum immunoglobin levels. Treatment consists of aggressive chemotherapy with bone marrow transplantation for disseminated disease. Focal lesions and spinal cord compression are treated with radiation therapy, with occasional ablative surgery for plasmacytomas. Bisphosphonates inhibit osteoclasts and prevent progression of osteoporosis. Serial radiography or MRI is used to follow tumor burden as well as to identify lesions at risk for pathologic fracture (i.e., large lesions or those involving greater than 50% of cortical width). Prophylactic placement of an intramedullary nail may be used to prevent an impending long bone fracture. Computed tomography (CT) can better quantify the degree of cortical destruction in an individual lesion. Vertebroplasty or kyphoplasty can stabilize painful spine fractures.

METASTATIC DISEASE OF BONE

Osseous metastasis occurs in 20% to 35% of malignancies. Metastases to bone are significantly more common (in a ratio of 25:1) than primary bone tumors. About 80% of bone metastases arise from primary tumors of the lung, breast, prostate, and kidney. Other common primary lesions metastasizing to bone include gastrointestinal, thyroid, and round cell malignancies.

Metastases are identified most frequently by radiographs, FDG PET, or bone scan. Bone scan is highly sensitive compared with radiography; 10% to 40% of metastatic lesions may be abnormal on bone scanning but normal radiographically. On the other hand, fewer than 5% of metastatic lesions are normal on bone scanning but are depicted by radiography. However, specificity of bone scanning is very poor. Therefore radiographs and MRI are used in a complementary fashion with bone scans in an effort to improve specificity. Furthermore, radiographs should be evaluated for signs of impending pathologic fracture that would warrant prophylactic surgical fixation. These signs include lesions that are 2.5 cm or larger, and those showing 50% or greater cortical width destruction. Magnetic resonance imaging is highly sensitive and specific for detection of metastases, but has several drawbacks. For example, it is more expensive and less practical than bone scanning,

and rib and small spine metastases can be difficult to detect with MRI. Nonetheless, selective use of MRI is very helpful in evaluating the oncologic patient with bone pain and in further evaluating abnormal bone scan findings. In the future it may serve as a whole-body screening examination.

Metastases usually have a moth-eaten or geographic pattern with an ill-defined or wide zone of transition, no sclerotic margin, and often little periosteal reaction or soft tissue mass (Fig. 35-10). Occasionally, a metastatic site may present as a geographic, bubbly, expansile mass (Fig. 35-11). Expansile solitary metastases are often due to renal cell or thyroid

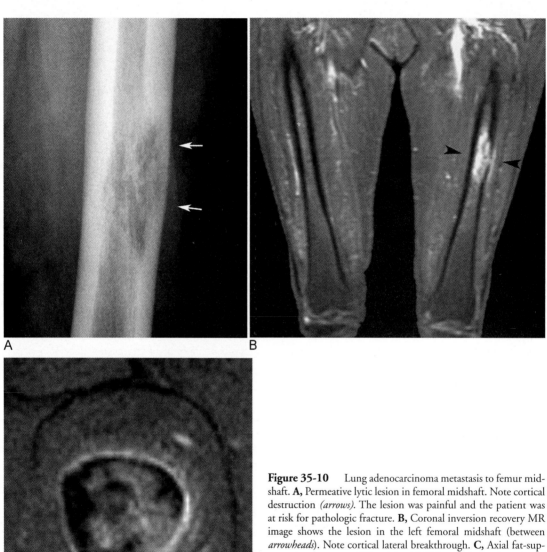

Figure 35-10   Lung adenocarcinoma metastasis to femur midshaft. **A,** Permeative lytic lesion in femoral midshaft. Note cortical destruction *(arrows)*. The lesion was painful and the patient was at risk for pathologic fracture. **B,** Coronal inversion recovery MR image shows the lesion in the left femoral midshaft (between *arrowheads*). Note cortical lateral breakthrough. **C,** Axial fat-suppressed, postcontrast T1-weighted MR image shows the enhancing tumor permeating through the normally low signal cortex.

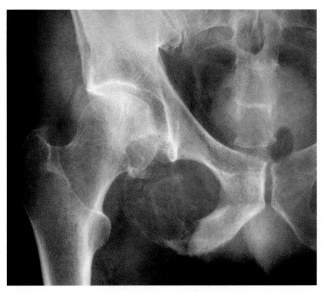

Figure 35-11   Bubbly lytic metastasis. AP radiograph of the pelvis in a 50-year-old man demonstrates an expanded lytic renal cell carcinoma metastasis in the right ischium. Renal cell and thyroid metastases are often highly vascular and may bleed significantly after biopsy. When presented with a lytic lesion and a request for percutaneous biopsy, many experts advise a search for a primary tumor with physical examination, chest radiography, and abdomen CT before biopsy. Because this patient had a renal mass at CT (not shown), a smaller biopsy needle would be used to reduce the risk of hemorrhage.

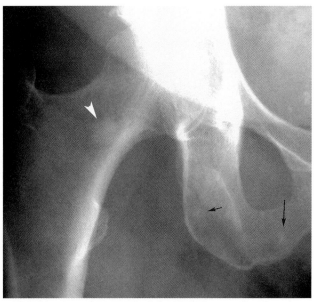

Figure 35-12   Blastic prostate metastases in a 45-year-old man with small blastic lesion in the right femoral neck *(arrowhead)* and subtle sclerotic areas in the ischium *(arrowheads)*. These lesions are not clearly bone islands because they do not blend into surrounding trabeculae. Bone scan (not shown) showed high tracer uptake in these lesions, excluding bone islands. The prostate-specific antigen (PSA) level was elevated, and biopsy of a bone lesion showed prostate cancer. The PSA level is frequently, but not necessarily, elevated with metastatic prostate cancer.

Key Concepts	Metastases

Purely lytic: Lung most frequent, followed by kidney, breast, thyroid, gastrointestinal (GI), neuroblastoma.
Blastic: Prostate, breast, bladder, GI (adenocarcinoma and carcinoid), lung (usually small cell), medulloblastoma.
Mixed lytic and blastic: Breast, lung, prostate, bladder, and neuroblastoma.
Therapy or radiation necrosis can change the lesion density (e.g., lytic metastases heal to more normal density).

carcinoma. The density of metastases varies. Purely lytic metastases are most frequently of lung origin, but are also seen with kidney, breast, thyroid, gastrointestinal, and neuroblastoma. Blastic metastases include prostate (Fig. 35-12), breast, bladder, gastrointestinal (adenocarcinoma and carcinoid), lung (usually small cell), and medulloblastoma. Mixed lytic and blastic metastases can be seen in breast (Fig. 35-13), lung, prostate, bladder, and neuroblastoma metastases. With therapy or radiation necrosis, one may see changing patterns of density.

Most metastases occur where red bone marrow is found; therefore, 80% of metastases are located in the axial skeleton (ribs, pelvis, vertebrae, and skull) (Figs. 35-13, 35-14), and proximal humerus and femur (see Figs. 35-1, 35-13). The epiphyses and mandible are rarely involved. Lesions distal to the elbows or knees are usually due to primary lung cancers. Although most metastases are central lesions found within the distribution of bone marrow, occasionally a cortically based metastasis can occur, most often of lung or breast origin (Fig. 35-15). Metastases are frequently found in the spine, where they may appear as nonspecific compression fractures due to vertebral body destruction. Bone or PET scan and MRI are the preferred modalities for detection of vertebral metastases. The latter also provides assessment of spinal cord compression.

Two specific sites are worthy of mention with respect to metastatic disease. First, a lesser trochanter avulsion fracture in an adult should be considered pathologic until proven otherwise (Fig. 35-16). Second, in patients with known breast cancer, a solitary sternal lesion is rare but, if present, has an 80% probability of being due to metastatic disease. Finally, the presence of a *transverse* fracture in a long bone, especially without significant prior trauma, should alert the radiologist to the possibility a pathologic fracture.

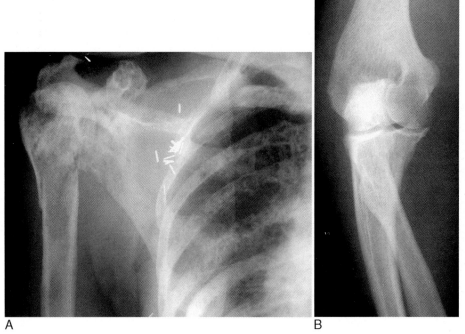

Figure 35-13   Mixed density metastases and distribution of metastatic disease. **A,** Lytic and blastic destructive lesions involving the ribs and shoulder girdle bones in this 45-year-old woman with widespread metastatic breast carcinoma. **B,** In contrast, the elbow and adjacent bones in the same extremity are normal. This case typifies the distribution of the metastases to sites of hematopoietic marrow, which in an adult are the axial and proximal appendicular skeleton.

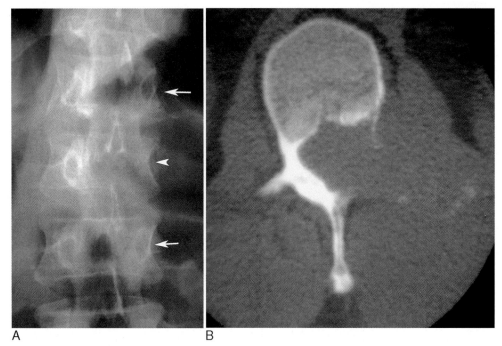

Figure 35-14   Spinal metastasis with absent pedicle. **A,** AP radiograph shows absent left L1 pedicle *(arrowhead)*. Contrast with the normal ovoid densities of the T12 and L2 pedicles *(arrows)*. **B,** Axial CT image shows the destroyed left L1 pedicle and associated soft tissue mass. Most metastases to the spine occur in the vertebral body and are very difficult to detect on radiographs until bone loss is extensive.

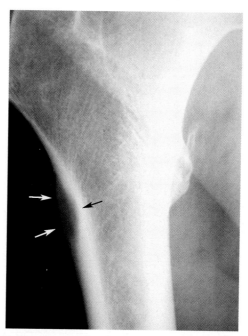

Figure 35-15   Unusual site of metastasis. AP radiograph of the proximal femur in this 65-year-old man demonstrates a cortically based lytic lesion *(arrows)*. Cortical metastases are uncommon, but when they occur are most likely due to pulmonary or breast primary lesions.

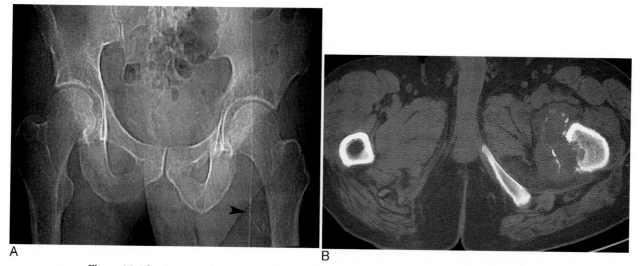

Figure 35-16   Lesser trochanter metastasis. Frontal scout image (A) and axial CT image (B) show destruction of the lesser trochanter *(arrowhead* in A). This is a classic presentation for lung cancer, but myeloma, renal cell carcinoma, or aggressive tumors could also present this way.

CHAPTER 36

Neural and Synovial Tumors

TUMORS ASSOCIATED WITH PERIPHERAL NERVES
  Peripheral Nerve Sheath Tumors
  Morton's Neuroma
  Neural Fibrolipoma (Fibrolipomatous Hamartoma)
SYNOVIAL TUMORS
  Pigmented Villonodular Synovitis
  Giant Cell Tumor of the Tendon Sheath
SYNOVIAL CELL SARCOMA

TUMORS ASSOCIATED WITH PERIPHERAL NERVES

Peripheral Nerve Sheath Tumors

Peripheral nerve sheath tumors (PNSTs), whether benign or malignant, are most classically distinguished by their fusiform shape. The mass tapers at one or both ends to accommodate the nerve entering and exiting the tumor. Together, neurofibromas and schwannomas represent about 10% of all benign soft tissue tumors. Both types of benign peripheral nerve sheath tumors most frequently affect patients 20 to 30 years of age. Both show initial slow growth and usually are small when detected. When large, these tumors can be exquisitely painful.

Key Concepts	Benign Peripheral Nerve Sheath Tumors

Neurofibroma, schwannoma.
Often fusiform shape.
Entering and exiting nerve.
MRI: Target sign, split-fat sign.
Neurofibromas are usually found in cutaneous nerves, with the fascicles separated and intimately involved with tumor.
Schwannomas most frequently involve the ulnar and peroneal nerves, with the tumor lying on the surface of the nerve.

Neurofibromas are composed of Schwann cells, fibroblasts, and collagen that surround and engulf the fibers of the associated nerve (Fig. 36-1). Neurofibromas may be localized, plexiform, or diffuse. Ninety percent of neurofibromas are solitary, and are not associated with neurofibromatosis type 1 (NF1). These most often arise in the superficial cutaneous nerves. Patients with NF1 may have hundreds of neurofibromas (Fig. 36-2). Although fusiform enlargement may not be seen in superficial cutaneous neurofibromas, it is a common feature of deeper lesions. Neurofibromas invade the nerve fascicles, which become separated and intimately involved with tumor. Computed tomography (CT) typically shows a near-water density mass. Magnetic resonance imaging (MRI) shows low signal intensity on T1-weighted images and heterogeneously increased signal intensity on T2-weighted images. The nerve fascicles may be visible within the tumor, seen on MRI as multiple small ring-like structures, known as the "fascicular sign" (see Fig. 36-1). The more frequently seen "target sign" is low signal intensity centrally with a ring of higher signal intensity peripherally on T2-weighted MR images (see Fig. 36-1C). This pattern reflects the histologic features of the tumor, with peripheral myxomatous tissue (with high T2 signal) surrounding a fibrocollagenous core. Enhancement may follow a reverse or similar pattern. The "split fat sign" is the finding of fat separating the tumor from adjacent muscles, best seen at a tapering margin of the tumor. Note that the split fat and target signs can also be seen in schwannomas and even occasionally in malignant peripheral nerve sheath tumors. Cutaneous neurofibromas are less likely to demonstrate these signs than are deeper lesions.

Schwannoma, also known as neurilemoma, neurinoma, perineural fibroblastoma, and peripheral glioma, is the other common benign peripheral nerve sheath tumor. Histologically, schwannomas are composed of Schwann cells and variable amounts of myxoid material and collagen, and are positive for S-100 protein. In contrast with neurofibromas, schwannomas do not engulf the associated nerve and therefore often can be "peeled off" of the associated nerve at surgery. Schwannomas

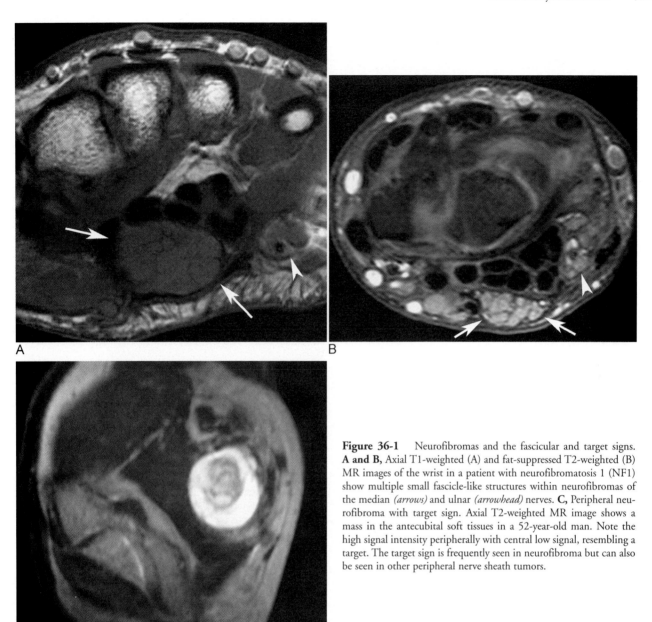

Figure 36-1 Neurofibromas and the fascicular and target signs. **A and B,** Axial T1-weighted (A) and fat-suppressed T2-weighted (B) MR images of the wrist in a patient with neurofibromatosis 1 (NF1) show multiple small fascicle-like structures within neurofibromas of the median *(arrows)* and ulnar *(arrowhead)* nerves. **C,** Peripheral neurofibroma with target sign. Axial T2-weighted MR image shows a mass in the antecubital soft tissues in a 52-year-old man. Note the high signal intensity peripherally with central low signal, resembling a target. The target sign is frequently seen in neurofibroma but can also be seen in other peripheral nerve sheath tumors.

are most commonly found in spinal and sympathetic nerve roots, and in the extremities usually affect nerves in the flexor surfaces of the upper and lower extremities, particularly the ulnar and peroneal nerves. Schwannomas, like neurofibromas, are usually solitary. If there are multiple schwannomas, they generally occur in a cutaneous distribution, with a very small proportion of these associated with NF1. (Note that intracranial schwannoma is associated with NF2.) Schwannomatosis is a rare syndrome of multiple peripheral schwannomas. As with neurofibromas, fusiform shape, association with a nerve, and the target and split fat signs are variably seen at MRI (Fig. 36-3). Some schwannomas have fairly uniform intermediate-low signal on T2-weighted images, and some contain cystic degeneration ("ancient schwannomas").

Malignant peripheral nerve sheath tumors (also called neurofibrosarcoma or malignant schwannoma) make up 5% to 10% of all soft tissue sarcomas. They are generally seen in patients 20 to 50 years of age and are much more common in men. Malignant PNST is frequently associated with NF1 (roughly half of cases). Although some of these lesions arise from a preexisting neurofibroma, it should be emphasized that the malignant potential of a neurofibroma is very low. Malignant PNSTs are usually deep lesions, involving the major nerve trunks such as the sciatic nerve, brachial plexus, and sacral plexus (Fig. 36-4). These lesions may be fusiform in shape and intimately associated with a large nerve, suggesting the diagnosis. The large size, irregular margins, and heterogenous signal intensity of many malignant PNSTs may suggest a malignant lesion, although these findings

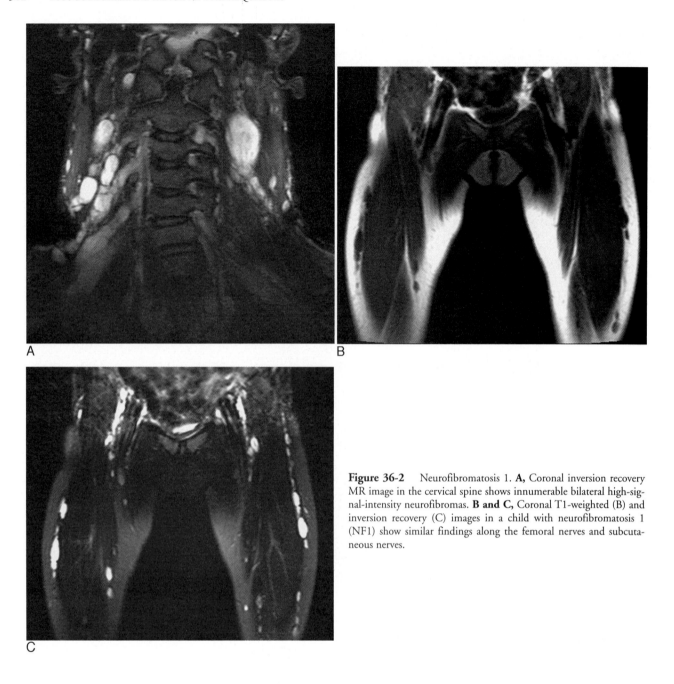

Figure 36-2   Neurofibromatosis 1. **A,** Coronal inversion recovery MR image in the cervical spine shows innumerable bilateral high-signal-intensity neurofibromas. **B and C,** Coronal T1-weighted (B) and inversion recovery (C) images in a child with neurofibromatosis 1 (NF1) show similar findings along the femoral nerves and subcutaneous nerves.

are not specific. A target sign is occasionally present. Rapid growth in a previously stable neurofibroma and invasion or destruction of adjacent tissues may be present are more specific signs. Malignant PNSTs are aggressive lesions, requiring wide surgical excision, chemotherapy, and often radiation therapy. Local recurrence and distant metastases to lung, bone, and lymph nodes is common.

Morton's Neuroma

Morton's neuroma is not a neoplasm but rather perineural fibrosis and nerve degeneration occurring in the interdigital space of the foot between the metatarsal heads and necks. The

cause is thought to be repetitive trauma, with the digital nerve abraded by the intermetatarsal ligament that connects adjacent metatarsal heads. The association of Morton's neuroma with high-heeled shoes may account for the gender frequency (female-to-male, ratio, 18:1). The lesions are most frequently found between the second and third or third and fourth metatarsal heads. The diagnosis can be made clinically but may be confused with other lesions such as stress fractures, intermetatarsal bursitis, metatarsophalangeal arthrosis, and tendonitis. Magnetic resonance imaging is helpful in differentiating these possibilities. When performed with a small field of view oriented in the short axis of the forefoot, MRI shows a small dumbbell-shaped mass between the distal

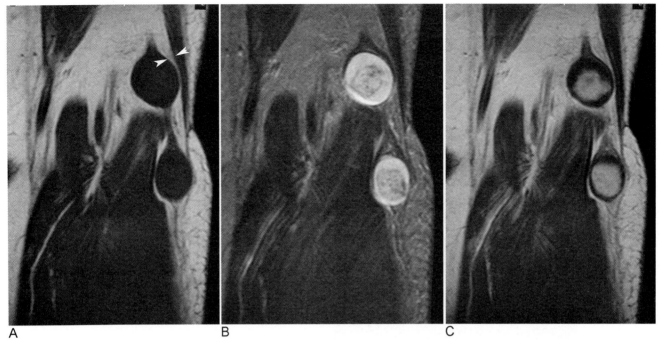

Figure 36-3   Peripheral schwannomas. **A–C,** Coronal T1-weighted (A), T2-weighted (B), and contrast-enhanced T1-weighted (C) MR images through the posterior knee region show two schwannomas in the peroneal nerve. Note the fusiform shape with tapering proximal and distal tumor margins, target appearance, and "split fat" between the tumors and adjacent muscles (*arrowheads* in part A).

metatarsal heads, usually demarcated from fat on T1-weighted images, occasionally with high T2 signal, and usually with intense enhancement (Fig. 36-5). The high vascularity of these lesions allows some to be detected with ultrasonography (US).

Neural Fibrolipoma (Fibrolipomatous Hamartoma)

Neural fibrolipoma is a tumor-like hamartomatous overgrowth of mesodermal and epidermal elements resulting in nerve enlargement, with fatty tissue interposed between thickened nerve bundles. The lesion is usually seen in children or young adults, and there is a marked predilection for the median nerve. The MRI appearance is pathognomonic, with high T1 and T2 signal lipomatous tissue surrounding longitudinally oriented low signal thickened nerve bundles (Fig. 36-6). This lesion may be associated with macrodactyly and macrodystrophia lipomatosa (see Chapter 47).

SYNOVIAL TUMORS

Pigmented Villonodular Synovitis

Pigmented villonodular synovitis (PVNS) is a monoarticular tumor-like proliferation of synovium that occurs in joints, bursae, and tendon sheaths. The condition is termed giant cell tumor of the tendon sheath when found in a tendon sheath. The cause of PVNS is unknown.

Key Concepts	Pigmented Villonodular Synovitis (PVNS)

Monoarticular mass-like synovial proliferation; hemorrhages. May be focal or diffuse.

Occurs more frequently in knee than in hip or ankle.

Radiographs: Monoarticular, effusion, well-circumscribed bone erosion and subchondral cysts; cartilage space preserved.

MRI: Typical—low signal on all sequences, especially gradient echo, because of hemosiderin deposition in synovium. Early cases may not have such extensive hemosiderin deposition.

Differential diagnosis: Hemophilia (PVNS is monoarticular), synovial chondromatosis, gout, amyloidosis, tuberculosis.

The synovial proliferation of PVNS begins as a focal mass. The abnormal synovium is prone to hemorrhage with minor trauma, resulting in hemorrhagic effusions. Thus, radiographs or MRI of early disease may show only a focal mass and a joint effusion. Magnetic resonance imaging also demonstrates subtle, early erosions when present. Over time, the process may enlarge to involve the entire joint and invade adjacent bones, resulting in large erosions and sometimes large subchondral cysts (Fig. 36-7). Radiographs at this more advanced stage thus may show radiodense synovial hypertrophy and large erosions. Bone density is normal and cartilage spaces are preserved until

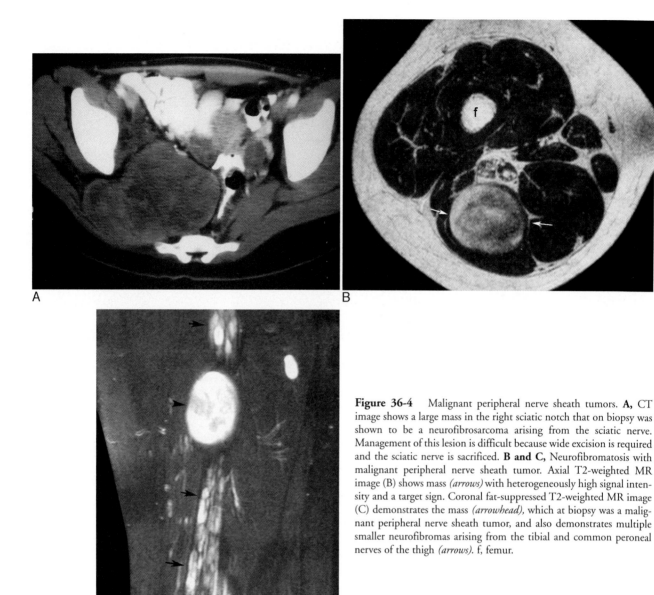

Figure 36-4 Malignant peripheral nerve sheath tumors. **A,** CT image shows a large mass in the right sciatic notch that on biopsy was shown to be a neurofibrosarcoma arising from the sciatic nerve. Management of this lesion is difficult because wide excision is required and the sciatic nerve is sacrificed. **B and C,** Neurofibromatosis with malignant peripheral nerve sheath tumor. Axial T2-weighted MR image (B) shows mass *(arrows)* with heterogeneously high signal intensity and a target sign. Coronal fat-suppressed T2-weighted MR image (C) demonstrates the mass *(arrowhead)*, which at biopsy was a malignant peripheral nerve sheath tumor, and also demonstrates multiple smaller neurofibromas arising from the tibial and common peroneal nerves of the thigh *(arrows)*. f, femur.

very late in the disease process. The single most classic MRI finding is synovial masses with variably low signal intensity on all MRI sequences due to hemosiderin deposition related to prior hemorrhages (Figs. 36-8, 36-9). Gradient echo images demonstrate the "blooming" paramagnetic effect of hemosiderin deposition. T2 signal is more variable owing to inconsistent proportions of fat, fibrous tissue, blood products, and edema. Intravenous gadolinium may more completely define the extent of the lesion but is not required for diagnosis.

Pigmented villonodular synovitis presents in a wide age range, from adolescents to elderly patients. Eighty percent of cases of PVNS are found in the knee. Other commonly affected joints include the hip and elbow. The differential diagnosis includes infection and other monoarticular arthritides such as gout. The signal intensity on MRI is not specific to PVNS and may be similar to that in gout, amyloid, or prominent synovitis in chronic low-grade infection, or in conditions with multiple prior intra-articular hemorrhages such as hemophilia or trauma. Also, synovial chondromatosis also is a monoarticular and noninflammatory process with maintained radiographic cartilage space. Synovial chondromatosis often shows nodule calcifications on radiographs and chondroid nodules on MRI. Synovial calcification is a rare finding in advanced PVNS.

Usual therapy for PVNS is open surgical resection with total synovectomy. Incompletely resected PVNS is likely to recur. Lesions located posterior to the cruciate ligaments, superior to the femoral condyles, or inferior to the tibial plateau are not accessible to arthroscopic synovectomy and must undergo an open procedure. Radiation synovectomy is another treatment

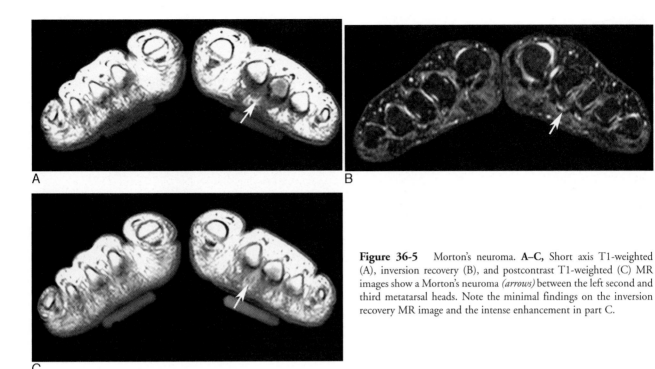

Figure 36-5   Morton's neuroma. **A–C,** Short axis T1-weighted (A), inversion recovery (B), and postcontrast T1-weighted (C) MR images show a Morton's neuroma *(arrows)* between the left second and third metatarsal heads. Note the minimal findings on the inversion recovery MR image and the intense enhancement in part C.

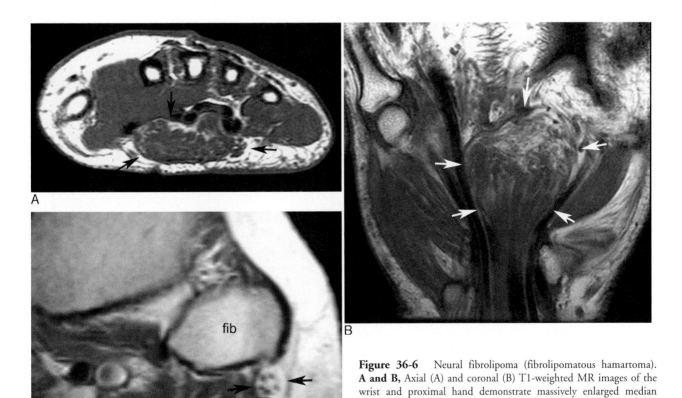

Figure 36-6   Neural fibrolipoma (fibrolipomatous hamartoma). **A and B,** Axial (A) and coronal (B) T1-weighted MR images of the wrist and proximal hand demonstrate massively enlarged median nerve with multiple nerve fascicles surrounded by bright lipomatous signal *(arrows)*. **C,** Axial T1-weighted MR image in the proximal left leg shows a similar lesion in the peroneal nerve *(arrows)*. fib, fibular head.

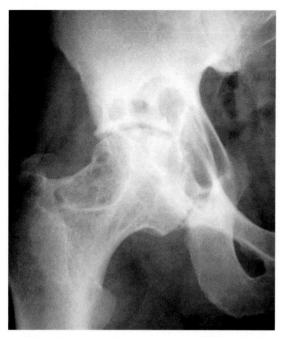

Figure 36-7   Pigmented villonodular synovitis (PVNS). AP radiograph of the hip in a 45-year-old woman demonstrates prominent cyst formation involving both sides of the joint. These cysts are large and well defined, yet the cartilage space remains intact. The findings are typical of PVNS.

option, which also requires accurate localization. Refractory cases with secondary osteoarthritis may require arthroplasty.

Giant Cell Tumor of the Tendon Sheath

Giant cell tumor of the tendon sheath is a painless, slow growing mass in a tendon sheath, usually of the finger. It is histologically identical to PVNS. Radiographs show a noncalcified soft tissue mass that is usually not centered on a joint. About 10% have an associated bony erosion (Fig. 36-10). Magnetic resonance imaging shows a low signal mass. Diagnosis is usually made by clinical and radiographic features. The lesion usually hemorrhages much less than does PVNS, and therefore tends to have less specific findings on MRI. However, if MRI is done, the lesion is typically hypointense to muscle on T1, and, like PVNS, is variably hypointense to hyperintense on T2, depending on the amount of hemosiderin present. Use of MRI can help localize the mass to the tendon sheath.

SYNOVIAL CELL SARCOMA

Synovial sarcoma represents only 5% of malignant soft tissue sarcomas, but it is one of the most common soft tissue sarcomas in younger adult patients (15 to 35 years of age). Although the

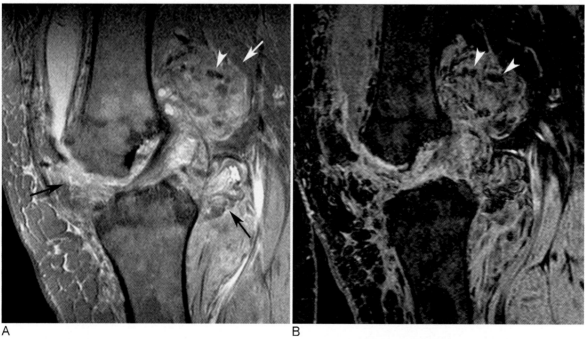

A   B

Figure 36-8   Pigmented villonodular synovitis (PVNS). **A and B,** Sagittal T2-weighted (A) and gradient echo (B) MR images shows massive knee synovial hypertrophy *(arrows)* with areas of low signal intensity that are more obvious on the gradient echo image *(arrowheads).* These represent areas of dense hemosiderin deposition.

(Continued)

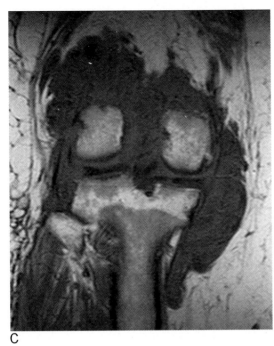

C

Figure 36-8—(Cont'd) **C,** Coronal T1-weighted image in the same patient shows intermediate signal intensity of synovium with areas of lower signal.

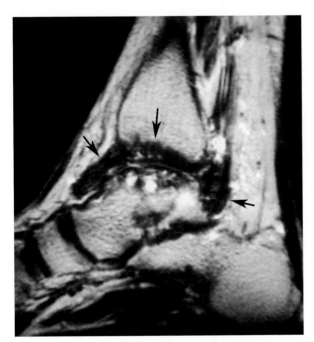

Figure 36-9 Pigmented villonodular synovitis (PVNS). Sagittal T2-weighted MR image in the ankle shows very-low-signal-intensity synovial proliferation *(arrows)*. Note cyst-like changes in the talar dome.

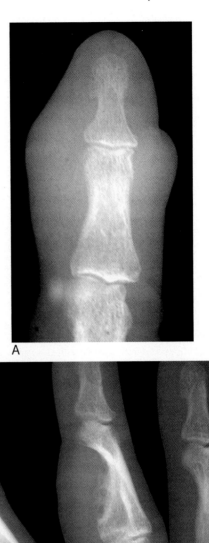

A

B

Figure 36-10 Giant cell tumor of the tendon sheath. **A,** AP radiograph of the finger in a 52-year-old woman demonstrates a nodular soft tissue mass with normal underlying bone. This is the most typical appearance for giant cell tumor of the tendon sheath. However, these lesions occasionally cause scalloping of adjacent bone, resulting in an appearance such as that seen in part B, a finger in a 20-year-old man.

name of the lesion suggests an articular process, and although this tumor is often found near a joint, 90% of synovial cell sarcomas do not originate from a joint. Rather, as with all sarcomas, the tumor is named by the predominant histologic differentiation, in this case tumor cells that resemble syn-

ovioblastic cells. Most occur in the lower extremity, especially at or distal to the knee. Synovial cell sarcomas have a higher prevalence of dystrophic calcification than do the other soft tissue sarcomas (20% to 30%). Thus, the age, location, and calcification, if present, can suggest this tumor (Fig. 36-11).

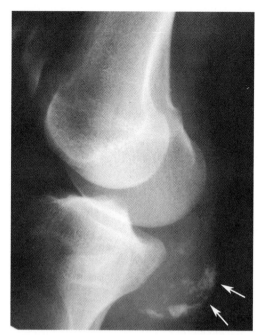

Figure 36-11 Synovial cell sarcoma with dystrophic calcification. Oblique radiograph of the knee in an 18-year-old man, demonstrating a soft tissue mass containing dystrophic calcification *(arrows)*. Synovial cell sarcoma calcifies more frequently than other soft tissue sarcomas. The location, calcification, and age of the patient should yield a strong suspicion of synovial cell sarcoma (Reprinted with permission from the American College of Radiology learning file.)

Key Concepts	Synovial Cell Sarcoma

Common soft tissue sarcoma in young adults.
Termed "synovial cell" because tumor cells resemble synovial cells, not because tumor is joint related. (Most are not!)
Most frequently occurs around or distal to knee, or around elbow.
Dystrophic calcification is relatively common.
MRI appearance can be deceptively nonaggressive.
  Intravenous contrast medium helps to show that the lesion is not a cyst.

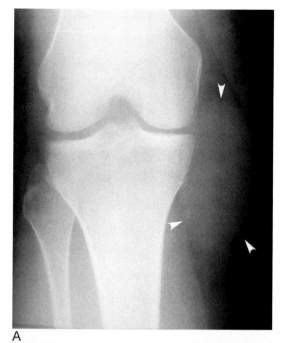

A

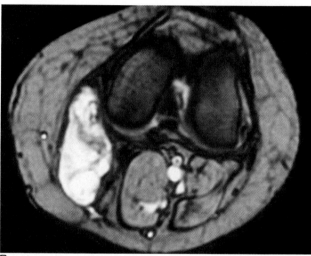

B

Figure 36-12 Synovial cell sarcoma without calcification. **A,** AP radiograph of the knee in a 17-year-old girl demonstrates a soft tissue mass adjacent to but not within the knee joint *(arrowheads)*. **B,** Axial gradient echo image of the lesion, demonstrated here to be juxta-articular. Despite the lack of calcification and the encapsulated appearance of this lesion, the age of the patient, location, and prevalence of the lesion lead one to suspect the diagnosis is synovial cell sarcoma, which was proven at biopsy.

The MRI appearance of synovial cell sarcoma is nonspecific, with T1 signal isointense with muscle, and heterogeneous high T2 signal intensity, often with areas of internal hemorrhage and occasional fluid-fluid levels. Most synovial sarcomas have well-defined margins without surrounding reactive edema. Some also have very bright signal intensity on T2-weighted images, which may falsely suggest a ganglion cyst (Fig. 36-12). It is important not to be misled by this appearance because this is an aggressive lesion and tumor microinvasion beyond the pseudocapsule is highly likely. Contrast enhancement can be helpful in distinguishing a solid mass from a ganglion cyst, as the latter enhances only faintly at the lesion margins.

Synovial cell sarcomas are treated with wide excision, often with adjuvant chemotherapy and occasional radiation therapy. Calcified tumors tend to have a better prognosis, but outcome is generally poor, with pulmonary metastasis frequent found, and local recurrence in about one quarter of patients despite aggressive local therapy.

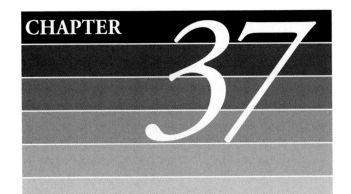

CHAPTER 37

Miscellaneous Tumors and Tumor-Like Lesions

GIANT CELL TUMOR OF BONE
SOLITARY BONE CYST (UNICAMERAL BONE CYST)
ANEURYSMAL BONE CYST
LANGERHANS CELL HISTIOCYTOSIS
BROWN TUMOR OF HYPERPARATHYROIDISM
MYOSITIS OSSIFICANS
CHORDOMA
ADAMANTINOMA
GANGLION CYST

GIANT CELL TUMOR OF BONE

Giant cell tumor (GCT) is a common, benign neoplasm constituting 5% of primary bone tumors. It consists of connective tissue, multinucleated osteoclastic giant cells, and a fibrous stroma. The tumor cell is not the giant cell but rather a spindle cell in the stroma, which helps to distinguish GCT from the many other lesions that may contain reactive giant cells. Giant cell tumors nearly always occur after epiphyseal fusion; 70% of them occur between the third and fifth decades of life. This is one of the few musculoskeletal tumors that is more common in women (female-to-male ratio, 2:1).

The typical radiographic appearance of GCT is a lytic geographic lesion with a narrow zone of transition and no marginal sclerosis (type 1B margin) at the end of a long bone, often with mild bone expansion (Fig. 37-1). A broader zone of transition (type 1C margin) can be seen, and areas of margin sclerosis are occasionally seen. (Remember to evaluate the aggressiveness of a lytic bone lesion by the most aggressive portion of the margin.) The lesion can also appear more aggressive, with cortical breakthrough and soft tissue mass (Fig. 37-2). The tumors are eccentric and arise in the metaphysis (Fig. 37-3), then enlarge (Fig. 37-4). In the skeletally mature, extension into the epiphysis is a hallmark feature, with extension typically seen to the articular margin (Fig. 37-5). Extension through the articular cartilage, however, is rare. Most occur about the knee, with

Key Concepts	Giant Cell Tumor (GCT)

Typical lesion lytic geographic at the end of a long bone, without margin sclerosis. In the skeletally mature, the lesion extends to the subchondral bone.

Most common sites: About the knee, distal radius. Spine: Sacrum or body of vertebra.

Originates in the metaphysis.

Rare before physeal fusion, most commonly between 20 and 40 years of age.

Most are benign, but may metastasize to lung.

Approximately 10% local recurrence rate; Can be higher with less aggressive surgery. Recurrent tumors behave more aggressively.

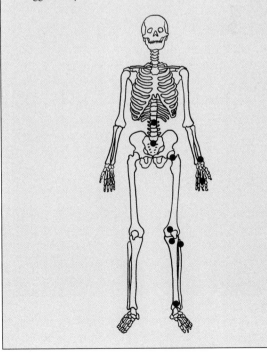

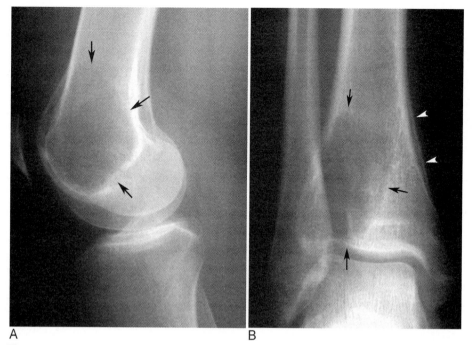

Figure 37-1   Giant cell tumor (GCT). **A,** Lateral knee radiograph shows a large lytic lesion in the distal femoral metaphysis *(arrows),* extending to the subchondral bone at the anterior portion of the femoral condyle and the roof of the intercondylar notch. There is no matrix, and the zone of transition is narrow and lacks a sclerotic margin (type 1B margin). This is a typical appearance of GCT, seen in a 31-year-old woman. **B,** GCT in the distal tibia of a 16-year-old boy *(arrows),* with similar features. Note the mature periosteal new bone formation *(arrowheads),* which is a normal stress response to structural weakening of the distal tibia rather than a direct response to the tumor.

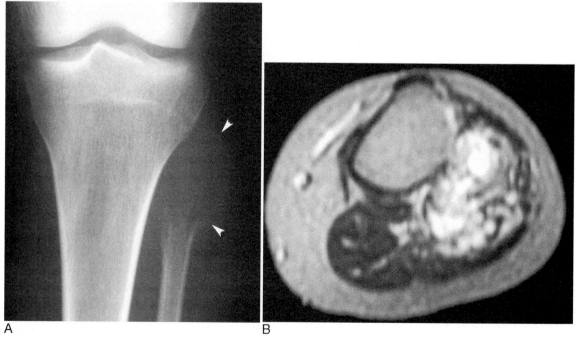

Figure 37-2   Aggressive giant cell tumor (GCT). **A,** AP radiograph demonstrates a lytic lesion in the proximal fibula *(arrowheads),* which is expanded and has a wide zone of transition (type 1C margin) in this 29-year-old woman. **B,** Axial T2-weighted spin-echo MR image shows a large soft tissue mass involving the anterior, lateral, and posterior compartments. This proved to be an aggressive GCT.

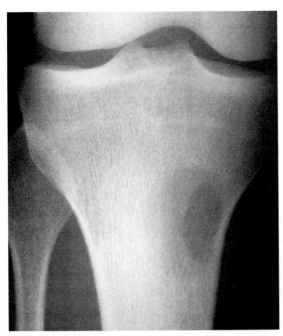

Figure 37-3   Metaphyseal giant cell tumor (GCT). AP radiograph of the proximal tibia in a 22-year-old woman demonstrates a lytic lesion arising eccentrically in the metaphysis having a narrow zone of transition but no sclerotic margin. Some might have a difficult time arriving at the diagnosis because the lesion does not extend all the way to the subchondral bone. It should be remembered that GCTs arise in the metaphysis and may only reach the subchondral bone when they are moderately large. (Reprinted with permission from the American College of Radiology learning file.)

most of the remainder at distal radius and ulna or proximal humerus. There is no calcified matrix. Giant cell tumors also occur in the spine, where they most often involve the sacrum or body of a vertebra (Fig. 37-6). Most GCTs are solitary. Multiple lesions can occur, especially in skull and facial bones affected by Paget's disease, mimicking metastatic disease.

The typical magnetic resonance imaging (MRI) appearance is uniform, intermediate-low signal intensity on T1-weighted images. The tumors enhance with intravenous gadolinium (Figs. 37-5, 37-7) High cellularity, hemosiderin, and collagen deposition often result in relatively low T2 signal in nodular, zonal, whorled, or uniform pattern. The appearance of areas of relatively low T2 signal intensity can help to distinguish GCT from other common subchondral lesions such as subchondral cyst or a Brodie's abscess, which are usually uniformly bright. Fluid-fluid levels also may be seen in GCTs.

The diagnosis is often made with radiography. In the long bones, differential diagnosis includes aneurysmal bone cyst, especially when fluid-fluid levels are present. These tumors may coexist, as discussed in the following section on aneurysmal bone cysts. A subchondral cyst or Brodie's abscess should not show bone expansion. Chondroblastoma also is a subchondral tumor, and also may contain fluid-fluid levels, but chondroblastoma is generally found in skeletally immature patients and arises from the epiphysis; it also typically has sclerotic margins and chondroid matrix calcification. Brown tumor of hyperparathyroidism may also have a radiographic appearance similar to that of GCT. However, these patients have appropriate clinical history and will

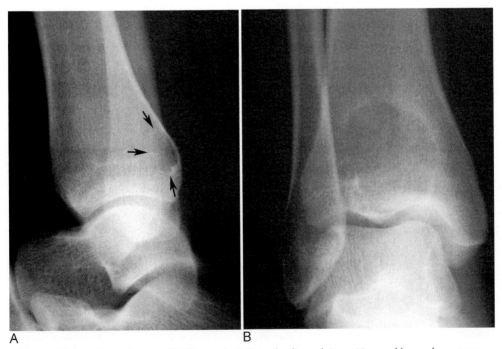

A   B

Figure 37-4   Giant cell tumor (GCT) growth. **A,** Lateral radiograph in an 18-year-old man shows a very subtle, small lytic lesion, with a narrow zone of transition lacking a sclerotic margin centered in the posterior distal tibial metaphysis extending into the epiphysis. **B–D,** Radiographs (B and C) and sagittal T1-weighted MR image (D) obtained 18 months later show the lesion has enlarged and now extends to the distal articular surface.

(Continued)

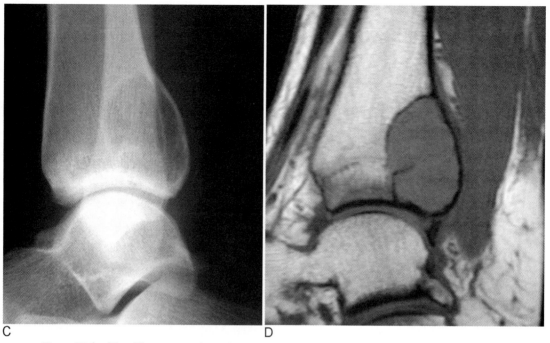

Figure 37-4—(Cont'd) **B–D,** Radiographs (B and C) and sagittal T1-weighted MR image (D) obtained 18 months later show the lesion has enlarged and now extends to the distal articular surface.

manifest typical radiographic features of hyperparathyroidism. Other lytic lesions, such as plasmacytoma, metastasis, or a sarcoma without matrix, may resemble GCT. Nonossifying fibroma is an eccentric metaphyseal lesion. Its slightly different location, as well as its sclerotic border, should easily differentiate this lesion from GCT. In the spine and sacrum, GCT could be confused most frequently with chordoma or chondrosarcoma because the location in the body of the sacrum or vertebra is similar. Spinal aneurysmal bone cyst and osteoblastoma usually occur in the posterior elements.

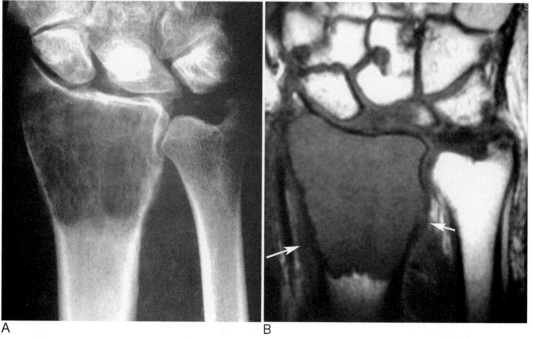

Figure 37-5 Giant cell tumor (GCT). **A,** Radiograph shows typical GCT of the distal radius in a 50-year-old man with cortical thinning and extension to the distal articular surface. **B and C,** Coronal T1-weighted (B) and fat-suppressed, contrast-enhanced, T1-weighted (C) MR images show subtle cortical breakthrough (*arrows* in part B and C).

(Continued)

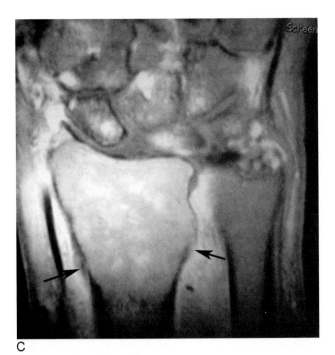

C

Figure 37-5—(Cont'd)   B and C, Coronal T1-weighted (B) and fat-suppressed contrast-enhanced T1-weighted (C) MR images show subtle cortical breakthrough (*arrows* in parts B and C).

Most GCTs are benign with low histologic grade; approximately 5% are malignant. The single most important predictor of clinical behavior of a giant cell tumor is the histologic appearance. However, clinical and radiologic features must be considered in evaluating the overall aggressiveness of a GCT. For example, both histologically malignant and benign GCT can metastasize to the lungs. The latter bizarre condition is known as "benign metastasizing giant cell tumor." Among patients with histologically benign lesions that metastasize, the prognosis may be good with surgical resection of the lung metastases.

Because GCTs that have recurred after surgical resection tend to behave more aggressively than the original tumor, surgical technique is important. Wide margins are preferred, but preservation of adjacent joint function also is desired, especially given the relatively young age of patients with GCT. The recurrence rate following curettage and bone graft can be as high as 50%. If cryosurgery is added, recurrence rates are lower. A lower recurrence rate also occurs with curettage and methacrylate injection. The methacrylate supports the thin residual overlying articular bone, and it cures at high temperature, enhancing tumor kill at the surgical margins. Follow-up radiographs after curettage will show a

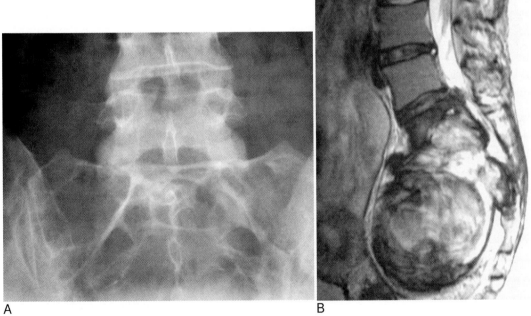

A   B

Figure 37-6   Giant cell tumor (GCT) in the spine. **A,** AP radiograph of the lumbar spine demonstrates an expanded lytic lesion occupying the superior sacrum. The extent of the lesion is seen better with MRI. **B,** Sagittal T2-weighted MR image demonstrates a very large mass with heterogenous signal intensity extending anteriorly from the sacrum. The spine and particularly the sacrum are favorite locations for GCT in the axial skeleton.

thin radiolucent halo around the methacrylate as a normal finding. New, enlarging, asymmetric lytic regions in the tumor bed or surgical margins indicate recurrence (Fig. 37-8). Magnetic resonance imaging can also be useful in evaluating these patients for tumor recurrence, as the methyl methacrylate is dark on all sequences and recurrent tumors are enhancing, intermediate-signal-intensity lesions often easily detected at the cement margins or in adjacent soft tissues. Aggressive surgical therapy with wide resection and replacement of the resected bone with an osteoarticular graft or a long-stem custom prosthesis also is a treatment option, but in a young patient, such a prosthesis might require multiple revisions throughout life, causing considerable morbidity. Moreover, tumors can recur despite such wide resection. Because of difficulty of resection, spine GCT may be treated with radiation.

Giant cell reparative granuloma is a nonneoplastic reactive lytic lesion that occurs primarily in the jaw, maxilla, hands, and feet. The radiographic features may be similar to those of GCT, but the lesion is otherwise unrelated to GCT (except of course that both contain giant cells at histology). The similarity in tumor names is a potential source of confusion.

SOLITARY BONE CYST (UNICAMERAL BONE CYST)

Solitary bone cyst (SBC), also termed simple or unicameral bone cyst, is a very common nonneoplastic lesion of childhood, most frequently discovered in the first and second decades of life. It is often found incidentally, or presents with a pathologic fracture. The most common sites are the proximal humerus (50%), followed by the proximal femur (20%). Solitary bone cyst is a geographic lytic lesion with sharp margins that typically are sclerotic (type 1A) but occasionally nonsclerotic (type 1B). It may be mildly expansile, and has no tumor matrix. The lesion does not cross the growth plate. Solitary bone cyst is a central lesion that initially is metaphyseal in location, abutting the growth plate. However, with advancing skeletal maturation, a solitary bone cyst "migrates" into the diaphysis. This "migration" actually represents growth of normal bone away from the cyst. As the name implies, the lesions are fluid-filled. Lesions may contain internal bone septations, but the lesion consists of a single communicating space, hence the terms "solitary" and "unicameral."

Lesions presenting with pathologic fracture may have the *fallen fragment sign,* which represents a fracture fragment that settles inferiorly in the dependent portion of the fluid-filled cyst (Figs. 29-1A, 37-9). In a young patient with a well-circumscribed lytic lesion in a typical location for SBC, this finding is pathognomonic.

Solitary bone cyst rarely can be found in adults, often in locations that are unusual for this lesion in children, such as the iliac wing, calcaneus, or talus (Figs. 37-10, 37-11).

Magnetic resonance imaging is rarely required for solitary bone cyst. However, the MRI appearance is typical of a cyst with low-signal T1 and high-signal T2 and occasional fluid levels if the cyst has been previously traumatized with internal hemorrhage (see Figs. 37-9, 37-11). Only a very fine rim of peripheral enhancement may be seen. Computed tomography (CT) or MRI can be helpful in evaluating lesions in unusual locations such as the spine.

The major radiographic differential diagnosis includes fibrous dysplasia (if there is no matrix present to give the typical ground-glass appearance of fibrous dysplasia), and Langerhans cell histiocytosis (eosinophilic granuloma). Aneurysmal bone cyst (ABC) is usually not part of this differential diagnosis because it is eccentrically located. Solitary bone cyst occurring in the adult calcaneus may resemble an

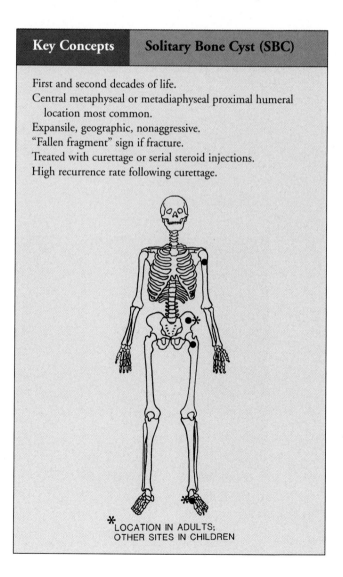

Key Concepts   **Solitary Bone Cyst (SBC)**

First and second decades of life.
Central metaphyseal or metadiaphyseal proximal humeral location most common.
Expansile, geographic, nonaggressive.
"Fallen fragment" sign if fracture.
Treated with curettage or serial steroid injections.
High recurrence rate following curettage.

*LOCATION IN ADULTS;
OTHER SITES IN CHILDREN

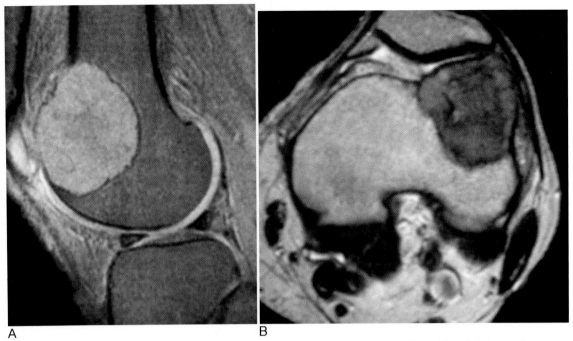

Figure 37-7   MRI of giant cell tumor (GCT). **A,** Sagittal fat-saturated contrast T1-weighted MR image of a metaphyseal GCT in a 63-year-old man. The fairly uniform and intense enhancement is typical. **B,** T2-weighted axial MR image demonstrates fairly low signal intensity, which may be a feature of GCTs and any other highly cellular tumor. GCTs may contain fluid-fluid levels as well.

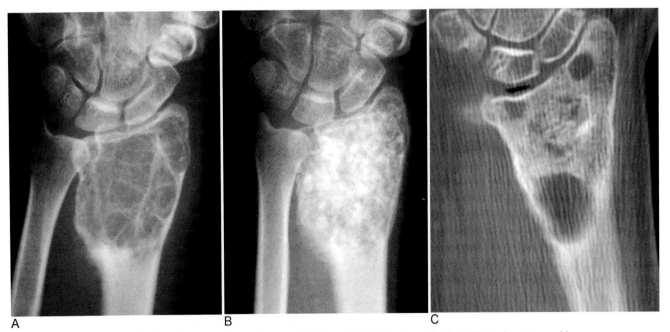

Figure 37-8   Recurrent giant cell tumor (GCT). **A,** Initial AP radiograph of a GCT in this 25-year-old woman. The distal radius is a common location for GCT, and this case is atypical only in the degree of pseudo-trabeculation seen. **B,** The lesion was treated with curettage and grafting, as shown in the radiograph. **C,** One year later, direct coronal CT demonstrates that although much of the bone graft has incorporated and matured, three separate sites of lucency are tumor recurrence within the distal radius.

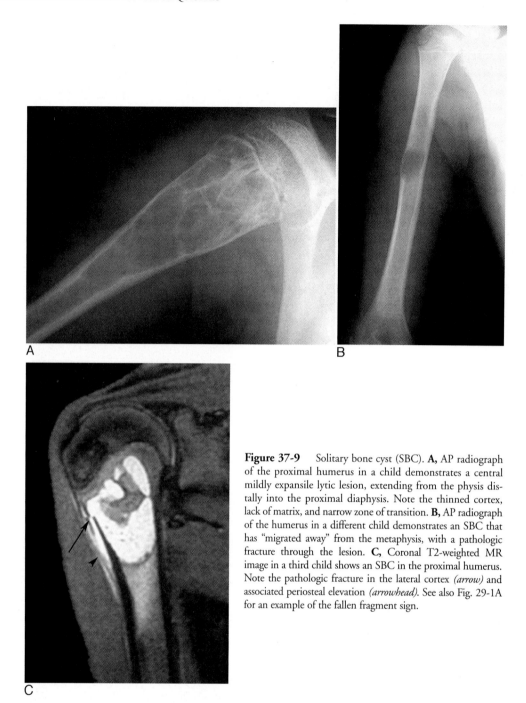

Figure 37-9 Solitary bone cyst (SBC). **A,** AP radiograph of the proximal humerus in a child demonstrates a central mildly expansile lytic lesion, extending from the physis distally into the proximal diaphysis. Note the thinned cortex, lack of matrix, and narrow zone of transition. **B,** AP radiograph of the humerus in a different child demonstrates an SBC that has "migrated away" from the metaphysis, with a pathologic fracture through the lesion. **C,** Coronal T2-weighted MR image in a third child shows an SBC in the proximal humerus. Note the pathologic fracture in the lateral cortex *(arrow)* and associated periosteal elevation *(arrowhead)*. See also Fig. 29-1A for an example of the fallen fragment sign.

intraosseous lipoma or a pseudocyst. (A pseudocyst is merely an area of relative lucency seen on a radiograph between areas of primary bone trabeculae.)

Solitary bone cysts are treated with curettage and bone grafting or direct injection of bone matrix biomaterial or corticosteroid into the cyst. Complications of treatment include acceleration or arrest of limb growth following curettage of a lesion adjacent to the growth plate. The recurrence rate is high (35% to 50%). The likelihood of recurrence relates predominately to patient age, with younger patients (those younger than age 10) having a much higher likelihood of recurrence. Solitary bone cyst may occasionally heal spontaneously following fracture.

ANEURYSMAL BONE CYST

An ABC is a benign, expansile (often extremely, hence the term "aneurysmal"), eccentric bone lesion consisting of blood-filled cystic cavities. It is found most frequently in the first through

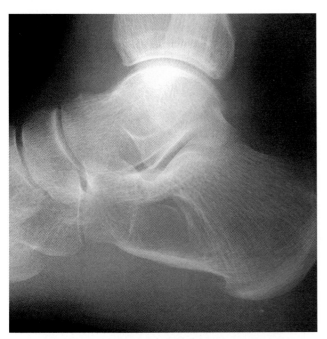

Figure 37-10 Adult solitary bone cyst (SBC). Lateral radiograph of the calcaneus in a 43-year-old man, demonstrating a lytic lesion in the anterior portion of the calcaneus. This is a typical location for either SBC or intraosseous lipoma. Biopsy in this case demonstrated SBC.

third decades of life, with 70% of cases occurring between 5 and 20 years of age. It may be primary or secondary. Secondary ABC arises within a pre-existing tumor, most frequently GCT, chondroblastoma, fibrous dysplasia, osteoblastoma, or nonossifying fibroma. These associations may be found in 30% to 50% of cases.

Key Concepts	Aneurysmal Bone Cyst (ABC)

Expansile (often extremely), lytic, narrow zone of transition, eccentric, metaphyseal in long bones. Thin, intact shell of expanded overlying bone.
Also found in posterior elements in the spine.
Generally under 30 years of age.
CT and MRI demonstrate fluid levels in most cases.
Occasionally it is rapidly progressive, simulating a more aggressive lesion.
May be post-traumatic (often cortically based), or secondary within a pre-existing tumor—look for a solid enhancing component that might represent the primary tumor.

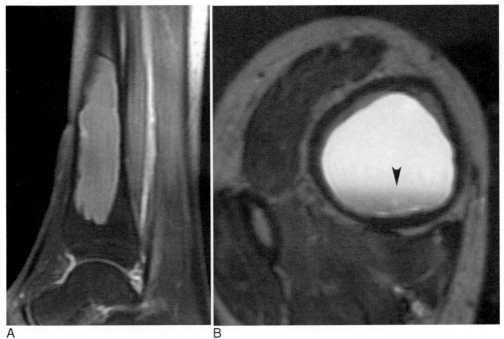

A   B

Figure 37-11 Adult solitary bone cyst (SBC). **A and B,** Sagittal fat-suppressed, postcontrast, T1-weighted (A) and axial fat-suppressed, T2-weighted (B) MR images show the typical features of a cyst, with uniform high T2 signal and fluid-fluid level in part B, and intermediate-low T1 signal and enhancement only of the rim of the tumor in part B. Absence of surrounding marrow or periosteal edema or enhancement suggests that despite the bone loss due to the lesion, there is no stress reaction in the surrounding bone.

One theory of the pathogenesis of ABC is that it is an intraosseous vascular anomaly induced by interference with venous drainage, caused either by trauma or a precursor lesion. It has been hypothesized, although not widely accepted, that *all* ABCs are secondary, and that the ABC obliterates the precursor lesion in many cases, leaving only a "primary" ABC. Regardless, these observations underlie the need for careful radiologic evaluation of ABCs so that the presence of an associated tumor is not missed during biopsy. Excisional biopsy is often preferred because it avoids this pitfall.

Aneurysmal bone cyst is usually a geographic lesion with a narrow zone of transition, often large with extreme ("aneurysmal") bone expansion, a narrow zone of transition, and a fine sclerotic rim (type 1A margin) (Fig. 37-12). This sclerotic rim may not be seen on radiographs (Fig. 37-13), but is more completely seen with CT. The shell of expanded bone may be very thin but should be uninterrupted. There is no tumor matrix. The lesion is monostotic and occurs in the metaphyses or metadiaphysis of long bones, where it is eccentrically located. Post-traumatic ABCs tend to be eccentric, often subperiosteal expansile lesions, whereas tumor-associated ABCs tend to be more central in location. Aneurysmal bone cysts also occur in the posterior elements of the spine and occasionally in the pelvis.

Both CT and MRI usually show fluid-fluid levels (Figs. 37-14–37-17), but it should be noted that such levels are not specific for ABCs; they also have been described in SBC, GCT, telangiectatic osteosarcoma, osteoblastoma, chondroblastoma, and rarely in other lesions (see Table 29-13). These are also some of the tumors associated with ABC, and thus a fluid-fluid level seen in these tumors may be within a secondary ABC. The presence of an associated tumor may be suggested by a thick rind, thick septations, or a peripheral nodule or mass. A solid variety of ABC (5%) does not show fluid levels.

The major differential diagnosis of ABC includes nonossifying fibroma, fibrous dysplasia, and SBC in the long bones; osteoblastoma in the spine; and lesions that may contain fluid-fluid levels as noted previously (see Table 29-13).

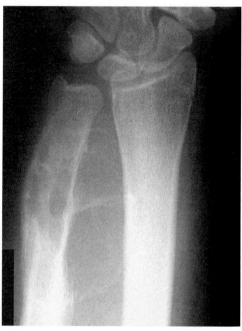

Figure 37-13 Aneurysmal bone cyst (ABC). AP radiograph of the distal forearm in a 16-year-old boy demonstrates an eccentrically located metaphyseal expansile lesion. This is a large but nonaggressive lesion, typical for ABC.

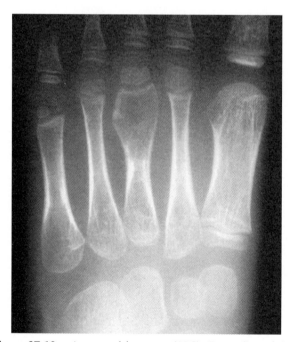

Figure 37-12 Aneurysmal bone cyst (ABC). Foot radiograph in a child shows an expansile lesion in the distal third metatarsal metadiaphysis. There is no matrix or cortical breakthrough. A solitary bone cyst (SBC) could be considered as well, although there is more bone expansion than usually seen with SBC.

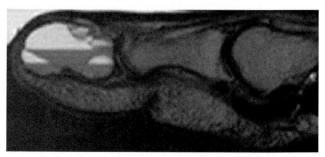

Figure 37-14 Aneurysmal bone cyst (ABC) of the great toe. Sagittal inversion recovery MR image shows an expansile lesion of the great toe distal phalanx with multiple fluid-fluid levels.

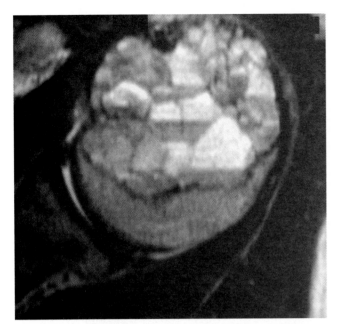

Figure 37-15 Aneurysmal bone cyst (ABC) of the proximal humerus. Axial T2-weighted MR image of the left shoulder shows an ABC in the proximal humerus of a 35-year-old woman, with the typical bone expansion and multiple fluid levels.

Treatment consists of curettage, often with cryosurgery because the recurrence rate is 20% to 50%. Low-dose radiation or ablative agent injection may be used for surgically inaccessible lesions (e.g., in the spine) (see Fig. 37-16). When evaluating an apparent recurrent ABC, keep in mind the possibility that the recurrence is of an associated tumor rather than of the ABC.

LANGERHANS CELL HISTIOCYTOSIS

Langerhans cell histiocytosis (LCH), formerly known as histiocytosis X, is a variety of rare disorders that occur predominantly in children, characterized by histiocytic infiltration of various organ systems. The defining infiltrating cell is the Langerhans cell, which is a specific type of immunologic cell. Neutrophils, eosinophils, and macrophages also are found in the infiltrates. The cause of LCH is poorly understood, and it is not agreed whether the condition is reactive or neoplastic. Overall, LCH is more common in males, and, although it can affect patients of any age, usually presents in patients younger than 15 years of age. The most common manifestation of LCH is eosinophilic granuloma, which is a localized, often solitary lytic bone lesion. More aggressive, clinical variations of LCH with multi-organ system involvement include Letterer-Siwe and Hand-Schüller-Christian disease, discussed later in this chapter. Other forms of LCH have been described, and many patients do not fit clearly into any category.

The most severe and least common (10%) clinical form of LCH is *Letterer-Siwe disease,* which is aggressive multisystem

Key Concepts	Langerhans Cell Histiocytosis (LPCH)

Rare spectrum of disorders in children related to histiocytic infiltration of various organ systems. Not all patients match the classic subtypes.

Letterer-Siwe disease: Aggressive multi-organ system disease, age 0–2 years, high mortality rate.

Hand-Schüller-Christian disease: Intermediate, chronic multi–organ system disease.

Eosinophilic granuloma of bone: Single organ system involvement in bone.

Bone lesions may have a variety of appearances. One classic pattern of long bone lesions begins with a highly aggressive appearance, with a permeative pattern and soft tissue mass, but usually heal spontaneously over 6–24 months.

10% to 20% are polyostotic.

Spine: Vertebra plana.

Skull: Beveled edge sharply defined lytic lesion.

Differential diagnosis depends on lesion appearance. Often includes Ewing's sarcoma, osteomyelitis, and metastatic neuroblastoma.

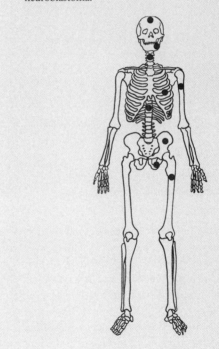

involvement in infants and toddlers younger than 2 years. Letterer-Siwe is more common in boys. Radiographic bone findings consisting of small lytic lesions primarily in the skull are present in only about half of children with Letterer-Siwe disease, although marrow infiltration is frequent. Clinical findings include hepatosplenomegaly, lymphadenopathy, pancytopenia (due to histiocytic infiltration of the marrow space), and skin infiltration. Mortality exceeds 50%.

Hand-Schüller-Christian disease is a clinically less aggressive, more common (20%) form of LCH, with chronic multiorgan

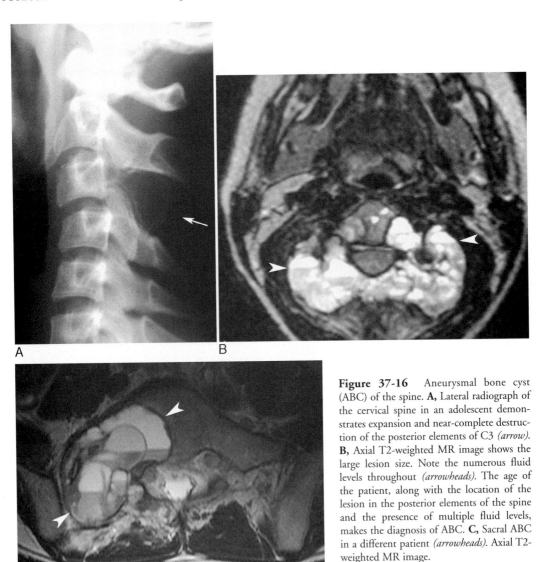

Figure 37-16 Aneurysmal bone cyst (ABC) of the spine. **A,** Lateral radiograph of the cervical spine in an adolescent demonstrates expansion and near-complete destruction of the posterior elements of C3 *(arrow).* **B,** Axial T2-weighted MR image shows the large lesion size. Note the numerous fluid levels throughout *(arrowheads).* The age of the patient, along with the location of the lesion in the posterior elements of the spine and the presence of multiple fluid levels, makes the diagnosis of ABC. **C,** Sacral ABC in a different patient *(arrowheads).* Axial T2-weighted MR image.

system involvement. Clinical onset is usually age 2 to 10 years. Classical clinical features include proptosis, diabetes insipidus, and lytic bone lesions. Thymus, liver, and lung involvement may occur. Spontaneous pneumothorax and eventual pulmonary fibrosis can occur. Mortality is low in the absence of pulmonary involvement.

Eosinophilic granuloma is the most common expression of LCH with single organ system bone involvement. Lesions may be single or multiple. Most occur at age 5 to 15 years, but it can present late into the 20s or in younger children, as an isolated lesion or as part of multiorgan system disease such as Hand-Schüller-Christian. Most cases of bone involvement present with a single lesion, but 10% to 20% develop polyostotic disease within 6 months of developing the first lesion. Those who present with a lesion at a young age are more likely to develop polyostotic disease. The skull is the most common site (50%), followed by the spine, jaw, and long bones (femur most common). Clinically, the lesions are painful and there may be a palpable lump.

The radiographic appearance of eosinophilic granuloma varies; thus it appears in the differential diagnosis of many types of lesions. Long bone lesions usually begin with a highly aggressive moth-eaten or permeative pattern. These lesions are usually central and metadiaphyseal, but any part of the bone may be involved. (Recall that eosinophilic granuloma is included in the short differential diagnosis of a lytic epiphyseal lesion in a child, along with infection and chondroblastoma.) There may be a soft tissue mass. When LCH is confined to bone, the lesions may heal spontaneously over months to 2 years. The margin becomes well defined, and periosteal reaction, which can be highly aggressive in appearance at presentation, becomes solid (Figs. 37-18, 37-19). Thus, depending on when a lesion is studied, the appearance can vary from aggressive to nonaggressive. Discordant findings of solid (nonaggressive) periosteal reaction around a permeative (highly aggressive) lesion in a long bone diaphysis in a child is a classic appearance in a spontaneously healing eosinophilic granuloma (Fig. 37-18).

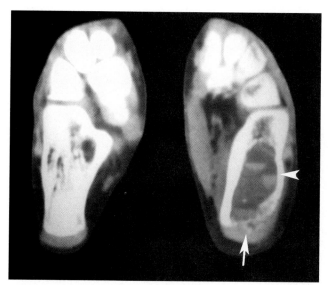

Figure 37-17 Secondary aneurysmal bone cyst (ABC). Axial CT shows a mass in the left calcaneus that contains areas with fluid-fluid levels *(arrowheads)*. Also note the posterior cortical destruction *(arrow)*. The appearance suggests telangiectatic osteosarcoma, but this was a giant cell tumor with a large secondary ABC that occupied most of the lesion.

Skull lesions have a narrow zone of transition with nonuniform involvement of the inner and outer skull tables, giving a beveled-edge appearance when viewed on edge, or concentric lytic discs when viewed en face. The lesions tend not to have a sclerotic margin. There is no tumor matrix, but, rarely, a fragment of bone may be left centrally, resembling a sequestrum. Periosteal reaction is common, and a soft tissue mass may be seen.

Langerhans cell histiocytosis can also involve the vertebral body. The vertebral body involvement can have a classic radiographic appearance of a compressed vertebral body *(vertebra plana)*, with intact posterior elements and disks and lack of an associated soft tissue mass (Fig. 37-20).

Key Concepts	Vertebra Plana
Eosinophilic granuloma (no associated soft tissue mass on cross-sectional imaging)	
Tumor (metastases, myeloma, leukemia, hemangioma)	
Fracture (osteoporosis, osteogenesis imperfecta)	
Infection	
Avascular necrosis (AVN)	

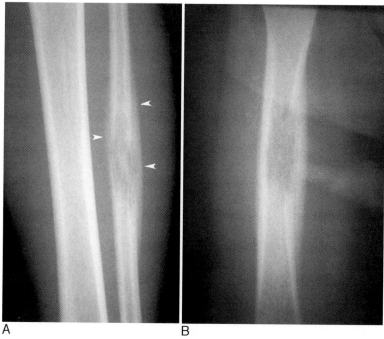

Figure 37-18 Langerhans cell histiocytosis (LCH): eosinophilic granuloma of bone. This condition can have a wide variety of appearances, ranging from highly aggressive to completely nonaggressive. **A,** AP radiograph showing a highly aggressive permeative lesion in the fibular mid-diaphysis of a 3-year-old girl, suggesting Ewing's sarcoma. However, there is a discordant finding of nonaggressive solid periosteal reaction *(arrowheads)*. This strange juxtaposition indicates a healing lesion, in this case a spontaneously healing eosinophilic granuloma. **B,** Similar pattern in the femur in of a 2-year-old.

(Continued)

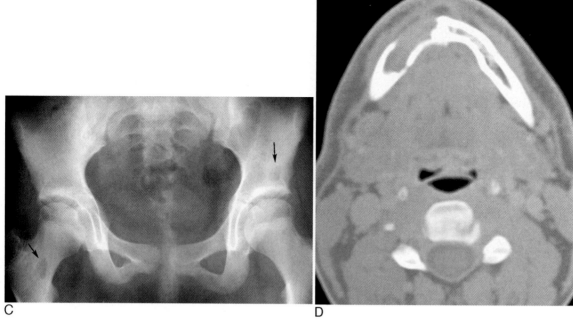

Figure 37-18—(Cont'd) **C,** Another pattern of LCH in a different patient, a 12-year-old girl. In this case, the disease is polyostotic and the lesions have narrow zone of transition, but lack sclerotic margins *(arrows)*. **D,** Lytic LCH lesion in the mandible of an adult, with cortical breakthrough but a narrow zone of transition.

Because LCH can be highly aggressive in its radiographic appearance as well as its rapid evolution, the differential diagnosis includes Ewing's sarcoma, lymphoma, osteomyelitis, and aggressive bone metastases. Although LCH can have a soft tissue mass and an aggressive appearance, it is a benign lesion.

Radiography may suggest the diagnosis, particularly when the lesion is polyostotic or has radiographic features noted previously, but biopsy may be required for definitive diagnosis.

Predictors of clinical outcome in children with LCH include the number of organ systems involved and the child's

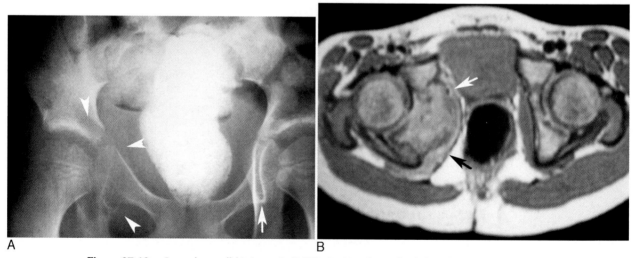

Figure 37-19 Langerhans cell histiocytosis (LCH). **A,** AP radiograph of the pelvis in a 6-year-old boy demonstrates a geographic lytic lesion with broad zone of transition involving the right acetabulum *(arrowheads)*. Note that the radiographic teardrop in the right hip has been destroyed, compared with the left side *(arrow)*. **B,** Axial proton density MR image demonstrates a large soft tissue mass *(arrows)*. With this aggressive pattern of osseous destruction and soft tissue mass in a patient of this age, Ewing's sarcoma should be most strongly considered, but it should be remembered that LCH can also have an aggressive appearance. This was proven to be LCH at biopsy. (Reprinted with permission from the American College of Radiology learning file.)

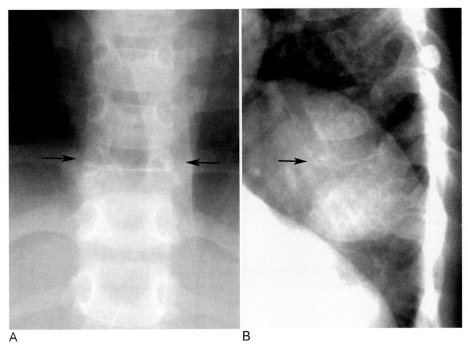

Figure 37-20   Vertebra plana in Langerhans cell histiocytosis (LCH). **A and B,** AP (A) and lateral (B) radiographs of the thoracolumbar spine in a 10-year-old patient, demonstrating complete flattening of the body of T10 *(arrows)*, although the posterior elements remain intact, as do the adjacent vertebral bodies. Note lack of paraspinal soft tissue mass.

age. Children with multiorgan system disease, especially with pulmonary disease, and those younger than 2 years of age fare more poorly. Many therapeutic regimens have been used, and therapy for LCH is not standardized. For single organ system bone disease with a single eosinophilic granuloma, curettage, wide excision, and intralesional steroid injection all have been effective. However, since eosinophilic granuloma often heals spontaneously, there is some debate as to whether any treatment is needed if the patient has no painful lesion or widespread bone disease. Optimal treatment for aggressive multisystem disease may include chemotherapy. Radiation may be used for vertebral disease with cord compression.

Erdheim-Chester disease is a rare, non-Langerhans histiocytosis that presents with painful sclerosis of the long bones sparing the epiphyses. Multi-organ system infiltration with lipid-laden macrophages, multinucleated giant cells, lymphocytes, and histiocytes bears some resemblance to LCH at histology. However, Erdheim-Chester is a disease of adults rather than children. This condition is fatal, causing organ failure such as cardiac or renal failure or pulmonary fibrosis.

BROWN TUMOR OF HYPERPARATHYROIDISM

Brown tumors are localized accumulations of osteoclasts that produce expanded lytic lesions in patients with hyperparathyroidism. Radiographically and pathologically a brown

tumor may be difficult to differentiate from a giant cell tumor. However, other manifestations of hyperparathyroidism are usually present as well, making possible the diagnosis (see Fig. 25-5). Brown tumors are thought to occur with greater frequency in primary hyperparathyroidism, but because secondary hyperparathyroidism is so much more common, most brown tumors occur in secondary hyperparathyroidism. Following treatment of hyperparathyroidism, a brown tumor may ossify, sometimes densely.

MYOSITIS OSSIFICANS

Myositis ossificans and the similar process of heterotopic ossification represent heterotopic formation of nonneoplastic bone and cartilage in soft tissue. Myositis ossificans generally denotes this process within skeletal muscle, while heterotopic ossification is a more general term for any soft tissue ossification. The cause is usually blunt trauma, sometimes only minor trauma. Myositis ossificans can occur in any muscle, but is most commonly found in the areas prone to blunt trauma, such as the thigh and around the elbow. Myositis ossificans also can be associated with burns and neurologic disorders, with greater than one third of paraplegic patients showing extensive myositis ossificans.

The histologic evolution of myositis ossificans parallels the radiographic evolution and MRI appearance. Histologically, during the first 4 weeks of evolution, myositis ossificans has a pseudosarcomatous appearance in its central zone, which may suggest malignant neoplasm. During weeks 4 through 8, histology shows a centrifugal pattern of maturation, where the periphery of the lesion is demarcated by immature osteoid formation that with time gradually organizes into mature bone. The radiographic evolution parallels this. In the first 2 weeks, only a soft tissue mass is present, which clinically may be painful, warm, and doughy. Weeks 3 to 4 begin to show amorphous density within the mass, often with periosteal reaction in the underlying bone. At this stage myositis may be mistaken for an early osteosarcoma because the calcification has the appearance of tumor osteoid. Over weeks 6 through 8, the amorphous osteoid matures into compact bone peripherally that surrounds a lacy pattern of less mature bone (Figs. 37-21, 2-17). Maturation proceeds centrifugally, as is seen histologically. Over ensuing months, the osseous mass reaches full maturity, often with reduction in size and migration toward the periosteum of the nearby bone. Thus, the history and timing are crucial in supporting the early diagnosis of myositis ossificans and avoiding a potentially disastrous diagnosis of osteosarcoma.

The MRI appearance of myositis ossificans relates to the age of the lesion, and is similar to the radiographic appearance. Early lesions show a mass that is isointense to muscle on T1-weighted imaging and high signal or heterogeneous on T2-weighted imaging (Fig. 37-22). Surrounding edema is prominent. Periosteal reaction and bone marrow edema may be seen if the myositis is located near bone. More mature lesions (over 8 weeks) are better defined. The center remains heterogeneous, but may be rimmed by a halo of decreased signal on all sequences. Thus, the zoning seen on radiographs and histology is mirrored on MRI (Fig. 37-23).

The differential diagnosis of myositis ossificans includes parosteal osteosarcoma. Parosteal osteosarcoma typically shows the reverse of the zonal phenomenon seen with myositis ossificans, with denser calcification in the center than in the periphery. Periosteal osteosarcoma might also be found in the differential diagnosis of myositis ossificans; periosteal osteosarcoma usually appears more aggressive, often scalloping the underlying cortex. Juxtacortical chondroma also often presents with scalloped underlying cortex and juxtacortical calcific densities. Early myositis ossificans could possibly mimic this appearance. An osteochondroma is easily distinguished from myositis ossificans because an osteochondroma arises from the underlying bone, with continuation of cortical and medullary bone into the lesion. Tumoral calcinosis presents as periarticular calcified soft tissue masses, usually around the hip, shoulder, and elbows. The masses, typically found in patients with renal failure, supposedly could appear similar to myositis ossificans. However, the calcifications in tumoral calcinosis are

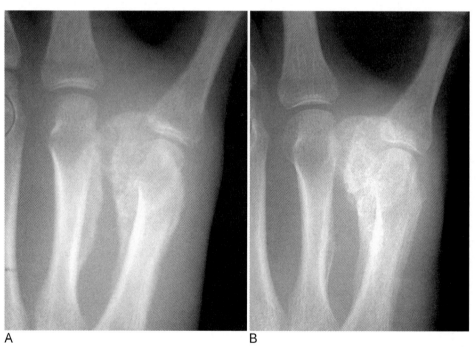

A   B

Figure 37-21 Myositis ossificans. **A,** PA radiograph of the hand in an 18-year-old man taken 7 weeks after crush injury demonstrates an immature myositis ossificans involving a hypothenar musculature. The matrix is clearly osteoid, but it does not yet show the mature periphery. **B,** PA radiograph of the same region taken 5 months after injury. At this time, the myositis has evolved to a more mature phase, having decreased in size adjacent to the fourth metacarpal and showing a defined rim adjacent to the fifth. This represents a mature myositis ossificans. (Reprinted with permission from the American College of Radiology learning file.)

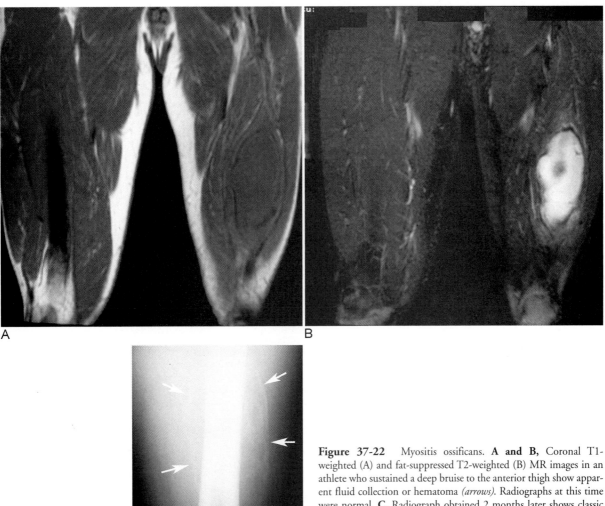

Figure 37-22 Myositis ossificans. **A and B,** Coronal T1-weighted (A) and fat-suppressed T2-weighted (B) MR images in an athlete who sustained a deep bruise to the anterior thigh show apparent fluid collection or hematoma *(arrows)*. Radiographs at this time were normal. **C,** Radiograph obtained 2 months later shows classic peripheral, mature ossification of myositis ossificans *(arrows)*. See also Fig. 2-17. (Reproduced with permission from: May DA, Disler DG, Jones EA, et al: Abnormal signal within skeletal muscle in magnetic resonance imaging: patterns, pearls, and pitfalls. Radiographics 20:S295–315, 2000.)

amorphous, and often show fluid-fluid levels on cross-sectional imaging.

Myositis ossificans progressiva is a hereditary mesodermal disorder characterized by progressive ossification of striated muscles, tendons, and ligaments. It has an autosomal dominant mode of inheritance with a wide range of expressivity, although it may appear as a spontaneous mutation. The target tissue in this disease is thought to be the interstitial tissues, with muscle involvement secondary to pressure atrophy. The pathologic abnormalities are similar to those of myositis ossificans. The most frequent presenting symptom and location is acute torticollis, with a painful mass seen in the sternocleidomastoid muscle. The process then progresses to the shoulder girdle, rib cage, upper arms, spine, and pelvis. The heterotopic bone often bridges between adjacent bones of the skeleton (Fig. 37-24) and eventually causes severe restriction of motion.

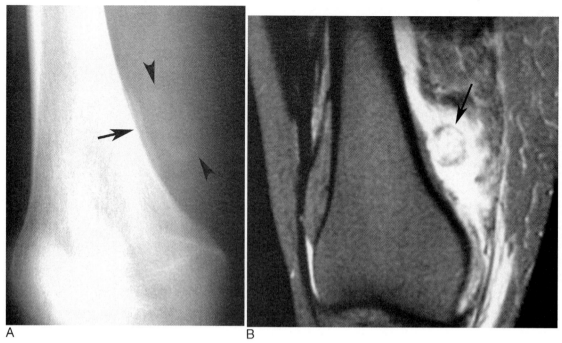

Figure 37-23 Myositis ossificans. **A,** Oblique radiograph of the distal thigh in a 15-year-old girl with a painful mass demonstrates faintly seen osteoid within a mass *(arrowheads),* as well as periosteal reaction along the adjacent femur *(arrow).* This is a nonspecific appearance and could represent either myositis ossificans or an early surface osteosarcoma. **B,** MRI is extremely helpful, with the T2 coronal image showing a ring of low signal *(arrow)* surrounding and surrounded by extensive soft tissue edema. The ring of low signal intensity represents maturing osteoid and is the zoning phenomenon of myositis ossificans.

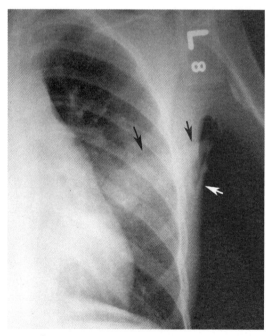

Figure 37-24 Myositis ossificans progressiva. AP radiograph of the chest demonstrates ossific masses in the latissimus dorsi *(white arrows)* and pectoralis muscles *(black arrow),* showing early bridging between the humeri and the thorax in this 6-year-old patient. Progressive ossification will occur.

CHORDOMA

Chordoma is a low-grade malignant neoplasm that arises from notochord remnants, most often in adults (fourth through seventh decades of life). It is more frequent in men (male-to-female ratio, 2:1). Because of the cell of origin, it is specifically restricted in location to the clivus, spine, and sacrum. The greatest number (50%) arise in the sacrum and coccyx; indeed, chordomas represent 40% of all sacrococcygeal tumors. Chordomas are next most frequently found in the clivus (35%), and 15% occur in the spine, most frequently the lumbar region (Fig. 37-25). Spine chordomas begin in the midline in the vertebral body but may extend into the posterior elements. Chordomas cause extensive local bone destruction, often with a large soft tissue mass, extending into either the spinal canal or the paraspinal soft tissues. Many tumors grow slowly and may have a narrow zone of transmission and a sclerotic margin, but the tumor size, predominant osteolysis, and location are clues to the diagnosis. The tumor infiltrates surrounding soft tissues, and may present with neurologic symptoms or, in the sacrum, rectal bleeding or bowel or bladder symptoms. Metastasis is uncommon (to the lung when it occurs), but chordoma is often a fatal tumor because of local neurologic involvement.

Computed tomography or, preferably, MRI with contrast medium is needed to define the extent of bone and soft tissue involvement. Internal hemorrhage and cyst formation may be seen. Sacrococcygeal chordomas are often large at presentation; frequently calcify in an amorphous pattern (not chondroid or osteoid matrix); and may resemble chondrosarcoma, GCT, or plasmacytoma. However, assessment of matrix may be difficult in the pelvis because of overlying structures, and a chondrosarcoma might be considered in some cases. Chondrosarcomas in the pelvis tend to occur off of the midline, whereas chordomas arise from the midline. Skull base chordomas are usually small when detected. A chondroid variant of chordoma that occurs in the skull base is similar to low-grade chondrosarcoma on imaging studies. In the vertebral body, metastatic disease, multiple myeloma, GCT, and lymphoma belong in the differential diagnosis. Chordomas may show little or no activity on bone scan.

Treatment is early wide resection, if possible, or surgical debulking, with radiation often used for recurrence. Five-year survival is 50%, but higher for the chondroid variant. Chordomas recur frequently in the surgical bed, and tumor seeding along biopsy tracts and surgical incisions also occurs. This can result in multicentric local recurrences.

ADAMANTINOMA

Adamantinoma is a rare epithelioid lesion of unknown pathogenesis, containing elements of squamous, alveolar, and vascular tissue (Fig. 37-26). Adamantinoma is a low-grade and sometimes multicentric malignant neoplasm. The most frequent location of adamantinoma is in the mid or proximal anterior tibial diaphysis (80% to 90%), usually eccentric or cortically based. This may be the most distinctive feature of adamantinoma. The early pattern of bone destruction is geographic, but may appear more aggressive with more advanced or recurrent disease. There is generally a sclerotic margin, and the lesion often has a bubbly lytic appearance. A soft tissue mass may occur as the lesion becomes larger. Although the lesion is monostotic, it may have satellite foci adjacent to the initial lesion in the tibia or even in the adjacent fibula.

The major differential diagnosis of adamantinoma is fibrous dysplasia and ossifying fibroma (osteofibrous dysplasia). In fact, many investigators believe there is a spectrum of all three of these disease processes. All may be cortically based and located in the tibia and appear somewhat aggressive (Fig. 37-27). These lesions are also similar but not identical

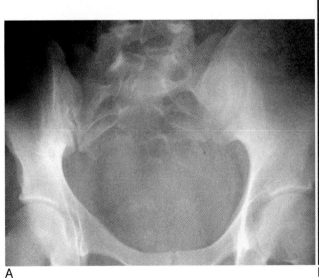

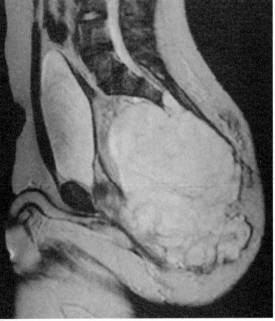

A   B

Figure 37-25   Chordoma. **A and B,** AP radiograph of the pelvis (A) and sagittal T2-weighted MR image (B) demonstrate how large and locally aggressive a chordoma can be. Note the extensive destruction of the distal sacrum and a large soft tissue mass. The radiograph shows subtle calcification in the mass that is difficult to reproduce in a textbook.

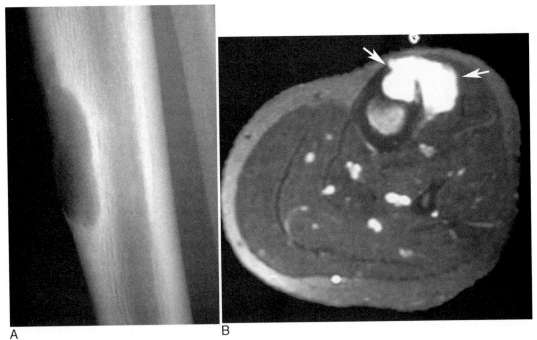

Figure 37-26 Adamantinoma. **A,** AP radiograph demonstrates a cortically based lytic lesion in the tibia in a 17-year-old girl. **B,** T2-weighted MR image confirms the cortical location of this lesion, as well as cortical breakthrough with a soft tissue mass *(arrows),* which indicates an aggressive lesion.

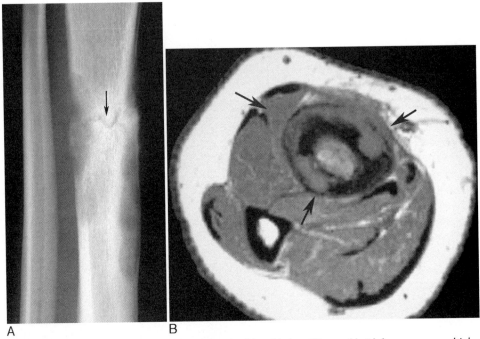

Figure 37-27 Adamantinoma. **A,** AP radiograph of the tibia in a 17-year-old girl demonstrates multiple cortically based lytic lesions with a pathologic fracture *(arrow).* **B,** T1-weighted MR image demonstrates that in fact this is a single cortically based lesion that wraps around the cortex *(arrows).* Although this cortically based tibial lesion is typical of an adamantinoma, it cannot be radiographically distinguished from osteofibrous dysplasia or cortically based fibrous dysplasia (see Fig. 30-11).

histologically, as the epithelial tumor cell will always be found with adamantinoma (see Fig. 30-11).

Adamantinoma is a malignant lesion; that 20% metastasize to the lung, lymph nodes, or skeleton. However, it is generally locally nonaggressive, and the lesion may be present for several years before developing metastatic lesions. It may also be quite large at presentation. Recurrence is common after surgery. The ideal treatment is wide excision; however, because the lesion is often mistaken as nonaggressive, the initial treatment is often an inadequate curettage. Lesions in older patients tend to be more aggressive. Overall 5-year survival is 60%.

Ameloblastoma is a histologically benign locally aggressive lytic lesion of the mandible that was formerly termed "adamantinoma of the mandible." This condition is unrelated to adamantinoma and is mentioned here only because the overlapping terminology may lead to confusion.

GANGLION CYST

Cyst-like masses are commonly found around the wrist, knee, and many other joints, and they are often described with the umbrella term "ganglion." Despite the name, these masses are unrelated to neural elements. Rather, they represent loculated accumulation of viscous fluid related to increased pressure in a tight joint or degeneration of a ligament or other collagenous structure. These lesions may be unilocular or multilocular; in the latter the locules typically communicate. Ganglion is the most common mass around the wrist. Most wrist ganglia originate from small capsular defects that act as a one-way valve, allowing fluid and debris to leave the joint but not return. Similar lesions occur in association with glenoid or acetabular labral or meniscal tears, termed *paralabral cysts* or *meniscal cysts,* respectively. Degenerated ligaments such as the ACL and PCL of the knee may have large associated adjacent or intrasubstance ganglion cysts. Intraosseous ganglia are common in the carpal bones.

Fluid-sensitive MR sequences typically show very bright, well-circumscribed unilocular or multilocular masses. Intravenous contrast shows enhancement only of the thin ganglion wall. Communication with the adjacent joint is sometimes demonstrated at arthrography. The connection of the ganglion to the joint, sometimes termed the "neck" of the ganglion, should be sought as successful resection of the ganglion requires resection of the neck, lest the lesion recur.

CHAPTER 38

Musculoskeletal Tumor Staging, Biopsy, and Follow-Up

SURGICAL STAGING OF SOLITARY BONE TUMORS
   AND SOFT TISSUE SARCOMAS
SUGGESTED ALGORITHMS FOR MUSCULOSKELETAL
   TUMOR WORK-UP
TUMOR BIOPSY
ASSESSING TUMOR RESPONSE TO PREOPERATIVE
   THERAPY
SURGICAL TREATMENT OPTIONS
TUMOR FOLLOW-UP
CONCLUSION

The material in this chapter is advanced for an introductory text, but this is essential practical information for radiologists who encounter musculoskeletal tumors.

SURGICAL STAGING OF SOLITARY BONE TUMORS AND SOFT TISSUE SARCOMAS

The Musculoskeletal Tumor Society has developed a staging system based on a combination of radiologic and histologic criteria in an attempt to reach an accurate prognosis and appropriate treatment for each individual lesion. This system, or a close variant, is universally used and relies on histologic features (grade), presence or absence of metastases, and evaluation of local site of involvement. Imaging is the crucial common denominator required for adequate staging, as it is used to evaluate the primary tumor site, detect metastases, and determine the best location for obtaining representative tissue for biopsy. The staging is commonly referred to as the Enneking method, in honor of the orthopedic oncologist. Note that this staging does not apply to bone lesions that turn out to be metastases or lymphoma, although it does include Ewing's sarcoma. It is outlined in Table 38-1. A key concept is tumor involvement of *compartments*. If tumor has entered a compartment, the *entire* compartment is considered to be potentially contaminated. Local tumor staging evaluates lesion size, skip lesions within the same bone, compartmental spread, neurovascular encasement, extension through growth plates, and extension into joints.

SUGGESTED ALGORITHMS FOR MUSCULOSKELETAL TUMOR WORK-UP

On the basis of the information that the treating clinician needs, algorithms can be suggested for the work-up of osseous as well as soft tissue masses. These algorithms produce the information required of the work-up, and help make the work-up as cost-efficient as possible. A suggested osseous lesion work-up is outlined in Fig. 38-1. Note that it always starts with a radiograph and with the evaluation of whether the lesion features are aggressive or nonaggressive. If the lesion is not aggressive, it is both logical and cost-efficient to stop the work-up before performing magnetic resonance imaging (MRI) or any other imaging. If the lesion is aggressive by plain radiography parameters, the algorithms work through the question of whether bone scanning is necessary, the timing of acquisition of chest computed tomography (CT) to evaluate for metastatic disease, and the timing of MRI for local staging. The algorithm for soft tissue musculoskeletal lesion work-up is shown in Fig. 38-2. This is a much simpler algorithm. It also starts with plain radiography, with the recognition that this modality will usually not add much information. It proceeds directly to MRI, followed by biopsy. The reason for delaying the work-up for metastatic disease (chest CT) until after the biopsy relates to the fact that MRI parameters rarely are specific in predicting whether the primary tumor is benign or malignant.

TUMOR BIOPSY

Both tumor staging and treatment decisions require confidence that representative tissue is obtained in the biopsy. Whether the biopsy is performed percutaneously by the

---

Table 38-1   Surgical Staging of Solitary Bone Tumors and Soft Tissue Sarcomas

G: Grade (histologic). Appropriate grading requires representative tissue sampling at biopsy, often guided by imaging.
  (1) G_0—benign
  (2) G_1—low-grade, malignant
  (3) G_2—high-grade, malignant

S: Site (radiographic and clinical features). This is determined by cross-sectional imaging (usually MR).
  (1) T_0—true capsule surrounds lesion (reactive rim of tissue).
  (2) T_1—extracapsular, intracompartmental; compartments are defined as follows:
    a Skin—subcutaneous.
    b Paraosseous—a potential compartment is seen when a lesion pushes muscle away from bone without invading either muscle or cortex.
    c Bone—intracortical; also a lesion in ray of the hand or foot is considered intracompartmental.
    d Muscle compartments—may contain more than one muscle if the muscle group is limited by a fascial plane:
      i Posterior compartment calf.
      ii Anterior compartment calf.
      iii Anterolateral compartment calf.
      iv Anterior thigh.
      v Medial thigh.
      vi Posterior thigh.
      vii Buttocks.
      viii Volar forearm.
      ix Dorsal forearm.
      x Anterior arm.
      xi Posterior arm.
      xii Deltoid.
      xiii Periscapula.

  (3) T_2—extracapsular, extracompartmental extension from any of the above named compartments or abutment of major neurovascular structures; in addition, some sites are extra-compartmental by origin:
    a Midhand, dorsal or palmar.
    b Midfoot or hindfoot.
    c Popliteal fossa.
    d Femoral triangle.
    e Obturator foramen.
    f Sciatic notch.
    g Anticubital fossa.
    h Axilla.
    i Periclavicular.
    j Paraspinal.
    k Periarticular, elbow or knee.

M: Metastases, usually bone or lung.
  (1) M_0—no metastases
  (2) M_1—metastases present.

Staging: Uses grade, site, and metastases as follows.
  (1) *Benign:*

1 (Inactive)	2 (Active)	3 (Aggressive)
G_0	G_0	G_0
T_0	T_0	T_{1-2}
M_0	M_0	M_{0-1}

  (2) *Malignant:*

Ia:	Low-grade without metastases, intracompartmental.
Ib:	Low-grade without metastases, extracompartmental.
IIa:	High-grade without metastases, intracompartmental.
IIb:	High-grade without metastases, extracompartmental.
III:	Low- or high-grade with metastases.

Ia	Ib	IIa	IIb	III
G_1	G_1	G_2	G_2	G_2
T_1	T_2	T_1	T_2	T_2
M_0	M_0	M_0	M_0	M_1

---

radiologist or by surgical incision, imaging contributes significantly to the biopsy planning process. Imaging should help to direct biopsy away from necrotic or less aggressive areas of tumor to obtain optimal tissue sampling. In addition, consideration of needle approach is crucial. One must work with the surgeon to determine the needle approach that will avoid contaminating more than one compartment or any of the soft tissues that the surgeon may require for reconstruction. Two regions in the body are frequently biopsied in a careless manner, compromising optimal treatment. The first is the region around the knee, where those obtaining a percutaneous biopsy specimen may not recognize that the suprapatellar bursa extent is quite large, often resulting in contamination of the knee joint during placement of the needle for a biopsy. The second site is the region of the pelvis. It is important to avoid placing the biopsy needle through the gluteal musculature if this soft tissue will be needed for coverage following resection of a pelvic lesion. Therefore, consultation with the surgical oncologist, combined with careful and thoughtful MRI, is a prerequisite to biopsy and eventual treatment of these musculoskeletal lesions.

ASSESSING TUMOR RESPONSE TO PREOPERATIVE THERAPY

Imaging assessment is difficult during the initial treatment phase of tumors treated with chemotherapy to determine their response. The most important indicator of response is a high percentage of tumor necrosis. Because imaging studies do not provide reliable quantitative assessment of tumor kill, rebiopsy of the tumor for histologic evaluation often is necessary. Some imaging findings are associated with a good response to chemotherapy. Decrease in tumor size, indicated by a 50% decrease in the product of the two largest diameters, suggests a good response. However, note that osteosarcoma often shows little change in size even if a good response has occurred. Dynamic, contrast-enhanced MRI, which evaluates the rate of contrast enhancement after an intravenous gadolinium bolus, has been advocated to assess tumor response to chemotherapy because malignant tumors tend to enhance more rapidly than other tissues. Positron emission tomography is a promising

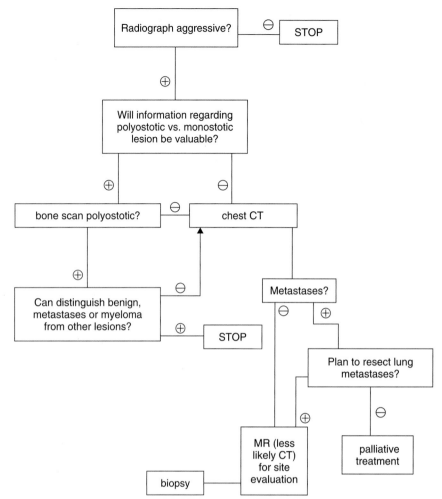

Figure 38-1 Suggested algorithm for osseous lesion work-up. CT, computed tomography; MR, magnetic resonance. (Adapted with permission from Manaster, BJ: Handbook of Skeletal Radiology, ed 2,. St. Louis, Mosby, 1997.)

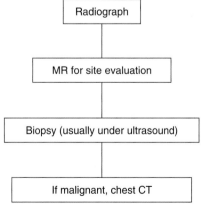

Figure 38-2 Suggested algorithm for soft tissue musculoskeletal lesion work-up. CT, computed tomography; MR, magnetic resonance. (Adapted with permission from Manaster BJ: Handbook of Skeletal Radiology, ed 2. St. Louis, Mosby, 1997, p 13.)

modality for this assessment, but has not yet been validated. Thalium-201 imaging is used in some centers for osteosarcoma.

During chemotherapy, reconversion to hematopoietic marrow in nonirradiated bones is often seen, especially if granulocyte/monocyte colony-stimulating factor is given concurrently. This may be potentially confusing because regions of previously normal-appearing fatty marrow develop low signal intensity on T1-weighted MR sequences. This must not be misinterpreted as widespread metastatic disease.

SURGICAL TREATMENT OPTIONS

Although chemotherapy and radiation are frequently used as adjuvant therapy, resection of the primary lesion is considered for almost all musculoskeletal sarcomas. There are four surgical treatment options. The first is intralesional excision (curettage). With this treatment, tumor is incompletely (partially) resected and tumor cells are found at the margin at histologic evaluation. This may be adequate for many benign tumors and, because of functional consideration, may rarely be considered in more aggressive lesions. The second option is marginal excision (excisional biopsy). With a marginal excision, the plane of dissection passes through the reactive tissue or pseudocapsule of the lesion. Satellites of residual tumor may be left behind. This is an inadequate treatment for malignant tumors or lesions with a high recurrence rate, but may occasionally be chosen for reasons of functionality if combined with radiation or chemotherapy. The third treatment option is wide excision. With wide excision, the entire lesion is removed, surrounded by an intact cuff of normal tissue. The plane of dissection is well beyond the reactive tissue surrounding the lesion as depicted on imaging studies, but the entire muscle or bone is not removed. This treatment is considered adequate for recurrent, aggressive benign tumors as well as most sarcomas. The fourth treatment option is radical resection, in which the lesion is removed along with the entire muscle, bone, or other involved tissues in the compartment. Radical resection is not commonly required for treatment of musculoskeletal tumors. Although wide excision is required for optimal treatment of aggressive tumors, compromises may be made to retain limb functionality, by achieving only a marginal excision but supplementing it with radiation or chemotherapy. Please note that the term "limb salvage" is not a specific treatment option. Rather, limb salvage procedures are simply those that offer tumor control without sacrifice of the limb. Most fall into the category of wide excisions. Consideration of limb salvage is based on the staging of the lesion, anatomic location, age, and expected growth of the patient; extent of local disease; and expected function after the procedure.

For further discussion of tumor biopsy, see Chapter 49.

TUMOR FOLLOW-UP

Timing and type of imaging used for follow-up examination is a crucial issue and ideally should be individualized for each tumor type and indeed each patient. It should relate to the hazard rate (i.e., the likelihood of timing of recurrence) of the tumor recurrence in that individual; the individual hazard rate is related to tumor type, grade, size, location; patient age and sex; tumor stage; type of treatment; and surgical margins. The goal of a follow-up imaging protocol is to concentrate testing when the relapse is most likely to occur. However, models relating to the hazard rate and utility/risk analysis do not exist for most individual extremity tumor types, and the best the literature offers is to consider the sarcomas as a group. Most reports agree that approximately 80% of sarcomas that recur locally or systemically will do so within 2 years of primary treatment. This suggests that the most frequent follow-up should occur in the first 2 years, with tapering of imaging frequency after that time. After an extensive review of the literature and development of a consensus, the American College of Radiology Appropriateness of Care Committee concluded that local recurrence imaging should, for routine malignant musculoskeletal tumors, start with a baseline MRI evaluation 3 months after surgery, followed by sequential 6-month follow-up evaluation for the first 5 years. After the first 5 years of follow-up, it is recommended that imaging surveillance for local recurrence may decrease in frequency to yearly examinations and that follow-up examination beyond 10 years might occur only if the patient becomes symptomatic. Note that follow-up examination for systemic disease includes chest CT and often bone scan, whereas follow-up for local recurrence uses MRI if possible. However, the presence of orthopedic hardware may preclude the use of MRI, in which case combinations of radiography, CT, and ultrasonography (US) may be necessary.

When MRI is used to follow treated tumors, it is important to recognize that high signal intensity on T2-weighted MRI can be seen in several nonneoplastic lesions. These include postoperative seroma, hematoma, changes related to radiation therapy, fat necrosis, the presence of packing material, scar tissue, or even herniation of other tissue into the tumor bed. Narrowing the search to enhancing nodules improves specificity for recurrent tumor. Dynamic contrast-enhanced MRI has been advocated, as recurrent tumor in general tends to enhance more rapidly than benign lesions. Positron emission tomography also is a promising technique for detection of recurrent tumor, but much more experience will be needed before its true reliability is known. In many cases, biopsy of suspicious postoperative lesions will be necessary to rule out tumor recurrence.

In addition to tumor recurrence, the radiologist must be aware of other potential complications of tumor therapy (Table 38-2). Radiation therapy in a skeletally immature patient can result in growth cessation or deformities if the epiphyses or apophyses are included in the field of radiation (Fig. 38-3A). Before the early physeal fusion, epiphysial plate widening and metaphysial fraying may be seen, resembling rickets. In addition, skeletally immature patients undergoing radiation can develop radiation-induced osteochondromas (Fig. 38-3A). A patient of any age can develop radiation osteonecrosis, with the appearance of a permeative change, often with some sclerosis in the bones, which is restricted to the radiation port (Fig. 38-3B). Radiation osteonecrosis often appears aggressive and may result

Table 38-2	Complications of Radiation Therapy for Musculoskeletal Tumors

Tumor recurrence
Early growth cessation
Growth deformities
Radiation-induced osteochondroma
Infection
Radiation osteonecrosis
Radiation-induced sarcoma

in pathologic fracture. This necrotic bone is also more susceptible to infection. Therefore, it may be quite difficult to differentiate radiation necrosis from infection or tumor recurrence. Furthermore, radiation-induced sarcomas can occur (Fig. 38-3B, C). These most commonly are high-grade osteosarcoma, malignant fibrous histiocytoma, fibrosarcoma, or chondrosarcoma, which arises in a previously radiated field, usually 4 to 20 years after therapy. When such tumors arise within bone, they may be difficult to differentiate initially from radiation osteonecrosis, but a soft tissue mass and other aggressive features are soon demonstrated. The prognosis is very poor for patients with radiation-induced sarcomas. Finally, lesions treated only with chemotherapy may heal with a bizarre appearance suggestive of Paget's disease.

Follow-up examination of a limb salvage with allograft is an art form. Because hardware is present, effective MRI may not be possible. If that is the case, tumor recurrence must be watched for on radiographs as a soft tissue mass, or formations of subtle matrix calcifications. Computed tomography with contrast or US may be useful in individual cases. Allografts are prone to an increased incidence of infection because of the presence of a large nonvascular piece of bone, in combination with hardware and an immunocompromised patient. Infection

that can retard postoperative healing must be differentiated from tumor recurrence. Complications of limb salvage also include hardware failure. Graft resorption often occurs. Large osteoarticular allografts may show a pattern of early cortical graft resorption, followed by slow thickening over several months. Resorptive "cysts" may be prominent for the first 2 years. Late remodeling may manifest as a subcortical sclerotic rim. Late articular collapse may occur. The allografts themselves may show a late fracture in 15% to 20% of cases. These insufficiency fractures can be difficult to detect. Even with the presence of hardware, CT with reconstruction can be helpful. It may take up to 2 years for union with the graft to be demonstrated. Such "delay" should be expected, although vascularized fibular grafts may progress to union considerably faster.

CONCLUSION

Careful thought and planning are required in the work-up and follow-up of musculoskeletal lesions. Consultation with the oncologist and surgeon is necessary to provide optimal imaging and assist in optimal planning for these patients.

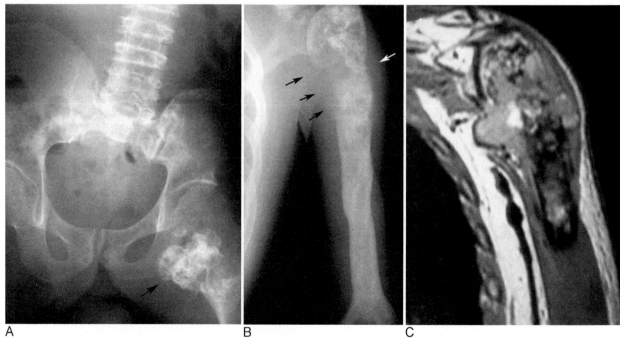

Figure 38-3   Complications of radiation. **A,** AP radiograph of the pelvis in a 20-year-old man who was treated with radiation for a left Wilms' tumor several years earlier. The hypoplastic left hemipelvis and the lumbar spine were in the radiation port. Note the large exostosis *(arrow)* arising from the proximal left femur. Hypoplasia and exostoses can be seen as a complication of radiation to the growing skeleton. **B,** AP radiograph of the humerus in a 25-year-old man who had undergone whole-bone radiation for Ewing's sarcoma 12 years earlier. Note the mixed lysis and sclerotis in the proximal half of the humerus, which is typical of radiation osteonecrosis. The bone is short relative to the patient's thorax owing to arrested growth that occurred because the bone was radiated before skeletal maturity. In addition, there is destruction of the bone at the proximal metaphysis, with a soft tissue mass *(arrows).* **C,** This mass is confirmed on the coronal proton density MR image. This is a radiation-induced sarcoma superimposed on the radiation necrosis. (Part A reprinted with permission from the American College of Radiology learning file.)

Part VI Sources and Suggested Readings

Aoki J, Tanikawa H, Ishii K, et al: MR findings indicative of hemosiderin in giant cell tumor of bone: Frequency, cause, and diagnostic significance. AJR 166:145–148, 1996.

Axoux EM, Saigal G, Rodriquez MM, Podda A: Langerhans cell histiocytosis: Pathology, imaging and treatment of skeletal involvement. Pediatr Radiol 35:103–115, 2005.

DeSchepper AM (ed): Imaging of Soft Tissue Tumors. Berlin, Springer, 1997.

DeSchepper AM, Ramon F, Degryseh P: Statistical analysis of MRI parameters predicting malignancy in 141 soft tissue masses. Fortschr Roentgenstr 156:587–591, 1992.

Enneking WF: Staging of musculoskeletal neoplasms. Skel Radiol 13:183–194, 1985.

Feldman F, Van Heertum R, Saxena C, Parisien M: 18FDG-PET applications for cartilage neoplasms. Skel Radiol 34:367–374, 2005.

Geirnaerdt M, Hermans J, Bloem J, et al: Usefulness of radiography in differentiating enchondroma from central grade one chondrosarcoma. AJR 169:1097–1104, 1997.

Geirnaerdt M, Hogendoorn P, Bloem J, et al: Cartilaginous tumors: Fast contrast enhanced MR imaging. Radiology 214:539–546, 2000.

Griffith LK, Dehdashti F, McGuire A, et al: PET evaluation of soft tissue masses with FDG. Radiology 182:185–194, 1992.

Hopper K, Moser R, Haseman D, et al: Osteosarcomatosis. Radiology 175:233–239, 1990.

Hosono M, Kobayashi H, Fujimoto R, et al: Septum like structures in lipoma and liposarcoma: MR imaging and pathologic correlation. Skel Radiol 26:150–154, 1997.

Huvos A: Osteogenic sarcoma of bones in soft tissues of older persons. Cancer 57:1442–1449, 1986.

Janzen L, Logan P, O'Connell J, et al: Intramedullary chondroid tumors of bone: Correlation of abnormal peritumoral marrow and soft tissue MRI signal with tumor type. Skel Radiol 26:100–106, 1997.

Jelinek J, Kransdorf M, Shmookler B, et al: Giant cell tumor of the tendon sheath: MR findings in nine cases. AJR 162:919–922, 1994.

Jelinek J, Murphey M, Kransdorf M, et al: Parosteal osteosarcoma: Value of MR imaging and CT in the prediction of histologic grade. Radiology 201:837–842, 1996.

Jones B, Sundaram M, Kransdorf M: Synovial sarcoma: MR imaging findings in 34 patients. AJR 161:827–830, 1993.

Kormaz M, Kim F, Wong F, et al: FDG and methionine PET in differentiation of recurrent or residual musculoskeletal sarcomas from post-therapy changes (abstract). J Nucl Med 34:33, 1993.

Kransdorf M: Malignant soft tissue tumors in a large referral population: Distribution of specific diagnosis by age, sex, and location. Am J Roentgenol 164:129–134, 1995.

Kransdorf M: Benign soft tissue tumors in a large referral population: Distribution of specific diagnosis by age, sex, and location. Am J Roentgenol 164:395–402, 1995.

Kransdorf M, Meis J, Jelinek J: Myositis ossificans: MR appearance with radiologic pathologic correlation. AJR 157:1243–1248, 1991.

Kransdorf M, Murphey M: Imaging of soft tissue tumors. Philadelphia, W.B. Saunders, 1997.

Kransdorf MJ, Murphey MD, Sweet DE: Liposclerosing myxofibrous tumor: A radiologic-pathologic-distinct fibro-osseous lesion of bone with a marked predilection for the intertrochanteric region of the femur. Radiology 212:693–698, 1999.

Manaster BJ, Dalinka M, Alazraki N, et al: Follow-up examinations for bone tumors, soft tissue tumors, and suspected metastasis post therapy. American College of Radiology ACR Appropriateness Criteria. Radiology 215(Suppl):379–387, 2000.

Manaster B, Doyle A: Giant cell tumor of the bone. Radiol Clin North Am 31:299–323, 1993.

Methta M, White L, Knapp T, et al: MR imaging of symptomatic osteochondromas with pathological correlation. Skel Radiol 27:427–433, 1998.

Moulton J, Blebea J, Dunco D, et al: MR imaging of soft tissue masses: Diagnostic efficacy and value of distinguishing between benign and malignant lesions. Am J Roentgenol 164:1191–1199, 1995.

Mulligan M, McRae G, Murphey M: Imaging features of primary lymphoma of bone. AJR 173:1691–1697, 1993.

Murphey M, Arcara L, Fanburg-Smith J: From the archives of the AFIP: Imaging of musculoskeletal liposarcoma with radiologic-pathologic correlation. Radiographics. 25:1371–1395, 2005.

Murphey M, Flemming D, Boyea S, et al: Enchondroma vs chondrosarcoma in the appendicular skeleton: Differentiating features. Radiographics 18:1213–1237, 1998.

Murphey M, Gross T, Rosenthal H: Musculoskeletal malignant fibrous histiocytoma: Radiologic pathologic correlation. Radiographics 14:807–826, 1994.

Murphey M, Robbin M, McRae G, et al: The many faces of osteosarcoma. Radiographics 17:1205–1231, 1997.

Murphey M, Smith W, Smith S, et al: Imaging of musculoskeletal neurogenic tumors: Radiologic pathologic correlation. Radiographics 19:1253–1280, 1999.

Murphey MD, Carroll JF, Flemming DJ, et al: From the Archives of the AFIP. Benign musculoskeletal lipomatous lesions. Radiographics 24:1433–1466, 2004.

Murphey MD, Jelinek JS, Temple HT, et al: Imaging of periosteal osteosarcoma: Radiologic-pathologic comparison. Radiology 233:129–138, 2004.

Nieweg O, Pruins J, Von Ginkel R, et al: FDG-PET imaging of soft tissue sarcoma. J Nucl Med 37:257–261, 1996.

Resnick D (ed): Diagnosis of Bone and Joint Disorders, ed 4. Philadelphia, W.B. Saunders, 2002.

Ryu K, Jaovisidha S, Schweitzer M, et al: MR imaging of lipoma arborescens of the knee joint. AJR 167:1229–1232, 1996.

Shapeero L, Vanel D, Couanet D, et al: Extra skeletal mesenchymal chondrosarcoma. Radiology 186:819–826, 1993.

Springfield D, Rosenberg A, Mankin H: Relationship between osteofibrous dysplasia and adamantinoma. Clin Orthop 309:234–244, 1994.

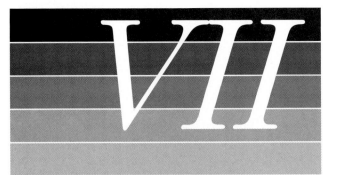

MARROW, INFECTION, AND HEMATOLOGIC IMAGING

CHAPTER 39

Bone Marrow

BONE MARROW IMAGING
MYELOFIBROSIS
GAUCHER'S DISEASE

Key Concepts	Bone Marrow

Components: Red (cellular, hematopoietic), yellow (fatty), trabecular bone
Symmetric left-right
Newborns: Widely distributed red marrow
Infants: Epiphyses and epiphyseal equivalents (apophyses) fatty conversion during first few months.
Children: Progressive replacement of red by fatty marrow, distal to proximal, and diaphyseal to metaphyseal.
Adults: Red marrow is normally found in the axial skeleton and the proximal portions of the appendicular skeleton; red marrow is more widely distributed in women, smokers, endurance athletes, patients with chronic anemia, obese patients, and persons living at high altitudes.
Marrow reconversion (yellow to red): Acquired anemia, medication, marrow infiltration.

BONE MARROW IMAGING

Bone marrow is a highly dynamic part of the musculoskeletal system that changes during growth and in response to local and systemic conditions. The basic components of the marrow cavity from an imaging standpoint are yellow (fatty) marrow; red (hematopoietic) marrow; trabecular bone; and, occasionally, tumor, pus, or deposition of products of abnormal metabolism. Yellow marrow is not entirely fat, but this is the main component and thus has magnetic resonance imaging (MRI) signal intensity similar to that of fat on all sequences. Red marrow contains cellular elements, but also some fat, and is vascular. Red marrow has intermediate signal on T1- and T2-weighted MRI sequences, and high signal intensity relative to the suppressed adjacent marrow fat on fluid-sensitive sequences (Fig. 39-1). Red marrow may fill the entire marrow cavity, have a "wispy," ill-defined configuration, or may be occasionally rounded and well circumscribed, simulating a metastasis. Trabecular bone contributes to marrow signal intensity by causing susceptibility artifact. This is most evident on gradient echo sequences, which show signal loss in regions of extensive trabecular bone.

The pattern of red marrow distribution varies with age, sex, and hormonal and other factors. Red marrow is more widely distributed in children than in adults. Red marrow is widely distributed at birth, but becomes progressively concentrated in the axial and proximal appendicular skeleton during early growth. The local process of change from one kind of marrow to the other is termed "conversion." There is normally a predictable pattern of conversion from red marrow to fatty marrow during growth. The earliest conversion to fatty marrow occurs in the epiphyses and apophyses, within the first few months after these centers begin to ossify. The terminal phalanges convert next. In the long bones, conversion begins in the diaphysis and progresses toward the metaphyses, beginning in early childhood (Fig. 39-2). Conversion of marrow in the flat bones lags behind that of the long bones. Conversion to fatty marrow is mostly complete by age 25, when red marrow is concentrated in the axial skeleton, proximal humeral and femoral metaphyses, and occasionally humeral heads. However, women often retain residual spotty red marrow more widely in the femurs and the pelvis, probably related to the demands of menstruation. With further aging beyond 25 years, there is a slower continuation of the fatty conversion process. By the eighth decade of life, even the pedicles and posterior elements of the vertebrae contain fatty marrow. This normal progression may be delayed or arrested in women or in persons with chronic anemia, obesity, cigarette smoking, or other causes of hypoxia.

Fatty marrow is quite labile and reconverts to hematopoietic marrow with any stress (Fig. 39-3). Reconversion to

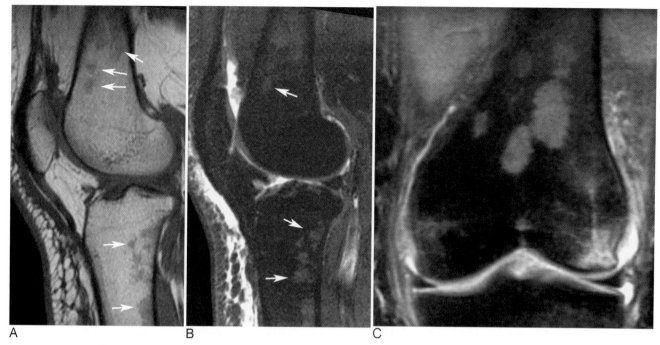

Figure 39-1   MRI of bone marrow. **A and B,** Sagittal T1-weighted (A) and fat-suppressed, T2-weighted (B) MR images of the knee in an obese 39-year-old woman with heavy menses due to fibroids. The hematopoietic (red) marrow has intermediate T1 and T2 signal intensity, in this case in a nodule-like configuration *(arrows)*. The fatty (yellow) marrow has typical fat signal intensity. This is a normal pattern. **C,** Another example of normal marrow simulating metastatic deposits, in this case also in the distal femur.

hematopoietic marrow usually follows an orderly pattern that is the reverse of the original conversion, beginning in the spine and flat bones and extending toward the appendicular skeleton. Reconversion may be spotty or complete, especially in the femora and humeri. Reconversion is often detected on MRI. Conditions in which one sees extensive marrow reconversion include anemias (whether hemolytic, related to chronic disease, or related to chronic blood loss), heavy cigarette smoking, hypoventilation hypoxia, poorly compensated heart disease, AIDS, and "sports anemia" (most frequently seen in endurance athletes such as marathon runners). Marrow-stimulating medications such as erythropoietin or granulocyte colony-stimulating factor can cause extensive marrow reconversion.

Marrow infiltration occurs with many processes, and is not specific by imaging criteria. The potential causes are many, and may include polycythemia vera, hemochromatosis, amyloidosis, Gaucher's disease, lymphoma, myelofibrosis, myeloma, and metastases (recall that metastases almost invariably are found in red marrow). Pathologic marrow infiltration can mimic marrow reconversion. With the marrow packing disorders such as Gaucher's disease there may be a significant amount of fibrous content and signal intensity may be intermediate on T1- and T2-weighted MR images. With infection or neoplastic infiltration, T1-weighted MR images are low signal and T2 weighted images usually have high signal.

Differentiating reconverted red marrow from a tumor or pathologic marrow infiltration can occasionally be difficult.

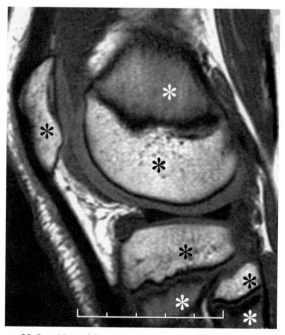

Figure 39-2   Normal hematopoietic marrow distribution in an older child. Sagittal T1-weighted MR image of the lateral aspect of the knee in a 12-year-old boy shows uniform high signal intensity of fatty marrow in the epiphyses and the patella *(black asterisks)*, and uniform intermediate signal intensity of hematopoietic marrow in the metaphyses *(white asterisks)*. This amount of hematopoietic marrow would be unusual in a man, suggesting the presence of chronic anemia or a marrow infiltrating process such as leukemia.

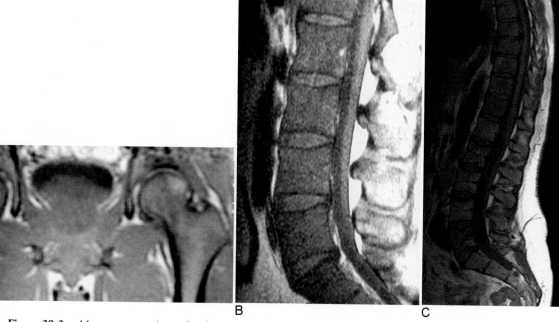

Figure 39-3   Marrow reconversion and replacement. **A,** Marrow reconversion in chronic anemia. Coronal T1-weighted MR image in a 23-year-old man with sickle cell disease demonstrates replacement of normal fat signal abnormality in the femoral heads and greater trochanters with the lower signal intensity of hematopoietic marrow. There are no findings of avascular necrosis, which is a frequent finding in sickle cell anemia. **B,** Marrow replacement due to acute myeloid leukemia. Sagittal T1-weighted MR image in a 30-year-old man who had severe low back pain but normal plain radiographs shows diffuse vertebral low signal intensity. A rule of thumb is that on a T1 image the vertebral body should have higher signal than the disk. The patient was not known to have a chronic anemia, so a peripheral blood smear was recommended, which showed acute myeloid leukemia. **C,** Sagittal T1-weighted image of a 45-year-old man shows less uniform marrow infiltration due to widespread non-Hodgkin's lymphoma. The areas of low marrow signal are abnormal.

A pathologic process may show T1 signal intensity lower than skeletal muscle or normal disk. Exceptions include repetition time (TR) greater than 700 ms (not a true T1), the spine in infants, and conditions associated with extensive marrow reconversion (e.g., patients with profound anemia, patients who have received a bone marrow transplant, and patients with AIDS who have undergone transfusion) in which the marrow changes are reactive but do not represent the primary pathologic process. Unusually high or low signal intensity on fluid sensitive sequences can suggest a pathologic marrow process. Evidence of bone destruction or extraosseous mass is never normal. Because normal red marrow contains a mixture of fat and cellular elements, it will show signal loss on the opposed phase of in and out of phase MRI, but a tumor will not (Fig. 39-4). Technetium-99m sulfur colloid is taken up by the red marrow, and therefore also can be used to distinguish infiltration from reconversion. However, this is not commonly performed.

Myeloid depletion occurs when the marrow space is devoid of hematopoietic elements (Fig. 39-5). The marrow signal is that of fat on all sequences. Myeloid depletion is seen in patients with aplastic anemia, in regions treated with radiation therapy, and with some chemotherapy regimens.

Marrow edema is often used as a generic term for increased marrow T2 signal on fluid-sensitive sequences in a localized or regional pattern. Marrow edema is seen in a variety of clinical settings, including trauma, infection, transient osteoporosis, and at the periphery of tumors. In fact, not all such signal change reflects true extracellular edema, so some authors therefore prefer to use the term "edema-like."

Osteonecrosis tends to occur more frequently in fatty marrow than hematopoietic marrow. (For a more in depth discussion of osteonecrosis, please see Chapter 22.) Osteonecrosis has many different causes, but the pattern of injury and osseous response is predictable. Following ischemic insult, myeloid cell death occurs within the first 12 hours. The bone responds with increased blood flow and inflammation. Granulation tissue forms and fibrosis develops in the area of injury. Bone resorption follows, itself followed by osteoblastic reinforcement. At a stage where an interface is formed between areas of osseous resorption and healing, the MRI "double-line" sign may be seen. This consists of a high-signal-

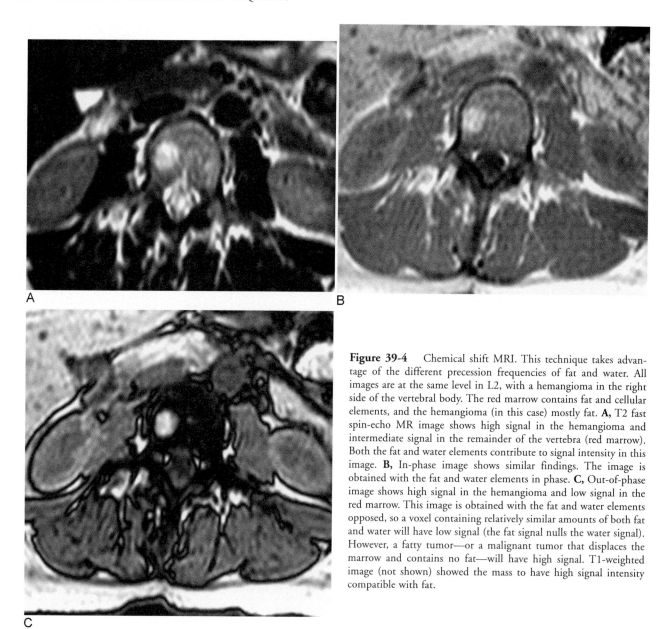

Figure 39-4   Chemical shift MRI. This technique takes advantage of the different precession frequencies of fat and water. All images are at the same level in L2, with a hemangioma in the right side of the vertebral body. The red marrow contains fat and cellular elements, and the hemangioma (in this case) mostly fat. **A,** T2 fast spin-echo MR image shows high signal in the hemangioma and intermediate signal in the remainder of the vertebra (red marrow). Both the fat and water elements contribute to signal intensity in this image. **B,** In-phase image shows similar findings. The image is obtained with the fat and water elements in phase. **C,** Out-of-phase image shows high signal in the hemangioma and low signal in the red marrow. This image is obtained with the fat and water elements opposed, so a voxel containing relatively similar amounts of both fat and water will have low signal (the fat signal nulls the water signal). However, a fatty tumor—or a malignant tumor that displaces the marrow and contains no fat—will have high signal. T1-weighted image (not shown) showed the mass to have high signal intensity compatible with fat.

intensity line of hyperemic tissue immediately adjacent to a low-signal-intensity line of sclerotic bone as seen on T2-weighted MRI.

Hemosiderin deposition due to chronic hemolytic anemias or transfusions can cause decreased marrow signal intensity on all sequences. Other reticuloendothelial sites (i.e., the liver and spleen) will show similar changes.

MYELOFIBROSIS

Myelofibrosis is in the spectrum of myeloproliferative disorders, and results in fibrosis in areas of the skeleton that are normally involved in hematopoiesis. Because of the resultant restriction in hematopoiesis in the usual locations (axial skeleton and proximal femoral and humeral diaphyses), patients develop compensatory reconversion in the fatty marrow of large tubular bones and extramedullary hematopoiesis. The reconverted marrow sites, in turn, may become fibrotic. The patients who develop extramedullary hematopoiesis show hepatosplenomegaly and paraspinous masses.

Radiographic findings include symmetric sclerotic trabeculae (either diffusely or as a patchy increased density with cortical thickening) in the hematopoietic bones (vertebrae, pelvis, ribs, and the long tubular bones) without bone expansion (Fig. 39-6). Magnetic resonance imaging shows low signal on both T1- and T2-weighted images from fibrosis in the hematopoietic bones, with reconversion of fatty marrow to red

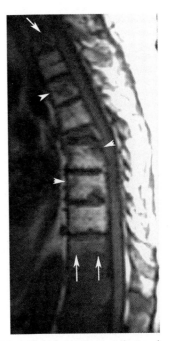

Figure 39-5   Myeloid depletion due to radiation therapy in a 50-year-old woman with history of breast cancer. The patient had previously received radiation treatment of metastatic disease to the midthoracic spine. Sagittal T1-weighted MR image shows fatty replacement in the radiation field (between *arrows*). The areas of low signal intensity within the treated vertebrae *(arrowheads)* could represent treated, healed blastic metastases or active metastases. In this case, the lesions were recurrent metastatic disease.

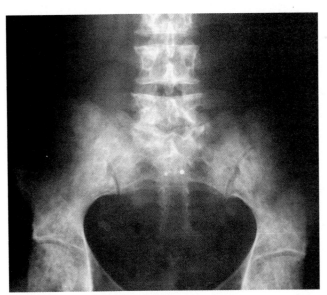

Figure 39-6   Myelofibrosis. This condition presents in the skeleton with fibrosis in the regions normally involved in hemopoiesis (axial skeleton), with subsequent compensatory hematopoiesis in the fatty marrow of the large tubular bones. The latter sites may in turn become fibrotic. The involved bones show mixed sclerosis and lucency, as do all the bones on this AP radiograph.

marrow in the shafts and more distal portions of the large tubular bones. The appearance varies according to the severity and stage of the disease.

GAUCHER'S DISEASE

Gaucher's disease is a familial sphingolipid storage disorder with accumulation of lipid-laden macrophages called Gaucher cells in the reticuloendothelial system including the marrow. The enzyme defect is glucocerebroside hydrolase or β-glucosidase. There are infantile and juvenile forms that involve the central nervous system and produce mental retardation and early death. The more common form develops in later childhood or young adulthood and is associated with a normal life span. The most frequently noted radiographic osseous abnormality is expansion of the distal femur, termed the Erlenmeyer flask deformity (Fig. 39-7). This expansion is due to marrow infiltration, and is present in 40% to 50% of patients. Because of the marrow replacement, the patients may show generalized osteoporosis and be susceptible to both fracture and osteomyelitis. The vertebral endplates may fracture in an H-shaped pattern, as is seen in sickle cell disease. Another common radiographic finding of Gaucher's disease is bone infarction, with focal sclerosis and occasional bone-within-bone appearance, or focal "cystic" lesions. Femoral head avascular necrosis is common. Any of these abnormalities, seen in conjunction with hepatosplenomegaly, should suggest the diagnosis of Gaucher's disease.

Magnetic resonance imaging of Gaucher's disease shows low T1 and T2 signal in the infiltrated marrow. The infiltration may be patchy or dense. Severe cases may show transcortical extension of the Gaucher cell infiltration. Avascular necrosis, especially of the hip, is frequent. Magnetic resonance imaging can be used to monitor response to enzyme replacement therapy. The marrow, liver, and spleen of successfully treated patients show dramatic response, attaining a near-normal appearance.

There is a differential diagnosis for the Erlenmeyer flask deformity of the distal femurs. Many of the severe anemias may expand marrow. In Niemann-Pick disease, sphingomyelin may accumulate with similar infiltrative bony findings, and there is hepatosplenomegaly. Finally, Pyle's disease is a metaphyseal dysplasia that results in expanded metaphyses of the tubular bones, especially about the knee, with normal diaphyses. Pyle's disease, however, does not show a true marrow infiltration. Osteoclast poisons, notably heavy metals such as lead, can cause failure of tubulation during skeletal growth, leaving a wide metaphysis.

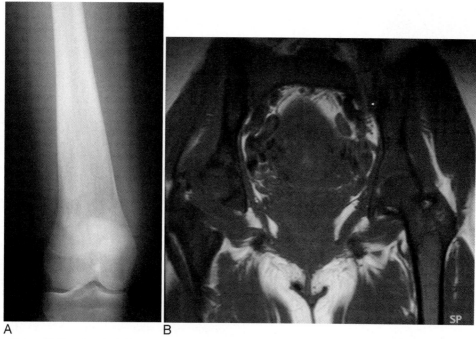

A   B

Figure 39-7   Gaucher's disease. **A,** AP radiograph of the femur in an 18-year-old woman with Gaucher's disease shows widening of the distal femur metadiaphysis (Erlenmeyer flask deformity) due to marrow packing with Gaucher cells, which are reticuloendothelial cells filled with the abnormal metabolites of Gaucher's disease (glucocerebrosides). Note the cortical thinning, also a typical finding. **B,** Coronal T1-weighted MR image in a different patient shows diffuse marrow low signal, also due marrow packing. MR imaging is so sensitive to the marrow disease burden that it can be used to guide enzyme replacement therapy. Successful therapy with enzyme replacement will return the marrow signal to normal.

Musculoskeletal Infection

SOFT TISSUE INFECTION

OSTEOMYELITIS

SEPTIC ARTHRITIS

AIDS

SARCOIDOSIS

Musculoskeletal infections, whether they involve the soft tissues, bones, or joints, can be highly aggressive yet extremely subtle to diagnose clinically and radiologically.

SOFT TISSUE INFECTION

Soft tissue infection may be initiated by direct inoculation by a penetrating injury, spread from adjacent osteomyelitis or septic joint, or hematogenous seeding. Radiographic signs of soft tissue infection are generally nonspecific, showing only a mass or swelling, often with blurring or obliteration of the soft tissue fat planes. Soft tissue gas, often sought, is rarely present (Fig. 40-1). Computed tomography (CT) and magnetic resonance imaging (MRI) with contrast enhancement can be more specific. An enhancing rim surrounding a water density mass is the classic appearance of an abscess. However, it should be noted that in parts of the extremities where the muscles are tightly packed, without loose fascial planes surrounding them (particularly the forearm and leg), soft tissue infections rarely have the classic appearance of an abscess. Findings of edema and compartmental swelling are more typical. Both CT and MRI may also demonstrate a draining sinus tract, deep venous thrombosis, or bone destruction suggestive of osteomyelitis. Magnetic resonance imaging is highly sensitive to the detection of soft tissue infection (Figs. 2-21, 40-1–40-3), and it may show nonspecific edema on water-sensitive sequences. Contrast enhancement may better demonstrate an abscess or regions of devitalized tissue that may progress to abscess (see Figs. 40-1, 40-2). Sinus tracts, the presence of multiple abscesses, and extensive inflammatory change contribute specificity in diagnosing soft tissue infection. There may be associated reactive change seen in

adjacent osseous structures (see Fig. 40-2). Inflammatory changes centered along fascial planes suggests fasciitis (i.e., inflammation of fascia) (see Fig. 40-3). Fasciitis is in general a more serious process that often requires surgical debridement. *Necrotizing fasciitis* is an extremely virulent form of infectious fasciitis, often due to *Clostridium* species or aggressive gram-positive organisms. Patients are extremely sick. Radiographs may show soft tissue gas bubbles along fascial planes. Necrotizing fasciitis is a true surgical emergency, and imaging beyond radiographs is generally not indicated.

Abscess may be simulated at imaging by necrotic tumors, myonecrosis due to severe trauma or extreme overuse, or ischemia (e.g., as can occur in patients with diabetes or sickle cell anemia). Both MRI and clinical features may provide clues to the diagnosis. Tumors with central necrosis usually show enhancing mural nodules. Traumatic myonecrosis will have an appropriate history. These patients are at risk for development of compartment syndrome. Diabetic myonecrosis occurs in the setting of poorly controlled diabetes mellitus, and is exquisitely painful (see Fig. 2-22). This condition most often occurs in the thigh, and also in the calf. Patients with sickle cell anemia may have similar muscle infarcts that simulate abscess on cross-sectional imaging studies.

OSTEOMYELITIS

Osteomyelitis is infection of bone or, more precisely, bone marrow. As with soft tissue infection, infection of bone may be caused by hematogenous seeding, penetrating injury, or surgery, or contiguous spread from an adjacent joint or soft tissue infection. A direct penetrating injury or adjacent infection can result in osteomyelitis at any site. Infection by contiguous spread begins with infection of the periosteum (truly, *periostitis*), followed by infection of the cortex *(osteitis)*, then infection of the marrow cavity *(osteomyelitis)*. Osteomyelitis may be classified as acute or chronic. Chronic osteomyelitis is bone infection of more than 6 weeks' duration.

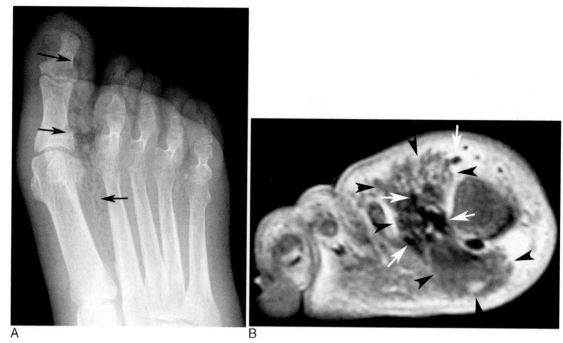

Figure 40-1   Soft tissue gas due to infection. **A,** Frontal radiograph of the foot of a diabetic patient shows mottled gas density centered between the first and second metatarsal heads, extending into the lateral first toe *(arrows)*. **B,** Short axis fat-suppressed, contrast-enhanced T1-weighted MR image through the metatarsal heads shows the gas bubbles seen as signal voids *(white arrows)* within a large nonenhancing abscess *(black arrowheads)*.

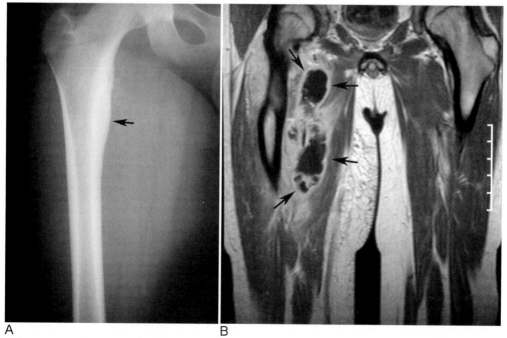

Figure 40-2   Soft tissue infection. **A,** AP radiograph of the thigh in a 16-year-old patient who had reported pain for 6 months. The radiograph demonstrates diffuse soft tissue swelling and thick, solid periosteal new bone formation in the medial subtrochanteric femur *(arrow)*. **B,** Coronal T1-weighted MR image following intravenous administration of gadolinium demonstrates a multiloculated intramuscular abscess with thick enhancing rim and adjacent edema *(arrows)*. The underlying bone was normal with the exception of thick cortical reaction as seen on the radiograph. This is the usual appearance of a soft tissue abscess, but the bone reaction is more exaggerated than usually is seen because the condition had been present for so long.

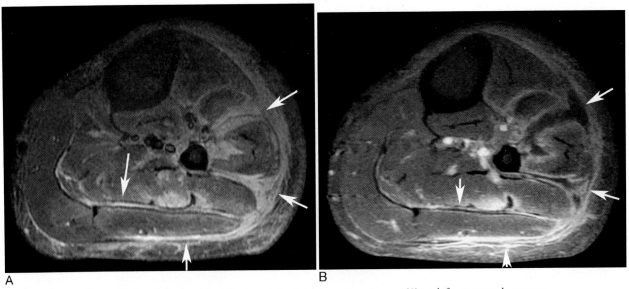

Figure 40-3   Infectious fasciitis. **A and B,** Axial inversion recovery (A) and fat-suppressed, contrast-enhanced T1-weighted (B) MR images show edema, fluid, and enhancement along fascial planes *(arrows)* of the lateral and posterior leg.

Key Concepts	Osteomyelitis Terminology

Sequestrum: Fragment of infected necrotic bone. Potential source of chronic infection.

Involucrum: New bone formed around sequestrum.

Sinus tract: Soft tissue channel between bone and skin. Pus drains through it.

Cloaca: Cortical and periosteal defect. Pus drains through it.

Abscess: Pus-filled cavity lined with granulation tissue.

Phlegmon: Solid infected/inflamed tissue. Vascular supply intact. May progress to abscess.

Radiography is often the first-line test for osteomyelitis, although it is not sensitive. Acute osteomyelitis is first demonstrated radiographically by blurring or obliteration of soft tissue fat planes. Even this radiographic change lags behind the clinical onset of infection by 1 to 2 weeks. Soft tissue changes are followed by signs of bone destruction. This can be seen as an extremely subtle permeative pattern within the bone or merely as indistinctness of the cortex (Fig. 40-4). These early changes are then followed by more obvious cortical destruction, endosteal scalloping, and periosteal as well as occasional endosteal new bone formation (Fig. 40-5). These osseous changes may appear highly aggressive in the acute phase of osteomyelitis and may be difficult to differentiate from an aggressive neoplasm (Figs. 40-6, 29-3). Knowing the time course of the disease may be helpful, as an acute osteomyelitis causes osseous destruction much more rapidly than does a tumor. Healing fractures and acute osteomyelitis may have

similar radiographic features, with bone resorption, soft tissue swelling and periosteal new bone formation. Moreover, bone destruction due to osteomyelitis increases the risk of fracture (Fig. 40-7). Clinical evaluation and laboratory evaluation usually are adequate to identify the presence of osteomyelitis, although in some situations, such as the feet of diabetic patients with coexisting neuropathic change, advanced imaging may be needed. This is discussed later in this chapter.

Computed tomography usually mirrors the appearance of the radiograph, but destructive osseous changes with serpiginous tracking may be more apparent. A serpiginous permeative pattern is specific for osteomyelitis (Fig. 40-8). Increased marrow attenuation may be seen because of inflammatory infiltration replacing fatty marrow. As with radiography, the soft tissue fat planes are obliterated on CT and the soft tissue abnormality may involve several muscle groups and be less discrete than many soft tissue tumor masses. Contrast enhancement may be nonuniform, but a thin enhancing rim helps to make the diagnosis of abscess (Fig. 40-9).

Multiphase bone scanning with diphosphonate classically shows increased tracer uptake on all phases in acute osteomyelitis. However, osteomyelitis may be "cold" on the delayed images, especially in children early in the acute phase. Gallium-67 scanning is almost 100% sensitive for osteomyelitis but is nonspecific. Tagged leukocyte scans have greater specificity than does gallium scanning.

At present, MRI is the imaging gold standard for evaluation of suspected osteomyelitis (Figs. 40-4, 40-5, 40-10). The combination of fluid-sensitive sequences (STIR or fat-suppressed T2), T1-weighted, and postcontrast T1-weighted

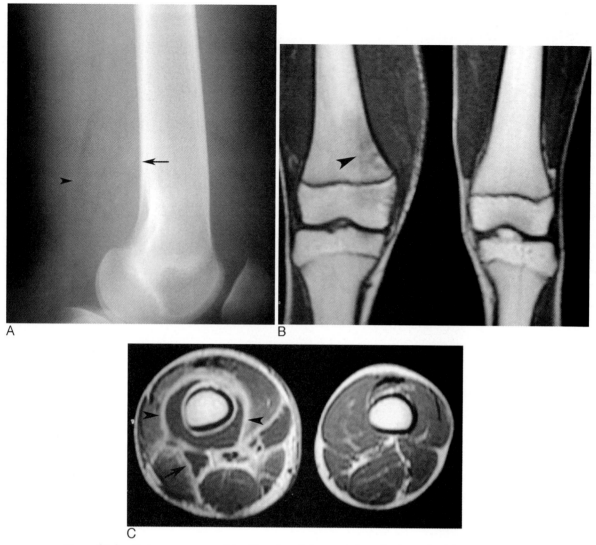

Figure 40-4   Early acute osteomyelitis with periosteal abscess. **A,** Lateral radiograph of the thigh in a 16-year-old boy shows obliteration of fat planes *(arrowhead)* and periosteal reaction at the posterior cortex *(arrow)*. **B,** Coronal T1-weighted MR image shows subtly decreased marrow signal intensity in the medial femur metaphysis *(arrowhead)*. **C,** Postgadolinium T1-weighted axial MR image shows periosteal abscess *(arrowheads)* and adjacent soft tissue abscess *(arrow)*, each with thick enhancing rim. This was a staphylococcal osteomyelitis.

imaging is highly sensitive and specific in diagnosing the presence and extent of osteomyelitis. This combination also allows detection of abscess, sinus tract, and devitalized tissues. Osteomyelitis causes marrow edema and enhancement. Specificity is increased if unequivocal decreased signal is present on unenhanced T1-weighted images. Trauma and marrow infiltration may mimic osteomyelitis on MRI. History usually is adequate to distinguish these possibilities. The presence of a fracture line, which may be incomplete, usually seen on T1-weighted images as a low signal line, suggests trauma. The feet of diabetic patients often have extensive

marrow edema and enhancement due to neuropathic arthropathy, and diagnosing or excluding osteomyelitis can be very challenging in these patients. The presence of osseous or soft tissue abscesses, ulcers extending to the bone, and sinus tracts extending between bone and ulcers or abscesses helps to differentiate osteomyelitis from neuropathic changes (see Fig. 40-10).

Osteomyelitis resulting from hematogenous spread tends to follow patterns based on age-related vascular anatomy. In infants up to about 12 months of age, some of the metaphyseal vessels penetrate the physis and anastomose with epiphyseal vessels.

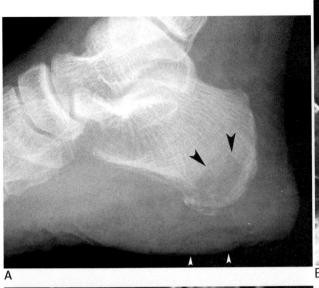

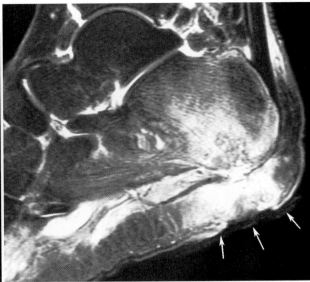

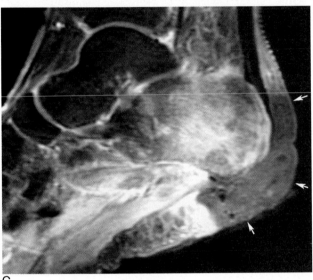

Figure 40-5   Osteomyelitis. Diabetic patient with plantar heel ulcer. **A,** Lateral radiograph of the calcaneus shows plantar ulcer *(small white arrowheads),* bone loss in the adjacent calcaneus *(black arrowheads),* and destruction of the adjacent cortex. **B and C,** Sagittal fat-suppressed, T2-weighted (B) and fat-suppressed, contrast-enhanced T1-weighted (C) MR images show intense marrow edema and enhancement in the posterior calcaneus. T1-weighted images (not shown) showed low signal intensity, also consistent with osteomyelitis. Also note lack of soft tissue enhancement plantar and posterior to the calcaneus *(arrows* in part C) that is more extensive than the pus and edema in and around the plantar ulcer *(arrows* in part B). This was devitalized tissue, not yet liquefied, that was débrided at surgery.

Key Concepts	Imaging of Acute Osteomyelitis

Plain radiography useful but insensitive
Nuclear imaging: Three-phase bone scanning, tagged leukocyte scanning
MRI with contrast usually best test
    Marrow edema and enhancement
    Search for: Abscesses, sinus tract, skin ulcers

Therefore, infections in infants often involve the metaphysis, epiphysis, and joint, and may result in osteonecrosis, slipped epiphyses, and growth deformity (Fig. 40-11). In toddlers and older children, blood vessels do not cross the physis. Rather, metaphy-

seal vessels terminate in loops with sluggish blood flow. As a result of this vascular anatomy, combined with the relative lack of phagocytes in the metaphysis, the metaphases of long bones are the most common site of infection in the child (Fig. 40-12). Epiphyseal and joint involvement are much less common in children than in infants, but does occur (Figs. 40-13, 40-14). Some cases may be detected only with MRI. In the adult, the terminal metaphyseal vessels anastomose with epiphyseal vessels across the physeal scar. Thus, joint involvement secondary to osteomyelitis is more common in the adult than in the child. In addition, adults tend to have osteomyelitis involving the spine and small bones more frequently than the large tubular bones.

Acute osteomyelitis is usually caused by pyogenic organisms. Common pathogens of acute osteomyelitis vary with the age of the patient. In neonates, *Staphylococcus aureus,* group B *Streptococcus,* and *Escherichia coli* are most common.

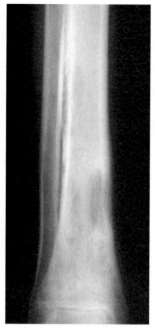

Figure 40-6   Osteomyelitis mimicking aggressive neoplasm. The osseous destruction is highly aggressive in this case, with a permeative pattern involving both the marrow and cortex, and periosteal reaction. Remember that osteomyelitis can have a radiographic appearance that is highly aggressive and not always differentiable from tumor. See also Fig. 29-3.

In normal children, *Staphylococcus* is most common. Children with sickle cell disease may also be infected with *Salmonella.* In adults, *Staphylococcus* and enteric pathogens predominate. Intravenous drug users, however, are often infected with gram-negative species such as *Pseudomonas* and *Klebsiella.*

Chronic osteomyelitis has varied appearances. Chronic osteomyelitis may demonstrate a prominent host reaction, including a thickened cortex and variable mixtures of lucency and density. Eventually, if the infection is not treated, a sequestrum and involucrum may develop. A *sequestrum* is necrotic bone isolated from living bone by granulation tissue. It appears relatively dense because it has no blood supply, whereas the surrounding bone is hyperemic and loses its mineralization (Fig. 40-15). A sequestrum may harbor bacteria, leading to chronic osteomyelitis. *Involucrum* is a shell of bone that surrounds a sequestrum. *Cloaca* (literally, "sewer") is a cortical and periosteal defect through which pus drains from an infected medullary cavity (see Fig. 40-9).

Chronic osteomyelitis may remain clinically silent for years, then reactivate. Such reactivation generally implies the presence of a sequestrum of necrotic, infected bone as the nidus of reactivation. Serial radiographs of reactivated chronic osteomyelitis may show a change in bone density or development of periosteal reaction. If radiographs do not help to localize a sequestrum, bone scanning or tagged leukocyte nuclear medicine scanning may improve specificity. Magnetic

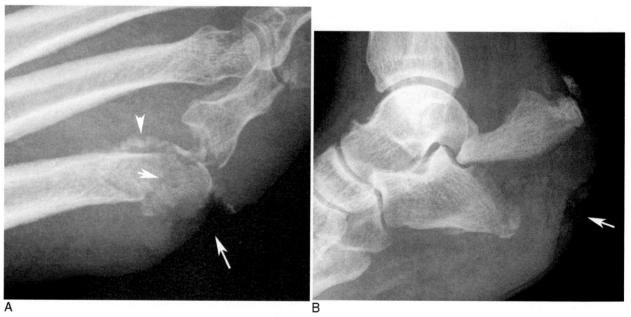

A   B

Figure 40-7   Osteomyelitis complicated by fracture. **A,** Diabetic patient with bone lysis of the fifth metatarsal head, pathologic fracture *(short arrow),* periosteal new bone formation *(arrowhead),* and an adjacent ulcer *(long arrow).* There are similar changes in the fifth toe proximal phalanx. **B,** A different diabetic patient with calcaneal osteomyelitis complicated by fracture. The superior displacement of the superior fragment is due to traction from the Achilles tendon. Note the soft tissue gas in the gap between the fracture fragments and posterior ulcer *(arrow).*

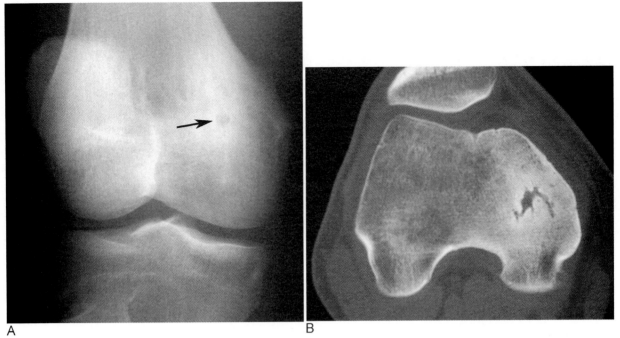

Figure 40-8   Serpiginous intraosseous tract of osteomyelitis. **A,** Oblique radiograph demonstrating a lytic, ill-defined lesion with surrounding sclerosis in the medial femoral condyle *(arrow).* **B,** Axial CT demonstrates serpiginous branching pattern of the lytic area, surrounded by reactive bone. This pattern is typical for osteomyelitis.

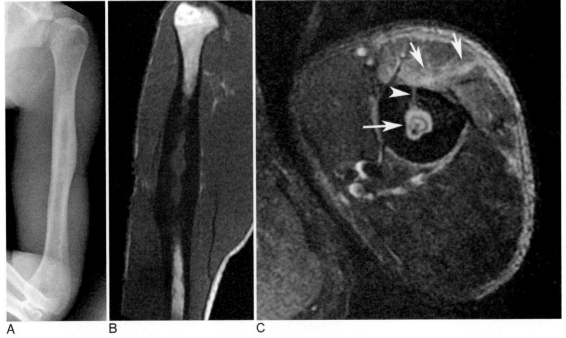

Figure 40-9   Chronic osteomyelitis with draining sinus tract. **A–C,** 29-year-old man who had sustained an open humerus fracture several years previously, now with a draining sinus in the upper lateral arm. Radiograph (A) shows cortical thickening and mild expansion of the humeral midshaft. Sagittal T1-weighted MR image (B) shows similar findings, as well as abnormal, low marrow signal intensity in the humeral midshaft. Axial fat-suppressed, contrast enhanced, T1-weighted MR image (C) shows intense enhancement in the marrow cavity *(long arrow),* cloaca *(arrowhead),* and sinus tract *(short arrows)* in the deltoid.

(Continued)

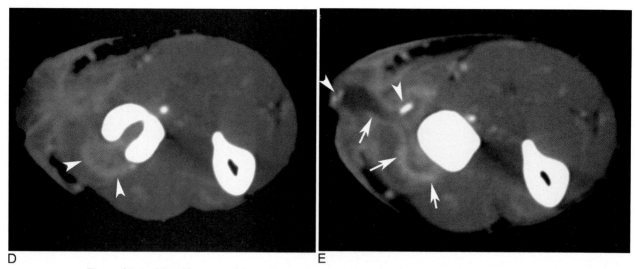

D   E

Figure 40-9—(Cont'd)   D and E, Axial CT images in the forearm of a different patient who developed osteomyelitis at the site of a radial shaft external fixation pin. Image at the pin tract (D) shows enhancing periosteal abscess margin *(arrowheads)*. The pin tract is functioning as a cloaca. Adjacent image (E) shows draining sinus tract *(arrows)*. Also note the fragments of infected, necrotic bone *(arrowheads)* that are expressed through the tract.

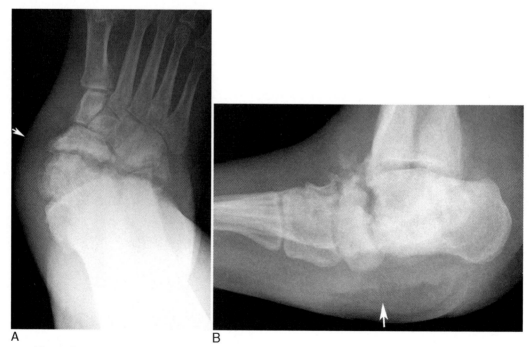

A   B

Figure 40-10   Osteomyelitis in diabetic neuropathic foot. **A and B**, AP (A) and lateral (B) radiographs show classic neuropathic changes in the midfoot and hindfoot with increased bone density, collapse of the arch, and severe degenerative changes. There is a medial plantar ulcer adjacent to the medially subluxed talar head *(arrow)*.

(Continued)

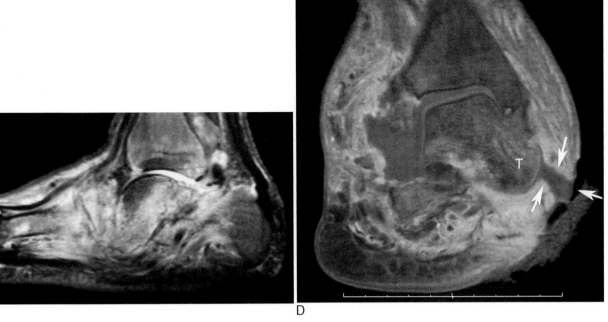

Figure 40-10—(Cont'd)   **C,** Sagittal inversion recovery MR image shows diffuse marrow edema and effusions, which are an expected finding given the severe neuropathic change and are not specific for osteomyelitis. **D,** Short axis, contrast-enhanced, fat-suppressed, T1-weighted MR image obtained through the distal hindfoot shows marrow enhancement, large fluid collection, and a sinus tract extending from the talar head to the lateral ulcer *(arrows)*. The sinus tract increases the MR imaging specificity for diagnosis of osteomyelitis. T, talar head.

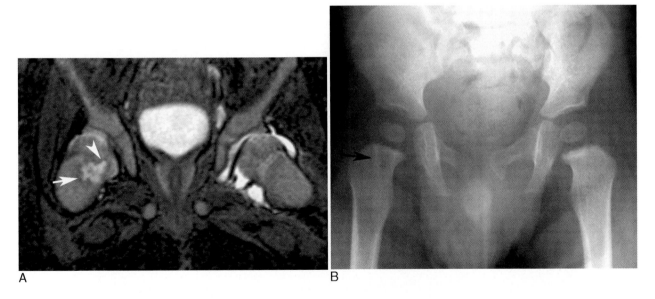

Figure 40-11   Osteomyelitis in an infant. **A,** Coronal inversion recovery MR image shows right proximal femur osteomyelitis. Note increased signal intensity in the epiphysis *(arrowhead)* and proximal metaphysis *(arrow)*. Also note the left hip joint effusion, which required diagnostic aspiration but did not show infection in this case. **B,** AP radiograph of the hips in a different child, a 13-month-old, shows a well-circumscribed lytic lesion in the proximal metaphysis *(arrow)*.

(Continued)

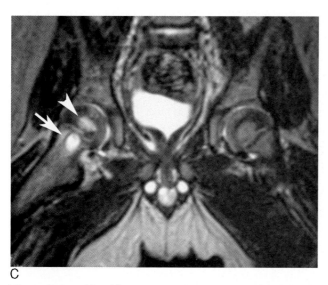

C

Figure 40-11—(Cont'd)   C, Coronal T2-weighted MR image in the same child shows high signal in the metaphyseal abscess *(arrow)* and in the epiphysis *(arrowhead)* due to osteomyelitis.

resonance imaging may show an enhancing area or fluid collection, which may surround a sequestrum. It also may allow tracing of a draining sinus tract back to the source bone.

Chronic osteomyelitis of the tibia or femur is often associated with a chronically draining sinus tract. If the drainage occurs over many years (usually decades), the tract may develop a squamous cell carcinoma. This tumor may be super-

Key Concepts	Chronic Osteomyelitis

Infection longer than 6 weeks
Sclerosis, cloaca, sequestrum
Sinus tract (may develop epidermoid carcinoma if present for many years)
May be quiescent for years, then reactivate
MRI for abscess, sinus tract, cloaca, and marrow edema and enhancement
Tagged leukocyte scanning for detection, localization

ficial and clinically apparent, or may be located deeper along the sinus tract and be suspected by new pain and detected by bone destruction on radiographs or visualization of the mass on MRI.

Subacute or chronic osteomyelitis in a child may be seen as a *Brodie's abscess.* This type of infection is usually found in the metaphysis. It is seen as a geographic lytic lesion with a well-defined, often broad sclerotic margin (Figs. 40-11, 40-16). It is usually oval, with the long axis parallel to the long axis of the bone, and typically borders the growth plate. Thus, a Brodie's abscess appears radiographically nonaggressive, unlike acute osteomyelitis. Clinically, patients with Brodie's abscess may not have associated fever or elevated erythrocyte sedimentation rate. A Brodie's abscess may be located in the epiphysis in a

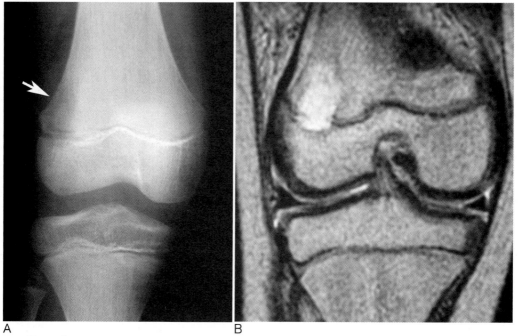

A   B

Figure 40-12   Osteomyelitis in an older child. **A,** AP radiograph and **B,** coronal T2-weighted spin-echo MR image demonstrate a typically located focus of osteomyelitis in the metaphysis of the lateral femoral condyle *(arrow* in part A), not crossing into the epiphysis, in this 8-year-old child.

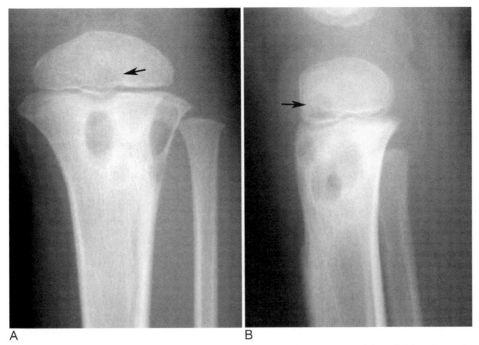

A   B

Figure 40-13   Epiphyseal osteomyelitis in a toddler. **A and B,** AP (A) and lateral (B) radiographs demonstrate multiple well-defined lytic lesions predominantly in the metaphysis, but also involving the epiphysis *(arrow)* in this toddler. Epiphyseal involvement with osteomyelitis can be seen, particularly in infants and toddlers.

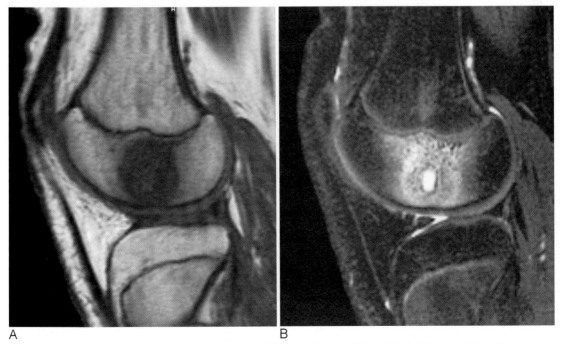

A   B

Figure 40-14   Epiphyseal osteomyelitis in a child. **A and B,** Sagittal T1-weighted MR image (A) and fat-suppressed, T2-weighted MR image (B).

(Continued)

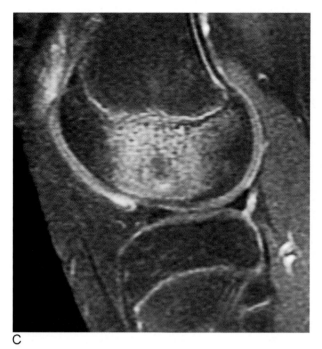

Figure 40-14—(Cont'd) **C,** Fat-suppressed, contrast-enhanced, T1-weighted MR image in a child with an epiphyseal abscess in the distal femur show small fluid signal intensity region surrounded by intense edema and enhancement.

young child and thus is included in the differential diagnosis of lytic epiphyseal lesions with chondroblastoma and eosinophilic granuloma (see Fig. 40-14). Occasionally, a Brodie's abscess is cortically based, where it may elicit significant sclerosis and periosteal reaction. These cortically based infections with significant reactive bone formation can have an appearance similar to that of a cortically based osteoid osteoma or reactive bone formation around a subacute stress fracture (see Fig. 1-17).

Some specific types of osteomyelitis, deserve separate mention. Congenital syphilis osteomyelitis initially demonstrates metaphyseal irregularity and a widened zone of provisional calcification, occasionally resulting in slipped epiphyses. It may progress to invade the diaphysis and elicit periosteal reaction. Congenital syphilis is in the extensive differential diagnosis for infants with generalized periosteal reaction (Fig. 40-17); other conditions to be considered include nonaccidental trauma, tumor, other infections, and metabolic diseases. Acquired syphilis presents as a chronic osteomyelitis, with periostitis and endosteal reaction resulting in an enlarged bowed bone with mixed lytic and sclerotic areas. The flat bones and cranium may be involved with syphilis osteomyelitis. When the tibia is involved, it tends to develop an anterior bowing deformity that has been termed the "saber shin" deformity. Another manifestation of syphilis is neuropathic arthropathy, especially involving the knees.

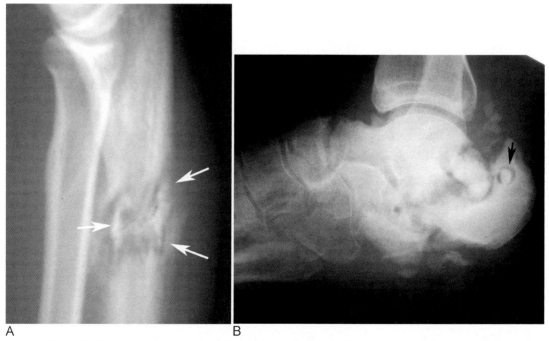

Figure 40-15 Sequestrum in osteomyelitis. **A,** Lateral radiograph of a proximal ulna shows osteomyelitis that has developed following an open fracture. There is permeative bone destruction, as well as an H-shaped dense fragment of necrotic bone *(arrow)*, termed a sequestrum. **B,** Lateral radiograph in a diabetic patient with neuropathic foot shows a round sequestrum *(arrow)* in the posterior calcaneus. (Part A reprinted with permission from the American College of Radiology learning file.)

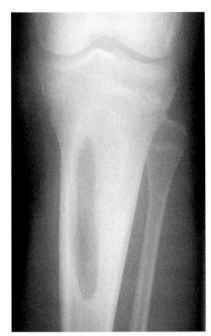

Figure 40-16 Brodie's abscess. This well-defined oval metaphyseal lytic lesion with a sclerotic margin and thick periosteal reaction represents chronic osteomyelitis, sometimes also termed Brodie's abscess. See also Fig. 40-11B.

In the hand, metacarpals and phalanges are at risk for infection from a human bite, usually acquired by punching an adversary in the mouth. A finger or toe may develop a felon or infection in the terminal pulp that may progress to osteomyelitis of the tuft. A stubbed great toe with a nail-bed

injury may result in osteomyelitis of the distal phalanx because the periosteum is immediately adjacent to the nail bed (Fig. 40-18). Soft tissue infection of the hand or foot may spread along tendon sheaths and fascial planes, so that a site of osteomyelitis may be distant from the site of soft tissue injury.

Foreign bodies in the hand or foot may lead to infection (Fig. 2-36).

Adult vertebral osteomyelitis often originates from hematogenous seeding, surgery, or a genitourinary infection via communication through the epidural venous plexus of Batson. In the adult spine, spontaneous infection starts in the subendplate region of the vertebral body and subsequently extends to the adjacent vertebral endplate and disk. The classic radiographic appearance of a disk space infection is irregularity and loss of disk height and loss of cortical density in the adjacent endplates (Figs. 40-19–40-21). A paravertebral mass or displaced psoas shadow in the lumbar region may be seen. Later, a sclerotic host reaction may evolve. Magnetic resonance imaging is needed to assess for epidural abscess and also can demonstrate the extent of osteomyelitis; neural compression; and epidural, paravertebral, or disk space abscess. Percutaneous disk aspiration for diagnosis is controversial because it may not be superior to blood cultures in identifying the causative organism. Dialysis-related amyloid deposition can simulate discitis (see Fig. 21-14).

Discitis in children tends to be less destructive and clinically aggressive than in adults. Childhood disk infection is thought to originate most often by hematogenous seeding

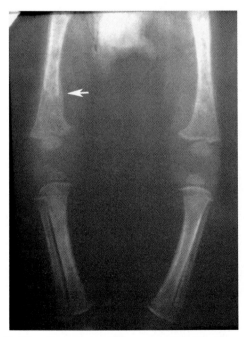

Figure 40-17 Congenital syphilis osteomyelitis. AP radiograph of the lower extremities shows periosteal reaction *(arrow)* and lucent metaphyses.

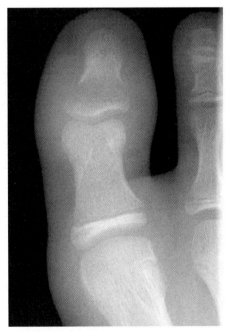

Figure 40-18 Osteomyelitis in the stubbed great toe. AP radiograph demonstrates soft tissue swelling about the great toe and lysis of the distal phalanx. This 13-year-old had a history of stubbed toe and nail bed injury. The great toe nail bed is contiguous with the proximal dorsal periosteum of the distal phalanx, which provides a route of bacterial entry. (Reprinted with permission from the American College of Radiology learning file.)

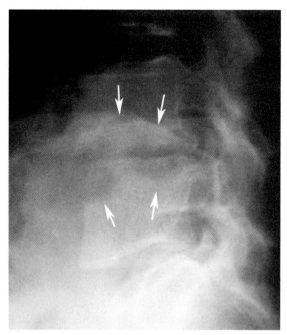

Figure 40-19   Discitis. Lateral radiograph shows endplate destruction at L4–L5 *(arrows)*.

of the disk, as the disk is still vascularized in children. Children with discitis present with malaise, back pain, low-grade fever, and elevated erythrocyte sedimentation rate, and may have a history of a pre-existing minor infection

such as an upper respiratory tract infection. Magnetic resonance imaging shows findings similar to but usually less severe than those seen in adult discitis, including decreased T1 signal intensity, edema, and enhancement in the infected disk and adjacent vertebral marrow. Paravertebral soft tissue mass may be minimal. The radiographic changes are delayed by 2 to 4 weeks and include a decrease in disk height, mild endplate irregularities, and sclerosis of the endplates. Organisms are often not cultured, either from blood or biopsy of the disk. These infections often are nonpyogenic and are treated conservatively. The adjacent vertebral bodies may fuse spontaneously following successful treatment.

Tuberculosis of the spine *(Pott's disease)* tends to involve the thoracolumbar region. Tuberculosis shows a slow progression, with relative preservation of the disk height and lack of sclerotic response. Late in the disease process, the patient may develop an acute angular kyphosis, termed a gibbus deformity. In addition, a calcified psoas abscess may develop (Figs. 40-22, 40-23). The infection may spread under the longitudinal ligaments to involve several disk levels. Multilevel disk infection with paravertebral soft tissue mass is highly suggestive of tuberculosis.

Tuberculosis and fungal osteomyelitis tend to have a slower course and less host reaction than pyogenic osteomyelitis. In the child, tuberculosis may be demonstrated first as dactylitis, where the tubular bones of the hands and feet show periosteal reaction followed by expansion of the bone. The differential

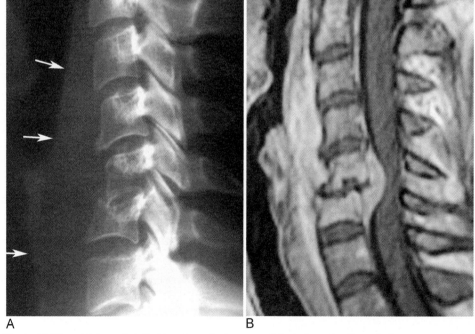

A   B

Figure 40-20   Adult cervical discitis and vertebral osteomyelitis. **A,** Lateral radiograph shows prevertebral soft tissue swelling *(arrows)* and destruction of the C5–C6 disk space and portions of the adjacent endplates. This is a classic radiographic appearance of a disk space infection. **B,** Postgadolinium T1-weighted MR image shows enhancement of C5 and C6, epidural mass with cord compression, and prevertebral phlegmon. Note lack of enhancement in the C5–C6 disk.

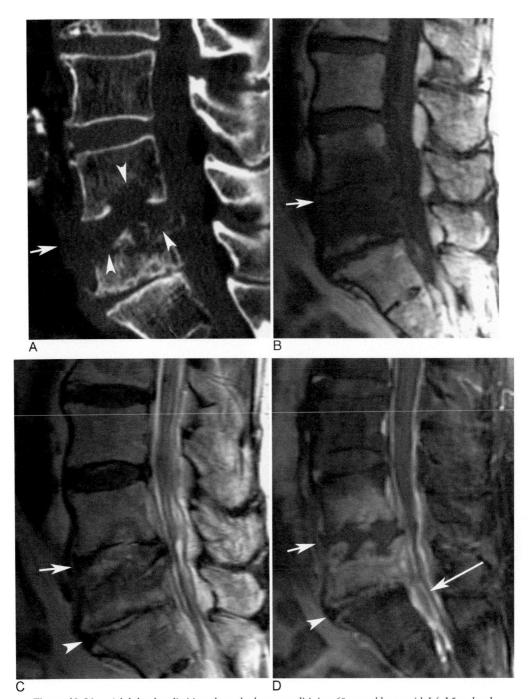

Figure 40-21   Adult lumbar discitis and vertebral osteomyelitis in a 60-year-old man with L4–L5 and early L5–S1 discitis. **A,** Sagittal CT reconstruction shows endplate destruction at L4–L5 *(arrowheads)* and anterior soft tissue attenuation *(arrow)*. **B–D,** Sagittal T1-weighted (B); T2-weighted (C); and postgadolinium fat-suppressed, T1-weighted (D) MR images show edematous L4–L5 *(arrow)* and L5–S1 *(arrowhead)* disks, intense marrow edema and enhancement in L4 and L5 adjacent to the L4–L5 disk, and loss of the normal low-signal cortical line of the vertebral endplates. Also note intense enhancement around an epidural abscess posterior to S1 in part D *(long arrow)*.

diagnosis for this appearance includes juvenile rheumatoid arthritis, sickle cell dactylitis, and other infections.

Chronic recurrent multifocal osteomyelitis (CRMO, plasma cell osteomyelitis) is a poorly understood condition of children and adolescents. The children sustain repeated episodes of pain and soft tissue swelling over bones that show radiologic and

histologic findings suggestive of osteomyelitis. No infectious agent is identified. Frequent sites are the metaphyses of the long bones of the lower extremity and the medial clavicle, but any bone can be involved. Because no organism is identified, a viral cause has been hypothesized. However, current understanding is that CRMO may be related to the SAPHO (synovitis, acne,

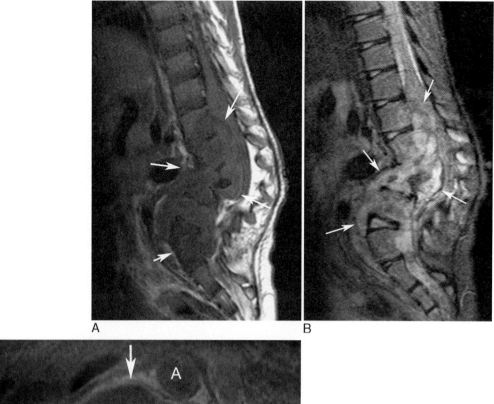

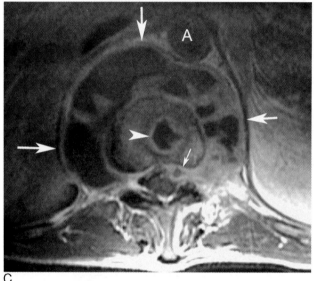

Figure 40-22 Spine tuberculosis. MR image of active disease. **A and B,** Sagittal T1-weighted (A) and inversion recovery (B) MR images show multilevel vertebral body and disk infiltration with a large surrounding mass *(arrows)*, representing diskitis, osteomyelitis, and large phlegmon. Note the lumbar kyphosis (gibbus deformity). **C,** Pott's disease in a different patient. Axial contrast-enhanced, T1-weighted MR image at L1 shows a massive abscess *(large arrows)*, small vertebral abscess *(arrowhead)*, and epidural abscess *(small arrow)*. A, aorta.

pustulosis, hyperostosis, osteitis) syndrome (see Chapter 19). This implies that CRMO it is a reactive process (i.e., that it is caused be a secondary autoimmune response, in this case involving bone) due to antigenic similarity to a previously encountered pathogen.

SEPTIC ARTHRITIS

Most joint infections are diagnosed clinically, without radiographs or other imaging. Joint aspiration is the gold standard test. However, imaging studies are sometimes requested. Joint effusion is the first radiographic sign of septic arthritis. With time, hyperemia may lead to periarticular osteoporosis, and cartilage destruction is seen as a decreasing joint space width. Bone erosion and destruction may follow rapidly (Fig. 40-24) and osteomyelitis may develop by means of contiguous spread. The patient may show sclerotic host reaction if the septic arthritis is bacterial in origin. Eventually, ankylosis may occur.

In the child, the hip is a common site of septic arthritis because of extension of osteomyelitis from the metaphysis of the femur, which is within the hip joint capsule. Two dilemmas are frequently encountered when a child presents with a clinically suspected septic hip. The first issue is whether a joint effusion is present, since joint infection by pyogenic organisms is almost invariably associated with an effusion. Radiographs may show an increased distance between the teardrop and the femoral meta-

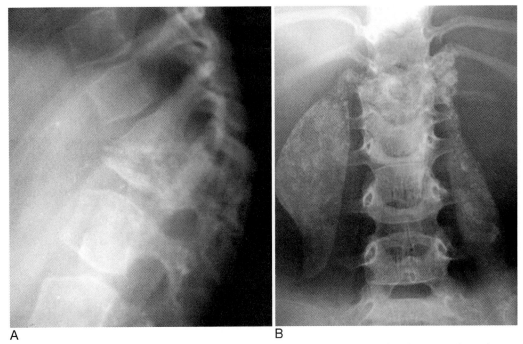

Figure 40-23   Tuberculosis of the spine, late radiographic findings. **A,** Lateral and **B,** AP radiographs demonstrate destruction of much of the vertebral bodies and disk spaces of T11, T12, and L1. There is a gibbus deformity, as well as densely calcified abscesses in the psoas muscles bilaterally, as seen on the AP view. (Reprinted with permission from the American College of Radiology learning file.)

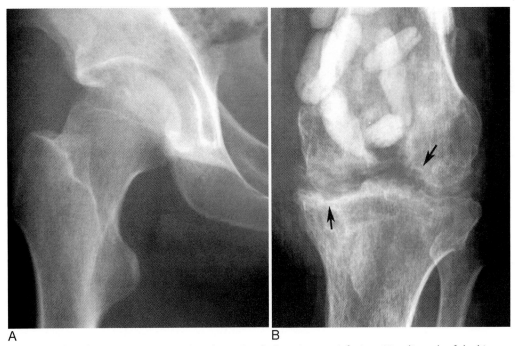

Figure 40-24   Septic joint. **A,** Early radiographic findings in acute infection. AP radiograph of the hip shows loss of cortical distinctness of the femoral head. **B,** Late radiographic findings in chronic infection. AP radiograph of the knee in a 40-year-old man with chronic recurrent methicillin-resistant staphylococcal septic arthritis. Note the sclerotic margins along the subchondral erosions *(arrows),* a finding suggestive of healing. The radiodense bodies are intra-articular antibiotic-impregnated methacrylate beads.

(Continued)

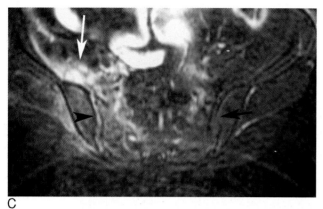

C

Figure 40-24—(Cont'd)   C, Septic sacroiliac (SI) joint. Axial inversion recovery MR image in a patient with AIDS shows high signal intensity in the right SI joint (*black arrowhead;* contrast with the normal left SI joint, *black arrow*). Also note the abscess *(white arrow)* anterior to the right SI joint *(white arrow)*. Spontaneous SI joint infection is more common in intravenous drug abusers and immunocompromised patients.

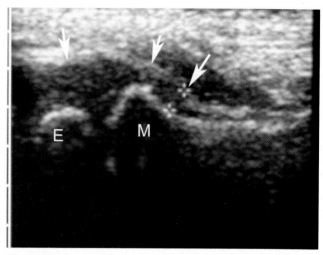

Figure 40-25   Septic hip in a child. Sagittal US image of the hip in a 13-month-old with septic hip shows low-echogenicity joint effusion with elevation of the anterior joint capsule *(arrows)*. Note the capital femoral epiphysis and the proximal femur metaphysis separated by the hypoechoic physis. E, epiphysis; M, metaphysis.

physis or bulging fat planes in a perfectly aligned anteroposterior (AP) radiograph. Producing a vacuum phenomenon in the joint with traction on the hip rules out an effusion and septic hip. However, ultrasonography (US) is far more sensitive and specific in diagnosis of a hip effusion in a child (Fig. 40-25). Magnetic resonance imaging also is very accurate and allows detection of osteomyelitis, but often requires sedation (see Fig. 40-11). The second dilemma arises if a hip effusion is present. Not all effusions indicate joint infection. *Toxic synovitis* is a noninfectious hip joint inflammation with clinical and imaging findings that may be indistinguishable from those of a septic hip. Toxic synovitis is self-limited and requires no therapy. If there is any real clinical suspicion of a septic hip, it should be regarded as an emergency and hip aspiration should be performed.

Tuberculosis and fungal septic arthritides are more chronic processes than bacterial arthritis. They therefore may elicit little or no host bone reaction. Cartilage destruction is often much slower and joint space width remains normal. The joint may demonstrate osteoporosis with minimal cartilage destruction. (Recall that other arthritides with preserved cartilage space include amyloid, pigmented villonodular synovitis, and silastic arthropathy.) Erosions are slow to progress and may appear particularly well delineated (Fig. 40-26A). The hip and knee are the most common sites of tuberculous arthritis, followed by the wrist and elbow. Fungal arthritis has a similar pattern of distribution, and also frequently involves the hand, perhaps due to direct inoculation (Fig. 40-26B).

AIDS

Patients with AIDS may demonstrate a variety of musculoskeletal abnormalities. These include development of lym-

phoma or Kaposi sarcoma, either in bone or soft tissue. Infection can occur with common or opportunistic organisms. Septic arthritis, osteomyelitis, and pyomyositis are more common than in the general population (see Figs. 2-21, 40-24C). In addition, bacillary angiomatosis, caused by the gram-negative agent *Bartonella henselae,* may be seen. This is usually a multifocal process that produces osteolytic lesions, variable bone sclerosis, periosteal reaction, and intramuscular soft tissue masses. Magnetic resonance imaging shows high T2 signal intensity in the lytic lesions and soft tissue masses. These masses have intermediate T1 signal intensity, generally higher than normal muscle.

Patients with AIDS also may demonstrate low signal intensity in the marrow related to reconversion anemia of chronic disease as well as hemosiderin deposition due to chronic transfusions. Arthritic-like changes may be seen in patients with AIDS, resembling psoriatic and reactive arthritis as well as secondary hypertrophic osteoarthropathy. Finally, treatment for AIDS places the patient at risk for avascular necrosis.

SARCOIDOSIS

Sarcoidosis is a systemic granulomatous disorder. Sarcoidosis is not known to be an infectious process but is included in this chapter because it has similar features. Patients with sarcoidosis frequently have muscle and joint pain. Lung abnormalities, including hilar adenopathy, pulmonary infiltrates and fibrosis, and apical bullous disease are present in most patients (80% to 90%). Nodular liver disease with hepatosplenomegaly may be present as well, as may ocular abnormalities such as uveitis and iritis. Sarcoidosis is seen in young adults without sex predominance. Black patients are affected more frequently than either white or Asian patients.

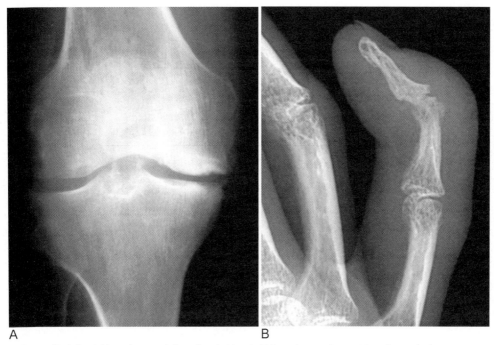

A   B

Figure 40-26   Tuberculosis and fungal arthritis. **A,** Tuberculous arthritis. AP radiograph demonstrates osteopenia and small cortical erosions but nearly normal cartilage width. This combination is typical of tuberculosis or fungal arthritis. **B,** Coccidioides septic arthritis in a 40-year-old man. In both cases, the joint infection was by hematogenous spread of a primary pulmonary infection. Fungal infections also can occur from direct inoculation.

Radiographic osseous abnormalities are seen in about 10% of patients with sarcoidosis, most frequently lacy lytic lesions usually found in the middle or distal phalanges, due to granulomatous infiltration (Fig. 40-27). Other, less frequent, radiographic osseous manifestations include generalized osteopenia, sclerosis of phalangeal tufts, and focal or generalized sclerosis. Magnetic resonance imaging shows that widespread marrow involvement by granulomas is much more common than suggested by radiographs or bone scans (Fig. 40-28). The granulomas are seen as nodules of various sizes, or infiltration, with high T2 signal, intermediate T1 signal, and enhancement with gadolinium. This is appearance can easily lead to a false diagnosis of metastatic disease.

Patients with sarcoidosis experience polyarticular arthralgias. Early in the disease, this is reactive, and imaging studies are normal or may show only an effusion. Chronic sarcoidosis causes granulomatous arthritis. Magnetic resonance imaging may show synovial thickening and enhancement in joints and tendon sheaths.

Muscular sarcoidosis is common, although many cases are asymptomatic (Fig. 40-29). Discrete enhancing nodules are occasionally seen on MRI, classically with a low-signal-intensity spiculated central region. Generalized sarcoid myositis is more common. This resembles polymyositis clinically and on MRI, and can lead to proximal muscle fatty atrophy if not controlled with steroids. Steroid therapy for sarcoidosis also can cause fatty atrophy.

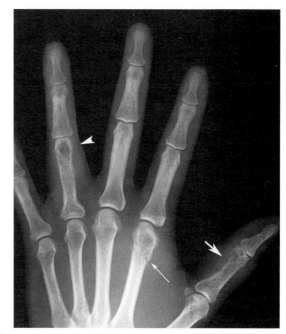

Figure 40-27   Sarcoidosis. PA hand radiograph shows lytic lesions *(arrowhead),* some so small that they produce a "lace-like" appearance in the thumb proximal phalanx *(large arrow).* Note the pathologic fracture through a lesion in the distal second metacarpal *(small arrow).*

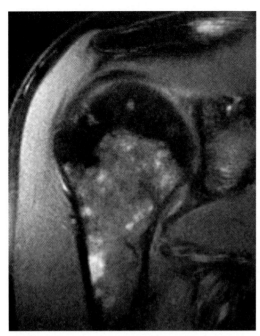

Figure 40-28 Sarcoidosis, marrow disease. Coronal fat-suppressed, T2-weighted MR image shows multiple small high-signal masses that are sarcoid granulomas. Marrow involvement with sarcoidosis is often extensive, but may be detected only with MR imaging or biopsy. (Courtesy of Sandra Moore, MD.)

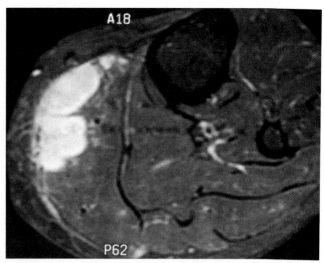

Figure 40-29 Sarcoidosis, muscle disease. Axial fat-suppressed, T1-weighted, contrast-enhanced MR image of the leg in a patient with sarcoidosis shows well-defined enhancing masses in the medial head of the gastrocnemius. Muscle sarcoidosis can cause regional muscle edema due to infiltration, or can cause discrete enhancing masses, as in this example. (Courtesy of Shigeru Ehara, MD. Reprinted with permission from May DA, Disler DG, Jones EA, et al: Abnormal signal within skeletal muscle in MRI: Patterns, pearls, and pitfalls. Radiographics 20:S295–S315, 2000.)

Hematologic Disorders

HEMOPHILIA

THALASSEMIA

SICKLE CELL ANEMIA

MASTOCYTOSIS

LEUKEMIA

HEMOPHILIA

Hemophilia is a group of related bleeding disorders resulting from clotting factor deficiencies. The two most common types of hemophilia, hemophilia A (factor VIII deficiency) and hemophilia B (factor IX deficiency, Christmas disease) are inherited through an X-linked recessive pattern and therefore are only found in males. Musculoskeletal manifestations include hemarthroses, growth deformity, arthropathy, and tumor-like hematomas.

Key Concepts	Hemophilia

Males
Joints
    Dense effusions, erosions, bony overgrowth, and early physeal closure due to hyperemia
    Knees, elbows, ankles most common locations
    May be indistinguishable from juvenile rheumatoid arthritis (JRA) on radiographs
    May resemble pigmented villonodular synovitis (PVNS) on MRI because of hemosiderin deposition and erosions
Pseudotumor
    Hematoma (interosseous, subperiosteal, or soft tissue), with bizarre MRI signal
    Erodes surface of adjacent bone, may resemble an aggressive neoplasm
    Femur, pelvis, tibia, calcaneus most common locations

Hemarthroses may occur in several joints, are often asymmetric, and can be caused by trivial trauma. The most commonly involved joints are the knee, elbow, and ankle, followed by less frequent occurrences in the hip and shoulder. Multiple episodes of hemarthrosis result in hypertrophied synovium, which often contains hemosiderin deposits. The hemarthroses may be seen on radiographs as unusually dense (Fig. 41-1), and the hemosiderin-laden synovium can be seen on magnetic resonance imaging (MRI) as having low signal intensity on T1-weighted and intermediate to low signal intensity on T2-weighted images. This is often accompanied by the "blooming" effect on gradient echo imaging of very low signal intensity (Fig. 41-2), similar to pigmented villonodular synovitis.

The hemarthroses cause synovial inflammation that, in turn, causes hyperemia. With hyperemia, the adjacent bones become osteoporotic. Because hemarthroses usually occur in skeletally immature patients, the hyperemia also results in epiphyseal overgrowth, which is seen radiographically as flared metaphyses and enlarged epiphyses, with comparatively gracile diaphyses (Figs. 41-1 and 41-3). The hyperemia can also result in early physeal fusion and resultant skeletal shortening. The inflammatory synovitis causes articular cartilage destruction, with erosions and subarticular cysts. Eventually, secondary degenerative arthritis develops. Thus, the joints in hemophilia can appear quite distinctive, with flared metaphyses and enlarged epiphyses, enlarged radial head in the elbow, wide intercondylar notch in the knee and trochlear notch in the elbow, and variable articular joint space narrowing and subchondral erosion (see Fig. 41-3). Juvenile rheumatoid arthritis may have an identical pattern of overgrowth and destructive change, which is not surprising as both are caused by inflammatory synovitis in a growing skeleton. The two processes may not be distinguishable radiographically. Clinically, however, the two diseases are distinct.

Pseudotumor of hemophilia is a nonneoplastic mass lesion that occurs with an intraosseous, subperiosteal, or soft tissue bleeding. With repeated bleeding in the same area, extrinsic or

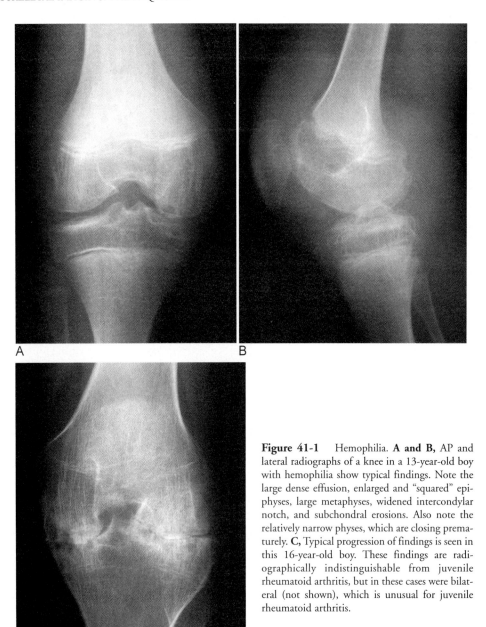

Figure 41-1   Hemophilia. **A and B,** AP and lateral radiographs of a knee in a 13-year-old boy with hemophilia show typical findings. Note the large dense effusion, enlarged and "squared" epiphyses, large metaphyses, widened intercondylar notch, and subchondral erosions. Also note the relatively narrow physes, which are closing prematurely. **C,** Typical progression of findings is seen in this 16-year-old boy. These findings are radiographically indistinguishable from juvenile rheumatoid arthritis, but in these cases were bilateral (not shown), which is unusual for juvenile rheumatoid arthritis.

intrinsic scalloping and pressure erosion occurs at the cortical margin of adjacent bone. Bone destruction and expansile periosteal reaction may be extensive, but the margins are generally sharply circumscribed and sclerotic, which may suggest the correct diagnosis. There may be a large soft tissue mass. The MRI appearance may be quite bizarre because of the presence of blood products of varying ages (Fig. 41-4). Magnetic resonance imaging may show a hypointense rim due to a fibrous capsule and to hemosiderin deposits, whereas the central signal will vary according to the age of the hematoma and the presence of clot contained therein. Usually, many different

combinations of signal intensities are seen, reflecting the process of remote and recurrent bleeding as well as clot organization. Pseudotumor of hemophilia is found most frequently in the femur, pelvis, tibia, and calcaneus.

THALASSEMIA

Thalassemia is a group of inherited hemoglobinopathies that occur most commonly in individuals of Mediterranean heritage, but also occurs in North Americans of African descent. The most

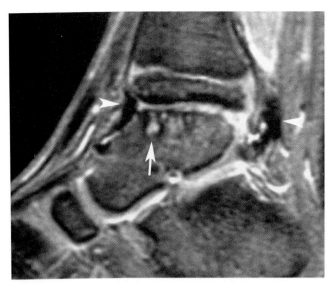

Figure 41-2   MR image of hemophilic arthropathy. Sagittal gradient echo image of the ankle in a 7-year-old boy with hemophilia demonstrates subchondral erosion in the talar dome *(arrow)*, and extremely low signal of thickened synovium *(arrowheads)*. The low signal intensity is due to susceptibility artifact caused by hemosiderin-laden macrophages in the synovium. The findings resemble pigmented villonodular synovitis. (Courtesy of Ray Kilcoyne, MD.)

severe form is thalassemia major (Cooley's anemia, β-thalassemia). It is clinically manifested early in life, and death often occurs during childhood. Marrow hyperplasia with an expanded marrow space is the major radiographic feature, and may be spectacular. The cranial diploic space is widened and may show dense striations with a hair-on-end appearance (Fig. 41-5). Marrow expansion obliterates the paranasal sinuses, alters dentition, and causes hypertelorism. Osteopenia and enlarged marrow cavities are seen in the appendicular skeleton. The distal femurs may show an Erlenmeyer flask deformity, like other marrow packing disorders. Multiple transfusions lead to hemochromatosis, potentially with associated calcium pyrophosphate dihydrate arthropathy and marrow hemosiderosis. Milder forms of thalassemia have milder or absent radiologic manifestations.

SICKLE CELL ANEMIA

Sickle cell anemia is an autosomal recessive inherited hemoglobinopathy found in 1% of the black population in North America. The radiographic findings reflect both the chronic hemolytic anemia and the consequences of microvascular occlusion created by sickled cells when exposed to low oxygen tension. The findings of marrow hyperplasia and extramedullary hematopoiesis are less severe than in thalassemia major, and may not be evident on radiographs.

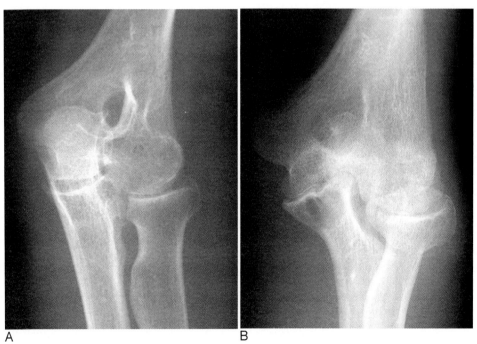

A   B

Figure 41-3   Hemophilia: elbow. **A,** Oblique radiograph of the elbow in an 18-year-old man demonstrates classic but mild changes of hemophilia, with a wide intercondylar notch, radial head overgrowth, and mild cartilage loss. **B,** Similar but more severe changes in a 34-year-old man. Note the enlarged radial head and much more advanced erosive change.

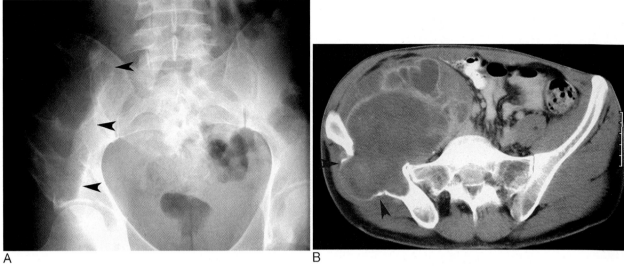

Figure 41-4   Pseudotumor of hemophilia. **A,** AP radiograph of the pelvis in a 35-year-old man demonstrates a well-defined lytic lesion in the right iliac wing *(arrowheads)*. There is pseudotrabeculation within the lesion and no matrix. **B,** CT demonstrates the large soft tissue mass with heterogeneous attenuation, enhancing margin, and well-defined lytic margins. The CT scan shows no trabeculae within the mass. The radiograph appearance is due to the shell of expanded bone at the posterior margin of the pseudotumor *(arrowheads)*.

Key Concepts	Sickle Cell Anemia (Hb SS)

Affects 1% of black population in North America
Chronic anemia: Usually much milder findings of marrow expansion than in thalassemia major
Thrombosis/infarction
  Renal papillary necrosis, cholelithiasis, splenic autoinfarction, cardiomegaly, pulmonary infarction, stroke
  Dactylitis (hand-foot syndrome): Digit swelling and periostitis in young children
  Bone infarcts
  H-shaped vertebrae
  Osteomyelitis. May be clinically indistinguishable from acute bone infarction or hand-foot syndrome
  Staphylococcus most common, followed by *Salmonella*

However, the consequences of microvascular thrombosis and infarction are dramatic and often pathognomonic. Nonmusculoskeletal radiographic findings include renal papillary necrosis, cholelithiasis (due to red cell lysis and bilirubinate stones), splenic autoinfarction, cardiomegaly, stroke, and pulmonary infarction. *Dactylitis,* also termed *hand-foot syndrome* is a common feature, occurring in 10% to 20% of young children with sickle cell disease. Ambient cold temperatures result in vasoconstriction in the persistent hematopoietic marrow of the digits. Radiographically, dactylitis is seen as periosteal reaction and soft tissue swelling (Fig. 41-6). Avascular necrosis of the femoral and humeral heads is extremely common. Marrow reconversion may be a prominent finding on MRI. Marrow infarcts are common, seen radiographically in older patients as patchy sclerosis or serpiginous calcified densities, sometimes with periosteal reaction, or as poorly marginated sclerotic regions (Figs. 41-7, 41-8). The central vertebral bodies collapse, resulting in an H-shape (Fig. 41-9). Diphosphonate bone scans often show diffusely increased tracer uptake, with focal "hot spots" in healing infarcts or at regions of infection.

Patients with sickle cell anemia are vulnerable to osteomyelitis, which radiographically may be indistinguishable from acute bone infarction or hand-foot syndrome. Radionuclide scanning with tagged leukocytes, MR imaging, and sometimes biopsy are necessary to distinguish between the two diagnoses. *Salmonella* osteomyelitis is more common than in the normal population, but *Staphylococcus* species are still the most common causative organisms for osteomyelitis in patients with sickle cell anemia.

Sickle cell trait causes few musculoskeletal findings. Bone infarcts are occasionally seen. Sickle cell hemoglobin C predominately shows marrow hyperplasia of the skull and subchondral avascular necrosis, without featuring metadiaphyseal bone infarcts. Splenomegaly rather than splenic infarction is a feature of this disease.

MASTOCYTOSIS

Mastocytosis is a rare proliferative disorder of mast cells. Clinical manifestations may be limited to the skin, usually without radiologic manifestation, or may be systemic. Systemic disease may result from a hyperplastic response to an unknown stimulus, or as an exceedingly rare variant of leukemia. Clinical features include the skin rash *urticaria pig-*

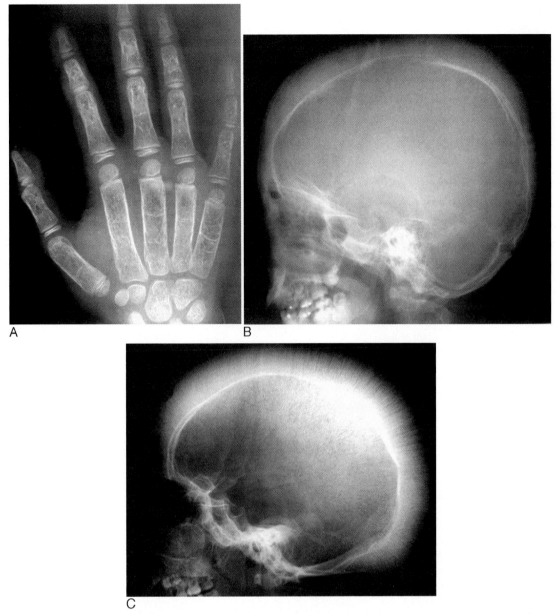

Figure 41-5   Thalassemia major: marrow space expansion. **A,** PA radiograph of a hand demonstrates diffuse osteopenia and widening and squaring of the metacarpals and phalanges. These features are seen in diseases where there is severe marrow hyperplasia with enlargement of the marrow space. **B,** Skull shows widened diploic space and obliteration of the maxillary sinuses. **C,** Similar findings in a different patient. Marrow expansion this profound is most often associated with thalassemia major. (Part C reprinted with permission of the American College of Radiology learning file.)

mentosa, and systemic findings related to histamine release include flushing, nausea, and vomiting. Marrow infiltration and histamine release by mast cells in the systemic form may result in generalized or localized osteoporosis, nonspecific lytic lesions, or focal or generalized sclerosis (Fig. 41-10, 41-11). Treatment is guided by the clinical aggressiveness, and includes histamine blockers. More aggressive forms also are treated with steroids and chemotherapy.

LEUKEMIA

The leukemias are a heterogeneous group of neoplastic proliferation of leukocytes. Leukemia is the most common malignancy of childhood. The clinical presentation may include bone or joint pain, the latter most often in the hip, that may clinically suggest juvenile rheumatoid arthritis. Potential radiologic manifestations

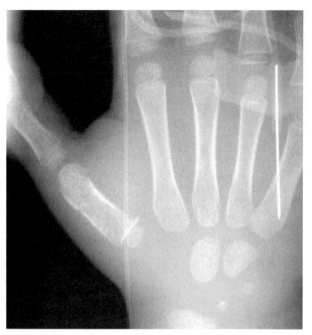

relate to hepatosplenomegaly, marrow infiltration, hemorrhage (due to low platelet counts) and opportunistic infections. Generalized osteoporosis is usually present, and the cranial sutures may be widened. Children of any age may develop non-specific metaphyseal lytic lesions. *Leukemic lines* are lucent transverse metaphyseal bands adjacent to the physis (Fig. 41-12). These usually occur in older children, and are thought to represent disturbed endochondral ossification with diminished mineralization of new bone rather than erosion of bone by leukemic infiltration. Growth recovery lines related to remissions and chemotherapy cycles are often pronounced.

Figure 41-6 Sickle cell dactylitis. Radiograph of the thumb in a 3-year-old girl with sickle cell disease and acute pain and swelling demonstrates subtle heterogeneous density and periosteal reaction in the first metacarpal. These findings could represent infection, but in this case represent the early changes of the bone infarct in this child with the clinical findings of hand-foot syndrome. (Reprinted with permission of the American College of Radiology learning file.)

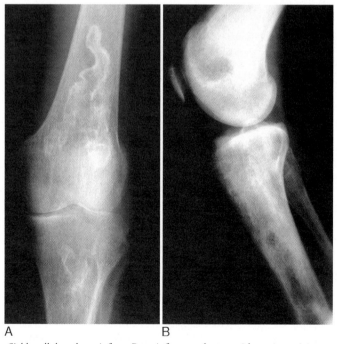

A   B

Figure 41-7 Sickle cell: long bone infarct. Bone infarct can be seen either as a serpiginous calcification (A) or as a generalized but patchy increase in bone density (B). The latter is the more common appearance of bone infarct in patients with sickle cell anemia.

(Continued)

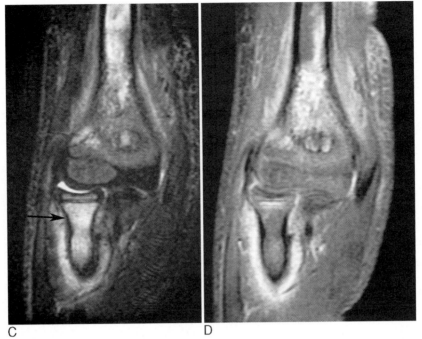

C   D

Figure 41-7—(Cont'd)   C and D, Coronal inversion recovery (C) and fat-suppressed, postcontrast, T1-weighted (D) MR images show acute bone infarcts in a child with sickle cell disease. Note the uniform marrow edema in the proximal radius (*arrow* in part C), yet only minimal enhancement in part D. Also note the intense periosteal edema and enhancement around the infarct. There are similar findings in the distal humeral metaphysis and diaphysis. These findings could represent infection, but in this case were acute infarcts. The classic serpiginous double-line sign of avascular necrosis is not seen early in the process.

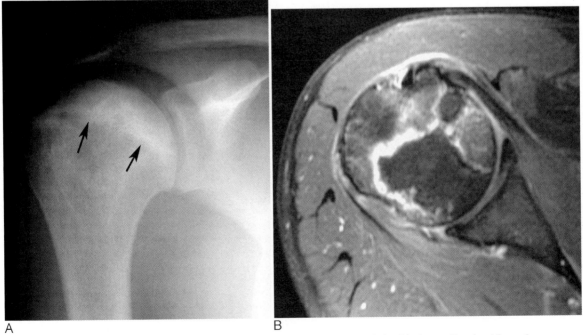

A   B

Figure 41-8   Sickle cell: avascular necrosis. Avascular necrosis, particularly of the humeral head and femoral head, is a typical finding of sickle cell disease. **A,** AP shoulder radiograph shows patchy sclerosis *(arrows)*. There is no collapse. **B,** Axial T2-weighted MR image in a different patient shows the classic serpiginous double-line sign of avascular necrosis.

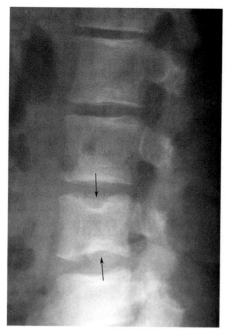

Figure 41-9 Sickle cell: spine. Lateral radiograph shows patchy increased density in all the vertebral bodies (typical finding in sickle cell disease). The sickled cells may sludge in the looping arcades at the endplates of the vertebral bodies, causing them to collapse in their central portion. This is seen on this radiograph *(arrows)*, where L4 is approaching what has been termed an H-shaped vertebra.

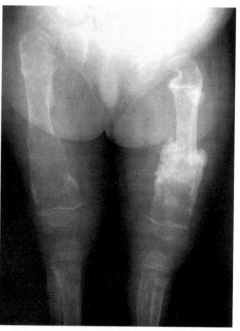

Figure 41-11 Mastocytosis. Radiographic manifestations of mastocytosis include diffuse osteopenia, as seen in this 4-month-old child who has already sustained multiple fractures. (Reprinted with permission from the American College of Radiology learning file.)

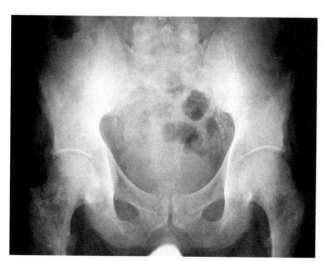

Figure 41-10 Mastocytosis. Mastocytosis can present with mixed osteopenia and sclerosis, as in this 50-year-old man. The sclerosis can be either diffuse (as in this patient) or focal.

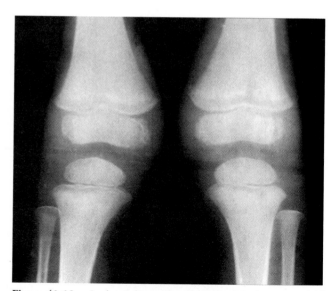

Figure 41-12 Leukemic lines. AP radiograph of the knees in a child with acute myeloid leukemia shows lucent metaphyseal bands.

Part VII Sources and Suggested Readings

Ahmadi ME, Morrison WB, Carrino JA, et al: Neuropathic arthropathy of the foot with and without superimposed osteomyelitis: MR imaging characteristics. Radiology 238:622–631, 2006.

Andrews C: Evaluation of the marrow space in the adult hip. Radiographics 20:s27–s42, 2000.

Blomlie V, Rofstad E, Skjonsberg A, et al: Female pelvic bone marrow: Serial MR imaging before, during, and after radiation therapy. Radiology 194:537–543, 1995.

Collins M, Schaar M, Wenger D, Mandrekar J: T1-weighted MRI characteristics of pedal osteomyelitis. AJR 185:386–393, 2005.

Matsuo M, Ehara S, Tomakawa Y, et al: Muscular sarcoidosis. Skel Radiol 24:535–537, 1995.

Moore SL, Teirstein AE: Musculoskeletal sarcoidosis: Spectrum of appearances at MR imaging. Radiographics 23:1389–1399, 2003.

Moore SL, Teirstein A, Golimbu C: MRI of sarcoidosis patients with musculoskeletal symptoms. AJR 185:154–159, 2005.

Morrison WB, Schwietzer ME, Batte WG, et al: Osteomyelitis of the foot: Relative importance of primary and secondary MR imaging signs. Radiology 207:625–652, 1988.

Morrison WB, Schwietzer ME, Bock GE, et al: Diagnosis of osteomyelitis: Utility of fat-suppressed contrast-enhanced MR imaging. Radiology 189:251–257, 1993.

Morrison WB, Schwietzer ME, Wapner KL, et al: Osteomyelitis in feet of diabetics: Clinical accuracy, surgical utility and cost effectiveness of MR imaging. Radiology 196:557–564, 1995.

Resnick D (ed): Diagnosis of Bone and Joint Disorders, ed 4. Philadelphia, W.B. Saunders, 2002.

Santiago Restrepo C, Lemos D, et al: Imaging findings in musculoskeletal complications of AIDS. Radiographics 24:1029–1049, 2004.

Sartoris D, Resnick D, Resnik C, et al: Musculoskeletal manifestations of sarcoidosis. Semin Roentgen 20:376–386, 1985.

Steinbach L, Tehrawzadeh J, Fleckenstein J, et al: Human immunodeficiency virus infection: Musculoskeletal manifestations. Radiology 186:833–838, 1993.

Stevens S, Moore S, Amylon M: Repopulation of marrow after transplantation: MR imaging with pathologic correlation. Radiology 175:213–218, 1990.

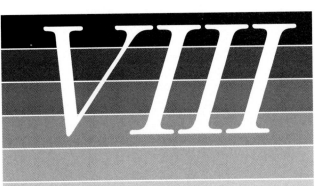

VIII CONGENITAL AND DEVELOPMENTAL CONDITIONS

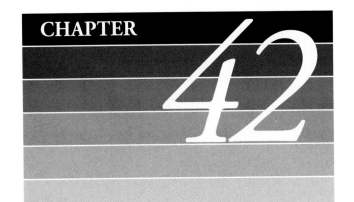

CHAPTER 42

Introduction to Congenital and Developmental Skeletal Conditions

A variety of disease processes and conditions may alter bone formation and growth and result in bone or joint deformity. This chapter reviews normal skeletal growth and development, then discusses several of the more common, distinctive, or otherwise important congenital and developmental musculoskeletal abnormalities. A complete review of this topic is beyond the scope of this book. When more information is needed, excellent sources include Taybi and Lachman's *Radiology of Syndromes, Metabolic Disorders, and Skeletal Dysplasias,* and the major pediatric radiology textbooks. Resnick's *Diagnosis of Bone and Joint Disorders* provides an encyclopedic discussion of many congenital and developmental conditions reviewed in this chapter. Keats and Anderson's *An Atlas of Normal Roentgen Variants that May Simulate Disease,* and Keats and Smith's *An Atlas of Normal Developmental Roentgen Anatomy* review many developmental variants, some seen only transiently during development, that may simulate pathologic conditions.

Development of the skeleton begins during the first trimester of gestation with aggregation of mesenchymal cells that subsequently become the bones and joints. The bones are formed by either of two processes, both of which involve replacement of connective tissues by bone. The calvaria of the skull, the mandible, most of the facial bones, and the central portion of the clavicles are formed by direct transformation of primitive mesenchyme into bone by a process termed *intramembranous ossification.* The remainder of the skeleton, including the skull base, the spine, the pelvis, and the extremities, is preceded by a continuously growing cartilage model that is continuously replaced by bone in a process termed *enchondral ossification.* The bone formed by either process is woven (immature) bone. The immature bone is subsequently extensively remodeled in a coordinated process of bone resorption by osteoclasts and bone formation by osteoblasts into the mature adult skeleton, which is composed of lamellar bone. After skeletal maturity is reached, further bone resorption and formation occur in response to mechanical stresses, hormonal regulation related to calcium homeostasis, or alterations in thyroid or sex hormones.

Long bones grow longitudinally by enchondral ossification at the *physis* (growth plate, epiphyseal growth plate; Fig. 42-1).

Key Concepts	Normal Skeletal Growth and Development: Bone Formation

Intramembranous ossification = direct conversion from mesenchyme to bone: Most of the skull and facial bones, mandible, central portion of clavicle.

Enchondral ossification = conversion of a cartilage model into bone: Skull base, spine, pelvis, extremities.

Physis produces longitudinal growth of long bones by enchondral ossification.

Injury to physis or its blood supply can cause growth arrest and deformity.

Tubulation: Process of remodeling the shaft of a long bone into normal configuration.

Overtubulation: Cylindrical portion of shaft is too long, with short and narrowed metaphysis (examples: absent weight bearing, neuromuscular conditions).

Undertubulation: Cylindrical portion of shaft is too short, with wide and long metaphysis (examples: osteopetrosis, Gaucher's disease).

The physis may be considered a rolling assembly line that pushes the epiphysis away from the metaphysis and diaphysis as it manufactures new bone. The process of new bone formation is initiated by chondrocytes located along the epiphyseal margin of the physis ("resting zone") that proliferate and produce a

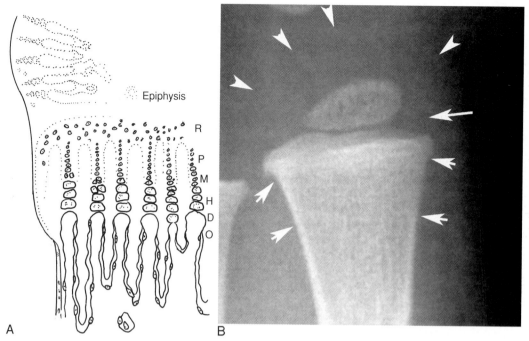

Figure 42-1   The physis. **A,** Diagram shows the histologic organization of the physis. The *resting zone (R)* adjacent to the epiphysis contains small clusters of cartilage cells. The *proliferation zone (P)* contains dividing and enlarging cartilage cells organized into longitudinal columns. Cell division ceases in the *maturation zone (M),* but the cartilage cells continue to enlarge. The cells greatly enlarge in the *hypertrophic zone (H)* and the surrounding cartilage becomes calcified (termed *provisional calcification* because it is not yet bone). The cartilage cells degenerate and die in the *cartilage degeneration zone (D)* and are replaced by osteoblasts. In the *osteogenic zone (O),* the osteoblasts begin the process of conversion of the calcified cartilage into bone. This zone marks the transition from the physis to the metaphysis. The term "bone bark" is sometimes used to describe the lateral margin of the physis, which occasional calcifies and is seen on radiographs as a small spicule of bone extending distally from the metaphysis. **B,** Radiograph of a child's distal radius shows the corresponding radiographic anatomy. The long arrow marks the physis. The convex contour of the metaphysis *(short arrows)* is the result of bone remodeling by osteoclasts and osteoblasts. If osteoclast activity is diminished, then this concave contour is not produced *(undertubulation,* see text and Fig. 42-3). The arrowheads mark the true margins of the epiphysis, which is composed mostly of cartilage in this young child.

cartilage template that becomes calcified, and subsequently invaded by osteocytes, finally to be ossified at the metaphyseal side of the physis. The new bone deposited along the metaphyseal side of the physis is immature and undergoes extensive remodeling to become mature trabecular bone. New cartilage is produced along the epiphyseal side of the physis at the same rate that it is converted to bone along the metaphyseal side. This equilibrium results in uniform width of the healthy physis throughout growth.

Direct trauma to the physis can result in osseous healing across the physis or injury to the chondrocytes that are needed to produce the cartilage model. Either complication can cause growth arrest or growth deformity. Intact metaphyseal blood vessels adjacent to the physis are essential to convert the cartilage model into bone. Loss of integrity of these vessels by trauma, infection, or other insult can result in widening of the physis, possibly focal, because the newly produced cartilage cannot be transformed into bone. Growth disturbance and deformity may result.

The rate at which a long bone is lengthened depends on circulating hormones, notably growth hormone, and poorly understood local factors that maintain proportional skeletal growth. The fastest longitudinal growth in the appendicular skeleton occurs at the distal femoral physis, where new bone is formed at up to 1 to 1.5 cm per year. As skeletal maturity is reached around puberty, the chondrocytes in the resting zone of the physis stop dividing. Consequently, no new cartilage is formed and longitudinal growth ceases. The remaining cartilage is converted to bone as the physis closes. A dense transverse line on radiographs, sometimes termed a physeal scar, marks the final position of the physis. The timing of physeal closure varies at different sites. The medial clavicle physes are among the last to close, typically in the third decade, years after adult stature has been achieved.

Stress lines, also termed *growth recovery lines, Park lines,* or *Harris lines,* are thin sclerotic lines within the metaphysis that are parallel to the physis (Fig. 41-2). They are associated with periods of childhood stress such as illness or trauma.

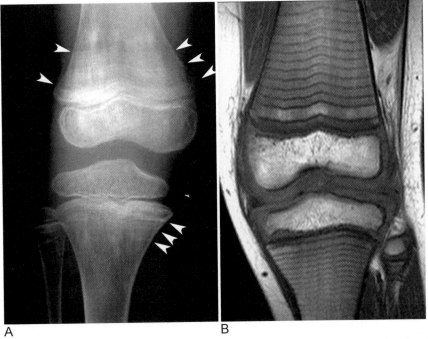

Figure 42-2   Growth recovery lines (Parke lines, Harris lines). **A,** AP radiograph of the knee shows thin, sharp lines parallel to the physes of the femur, tibia, and fibula *(arrowheads).* The other knee (not shown) had an identical appearance. The growth recovery lines are more widely spaced in the femurs than in the tibias because the femurs grow more rapidly. **B,** Coronal T1-weighted MR image in a different patient shows similar findings, although extraordinarily prominent. This child has osteogenesis imperfecta that has been treated with periodic bisphosphonate injections. The growth recovery lines are formed by impaired osteoclast function during therapy.

The lines appear to be formed during the recovery phase after such episodes. Stress lines often persist into adulthood, but are eventually removed by routine bone remodeling. Stress lines are narrow and sharply defined, and do not abut the physis. In contrast, broader, less well-defined sclerotic transverse metaphyseal bands that abut the physis can be seen as a normal finding when found only in weight-bearing bones, or as an abnormal finding when found in all bones as a consequence of heavy-metal poisoning (Fig 26-5). *Lucent* metaphyseal bands can occur in rickets, leukemia, and metastatic neuroblastoma.

Long bones also undergo lateral growth and remodeling that are due primarily to periosteal new bone formation and remodeling of the metaphysis into an approximately tubular shape. This process, termed *tubulation,* is mediated by coordinated function of osteoclasts and osteoblasts. Disorders of tubulation may result in a wide metaphysis *(undertubulation, Erlenmeyer flask deformity,* Figs. 39-7, 42-3, and Table 42-1), or a narrow, tubular metaphysis *(overtubulation,* Fig. 42-4 and Table 42-2). For example, the diminished osteoclastic activity associated with osteopetrosis and marrow packing in storage diseases result in undertubulation. Overtubulation is seen most commonly in neuromuscular conditions with absent or diminished weight bearing, such as cerebral palsy.

The process of skeletal maturation tends to follow an orderly progression, even when accelerated or delayed by endocrine

Table 42-1   Common Causes of Undertubulation

Bones of normal length
  Rickets
  Osteopetrosis
  Fibrous dysplasia
  Multiple osteochondromas
Short, often squat bones
  Dwarfism (numerous types, achondroplasia most common)
  Storage diseases
  Multiple osteochondromas

Table 42-2   Common Causes of Overtubulation (Long, Thin Bones)

Neuromuscular conditions (e.g., cerebral palsy, myelomeningocele)
Osteogenesis imperfecta
Juvenile rheumatoid arthritis
Marfan syndrome
Homocystinuria
Arthrogryposis

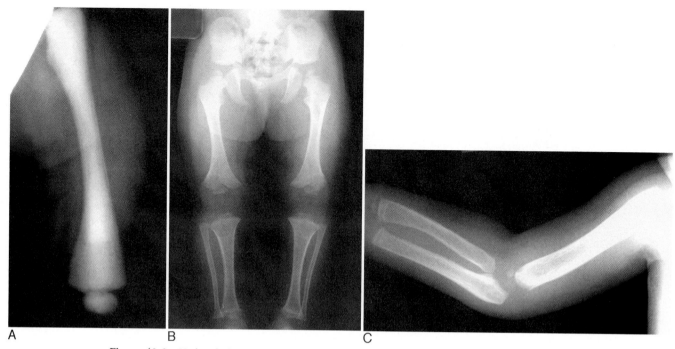

A B C

Figure 42-3 Undertubulation. **A,** Osteopetrosis. Failure of osteoclast function results in wide metaphyses. **B,** Achondroplasia. Note the short, squat bones with wide metaphyses. **C,** Hurler's syndrome (mucopolysaccharidosis 1H). The marrow is packed with abnormal metabolites, causing expansion of the diaphyses and metaphyses. (Part B courtesy of Stephanie Spottswood, MD.) See also Fig. 39-7.

conditions, nutritional deficiencies, or other disease states. Greulich and Pyle's *Radiographic Atlas of Skeletal Development of the Hand and Wrist* has been widely adopted as the standard reference for determining the skeletal age of children older than 1 year of age. The standard images of the maturing left hand used in this atlas were derived from a longitudinal study of healthy children of northern European decent living in the Cleveland area during the 1930s. This may not represent an optimal data set, but current appreciation of the potential harm of ionizing radiation makes it unlikely that a similar study will ever be performed in other racial or ethnic groups. Contemporary evaluations of this atlas have verified its accuracy, at least in children of European descent. As a general rule, children of African descent tend to skeletally mature faster than white persons. Girls mature faster than boys, and the difference becomes greater as they grow.

In infants and very young children up to about 1 year of age, the *method of Sontag, Snell, and Anderson* is a useful technique for determining skeletal age (Table 42-3). This method is based on tabulation of the number of secondary growth centers (epiphyses and apophyses) that have started to ossify and thus are visible on anteroposterior (AP) radiographs of one upper and one lower extremity. The appeal of this method is that it relies on a yes-or-no determination of the presence of visible ossification in each secondary growth center. There are

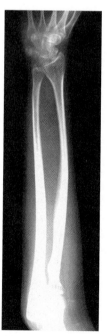

Figure 42-4 Overtubulation. Note the short transition from epiphysis to diaphysis in the forearm of this child with osteogenesis imperfecta. Also note the long, narrow diaphyses. This overall appearance is often described as "gracile bones" and is most commonly seen in neuromuscular conditions with chronic absence of weight bearing, such as cerebral palsy.

other systems for radiographic determination of skeletal age. One additional system is the *Elgenmark method,* which is similar to the method of Sontag, Snell, and Anderson in that it is based on the number of visible ossification centers, but it uses only unilateral carpal and tarsal bones. This system uses less ionizing radiation, but still maintains high precision.

The *Risser technique* is used to estimate skeletal maturity of the spine in adolescents with scoliosis. It is based on the radiographic appearance of the iliac crest apophyses (Fig. 42-5). This is wonderfully convenient because the iliac crests are easily included on frontal spinal radiographs. The iliac crest apophyses ossify in an orderly sequence from lateral to medial that begins roughly 4 years before spinal growth is complete. Soon after becoming completely ossified, the apophyses fuse with the iliac crests. This fusion is synchronous with completion of spinal growth.

The appearance of the bone marrow on magnetic resonance (MR) images also undergoes predictable changes during growth and development that reflect the shifting distribution of hematopoietic elements away from the peripheral skeleton. This was discussed in Chapter 39. Hematopoietic marrow may be present in all portions of the marrow in neonates. A useful rule of thumb is that anything other than fat signal intensity in an epiphysis or apophysis after age 6 months should be considered abnormal, with the exception of the medial humeral head, where hematopoietic marrow may be normally seen well into middle-age. Conditions that may cause abnormal signal intensity in the secondary growth centers are listed in Table 42-4. See Chapter 39 for addition discussion of marrow imaging.

Unossified epiphyseal cartilage, also called "growth cartilage" or the cartilaginous anlage (anlage means "that which will

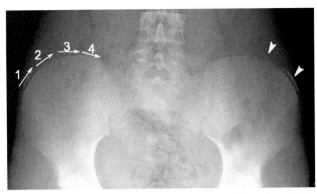

Figure 42-5   Risser classification for estimation of spinal maturity. This system is based on the ossification of the iliac crest apophysis, which begins laterally and proceeds medially, followed by fusion of the apophysis to the iliac wing. Stage 0: no ossification of the iliac crest apophysis; stage 1: ossification of the lateral one fourth of the iliac crest apophysis; stage 2: ossification of the lateral half of the iliac crest apophysis; stage 3: ossification of the lateral three fourths of the iliac crest apophysis; stage 4: ossification of the entire iliac crest apophysis, without fusion to the iliac crest; stage 5: fusion of the iliac crest apophysis (coincides with completion of spinal growth). This child is Risser stage 2 *(arrowheads).*

become"), is predominantly fibrocartilage and has lower signal intensity on T2-weighted MR images than articular cartilage. Growth cartilage is highly vascular and enhances after gadolinium administration. Because fractures through unossified growth cartilage, like the cartilage, are not visible on radiographs, detection of such fractures requires MRI, ultrasonography (US), or sometimes intraoperative arthrography (for intra-articular fractures).

Table 42-3	Skeletal Age in Infants: The Method of Sontag, Snell, and Anderson

Mean Total Number of Centers on the Left Side of Body Ossified at Given Age Levels

	Boys		Girls	
Age (months)	Mean No.	SD	Mean No.	SD
1	4.11	1.41	4.58	1.76
3	6.63	1.86	7.78	2.16
6	9.61	1.95	11.44	2.53
9	11.88	2.66	15.36	4.92
12	13.96	3.96	22.40	6.93
18	19.27	6.61	34.10	8.44
24	29.21	8.10	43.44	6.65

Table 42-4	Abnormal Epiphyseal Marrow Signal

Hematopoietic marrow
   Chronic anemia
   Marrow reconversion after chemotherapy
Neoplasm
   Child: Chondroblastoma, eosinophilic granuloma
Infection
Marrow packing with abnormal metabolites (e.g., Gaucher's disease)
Trauma (fracture, hemorrhage, edema)
Osteoarthritis (subchondral cyst, sclerosis, metaplasia)
Osteonecrosis
Bone island (low signal intensity on all sequences)
Orthopedic hardware

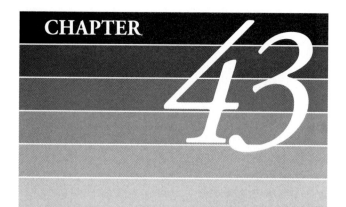

Spine Disorders

SCOLIOSIS
JUVENILE KYPHOSIS AND SCHEUERMANN'S DISEASE
SPONDYLOLYSIS
TRANSITIONAL SEGMENTATION AND KLIPPEL-FEIL
  SYNDROME
CAUDAL REGRESSION SYNDROME

SCOLIOSIS

The normal infant spine is straight. The adult pattern of cervical lordosis, thoracic kyphosis, and lumbar lordosis develops after infancy. *Scoliosis* is lateral curvature of the spine in the coronal plane. Rotatory deformity (vertebral rotation along the long axis of the spine) and abnormal kyphosis or lordosis may coexist. Abnormal spinal alignment can cause cosmetic deformities, and severe scoliosis may decrease the size of the thorax with consequent restriction of pulmonary and cardiac function. Management decisions are complex, but generally depend on the cause of the scoliosis (the single most important issue), the degree of abnormal curvature, the child's age and how much additional spinal growth may be expected, and whether the curvature is increasing over time. Radiographic assessment has an important role in each of these issues.

Key Concepts	Scoliosis

Most cases are idiopathic, but other potential causes must be evaluated: Vertebral body anomalies, neurofibromatosis, tumor, leg-length discrepancy, and neuromuscular condition.

Scoliosis in neurofibromatosis may progress rapidly and become unstable.

Causes of scoliosis are numerous (Tables 43-1, 43-2). Although idiopathic scoliosis is by far the most common

Table 43-1	Causes of Scoliosis

Idiopathic (85%)
Leg-length discrepancy
Congenital
Neuromuscular
Neurofibromatosis
Connective tissue disorders
Trauma
Tumors
Radiation therapy

Table 43-2	Clues That Scoliosis May Not Be Idiopathic

Present at birth
Deformities of vertebral bodies
Multiple limb deformities (arthrogryposis, chromosomal abnormalities)
Convex left thoracic curve (associated with syringomyelia and spinal cord tumors)
Long, C-shaped curve (neuromuscular conditions)
Focal, sharp curve (trauma; focal bony bar; neurofibromatosis, often with kyphosis and vertebral body dysplasia)
History of radiation therapy
Pelvic tilt (leg-length discrepancy)
Pain (osteoid osteoma or other tumor; fracture; infection)

form (85%), it is a diagnosis of exclusion and therefore is discussed last.

Leg-length discrepancy (i.e., unequal leg length) is considered to be significant if greater than 1 to 2 cm. A leg-length discrepancy may be suggested by pelvic tilt on a standing radiograph. Causes of leg-length inequality are numerous. Unilateral leg shortening may be caused by trauma, especially if the physis was injured; slipped capital femoral epiphysis; or congenital conditions, such as infantile coxa vara. Conversely, unilateral leg lengthening may also cause a leg-length discrepancy. Any condition that causes hyperemia near a physis has the potential to accelerate growth at that physis. Potential causes are inflammatory arthritis, high-flow vascular malformation, and fracture. Hemihypertrophy also may cause leg-length discrepancy.

Leg length can be radiographically assessed with a long-cassette, "sliding table" technique (Fig. 43-1), or with a frontal computed tomography (CT) scanogram. This test has the advantage of using the least amount of ionizing radiation. Regardless of the technique, radiographic assessment should be accomplished with gonadal shielding. The landmarks used for determining the length of the femurs and tibias are the tops of the femoral heads, distal medial femoral condyles, and the tibial plafond. Orthopedic intervention for leg-length discrepancy consists of unilateral lengthening of the short leg (Fig. 43-2) or shortening of the longer leg by *epiphysiodesis* (fusion of a physis to prevent further growth; Fig. 43-3).

WHAT THE CLINICIAN WANTS TO KNOW:
SCOLIOSIS RADIOGRAPHS

Position (standing, seated, etc.)
Wearing a brace? Fitted with a heel lift?
Curve location (specify vertebral levels), orientation,
  rotational component
Underlying vertebral body anomalies
Leg-length discrepancy
Report prior surgery if present
Risser stage

Congenital scoliosis is due to abnormalities of formation or segmentation of the vertebral bodies during the first trimester of gestation. Each vertebra (segment) is normally formed from three ossification centers: one for the vertebral body and one for each side of the posterior elements. One of these ossification centers may fail to form or may aberrantly fuse to a center from an adjacent segment. The resulting deformities include misshapen vertebrae, such as hemivertebrae, or a bone or fibrous bar that tethers part of one vertebral body to another (Fig. 43-4). The presence of vertebral body anomalies in a neonate warrants a careful search for associated abnormalities in the VACTERL spectrum (vertebral, anorectal, cardiac, tracheoesophageal fistula, renal, and limb anomalies; Fig. 43-4B) as well as spinal cord anomalies such as tethered cord or diastematomyelia. Spine magnetic resonance imaging (MRI) evaluation should be considered. Including a coronal inversion recovery or fat-suppressed, T2-weighted sequence helps to delineate the misshapen vertebrae from the disks, as the disks are very bright. Treatment of congenital scoliosis is frequently surgical in order to provide stabilization and to prevent further deformity due to asymmetric growth.

A variety of *neuromuscular conditions* cause paraspinal muscle imbalance due to spasticity or flaccidity with resulting scoliosis. Neuromuscular scoliosis tends to be long and

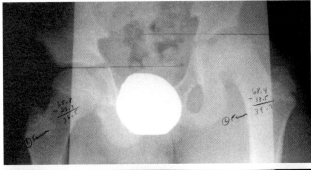
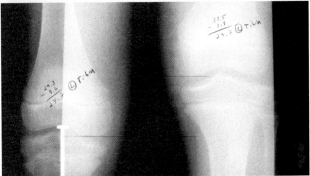
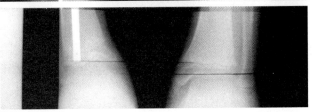

Figure 43-1   Leg-length discrepancy. Scanogram in a child with neurofibromatosis shows a short right tibia that causes a marked pelvic tilt and also caused scoliosis (not shown). The annotations on the film were made by the orthopedic surgeon. The right tibia was short owing to a chronic pseudarthrosis that required resection of the pseudarthroses and pin fixation. The ends of the pin are visible in the right tibia, but the pseudarthrosis is not shown.

C-shaped without compensatory curves above or below (Fig. 43-5). Cerebral palsy, muscular dystrophy, paralysis, and arthrogryposis are frequent causes of neuromuscular scoliosis. Dysplasia or dislocation of one or both hips is a frequently seen association.

Scoliosis associated with *neurofibromatosis* (Fig. 43-6) deserves special mention because of its potential for devastating rapid progression to severe angulation and subluxation that can lead to paralysis. These curves frequently include a kyphotic component and are most frequently seen in the midthoracic spine. Clues to the diagnosis include associated findings of dural ectasia (posterior vertebral body scalloping, enlarged neural foramina) and rib abnormalities (twisted, narrow "ribbon ribs"). The musculoskeletal manifestations of neurofibromatosis are further discussed later in Chapters 33 and 47.

Connective tissue disorders such as Marfan syndrome and Ehlers-Danlos syndrome frequently cause scoliosis. These conditions are reviewed in Chapter 47.

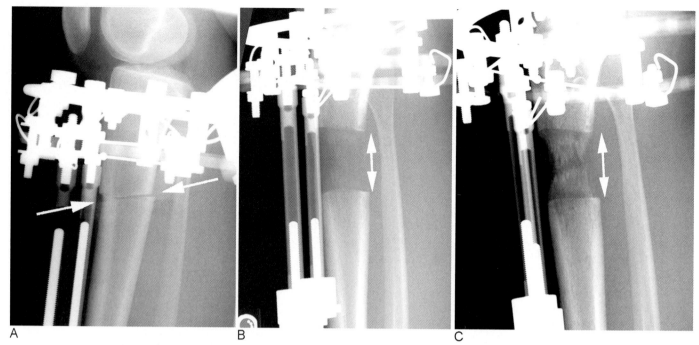

A   B   C

Figure 43-2   Surgical leg lengthening. **A,** Initial study shows a proximal tibial osteotomy *(arrows).* The periosteum was not completely divided. Note the external hardware (only partially shown) that is designed to allow the fragments to be distracted each day by a small amount, usually 1 mm or less because this is the maximal rate of growth of the nerves that are also being elongated. **B and C,** Follow-up views obtained 4 months (B) and 7 months (C) later show new bone formed by the periosteum that will eventually thicken and remodel into normal cortex. Arrows mark the amount of bone lengthening. (Courtesy of Tim Sanders, MD.)

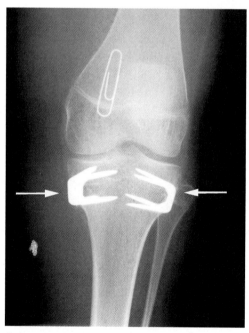

Figure 43-3   Leg shortening by epiphysiodesis. The proximal tibial physis was fused (epiphysiodesis) by fixation with staples *(arrows)* over 1 year previously to allow the shorter contralateral leg (not shown) to catch up. (The paper clip is an artifact.) Note that the distal femoral physis is closing, indicating the completion of growth of both legs. Limbs can also be shortened by resection of a segment of a long bone with plate fixation.

Spine trauma may result in scoliosis. Instrumentation may be required to maintain stability.

Painful scoliosis should prompt a search for an underlying tumor of the spine or spinal cord, stress fracture, or infection. Although a variety of tumors of the vertebrae or spinal canal may cause scoliosis, *osteoid osteoma* is the most common. Vertebral osteoid osteoma usually occurs in the posterior elements. The scoliosis is concave toward the side of the nidus because of ipsilateral muscle spasm. Associated sclerosis may be detected on radiography or CT. Radionuclide bone scanning will reveal intense tracer uptake around the tumor. Computed tomography is the preferred technique for characterization and precise localization of the nidus before resection.

Radiation therapy has the potential to arrest the growth of any portion of the spine included in the radiation field. If only one side of the vertebral column is included in a radiation field in a child, the nonirradiated side will continue to grow, and vertebral body deformity with scoliosis convex away from the radiated side will develop. Associated findings may include hypoplastic ribs on the concave (radiated) side of the curve and a previous history of a childhood Wilms' tumor or other neoplasm. Postradiation scoliosis is fortunately becoming rare as careful attention to radiation ports and effective alternative treatments for childhood tumors have become more common.

Idiopathic scoliosis is by far the most common form of scoliosis, but, as mentioned earlier, is a diagnosis of exclusion. This is a fairly

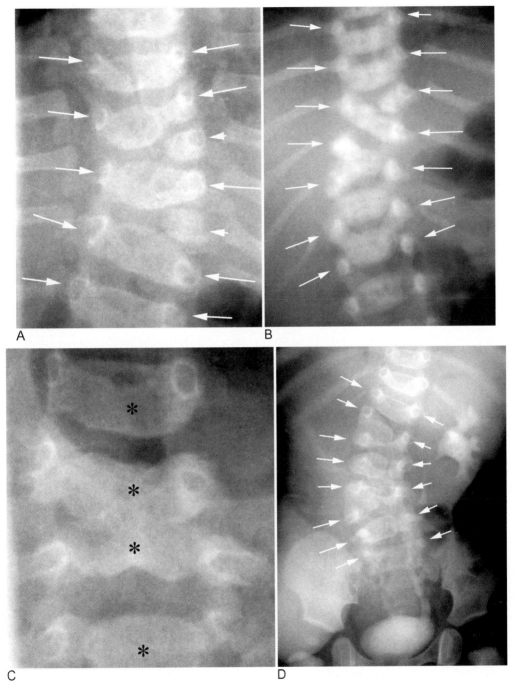

Figure 43-4   Vertebral segmentation anomalies. **A,** Hemivertebrae. The pedicles are marked with arrows. Note the hemivertebrae *(short arrows)* with associated scoliosis. **B,** Segmentation anomalies with fusion abnormalities, hemivertebrae, and scoliosis. The pedicles are marked with arrows. **C,** Failure of segmentation. The vertebral bodies are marked with asterisks. Note the fusion of the two bodies at the center of the image. **D,** Failure of formation and the VACTERL association (vertebral, anorectal, cardiac, tracheoesophageal fistula, renal, and limb anomalies). The pedicles are marked with arrows. Note the greater number of pedicles on the right than the left, with associated scoliosis. The intravenous urogram shows unilateral right renal agenesis. (Courtesy of Stephanie Spottswood, MD.)

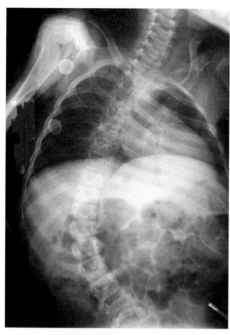

Figure 43-5 Long C-shaped scoliosis due to a neuromuscular condition. (Courtesy of L. Das Narla, MD.)

common condition: it has been estimated that nearly 5% of the population has a curve of 10 degrees or greater. Fortunately, most of these curves are less than 20 degrees. Idiopathic scoliosis is more common in girls (female-to-male ratio, 7:1), and also tends to be more severe in girls. The cause is unknown, although a genetic component has been noted in many cases and muscular imbalance is thought to play a role.

The spinal curvature is usually composed of a primary ("major") curve that may be thoracic, thoracolumbar, or lumbar. Secondary compensatory ("minor") curves are seen above and below the primary curve. A double major S-shaped thoracolumbar curve is seen in many cases (Fig. 43-7). Long-cassette radiographs are a cornerstone of diagnosis and surveillance. Scoliotic curves are measured by the Cobb method. The scoliosis is divided into individual components that are convex toward the right (dextroscoliosis, or simply "right scoliosis") or convex toward the left (levoscoliosis, or "left scoliosis"). The angle formed by the upper endplate of the most cephalad vertebral body and the lower endplate of the most caudad body of the curve is measured for each component. If the endplates are not well seen, then the pedicles are used. The vertebral body or disk space at the apex (midpoint of the angular deformity) of the curve is also noted. It is important to document whether a radiograph was obtained while the child was wearing a body brace, especially when comparing with previous radiographs, because the brace will tend to reduce the scoliotic curvature. Frontal radiographs, obtained with left and right lateral bending, demonstrate how much of a curve is fixed ("structural") from how much is flexible ("functional") and hence correctable by surgery (Fig. 43-8).

The initial radiograph may be obtained anteroposterior (AP) to allow for better assessment for underlying vertebral anomalies or tumors. (The vertebral bodies are closer to the film cassette on an AP radiograph and thus are more sharply rendered.) Follow-up radiographs should be obtained posteroanterior (PA) because the breast and thyroid radiation dose is dramatically reduced by this technique. Routine breast and gonadal shielding should also be used. By optimizing these techniques, radiation dose to the breast and thyroid may be reduced over 50-fold

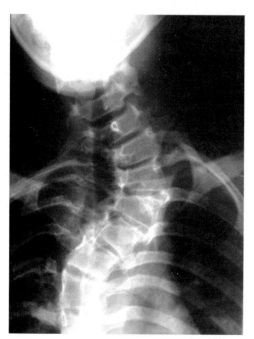

Figure 43-6 Scoliosis in neurofibromatosis. Note the wide interpediculate distance (transverse distance between pedicles) due to dural ectasia.

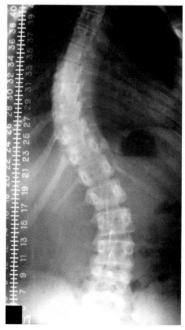

Figure 43-7 Idiopathic scoliosis with a double major curve.

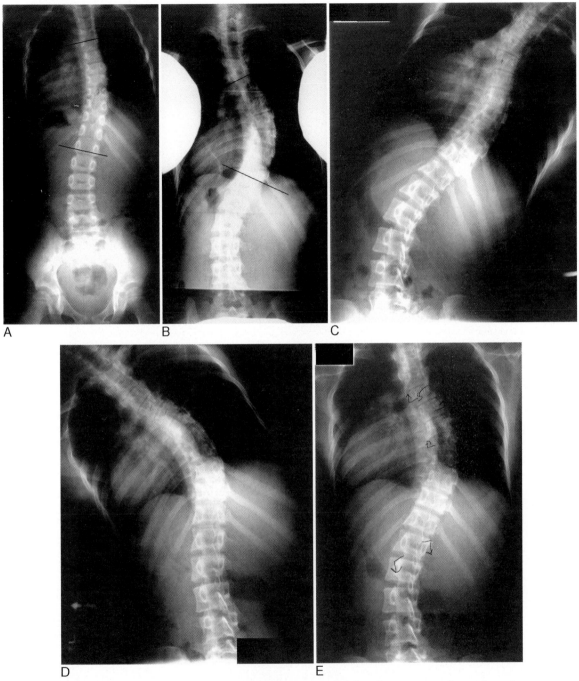

Figure 43-8   Idiopathic scoliosis: the surgeon's perspective. Orthopedic surgeons prefer to view spine radiographs the same way they examine the spine—from the back. Thus, they will view and mark the radiographs with the patient's right to the right. **A,** Standing view in an adolescent girl shows a convex right curve from T5 to L1 that measures 25 degrees. The child was treated with a brace. **B,** Standing PA view obtained 3 years later shows that the curve has progressed despite the bracing and now measures almost 50 degrees. **C and D,** Right (C) and left (D) bending views reveal that the primary curve is partially but not completely correctable. **E,** Preoperative standing radiograph shows the surgeon's planned placement of laminar hooks *(arrows drawn on the radiograph)* as part of spinal fixation.

(Continued)

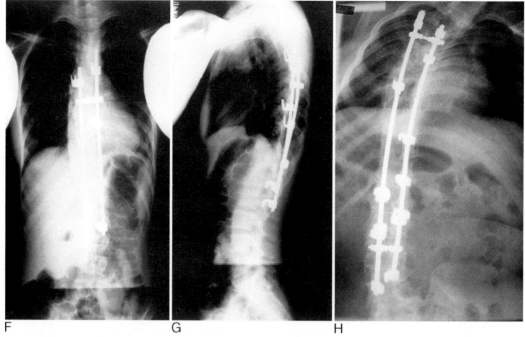

F   G   H

Figure 43-8—(Cont'd)   F and G, Postoperative AP (F) and lateral (G) views show Cotrel-Dubousset hardware with significant improvement in the scoliosis. Note that the primary curve was not corrected beyond the alignment revealed in the preoperative bending views (C). This is because further straightening of the spine would injure the paraspinal supporting soft tissues. H, Cotrel-Dubousset instrumentation in a different patient better demonstrates the appearance of this hardware.

when compared to conventional AP radiographs. This is an important consideration because many children will require dozens of radiographs during their treatment.

Management options in idiopathic scoliosis include observation, bracing, and surgical instrumentation and fusion. Important management decisions require knowledge of the skeletal maturity of the spine and specifically the anticipated completion of spinal growth. Because the ring apophyses of the spine (Fig. 43-9) do not contribute significantly to vertebral growth, their fusion is not a reliable indicator of completion of growth of the spine. Thus, the

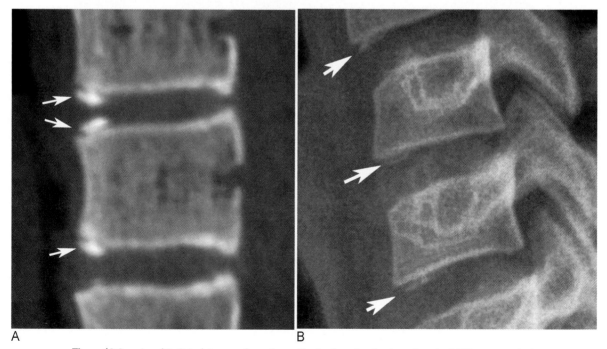

A   B

Figure 43-9   A and B, Spinal ring apophyses *(arrows)* in the thoracic spine (part A, sagittal CT reconstruction) and cervical spine (B).

Risser method described earlier in Chapter 42 is a preferred method for determining spinal maturity in adolescents (see Fig. 42-5). Many surgeons will also use bone age determination by Greulich and Pyle's technique. Less severe curvature tends not to progress after skeletal maturity is attained, and thus is often managed successfully with observation or bracing. A brace is used for a scoliosis of about 25 degrees or greater, or in a younger child with less severe curvature that is rapidly progressing. The goal of bracing is to halt progression of the scoliosis until spinal maturity is reached. Severe curves greater than 50 degrees generally require surgery to prevent respiratory and other complications. It is often preferred to delay surgery until after spinal growth is complete, but very severe or rapidly progressing curves that are not responding adequately to bracing may require earlier surgical intervention.

There are several surgical options, each designed to improve alignment and prevent further progression. The popular techniques combine fixation hardware with fusion of either the posterior elements (posterior fusion) or across the disk spaces (anterior fusion). The importance of the bony fusion must be emphasized because the hardware eventually may fail if spinal fusion is not achieved.

The basic hardware elements used in posterior fusion are rods or plates, hooks, and wires. The famous, early application of orthopedic fixation in management of scoliosis was the Harrington rod (Fig. 43-10). In this technique, a single straight spinal rod was placed along the concave side of the curve. The rod was fixed to the spine by two hooks: one under the inferior margin of the vertebral lamina at the upper end of the curve, and one over the superior margin of the vertebral lamina at the lower end of the curve. The hooks

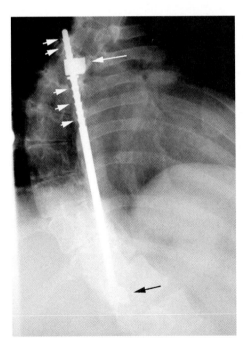

Figure 43-10 Harrington rod. Note the laminar hooks *(long arrows)* and the distinctive serrated contour of the superior portion of the rod *(short arrows).*

were distracted (spread apart), resulting in straightening of the curve, and fixed to the Harrington spinal rod. This system is simple, but it is limited by the amount of force that can be safely applied to just two laminae. In addition, the early Harrington rods were vulnerable to rod fracture owing to their distinctive shape. Current applications of the distracting rod technique tend to use smooth or threaded distracting rods that are less vulnerable to rod failure. Some techniques involve custom-fitted spinal rods, often in pairs, that are fixed to the posterior elements at multiple points. Spinal rods may be fixed to multiple laminae by wires (Luque [Fig. 43-11]) or hooks (Cotrel-Dubousset [Fig. 43-8] and Texas Scottish Rite), or they may be fixed to the spinous processes by wires (Drummond-Wisconsin). Pedicle screws also are frequently employed (Fig. 43-11C). These techniques distribute forces more widely than can be achieved with a single distracting rod, thereby allowing better correction of the curve, better fixation, and reduced risk of hardware failure and fracture. The basic hardware elements used in anterior spinal fusion are vertebral body screws and a cable or rod linkage. The screws are placed transversely in the vertebral bodies, with portions projecting laterally along the convex side of the scoliotic curve. The screws are linked together by a rod (Zielke) or a cable (Dwyer). These systems are used most often for treating neuromuscular or congenital scoliosis. Newer systems of spinal fixation are constantly being developed.

Each system has advantages and disadvantages, and the surgeon's preference often determines which system is used. Because surgical hardware and technique are constantly evolving, the reader is cautioned not to be dogmatic in naming the hardware system seen when interpreting radiographs. In particular, not all rods are Harrington rods! In fact, most are not. It is preferable to use generic terms such as "spinal rod" unless the radiologist is certain of the system that has been implanted.

JUVENILE KYPHOSIS AND SCHEUERMANN'S DISEASE

Juvenile kyphosis is greater than 40 degrees of kyphotic curvature from T3 to T12. Juvenile kyphosis may be caused by any of the many causes of scoliosis (see Table 43-1), or may be idiopathic. Idiopathic forms include postural kyphosis, in which case there are no associated abnormalities, and *Scheuermann's disease* (Fig. 43-12). In the latter condition, thoracic vertebral body wedging, disk space narrowing, and frequently pain and endplate irregularity are present. The cause is unknown but is believed not to be necrosis; it may be due to a congenital endplate weakness or repetitive microtrauma. Scheuermann's disease is seen equally in males and females and preferentially affects the lower thoracic spine. Some authorities consider Scheuermann's disease to be a type of osteochondrosis. This concept was discussed in Chapter 3.

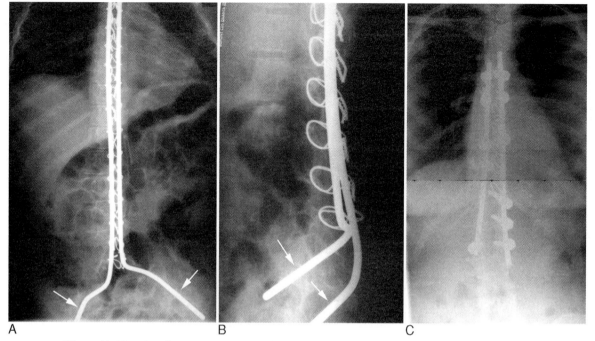

Figure 43-11 Spinal instrumentation. **A and B,** Luque fixation. AP (A) and lateral (B) radiographs show that custom curved spinal rods are fixed to the laminae at multiple levels by wires. Note the extension of the spinal rods into the iliac bones *(arrows),* termed the "Galveston technique." **C,** Many surgeons use hybrid systems with laminar wires, laminar hooks, and pedicle screws.

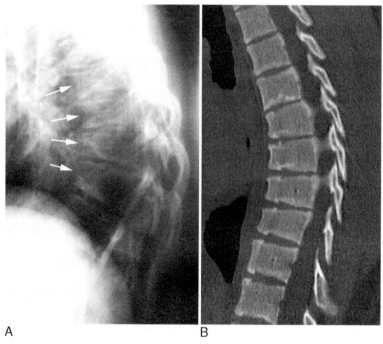

Figure 43-12 Scheuermann's disease. **A,** This teenage boy had painful, clinically evident kyphosis. Note the wedging of several adjacent midthoracic vertebral bodies *(arrows)* with irregular vertebral body endplates. **B,** Sagittal CT reconstruction in a different teenager shows similar findings.

SPONDYLOLYSIS

Spondylolysis is interruption of the pars interarticularis of the posterior elements (Fig. 43-13). Although the rare cervical spondylolysis is probably congenital, it is generally thought that the more common lumbar spondylolysis is acquired during childhood as a form of stress fracture. These fractures occur more frequently in children who participate in activities with extreme lumbar spine extension, such as gymnastics. There also appears to be a genetic predisposition in some cases. L5 is the most commonly affected level. Bilateral spondylolysis may result in *spondylolisthesis* (anterior displacement of the affected vertebral body relative to the body below) that is graded by the degree of displacement. Grade 1 spondylolisthesis is anterior displacement of the superior vertebral body by up to 25% of the AP dimension of the endplate. Grade 2 spondylolisthesis is displacement of 25% to 50%. Grade 3 is displacement by 50% to 75%, and grade 4, by 75% to 100%. Spondylolisthesis tends not to progress after about age 20, but may become painful after that age. Spinal fusion is sometimes required.

Spondylolysis may be detected with oblique radiographs, where the defect is seen as a break in the neck of the famous "scottie dog" (see Fig. 43-13). Bilateral spondylolysis often may be appreciated on a coned lateral radiograph centered at the affected level. Computed tomography is the optimal method with which to detect and characterize these lesions (see Fig. 43-13). Radionuclide bone scanning may reveal increased tracer uptake at the affected side in a subacute or healing defect, at the contralateral side due to increased mechanical stress or an additional impending spondylolysis, or bilaterally. Single photon emission CT (SPECT) imaging helps to localize the tracer uptake to the posterior elements. These lesions may be difficult to detect on routine MRI scans unless spondylolisthesis is present. Marrow edema may be seen in pars stress fractures on inversion recovery images, although this finding may be very subtle.

Incomplete formation of a pedicle is occasionally encountered and may suggest an aggressive process. Computed tomography will show intact cortex at the defect and no soft tissue mass (Fig. 43-14).

TRANSITIONAL SEGMENTATION AND KLIPPEL-FEIL SYNDROME

A spectrum of spinal abnormalities may result from abnormal formation and segmentation of the vertebral bodies, as noted earlier in the discussion of congenital scoliosis. Two common variations of congenital spinal segmentation anomalies that merit further discussion are transitional segmentation of the lumbosacral spine and the Klippel-Feil syndrome.

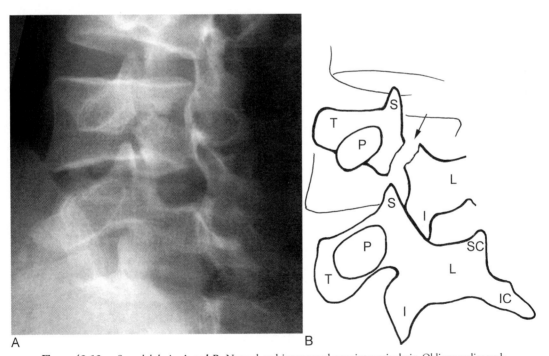

A   B

Figure 43-13   Spondylolysis. **A and B,** Normal and interrupted pars interarticularis. Oblique radiograph (A) and corresponding line drawing (B) show an intact pars interarticularis at L5 and a pars defect with a collar around the "Scottie dog's" neck at L4 (*arrow* in part B). P, pedicle (the Scottie dog's eye); T, transverse process (nose); S, superior articulating facet (ear); I, inferior articulating facet (front leg); L, lamina (body); IC, contralateral inferior articulating facet (rear leg); SC, contralateral superior articulating facet (tail).

(Continued)

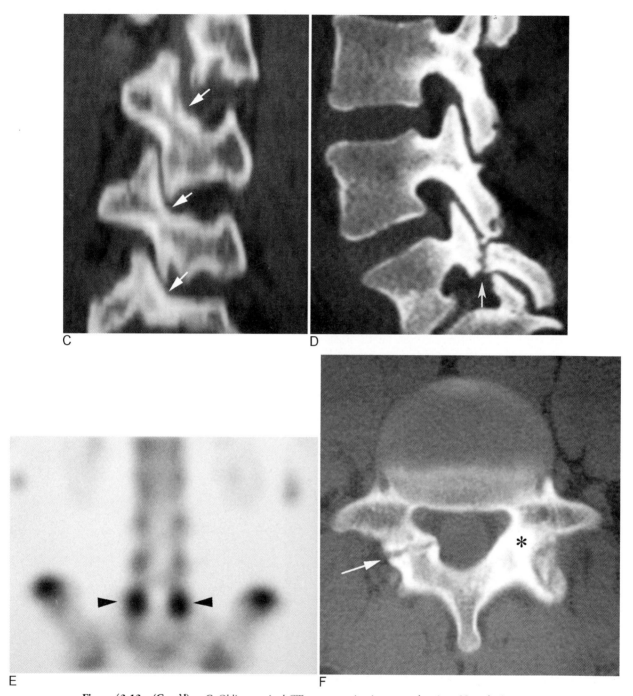

Figure 43-13—(Cont'd) C, Oblique sagittal CT reconstruction in a normal patient. Note the intact pars interarticularis *(arrows)*. D, Sagittal CT reformat shows a pars defect in L5 *(arrow)*. E, Radionuclide bone scan of bilateral L5 pars defects. Coronal single photon emission (SPECT) image obtained through the posterior elements shows increased tracer bilaterally at L5 *(arrowheads)*. A CT scan (not shown) was needed to confirm bilateral defects, as a unilateral defect with adaptive hypertrophy on the contralateral side could have similar bone scan findings. F, Axial CT image of unilateral spondylolysis. Note the spondylolysis on the right *(arrow)*. Also note the sclerosis of the contralateral pars interarticularis *(asterisk)*. This nonspecific finding may indicate that left-sided adaptive changes caused increased stress because of the right-sided pars defect, or an impending left pars stress fracture.

(Continued)

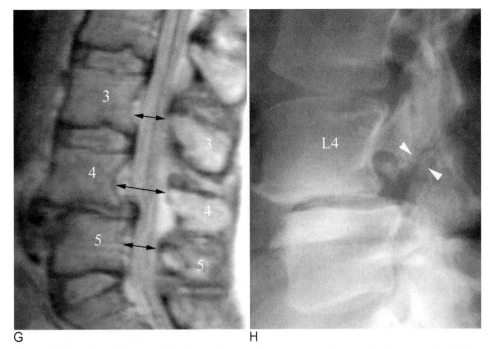

Figure 43-13—(Cont'd)   G and H, Bilateral L4 spondylolysis with grade 1 spondylolisthesis at L4–L5. The sagittal proton density weighted MR image (G) shows the spondylolisthesis, but, as is often the case, the pars defects could not be seen on the MR images. Because the most common cause of mild spondylolisthesis is disk degeneration, which is present in this case, it would be easy to overlook the pars defects. However, note the greater AP dimension of the spinal canal at L4 compared with the levels above and below *(arrows,* the numbers mark the vertebral bodies anteriorly and the corresponding spinous processes posteriorly). This focal widening is an important clue to the correct diagnosis of spondylolysis with spondylolisthesis. The lateral radiograph (H) clearly reveals the pars defects *(arrowheads).* Bilateral pars defects are often easy to see on a lateral view. (Part C courtesy of Fred Laine, MD.)

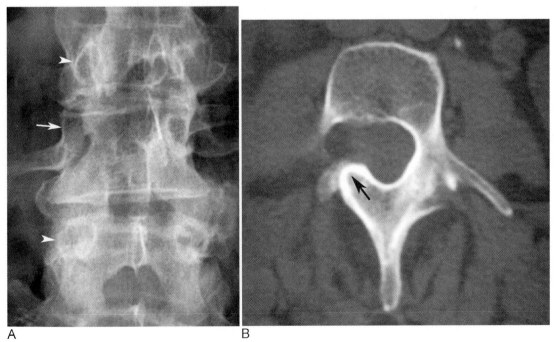

Figure 43-14   Congenital absence of a pedicle. **A,** AP radiograph shows absent right lumbar pedicle *(arrow).* Contrast with normal ring shadow of normal pedicles *(arrowheads).* **B,** Axial CT shows intact cortex *(arrow)* adjacent to the defect.

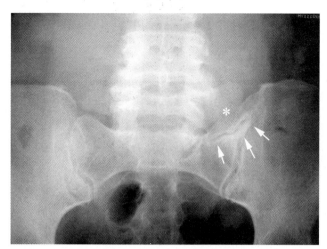

Figure 43-15   Transitional lumbosacral segmentation. AP radiographic view of the lower lumbar spine shows wide transverse process of the lowest lumbar segment *(asterisk)*, with a false joint formation with the sacrum. Note the sclerosis along this joint *(arrows)*.

Transitional segmentation refers to congenital variation from the standard arrangement of seven cervical, 12 thoracic, and five lumbar vertebrae and five sacral segments. Transitional segmentation occurs most frequently in the lumbosacral spine. Numerous variations may be seen. A common form of transitional segmentation is a transitional lumbosacral segment, with morphologic features intermediate between a lumbar vertebra and a sacral segment (Fig. 43-15). Assigning a numeric level to each vertebra (e.g., L1, L2) can be somewhat arbitrary. Consistency is essential when correlating different studies in order to direct spine surgery to the intended level. Guidelines to assist in assigning numbers to lumbar vertebra are based on findings in "normal" spines: a chest radiograph usually shows 12 rib pairs but may show 11 or 13 rib pairs; a line connecting the top of the iliac crests usually passes through L4–L5; the widest transverse processes usually occur at L3, and, on MRI, the left renal vein is usually located anterior to L1–L2.

Klippel-Feil syndrome is failure of cervical segmentation at multiple levels, with a short neck with low hairline (Fig. 43-16). Cervical motion is limited owing to the paucity of normally formed disks and facet joints. Associated findings may include renal; spinal cord; and inner-, middle-, and outer-ear abnormalities. The term Klippel-Feil is also often used less narrowly to describe any congenital fusion anomaly encountered in the cervical spine (Fig. 43-17). Such abnormalities most frequently are isolated to a single disk level and are asymptomatic. The congenitally fused segments tend to be short in the AP dimension.

Approximately one third of patients with Klippel-Feil syndrome have *Sprengel's deformity* (Fig. 43-18). Sprengel's

deformity is tethering of the scapula to the cervical spine by a fibrous band or an anomalous bone *(omovertebral bone)* that results in a high position of the scapula and reduced shoulder mobility.

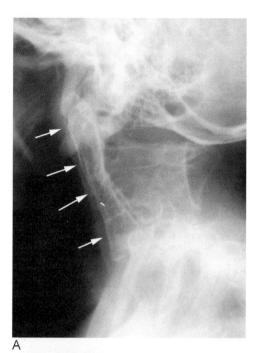

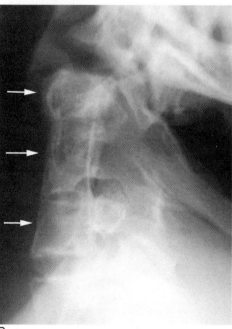

Figure 43-16   Klippel-Feil syndrome. **A,** Lateral cervical spine radiograph shows absent segmentation of several cervical segments *(arrows)*. **B,** Different patient with similar findings *(arrows)* on a lateral radiograph.

(Continued)

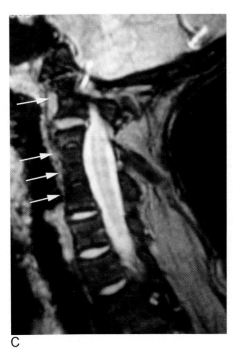

C

Figure 43-16—(Cont'd)   **C,** Different patient with similar findings *(arrows)* on a sagittal T2-weighted MR image.

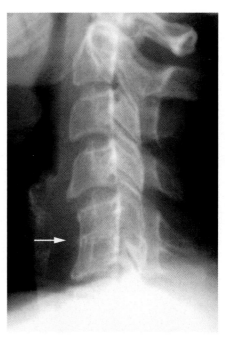

Figure 43-17   Absent segmentation at C5–C6 *(arrow)*. Note the narrow AP dimension of the fused vertebral bodies, which distinguishes this finding from a mature surgical fusion. Juvenile rheumatoid arthritis could have a similar appearance but would involve more levels.

CAUDAL REGRESSION SYNDROME

The *caudal regression syndrome,* also known as the caudal dysplasia sequence, is a spectrum of caudal axial skeletal and associated neurologic and soft tissue defects caused by an insult to the caudal mesoderm and ectoderm early in the first trimester. A wide spectrum of spinal defects may result, ranging from subtle partial sacral agenesis to complete absence of the sacrum, lumbar spine, and caudal thoracic spine (Fig. 43-19). Other axial skeletal findings may include spina bifida; spinal stenosis; an angular, wedge-shaped conus medullaris; and presacral (anterior) meningocele. Clinical findings also are highly varied, ranging from mild leg weakness to bowel and bladder control difficulties to anorectal atresia, renal aplasia, and pulmonary hypoplasia. Sagittal MRI in some cases reveals a characteristic angular contour of the malformed conus medullaris (Fig. 43-19B). The caudal regression syndrome is much more frequent in children of diabetic mothers, but most cases are sporadic.

Caudal regression syndrome has been associated with congenital fusion of the lower extremities (*sirenomelia,* Fig. 43-20), but these most likely are unrelated conditions. Sirenomelia is associated with severe oligohydramnios. This condition is named after the Greek mythical creatures called sirens or mermaids who, with their sweet songs, lured sailors to their deaths on rocky reefs and coastlines.

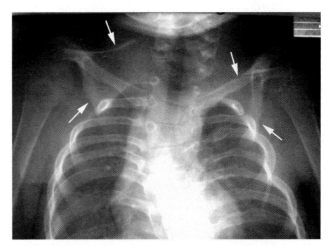

Figure 43-18   Sprengel's deformity. Compare the position of the scapulae *(arrows),* with the right higher than the left. Also note the upper thoracic spinal segmentation anomalies with associated scoliosis.

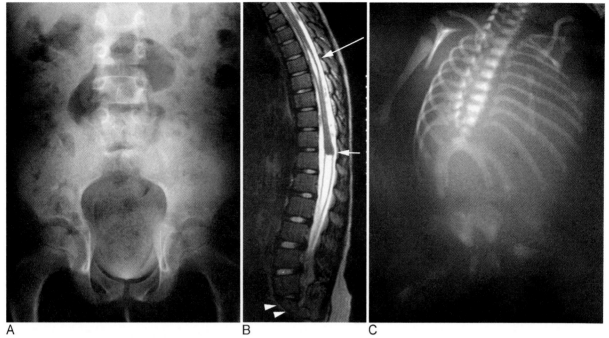

A   B   C

Figure 43-19   Sacral agenesis (caudal regression syndrome). **A,** This radiograph was obtained after intravenous urography (note the contrast medium in the bladder). Note the absence of the mid- and lower sacrum. Also note the large amount of stool in the colon due to related colon dysfunction. **B,** Sagittal T2-weighted MR image shows the characteristic angular contour of the conus medullaris *(short arrow)*. This finding is not always present in sacral agenesis, however. Note the syrinx *(long arrow)*, a finding that can occur in association with caudal regression. Also note the small sacrum *(arrowheads)*. **C,** Severe case. Note the complete absence of the lumbar spine and sacrum.

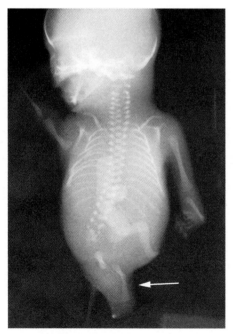

Figure 43-20   Sirenomelia. Note the fused, dysplastic lower extremities *(arrow)*.

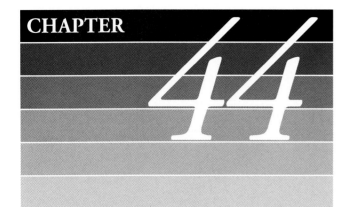

Congenital and Developmental Hip Disorders

DEVELOPMENTAL DYSPLASIA OF THE HIP
    Imaging of DDH
        Radiography
        Ultrasonography
        Arthrography, MRI, and CT
    Management of DDH
PROXIMAL FOCAL FEMORAL DEFICIENCY
COXA VARA AND COXA VALGA
PRIMARY PROTRUSIO OF THE ACETABULUM (OTTO PELVIS)

Legg-Calvé-Perthes disease (avascular necrosis [AVN] of the pediatric hip) is discussed in Chapter 22 (Avascular Necrosis). Slipped capital femoral epiphysis is discussed in Chapter 11 (Hip).

DEVELOPMENTAL DYSPLASIA OF THE HIP

Developmental dysplasia of the hip (DDH), congenital hip dislocation, and congenital dislocation of the hip are terms often used interchangeably, although each term reflects different nuances of what may be considered a diverse group of abnormalities of the newborn and infant hip. These conditions have in common hip dysplasia or dislocation at birth, or more frequently *the potential to develop dysplasia and possibly dislocation later in infancy and childhood.* True congenital hip dislocation is relatively infrequent. It may occur in association with severe congenital defects, such as Chiari II malformation or arthrogryposis, in which case it is termed *teratogenic* or *pathologic dislocation.* Pathologic dislocations are usually readily detected at birth by physical examination and confirmed with radiographs. Congenital hip dislocation may also occur as an isolated abnormality in otherwise normal neonates because of severe hip laxity. The hip dislocation in such neonates may be intermittent, and easy to reduce and redislocate. An experienced clinician usually reliably detects this condition, but radiographs are occasionally of some use (e.g., in

excluding an underlying teratogenic condition). The most insidious and most frequent form of neonatal hip dysplasia is merely mild hip laxity or a shallow acetabulum at birth. This seemingly innocuous situation has the potential to progress over a period of months and years to significant hip dysplasia, hip dislocation, and early osteoarthritis. Because the initial abnormalities are so minimal, they may not be detected by physical examination or by radiographs. The term *developmental dysplasia of the hip* is generally preferred to describe this progressive condition, as it emphasizes that dislocation was not present a birth.

Key Concepts	Developmental Dysplasia of the Hip (DDH)

Deformity and subluxation of the hip, usually developmental rather than congenital. Often completely curable if diagnosed and treated early.
Delayed diagnosis leads to decreased joint mobility, pain, and early osteoarthritis.
Radiographs are of limited utility in neonates.
US is highly sensitive, but usually is best performed after about age 3–4 weeks because of false-positive findings in neonates.

Developmental dysplasia of the hip is a frequent condition (1 case per 1000 births) and is bilateral in one third of cases. Several risk factors have been identified (Table 44-1). These include female gender (female-to-male ratio, 6:1, due to increased sensitivity to maternal hormones that relax ligaments); intrauterine positioning, such as breech presentation that tends to lever the femoral head out of the acetabulum, and genetic and cultural factors. The left hip is more frequently affected because the fetal spine is usually to the maternal left in a fetus in vertex presentation.

Table 44-1	Risk Factors for Development Dysplasia of the Hip (DDH)

Mechanical (In Utero "Packaging Problems")
Breech birth
Oligohydramnios
First born ("unstretched" uterus)
Large birth weight
Genetics
Females
Family history
Native Americans (may be entirely cultural)
White persons
Cultural: Papoosing, Swaddling
Native Americans
Lapps
Musculoskeletal Associations
Contralateral DDH
Torticollis
Scoliosis
Ehlers-Danlos syndrome (generalized joint laxity)
Neuromuscular imbalance (e.g., cerebral palsy)

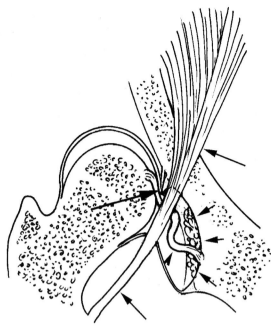

Figure 44-1 Chronic hip subluxation: associated soft tissue changes. Pulvinar *(short arrows)*. Elongated ligamentum teres *(arrowhead)*. Labrum flipped medially ("inverted limbus," *large long arrow*). Tight psoas tendon stretched across the anterior joint capsule *(small long arrows)*.

This places the fetal left knee against the unyielding maternal spine, which tends to displace the left knee anteriorly relative to the mother and medially relative to the fetus and lever the femoral head out of the acetabulum. The practice in some cultures of papoosing infants with the hips adducted and extended increases the risk of DDH. (In contrast, backpack-style child carriers do not carry this risk because they hold the hips in flexion and abduction.)

The ligamentous laxity that initiates DDH results in abnormal femoral head mobility. The femoral head may become "decentered" relative to the acetabulum. The acetabulum adapts to the abnormal femoral head mobility by becoming wider and shallower ("acetabular dysplasia") as it attempts to accommodate the abnormal range of motion of the femoral head. A vicious cycle, consisting of worsening ligamentous laxity, femoral head subluxation, and acetabular dysplasia, may ensue. Muscle pull and weight bearing tend to direct the femoral head out of the acetabulum in a superior and lateral direction. In advanced cases, the femoral head dislocates completely and flattens along its superomedial margin as it abuts the lateral aspect of the ilium.

A variety of soft tissue changes may occur in chronic hip subluxation that can impede or completely block hip reduction (Fig. 44-1). Fibrofatty tissue, termed *pulvinar* (pillow), can fill the acetabulum. The acetabular labrum may flip inferiorly against the medial margin of the subluxed femoral head, termed an *inverted limbus.* A tight psoas tendon may stretch across the hip joint medial to the laterally displaced femoral head, resulting in an hourglass configuration of the joint capsule. The adductor muscles also are shortened by the superior migration of the femoral head. The ligamentum teres, which extends from the femoral head to the center of the acetabulum, becomes elongated and redundant.

> **WHAT THE CLINICIAN NEEDS TO KNOW: DEVELOPMENTAL DYSPLASIA OF THE HIP (DDH)**
> Hip location (subluxed or dislocated?)
> Subluxable with stress maneuvers?
> Acetabular maturity (alpha angle, coverage of femoral head, acetabular angle on radiographs)

Superior femoral head migration is eventually halted by tightening of the surrounding connective tissues, which helps to alleviate the hip instability but is associated with loss of hip joint mobility. A broad shallow depression can develop in the lateral ilium adjacent to the dislocated femoral head, termed a *pseudoacetabulum,* as the body attempts to adapt to the abnormal position of the femoral head and form a stable hip joint (Fig. 44-2). Pain and early osteoarthritis are late complications, even in comparatively mild cases. Hip replacement surgery may be required as early as the fourth decade of life.

Imaging of DDH

Radiography and ultrasonography (US) are the cornerstones of imaging of DDH. Ultrasonography is ideally suited to assessment of the neonatal hip because it provides excellent visualization of the cartilaginous femoral head and unossified acetabulum without exposure to ionizing radiation, and it allows for dynamic assessment of hip joint stability. Radiography is of limited value in the newborn period

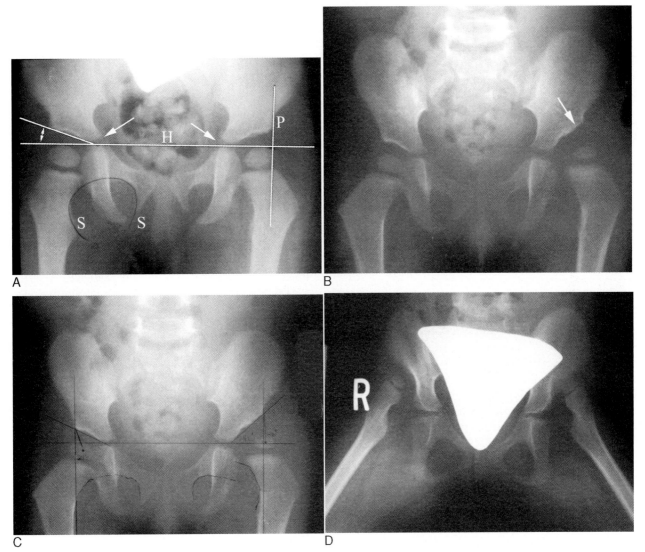

Figure 44-2   Radiography of developmental dysplasia of the hip (DDH). **A,** Normal hips. Arrows mark the triradiate cartilages. Double arrow marks the acetabular angle (acetabular index). Note that the femoral heads are symmetric in size and are nearly completely covered by the acetabular roofs. The acetabular angle is less than 30 degrees. H, Hilgenreiner's line; P, Perkin's line; S, Shenton's arc (arc drawn in black). **B,** Left DDH. Note the shallow acetabular roof, early pseudoacetabulum *(arrow),* superolateral subluxation of the left femoral head, and small size of the left femoral epiphysis compared with the normal right side. **C,** Same radiograph as in part B, after review by an orthopedic surgeon. The lines shown on part A have been marked on the film, as well as the center-edge angle. The normal right acetabular angle is 24 degrees. The dysplastic left hip acetabular angle is 42 degrees. The right center-edge angle is 21 degrees (normal), and the left is −3 degrees. Also note the discontinuity of Shenton's arc on the left. **D,** Bilateral hip dislocations in a child with cerebral palsy.

(Continued)

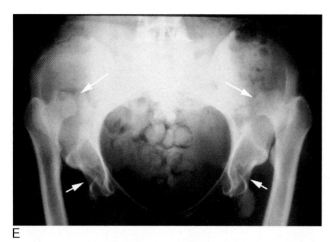

Figure 44-2—(Cont'd) E, Untreated DDH: late sequelae in 35-year-old woman with bilateral, severe, untreated DDH. Note the superior bilateral femoral head dislocations *(long arrows)*. Also note the dysplastic acetabula *(short arrows)*. This patient was able to ambulate but was developing progressive hip pain that required bilateral hip arthroplasties.

because the capital femoral epiphyses are not ossified at birth. In infants older than about 3 months of age, the capital femoral epiphyses begin to ossify and both techniques are useful. After about 6 months of age, shadowing from the increasing ossification of the capital femoral epiphyses obscures the acetabulum and limits the role of US to selected cases. Arthrography, computed tomography (CT), and magnetic resonance imaging (MRI) can be highly useful in specific situations that are discussed in the following paragraphs.

Radiography

Radiographic evaluation of DDH requires a well-positioned anteroposterior (AP) radiograph (see Fig. 44-2). The symphysis pubis and coccyx should be superimposed or very nearly superimposed on a properly positioned AP radiograph (assuming that neither is deformed). A series of lines and curves are drawn on the radiograph as part of the assessment of DDH. *Hilgenreiner's line* (think "H for horizontal," also called the Y-Y line) is drawn horizontally through the center or top of the bilateral radiolucent triradiate cartilages. The triradiate cartilage is the confluence of the ilium, ischium, and pubis slightly anterior to the center of the acetabulum. It is formed by cartilage of the three bones that make up the pelvis, hence its name. *Perkin's line* is drawn perpendicular to Hilgenreiner's line (think "P for perpendicular") through the superolateral corner of the acetabular roof. The ossified portion of the capital femoral epiphysis should be entirely or nearly entirely medial to this line. Compare each side. A difference in acetabular coverage of the ossified portion of the femoral heads by as little as 2 to 3 mm is considered by some authors to be significant. Lateral femoral

head subluxation may also be quantified by measuring the *center-edge angle* that is formed by Perkin's line and a line drawn through anterior inferior iliac spine and the center of the capital femoral epiphysis. A normal center edge-angle is about 20 degrees in infancy and 26 to 30 degrees in adolescence. A fourth line is drawn between the triradiate cartilage and the anterior inferior iliac spine of each hip. The angle formed by this line and Hilgenreiner's line is the *acetabular angle* or *acetabular index*. A useful rule of thumb is that the acetabular angle should be 30 degrees or less. The reader should note that 30 degrees is a useful oversimplification. In fact, the acetabular angle normally decreases as the child grows, and, on average, is about 2 degrees; it is greater in normal girls than boys. Also note that a nearly horizontal acetabular roof is abnormal. A nearly horizontal acetabular roof is seen in several syndromes and skeletal dysplasias, and is further discussed later in Chapter 46. *Reimer's migration index* is a common measurement of hip dysplasia in children with cerebral palsy, whose dysplasia is not DDH but rather due to muscle imbalance. The migration index is the percentage of the transverse width of the ossified capital femoral epiphysis lateral to Perkin's line. *Shenton's arc* is drawn along the medial and superior obturator foramen and medial-proximal femur. This arc is interrupted or elongated if the femoral head is subluxed. Finally, some hips with DDH have a smaller ossified capital femoral epiphysis on the affected side. This is a nonspecific finding, as some asymmetry may be normal.

Limitations of radiography in DDH include limited assessment of the hips of neonates because the capital femoral epiphyses are not ossified at birth, the potential for incorrect acetabular angle measurements if the radiograph is improperly positioned, the lack of dynamic imaging, and the use of ionizing radiation.

Ultrasonography

The initial application of US to infants with DDH emphasized static coronal imaging, simulating an AP radiograph. An elaborate system of measurements and categories was developed, termed the Graf system in honor of the Austrian orthopedic surgeon Reinhard Graf, MD, who developed this approach. The subsequent application of real-time US by the American pediatric radiologist H. Theodore Harcke, MD, and others pioneered the dynamic assessment of hip stability. Posteriorly oriented stress, similar to the Barlow maneuver used in screening newborns for hip dislocation, can detect hip laxity in infants with a subluxable or a dislocatable hip that might be normally located on static images. Current practice of hip US incorporates features of both approaches (Figs. 44-3 and 44-4), although some institutions prefer to emphasize the detailed morphologic assessment of the Graf system, while others emphasize the dynamic assessment of hip stability. An overview of a popular hybrid approach is described in Chapter 50.

Regardless of the radiologist's preferred technique, complete US assessment of the infant hip always includes documentation of the position of the femoral head relative to the acetabulum, the contour of the acetabular roof, hip stability, and the alpha angle. The osseous portion of the acetabular roof should cover at least half of the cartilaginous femoral head. The contour of the osseous acetabular roof should be straight or gently concave, matching the contour of the cartilaginous femoral head. The cortex of the roof of the acetabulum and the lateral ilium should meet at a sharp angle that is not rounded. The angle formed by the acetabular roof and the lateral ilium is the *alpha angle* (see Fig. 44-3D). *A normal alpha angle is 60 degrees or greater,* although lower values (as low as 55 degrees) may be accepted in newborns if there are no other findings to suggest DDH. The *beta angle,* a component of the Graf system, is the angle formed by the lateral ilium and the inferior surface of the labrum (see Fig. 44-3D). A normal beta angle is roughly 55 degrees or less. If the femoral head is subluxed laterally, the beta angle will be greater than 55 degrees. The beta angle is not routinely measured unless the complete Graf system is used.

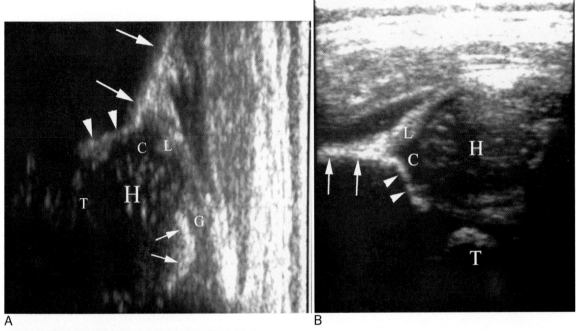

Figure 44-3 US of developmental dysplasia of the hip (DDH): Coronal images. **A,** Coronal image of the left hip oriented to simulate an AP radiograph. The lateral margin of the ilium *(large arrows)* is seen as an echogenic line with posterior acoustic shadowing. Note the osseous roof of the acetabulum *(arrowheads),* the unossified (cartilaginous) portion of the acetabular roof, and adjacent hyperechoic labrum, and the cartilaginous femoral head. The hypoechoic triradiate cartilage is located at the anterior margin of the center of the acetabulum. This image was obtained with the hip extended; note the lateral margin of the ossified portion of the proximal femur *(small arrows)* and a portion of the cartilaginous greater tuberosity. **B and C,** Normal standard coronal image (two different infants). Superior is to the viewer's left and lateral is toward the transducer. The transducer has been positioned to display the lateral margin of the ilium as a straight line parallel to the transducer *(long arrows),* with the center of the cartilaginous femoral head and the triradiate cartilage toward the right side of the image. Note that the osseous portion of the acetabular roof *(arrowheads),* which is straight in part B and slightly concave in part C, covers at least 50% of the femoral head (just barely in part A). Note the hypoechoic cartilaginous acetabular roof and the echogenic labrum and capsule. Also note the overlying muscle layers, labeled in part C: gluteus maximus, gluteus medius, and gluteus minimus.

(Continued)

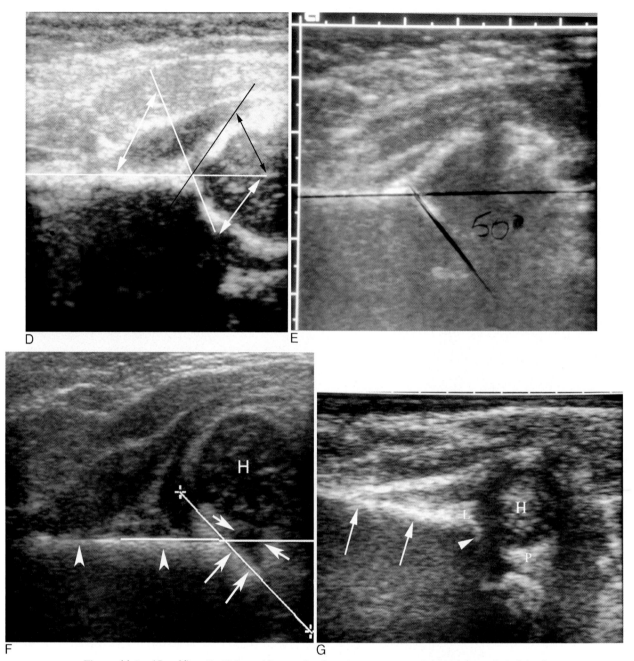

Figure 44-3—(Cont'd) D, Alpha and beta angles. Same image as in part C. The alpha angle is formed by the osseous acetabular roof and the lateral ilium *(white lines and arrows)*. The beta angle is formed by the lateral ilium and the inferior surface of the labrum *(black line, black arrows)*. The beta angle is not widely used. **E**, Mild DDH. The alpha angle is 50 degrees, and slightly less than 50% of the femoral head is covered by the acetabulum. **F and G**, Severe DDH (different infants). In both cases, the femoral head is subluxed superiorly and laterally (i.e., toward the transducer). Note the very shallow angle formed by the ilium *(arrows)* and the steep osseous acetabular roof *(arrowheads)*. **F**, Inverted limbus (between *short arrows*): the echogenic capsule and labrum are interposed between the femoral head and the acetabulum *(long arrows mark the acetabular roof, arrowheads mark the lateral ilium)*. **G**, Pulvinar as echogenic tissue filling the acetabulum medial to the femoral head. All images: *arrows* mark the lateral ilium; *arrowheads* mark the acetabular roof. C, cartilaginous portion of acetabular roof; H, femoral head; G, greater tuberosity; L, labrum; max, gluteus maximus; med, gluteus medius; min, gluteus minimus; P, pulvinar; T, triradiate cartilage.

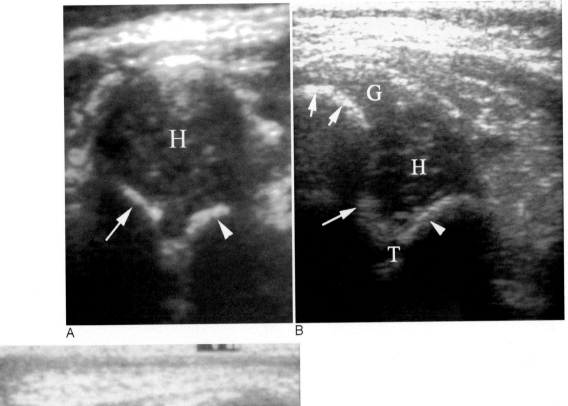

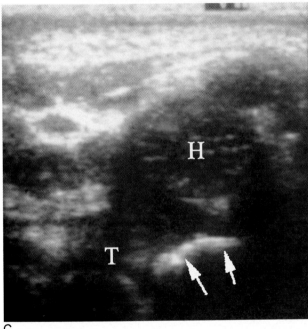

Figure 44-4   US of developmental dysplasia of the hip (DDH): axial images. **A and B,** Normal axial image (two different infants). The transducer is positioned to display the center of the femoral head centered over the triradiate cartilage, between the pubis anteriorly *(arrow)* and the ischium posteriorly *(arrowhead).* **B,** US image obtained approximately parallel to the flexed femur; note the cartilaginous apophysis of the greater tuberosity and the ossified portion of the proximal femur *(short arrows).* **C,** Severe DDH, oblique axial image. The transducer was angled to include the triradiate cartilage at the center of the acetabulum, and the subluxed femoral head. The femoral head is subluxed superiorly, laterally, and posteriorly over the ilium *(arrows).* G, greater tuberosity; H, femoral head; T, triradiate cartilage.

Limitations of US include operator dependence, limited visualization of the acetabulum in older infants due to shadowing from the ossifying capital femoral epiphysis, and potential for false-positive findings in the immediate neonatal period. The latter is due to transient, physiologic hip ligamentous laxity in neonates caused by residual maternal hormonal effects. False-positive neonatal scans can result in unnecessary follow-up examinations and overtreatment. Therefore, it is generally recommended that the first US examination be delayed until the child is 4 to 6 weeks old in order to avoid such false-positive results. However, if clinical findings are sug-

gestive of a dislocated or unstable hip, then earlier US may be appropriate.

Arthrography, MRI, and CT

Arthrography and MRI allow visualization of the femoral head, acetabular cartilage, and potential soft tissue impediments to reduction such as pulvinar, inverted limbus, tight psoas tendon, and redundant ligamentum teres. Arthrography is usually performed by an orthopedic surgeon at the time of closed or open reduction of a chronically subluxed or dislocated hip (Fig. 44-5). Computed tomography is often used to determine whether reduction with casting has successfully aligned the femoral head and acetabulum (Fig. 44-6). Low-dose technique should be used in this setting by obtaining only four or five slices with a low-mA technique (30 mAs). Both US and MRI may also be used to document hip joint alignment in this setting (Fig. 44-6C). In addition, gadolinium-enhanced MRI and possibly US may also allow assessment of the integrity of the femoral head blood supply after closed reduction. This is not a

trivial matter, as AVN of the femoral head is an infrequent but potentially catastrophic complication of hip reduction with casting. Early identification of femoral head ischemia allows this complication to be avoided. Finally, CT with three-dimensional reconstruction can be used to help the orthopedic surgeon assess the shape of a dysplastic acetabulum before surgical modification of the acetabulum (acetabuloplasty, see discussion later in this chapter). In the adult with hip dysplasia, MR arthrography is used to evaluate for labral deformity and tear, chondral defects, and pulvinar and hypertrophic ligamentum teres.

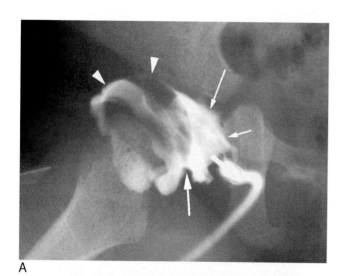

A

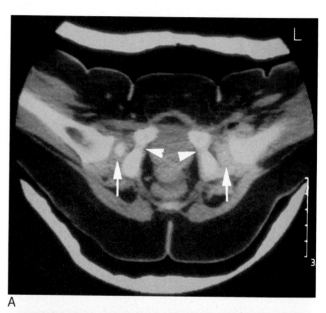

A

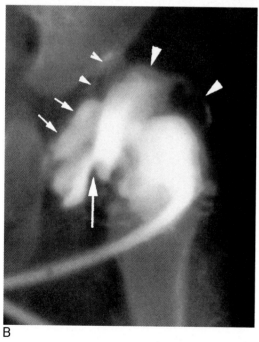

B

Figure 44-5 Developmental dysplasia of the hip (DDH): arthrography. Compare to Fig. 44-1. **A and B,** Both studies show the radiolucent cartilaginous femoral head *(arrowheads),* filling defect from pulvinar *(small arrows),* and hourglass shape of the capsule *(large arrow).* **B,** Arthrogram also shows an inverted limbus *(small arrowheads).*

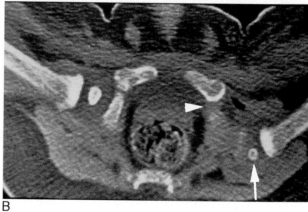

B

Figure 44-6 Developmental dysplasia of the hip (DDH): imaging after reduction and casting. **A,** Good reduction of left DDH. Axial CT through the hip joints shows both femoral heads *(arrows)* to be adjacent to the triradiate cartilages *(arrowheads).* The left capital femoral epiphysis ossification center is smaller than the normal right side, a frequent finding in DDH. **B,** Poor reduction of left DDH. The left femoral head *(arrow)* is subluxed posteriorly relative to the triradiate cartilage *(arrowhead).* The right hip is normal.

(Continued)

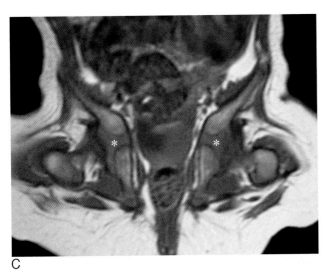

Figure 44-6—(Cont'd) C, Poor reduction of bilateral DDH. Coronal T1-weighted MR image obtained through the triradiate cartilages *(asterisks)* should also show both femoral heads, but neither is seen. Axial images (not shown) revealed both femoral heads to be posteriorly dislocated.

Management of DDH

Management of DDH depends on the age of the patient and the severity of the dysplasia. Very mild dysplasia may resolve spontaneously. A harness that holds the hips in flexion, mild abduction, and mild external rotation may be used (Pavlik harness, Fig. 44-7). This position keeps the femoral head within the center of the acetabulum, allowing healthy

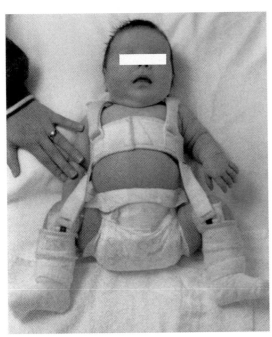

Figure 44-7 Pavlik harness.

acetabular growth. The infants and their parents tolerate this treatment well, and follow-up US can be performed with the harness in place. After a few months, the acetabulum will deepen and the hip joint capsule will tighten (Fig. 44-8). No further intervention will be needed.

Advanced dysplasia in older children requires aggressive therapy, and a completely normal outcome is often impossible. The main goal of the orthopedic surgeon is to return the femoral head to the center of the acetabulum and keep it there with a brace, cast, or surgical modification of the femoral neck or acetabulum. Closed reduction may be combined with casting or skeletal traction. Soft tissue impediments to closed reduction may require correction, including releasing tight adductor or psoas tendons. *Varus osteotomy* of the proximal femur (i.e., an osteotomy of the proximal shaft that produces varus alignment of the femoral neck) tends to enhance hip reduction and stability.

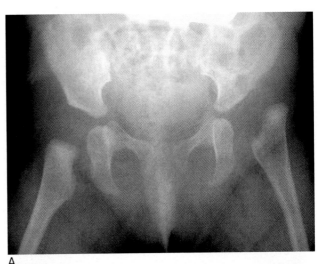

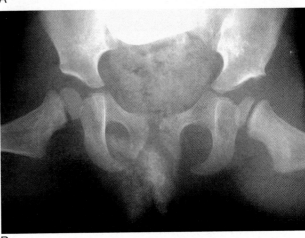

Figure 44-8 Successful treatment with a Pavlik harness. **A,** Radiograph during the first week of life shows a left hip dislocation and shallow left acetabulum. The right is normal. **B,** Radiograph at approximately age 8 months shows near-normal left hip.

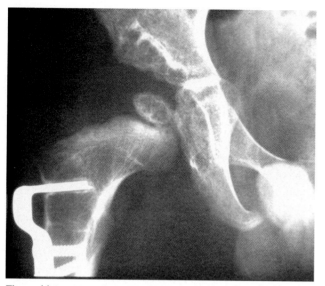

Figure 44-9 Varus derotation osteotomy. A blade plate and screws (not completely shown) were used to fix the varus-producing osteotomy. This procedure directs the femoral head more directly into the acetabulum.

Excessive femoral anteversion is a frequent complication of advanced DDH. Anteversion is defined and discussed further in the section on torsion at the end of this chapter. A "derotation osteotomy," also performed through the proximal femoral shaft, corrects excessive femoral anteversion and results in better containment of the femoral head within the acetabulum. These procedures are frequently combined (*varus derotation osteotomy;* Fig. 44-9). A variety of surgical modifications of the acetabulum have been developed (Fig. 44-10). All increase acetabular coverage of the femoral head and are used variably, depending on the patient age, morphology of the acetabulum, and preference of the surgeon.

Any procedure for treatment of DDH has the potential to compromise the blood supply to the femoral head. Some centers routinely image children placed in spica casts with gadolinium-enhanced MRI, searching for delayed contrast enhancement of the femoral heads as a sign of diminished blood supply.

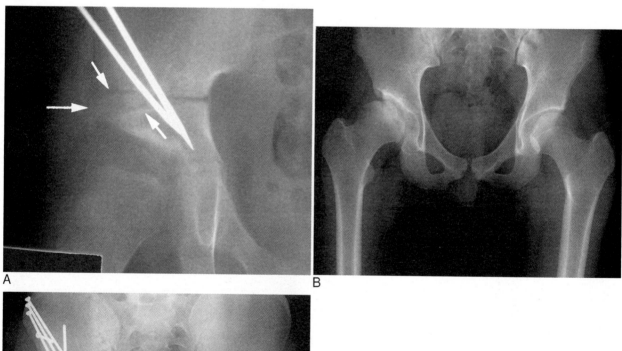

Figure 44-10 Acetabular osteotomy for developmental dysplasia of the hip (DDH). **A,** Salter osteotomy. The ilium has been divided transversely, a wedge opened and fixed with a bone plug *(arrows),* resulting in a more horizontal alignment of the acetabular roof. **B,** Woman with DDH and early secondary osteoarthritis. **C,** Ganz osteotomy was performed. This procedure rotates the entire acetabulum to contain the femoral head.

PROXIMAL FOCAL FEMORAL DEFICIENCY

Proximal focal femoral deficiency (PFFD) refers to a spectrum of congenital deficiency (hypoplasia or aplasia) of the proximal femur (Fig. 44-11). The condition may be bilateral. Curiously, the abnormalities in PFFD tend to be centered roughly at the intertrochanteric femur. Mild cases have only hypoplasia of a short segment of intertrochanteric femur, with a normal femoral head and hip joint. The hypoplastic segment may be composed of uncalcified cartilage or bone. More severe cases have hypoplasia of the femoral head with resulting acetabular dysplasia, or absence of the proximal femoral shaft, resulting in a gap (deficiency) in the femur between the head and shaft with overall femoral shortening. The most severe cases of PFFD involve absence of nearly the entire femur (Fig. 44-11C). Both US and MRI can assist in characterizing the femoral deficiency and the status of the hip joint. Associated abnormalities include congenital absence of the ipsilateral fibula and foot deformities. Most cases are evident at birth because the affected leg is short. The goal of treatment is to maximize function of the affected limb. Mild cases do not benefit from surgery.

COXA VARA AND COXA VALGA

The angle formed by the femoral neck and shaft is normally 150 degrees at birth. This angle decreases throughout development to reach an average angle of about 125 degrees in normal adults. Increase in this angle is coxa valga, and decrease is coxa vara.

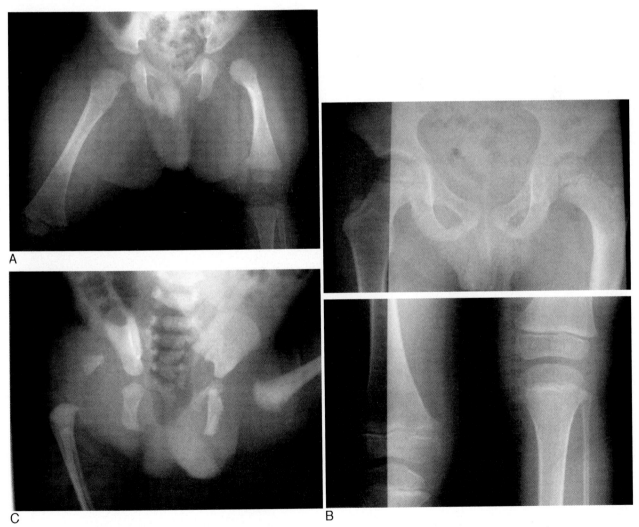

Figure 44-11   Proximal focal femoral deficiency: spectrum of abnormalities. **A,** Mild case in a 2-month-old. Note the normal left acetabulum, which indicates that the femoral head is present. **B,** Same patient at age 4 years. The proximal femur has ossified but is short and dysplastic. **C,** Severe case with presence only of the most distal right femur. Note the shallow acetabulum, which indicates that there is no right femoral head.

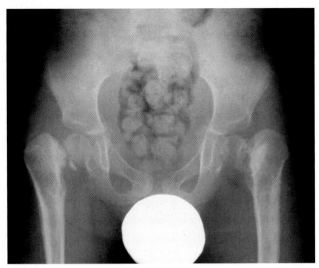

Figure 44-12   Congenital coxa vara. The findings in this 4-year-old were unchanged from birth.

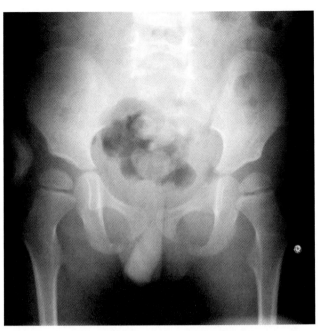

Figure 44-13   Bilateral coxa valga.

Coxa vara in children may be divided into congenital, infantile, and acquired forms. *Congenital coxa vara* probably results from a limb bud insult in the first trimester of gestation. In this manner it is similar to proximal focal femoral deficiency, and both may occur in the same patient. Congenital coxa vara tends to worsen little, if at all, after birth (Fig. 44-12). In contrast, *infantile coxa vara* (also termed developmental coxa vara) progresses as the child grows, with resulting limb-length discrepancy. Infantile coxa vara is often bilateral (up to 50%), but otherwise usually occurs as an isolated abnormality. Surgery is often required to manage this progressive condition. *Acquired coxa vara* may be caused by trauma to the proximal femoral physis, notably slipped capital femoral epiphysis, metabolic conditions that cause bone softening (notably rickets and osteomalacia), and tumors, skeletal dysplasias, and fibrous dysplasia and Paget's disease in adults.

Coxa valga in children usually reflects decreased tone of the muscles that cross the hip and decreased ambulation. Neuromuscular conditions such as cerebral palsy are the most frequent cause of coxa valga (Fig. 44-13).

PRIMARY PROTRUSIO OF THE ACETABULUM (OTTO PELVIS)

Protrusio acetabuli is abnormal medial position of the femoral head compared to the pelvis. Protrusio acetabuli is present if the medial margin of the femoral head touches or crosses a line connecting the lateral margins of the pelvic inlet and the obturator foramen on an AP radiograph of the pelvis (Fig. 44-14). Protrusio may occur transiently as a normal variant in preadolescents, and should not persist into adulthood. Unilateral or bilateral protrusio acetabuli can

occur *secondary to* rheumatoid arthritis and rheumatoid variants, osteoarthritis, Turner's syndrome, Marfan syndrome, pelvic fracture, and "bone softening" conditions such as osteogenesis imperfecta, Paget's disease, fibrous dysplasia, osteomalacia, and renal osteodystrophy. In contrast, *primary*

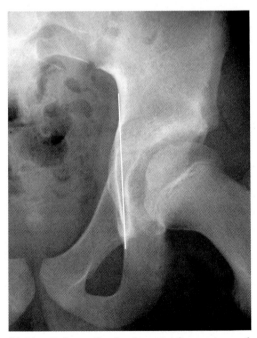

Figure 44-14   Reference line for diagnosis of protrusio acetabuli. The femoral head should not touch or cross the line drawn between the lateral margins of the pelvic inlet and the obturator foramen. This example is normal.

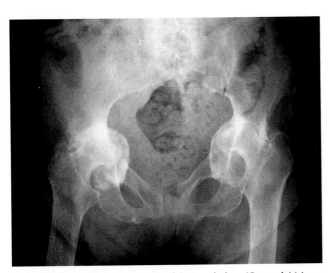

Figure 44-15 Primary protrusio of the acetabulum (Otto pelvis) in an adult with bilateral secondary osteoarthritis.

protrusio of the acetabulum (Otto pelvis) refers to severe bilateral protrusio acetabuli that appears to occur as a developmental malformation (Fig. 44-15), although this is controversial. The cause is unknown, but abnormal acetabular remodeling appears to contribute. Otto pelvis is more frequent in women and is often familial. It may not be discovered until adulthood. Mild protrusio is frequently incidental. Severe protrusio, such as an Otto pelvis, is associated with pain, obstetrical complications, and premature osteoarthritis.

CHAPTER 45

Common Congenital Foot Deformities and Tarsal Coalitions

COMMON CONGENITAL FOOT DEFORMITIES
TARSAL COALITION

COMMON CONGENITAL FOOT DEFORMITIES

The most common foot deformities can be described in a straightforward manner, using descriptors and occasional measurement of only three parameters: hindfoot equinus, hindfoot varus or valgus, and forefoot varus or valgus. This chapter first describes these parameters, and then relates them to the common foot deformities. Foot deformities should be evaluated on anteroposterior (AP) and lateral weight-bearing radiographs, or with equivalent position in infants.

Hindfoot equinus is the easiest concept of the three. It is evaluated only on a lateral weight-bearing radiograph. Normally, the calcaneus is dorsiflexed relative to the plantar surface of the foot. If measurement is desired, the angle between the longitudinal axis of the tibia and the calcaneus (measured along its base) ranges between 60 and 90 degrees (Fig. 45-1). Another way of measuring the alignment of the calcaneus is "calcaneal pitch," where on a lateral view a line drawn along the base of the calcaneus should slant upward from the horizontal surface by 20 to 30 degrees. The relationship of the calcaneus is abnormal if it is plantarflexed or excessively dorsiflexed. Plantarflexion of the calcaneus such that the calcaneal-tibial angle is greater than 90 degrees represents hindfoot equinus (see Fig. 45-1B). Hindfoot equinus is seen in clubfoot and congenital vertical talus. The opposite occurs with hindfoot calcaneus, where the calcaneus is excessively dorsiflexed such that the calcaneal-tibial angle is less than 60 degrees (Fig. 45-1C). Hindfoot calcaneus is seen in cavus and spastic deformities.

The second parameter in evaluating a foot deformity is the presence of *hindfoot varus or valgus*. Both AP and lateral weight-bearing radiographs are used for this evaluation. Conceptually, the talus may be considered the point of reference because it may be assumed to be fixed relative to the lower leg. Although this is

Key Concepts	Congenital Foot Deformities: Terminology

Weight-bearing radiographs.
Hindfoot equinus: Calcaneus plantarflexed.
Hindfoot calcaneus: Calcaneus is excessively dorsiflexed (calcaneal-tibial angle is less than 60 degrees).
Hindfoot varus: Talocalcaneal angle less than 15 degrees (AP radiograph)—talus and calcaneus look parallel.
Hindfoot valgus: Talocalcaneal angle greater than 40 degrees (AP radiograph).
Forefoot varus: Forefoot is inverted and often slightly supinated. Metatarsals parallel in AP and lateral radiographs.
Forefoot valgus: Forefoot is everted and often pronated. First metatarsal most plantar on lateral radiograph.
Clubfoot : Hindfoot equinus, hindfoot varus, and forefoot varus.
Congenital vertical talus (rocker bottom foot): Talus in extreme plantarflexion with dorsal dislocation of the navicular, hindfoot equinus, valgus hindfoot, dorsiflexed and valgus forefoot.
Flexible flatfoot deformity (pes planovalgus): Hindfoot valgus, forefoot valgus, but no equines. Weight-bearing radiographs definitely required!
Pes cavus: High arched foot (hindfoot calcaneus) with compensatory plantarflexion of the forefoot.
Metatarsus adductus: Forefoot adduction, normal hindfoot.

not exactly correct, for the purpose of this discussion, let us assume that the calcaneus rotates medially or laterally with respect to a fixed talus. On an AP view, the *talocalcaneal angle* is described by lines drawn through the longitudinal axis of the talus and calcaneus. The AP talocalcaneal angle normally measures 15 to 40 degrees (30 to 50 degrees in newborns). You might note also that in the normal foot the midtalar line passes through or slightly medial to the base of the first metatarsal. The midcalcaneal line passes through the base of the fourth metatarsal (Fig. 45-2). If you

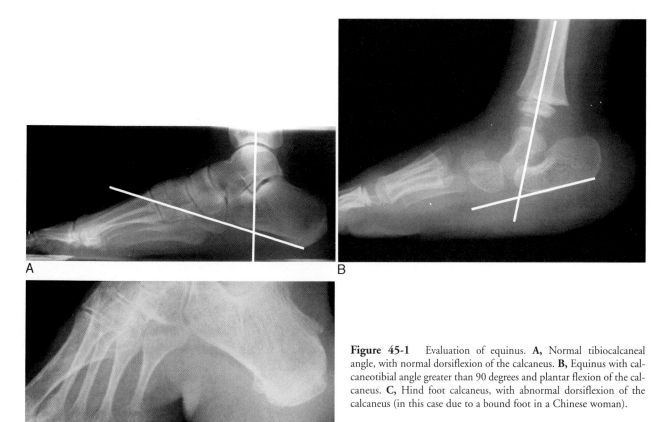

Figure 45-1   Evaluation of equinus. **A,** Normal tibiocalcaneal angle, with normal dorsiflexion of the calcaneus. **B,** Equinus with calcaneotibial angle greater than 90 degrees and plantar flexion of the calcaneus. **C,** Hind foot calcaneus, with abnormal dorsiflexion of the calcaneus (in this case due to a bound foot in a Chinese woman).

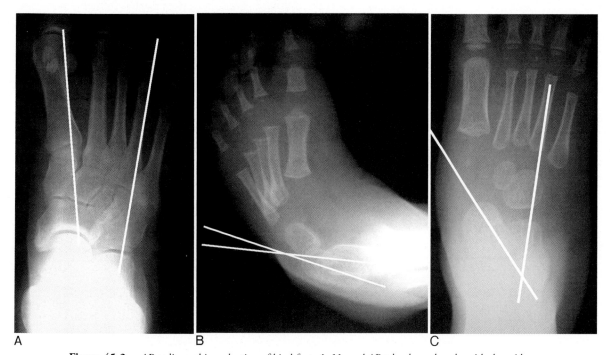

Figure 45-2   AP radiographic evaluation of hind foot. **A,** Normal AP talocalcaneal angle, with the midtalar line passing through the base of the first metatarsal and the midcalcaneal line passing through the base of the fourth metatarsal. **B,** AP evaluation of hindfoot varus, with a decreased talocalcaneal angle and the talus pointing lateral to the first metatarsal base. **C,** AP evaluation of hindfoot valgus, with an increased talocalcaneal angle and the talus pointing medially to the first metatarsal base.

presume, then, that the talus is fixed and the calcaneus internally rotates, the talocalcaneal angle decreases to less than 15 degrees, to the point that in some cases the talocalcaneal angle may approach 0 degrees or parallelism of those bones. A talocalcaneal angle less than 15 degrees is hindfoot varus (see Fig. 45-2B). In classic cases, the angle is 0 degrees. You might note that in a hindfoot varus deformity, the talus ends up pointing lateral to the first metatarsal because the entire foot is swung medially. The opposite occurs when the calcaneus externally rotates relative to the talus. A talocalcaneal angle greater than 40 degrees is hindfoot valgus. Note also that with this increased talocalcaneal angle, the talus points medial to the first metatarsal because the calcaneus and the entire foot swings laterally (Fig. 45-2C).

As noted previously, hindfoot varus or valgus is also evaluated on the lateral view. Normally, the lateral talocalcaneal angle (also termed *Kite's angle*) is measured by a line bisecting the talus and a line along the base of the calcaneus, measur-

ing 25 to 45 degrees (50 degrees in newborns). The calcaneus is dorsiflexed, as already discussed, and the talus is mildly plantarflexed to produce this angle (Fig. 45-3). Consider now the case when the calcaneus internally rotates (hindfoot varus). With the anterior portion of the calcaneus moving into a position beneath the head of the talus, the talus can no longer be as plantarflexed. This results in a decrease in the talocalcaneal angle on the lateral view, with the two bones approaching parallelism (see Fig. 45-3B). This is the appearance on the lateral view of a hindfoot varus. Thus, on both the AP and lateral views, with a hindfoot varus deformity the talocalcaneal angles decrease and the bones approach parallel. Consider now the situation where the calcaneus externally rotates, hindfoot valgus as seen on the AP view in Fig. 45-2C. With external rotation of the calcaneus, the anterior calcaneus no longer supports the head of the talus and the talus is allowed to further plantar flex. On the lateral view, then, we

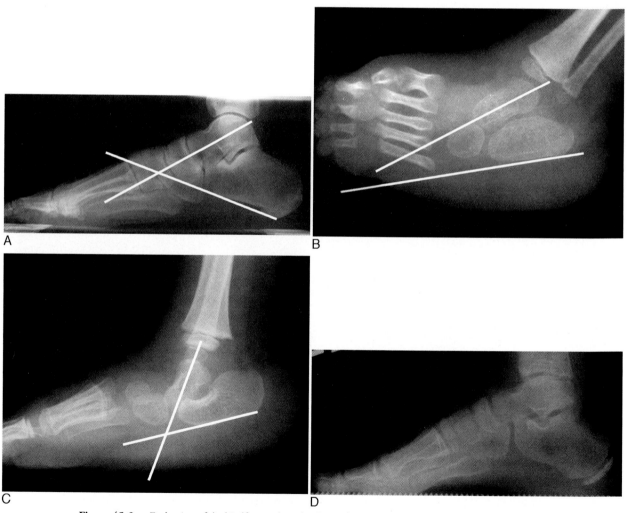

Figure 45-3 Evaluation of the hindfoot on lateral radiography. **A,** Normal hindfoot, with a normal lateral talocalcaneal angle. **B,** Varus hindfoot, with a decreased talocalcaneal angle. **C,** Valgus hindfoot, with an increased talocalcaneal angle. **D,** Pes cavus (hindfoot valgus, high longitudinal arch).

see increased plantarflexion of the talus, which results in an increased talocalcaneal angle (Fig. 45-3C). This is the appearance of hindfoot valgus on the lateral view. Thus, with hindfoot valgus there is an increased talocalcaneal angle on both AP and lateral radiographs.

With hindfoot equinus and hindfoot varus or valgus described, that leaves forefoot varus or valgus to be understood. This is a much more qualitative and subjective evaluation. On the AP radiograph, the metatarsals normally converge proximally with slight overlap at the bases (Fig. 45-4A). With forefoot varus, the forefoot is inverted and often slightly supinated. On the AP radiograph, then, the forefoot would appear narrowed, with an increased convergence at the bases of the metatarsals (Fig. 45-4B). With forefoot valgus, the forefoot is everted and often pronated. With this change in position, on the AP radiograph the forefoot is seen to be broadened with a decrease in overlap at the metatarsal bases (Fig. 45-4C). Consider now the appearance of the forefoot on the lateral view. Normally, the metatarsals are partially superimposed, with the fifth metatarsal in the most plantar position (Fig. 45-5A). With forefoot varus (inversion, often with supination), the metatarsals on the lateral view have a more ladder-like arrangement, with the first metatarsal in the most dorsal position and the fifth metatarsal in the most plantar position (Fig. 45-5B). On the other hand, with forefoot valgus (eversion and pronation), the metatarsals are usually more superimposed on one another on the lateral radiograph, and the first metatarsal is in the most plantar position (Fig. 45-5C).

We are now in a position to discuss the common foot deformities. The deformity most frequently studied with radiographs is *clubfoot* (talipes equinovarus; *talipes* means any deformity of the foot involving the talus). Clubfoot is seen in 1 in 1000 births, more frequently in males than females (male-to-female ratio, 2–3:1). The cause of the clubfoot deformity is unclear, but possible contributing factors include ligamentous laxity, muscle imbalance, intrauterine position deformity, and persistence of an early normal fetal relationship. The radiographic findings of a clubfoot deformity are hindfoot equinus, hindfoot varus, and forefoot varus (Fig. 45-6).

Congenital vertical talus (*rocker bottom foot*) is a deformity in which the talus is in extreme plantarflexion with dorsal dislocation of the navicular, locking the talus into plantarflexion. Radiographically, one sees an equinus deformity, valgus hindfoot, dorsiflexed and valgus forefoot, and abnormal talus with dislocated navicular (Fig. 45-7A, B). Congenital vertical talus clinically presents as a rigid flat foot and may occur in isolation or as part of a variety of syndromes, and frequently is associated with myelomeningocele.

Flexible flatfoot deformity (*pes planovalgus*) is relatively common, affecting 4% of the population. An important part of the diagnosis is that it is indeed flexible; the abnormality

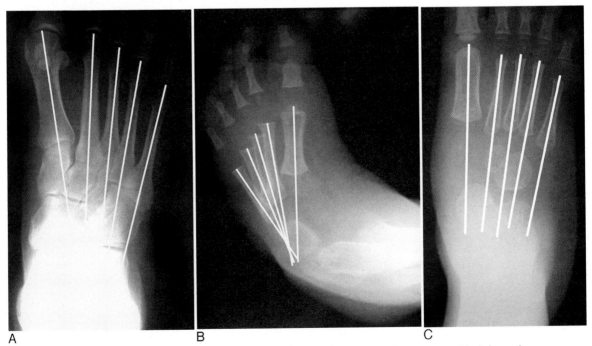

Figure 45-4   AP evaluation of the forefoot. **A,** The normal appearance of convergence with slight overlap at the bases of the metatarsals. **B,** Forefoot varus, with abnormally increased convergence at the bases of the metatarsals. **C,** Forefoot valgus, with divergence or at least a decrease in the overlap at the bases of the metatarsals.

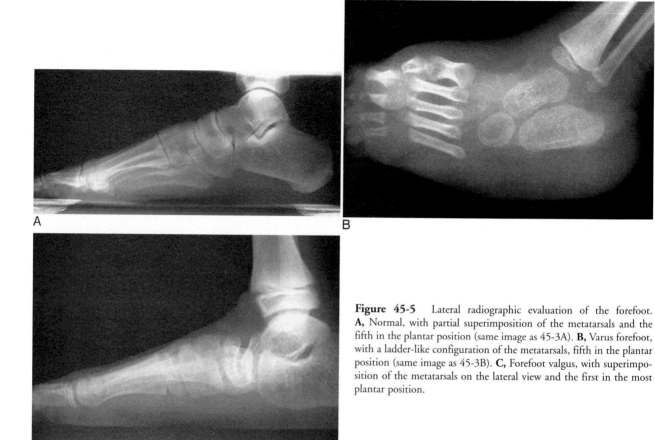

Figure 45-5 Lateral radiographic evaluation of the forefoot. **A,** Normal, with partial superimposition of the metatarsals and the fifth in the plantar position (same image as 45-3A). **B,** Varus forefoot, with a ladder-like configuration of the metatarsals, fifth in the plantar position (same image as 45-3B). **C,** Forefoot valgus, with superimposition of the metatarsals on the lateral view and the first in the most plantar position.

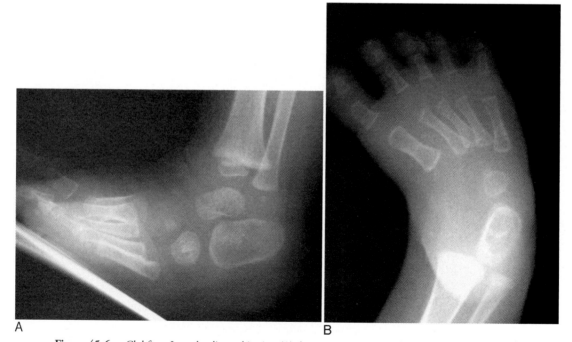

Figure 45-6 Clubfoot. Lateral radiographic view (A) demonstrates equinus of the hindfoot. Both the AP (B) and lateral views show a varus hindfoot (decreased talocalcaneal angle, with the bones nearly parallel). Both views show forefoot varus. The lateral view is obtained with dorsiflexion force (the equivalent of a weight-bearing view in an infant), which diminishes the apparent forefoot varus. See Fig. 45-5B for the appearance of the forefoot in clubfoot without application of dorsiflexion stress.

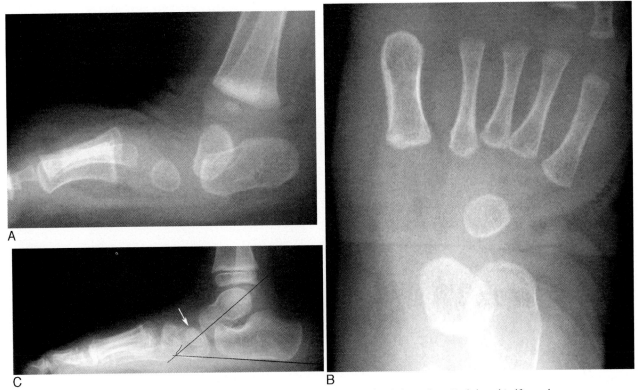

Figure 45-7   Congenital vertical talus (rocker bottom foot) and planovalgus. Both have hindfoot valgus. **A and B,** Congenital vertical talus. Note the hindfoot equinus and hindfoot valgus (increased talocalcaneal angle), with the talus being nearly vertical on the lateral view. Both views show forefoot valgus. Note that the navicular *(arrow)* is dorsal relative to the talar head. **C,** Planovalgus. Hindfoot valgus is present with forefoot valgus, like congenital vertical talus, but the hindfoot is not in equinus and the navicular *(arrow)* is aligned with the talus.

is seen only on weight-bearing radiographs and the deformity is reduced with non–weight-bearing radiographs. The flexible flatfoot deformity has a hindfoot valgus and forefoot valgus, but no equinus (Figs. 45-7C, 45-8). The valgus deformities are usually subtler than those of a congenital vertical talus.

Pes cavus is a high arched foot (hindfoot calcaneus) with compensatory plantarflexion of the forefoot. It is seen in patients with upper motor neuron lesions (Friedreich's ataxia), lower motor neuron lesions (polio), vascular ischemia as in Volkmann's contracture, and muscular dystrophy of the peroneal type (Charcot-Marie-Tooth disease).

Metatarsus adductus is the most common structural abnormality of the foot, seen in infancy 10 times more frequently than clubfoot. Radiologists do not see it as frequently because it usually is not imaged. Metatarsus adductus is usually bilateral and more common in females than males. The radiographic findings are of forefoot adduction, with a normal hindfoot (Fig. 45-9).

The commonly acquired bunion deformity is first metatarsal varus and hallux valgus. Although this is an adult condition, it probably begins in many cases during the teenage years. Ill-fitting shoes are a main cause, and women outnumber men.

Foot deformities that combine varus and valgus hindfoot and forefoot deformities are usually due to spastic neuromuscular conditions such as cerebral palsy.

TARSAL COALITION

Tarsal coalition is osseous, cartilaginous, or fibrous fusion between bones of the hindfoot or midfoot. Tarsal coalition occurs in 1% of the population, and is bilateral in about one fourth of these patients. Most are isolated and are due to a failure of segmentation of the bones of the foot in utero. Rarely, tarsal coalitions may be seen as a part of various syndromes, including hereditary symphalangism, Apert's syndrome (acrocephalosyndactyly), and hand-foot-uterus syndrome.

Key Concepts	Tarsal Coalition

Fibrous, cartilaginous, or osseous.
May be bilateral.
CT or MRI for diagnosis if radiographs negative or indeterminate, and for therapy planning.
Subtalar: Medial facet. Talar beak.
Calcaneonavicular coalition: "Anteater sign" on oblique or lateral radiograph.
Other patterns: Talonavicular, calcaneocuboid, cubonavicular.

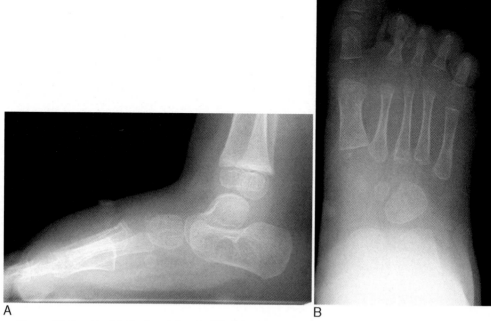

A   B

Figure 45-8   Flexible flat foot deformity. The lateral (A) and AP (B) weight-bearing radiographic views demonstrate no hindfoot equinus but do show hindfoot and forefoot valgus. Non–weight-bearing radiographs (not shown) would depict a normal alignment of both the hindfoot and forefoot. (Reprinted with permission from the American College of Radiology learning file.)

Symptoms of a tarsal coalition are generally first noted in the second decade of life, when a combination of greater activity and more advanced ossification makes a previously asymptomatic coalition painful. A teenager or young adult who

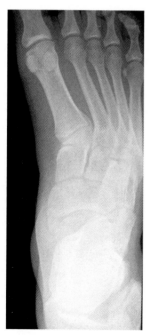

Figure 45-9   Metatarsus adductus. Mild case in an adult shows adduction of the forefoot.

presents with limited subtalar motion, pes planus, and shortening or persistent or intermittent spasm of the peroneal muscles should be imaged for tarsal coalition.

The coalition may be fibrous, cartilaginous, or osseous. Osseous coalition shows continuous bony bridging between the involved bones. Fibrous and cartilaginous coalition show close approximation of the bones with irregular cortical margin, bone deformity, sclerosis, and, on fluid-sensitive magnetic resonance imaging (MRI) sequences, adjacent marrow edema.

Calcaneonavicular and talocalcaneal (subtalar) coalitions are the two most common tarsal coalitions. Either may show a secondary sign of a large dorsal osteophyte at the distal talus, known as a "talar beak." The talar beak is caused by excess motion at the talonavicular joint resulting from restriction in the other hindfoot/midfoot joints. A talar beak is more frequently seen with subtalar coalitions than calcaneonavicular coalitions because of the greater mechanical restriction in the former type.

A *calcaneonavicular coalition* is best seen on an oblique radiograph where either the solid osseous coalition or the fragmented sclerotic abnormal joint is noted. The elongated anterior process of the calcaneus resembles the long snout of an anteater when seen on a lateral radiograph (Fig. 45-10). Computed tomography (CT) or MRI are generally not needed for diagnosis, but can better assess the anatomy before surgery (Fig. 45-10D, E).

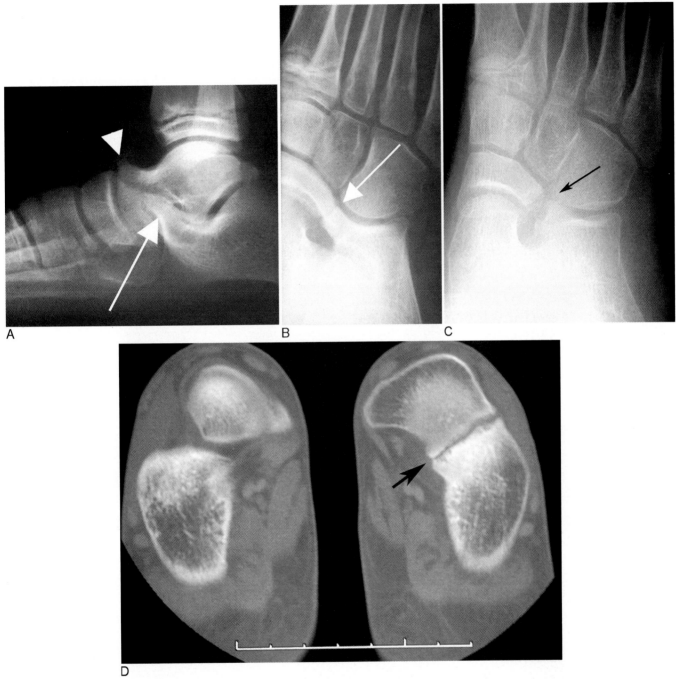

Figure 45-10 Calcaneonavicular tarsal coalition. **A,** Lateral radiograph in a 14-year-old boy demonstrates a small talar beak *(arrowhead)* and an elongated anterior extension of the calcaneus *(arrow,* "anteater" sign). **B,** The oblique view shows the calcaneonavicular coalition to be osseous *(arrow).* **C–E,** Fibrous coalitions. Oblique radiograph (C) shows irregularity and fragmentation at the calcaneonavicular joint *(arrow).* CT image (D) in a different patient shows broad and irregular left calcaneonavicular joint *(arrow).*

(Continued)

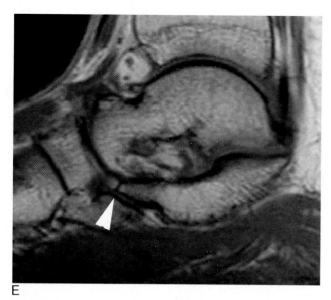

E

Figure 45-10—(Cont'd) **E,** Sagittal T1-weighted MR image in a third patient shows findings similar to those seen in part D.

Talocalcaneal (subtalar) coalition may be more complex than calcaneonavicular coalition (Fig 45-11, 45-12). A talocalcaneal coalition usually occurs at the middle facet between the talus and the sustentaculum tali of the calcaneus. More extensive cases also involve the posterior facet and occasionally the anterior facet. Subtalar coalitions can be difficult to detect on routine radiographs. The normal middle facet usually is seen on a weight-bearing lateral radiographic view, but failure to visualize this joint may be due to alignment rather than a coalition. A Harris (skier's) view can be useful when a subtalar coalition is suspected because this view profiles the sustentaculum and middle facet joint. Direct coronal CT and MRI provide the same orientation and therefore are preferred for detection and characterization of these coalitions. We routinely image both feet because tarsal coalitions of any type can be bilateral. Indirect radiographic signs of a subtalar coalition include the previously discussed talar beak and the C-sign. The C-sign is caused by bony continuity across the middle facet, resembling the letter C. It has been described but is regarded by many as unreliable (Fig. 45-13).

Coalitions also occur in other patterns: talonavicular, calcaneocuboid, and cubonavicular. Any or all of the hindfoot and hindfoot/midfoot joints may be fused. When there is a substantial coalition, with multiple fusions, the patient may develop a ball-and-socket ankle, as seen on the AP radiograph (Fig. 45-14). Converting the tibiotalar joint from a hinge joint to a ball-and-socket joint provides the inversion-eversion motion that is restricted at the coalesced talocalcaneal joint.

Treatment of tarsal coalitions is tailored to each case. Treatment options include casting, surgical resection of the coalition, or arthrodesis.

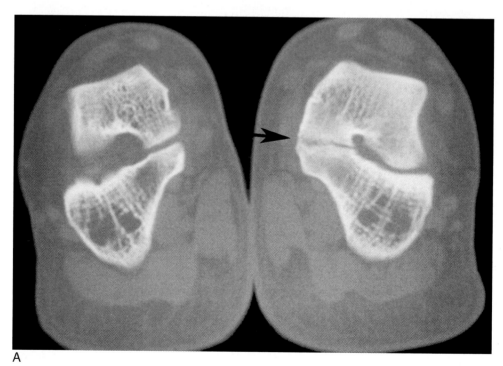

A

Figure 45-11 Fibrous talocalcaneal (subtalar) coalition. **A,** Direct coronal CT shows typical appearance of a fibrous coalition of the left medial facet joint *(arrow),* in contrast with normal medial facet joint on the right.

(Continued)

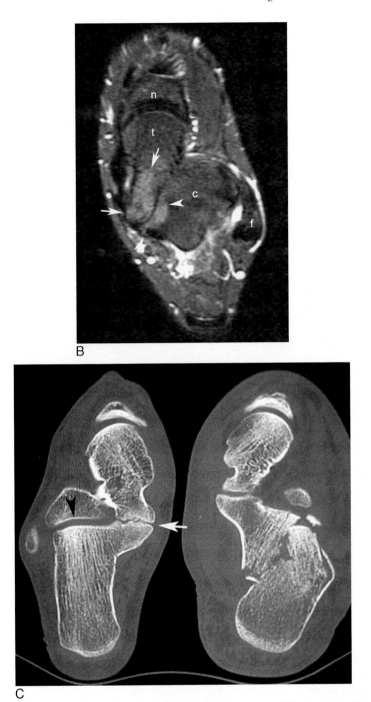

Figure 45-11—(Cont'd) **B,** Axial inversion recovery MR image in a different patient shows marrow edema in the calcaneus *(arrows)* and talus *(arrowheads)* around the narrow, deformed middle facet. c, calcaneus; f, distal tip of fibula; n, navicular; t, talar head. **C,** CT of right fibrous subtalar coalition in a different patient *(white arrow).* Note the normal right posterior facet joint *(black arrowhead)* and the left calcaneus fracture.

(Continued)

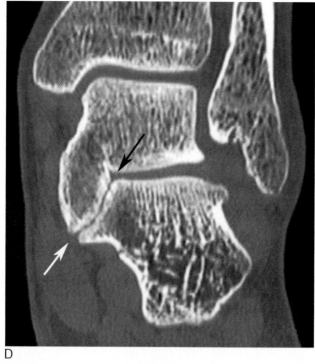

Figure 45-11—(Cont'd)   **D,** Coronal CT reconstruction in a different patient. Note the oblique orientation of the dysplastic middle facet *(arrows)*, which is a frequent finding in fibrous subtalar coalition.

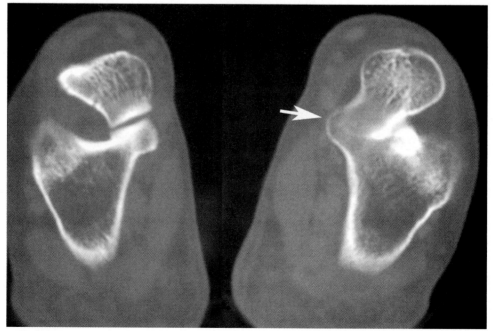

Figure 45-12   Osseous subtalar coalition. The left middle facet is fused *(arrow)*, in contrast with the normal right middle facet. The posterior facets (not shown) were normal bilaterally.

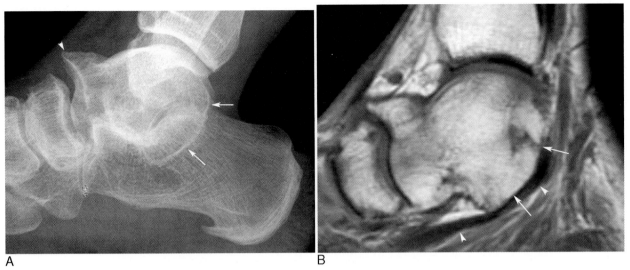

A   B

Figure 45-13   Talar beak and C signs in subtalar coalition. Both the middle and posterior facets are extensively fused in this young adult. **A,** Lateral radiograph shows a dorsal spur at the distal talus, known as a talar beak *(arrowhead).* This radiograph also shows the less common and less reliable C-sign, formed by continuous bone across the posterior margin of the middle facet *(arrows).* **B,** Sagittal T1-weighted MR image shows continuous marrow between the talus and calcaneus. *Arrows* mark the posterior cortex of the fused middle and posterior facets. Note the flexor hallucis longus tendon coursing below the sustentaculum tali *(arrowheads).* The talar beak finding is more commonly seen with subtalar coalition, but sometimes neither is present.

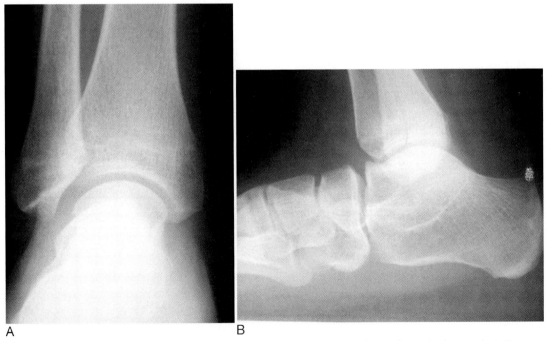

A   B

Figure 45-14   Tarsal coalition: ball-and-socket joint. AP (A) and lateral (B) radiographs show a spherical contour of the tibiotalar joint, allowing a ball-and-socket type of motion. The talus and calcaneus are completely fused, with no definition of the normal subtalar facets.

Skeletal Dysplasias

CLEIDOCRANIAL DYSPLASIA
OSTEOGENESIS IMPERFECTA
SCLEROSING BONE DYSPLASIAS
DWARFISM
    Achondroplasia and Clinical Mimickers
    Dwarfisms That Are Uniformly Fatal at Birth
    Dwarfisms with Short Ribs as a Main Finding
    Dwarfisms with Stippled Epiphyses as a Main Finding
    Miscellaneous Other Dwarfisms
OTHER SKELETAL DYSPLASIAS WITH SHORT STATURE
MUCOPOLYSACCHARIDOSES AND OTHER STORAGE
    DISEASES

Dozens of distinct skeletal dysplasias, or more precisely *osteochondrodysplasias,* have been identified. These are constitutional diseases of bones, caused by errors in bone formation or remodeling. This chapter emphasizes many of the more common or distinctive skeletal dysplasias, and includes a limited review of the more esoteric topics of dwarfism and the storage diseases. Excellent sources for more detailed information include Taybi and Lachman's *Radiology of Syndromes, Metabolic Disorders, and Skeletal Dysplasias;* Spranger, Brill, and Poznanski's *Bone Dysplasias;* Resnick's multivolume *Diagnosis of Bone and Joint Disorders;* and the major pediatric radiology textbooks. Shultz's algorithmic approach in Manaster's *Handbook of Skeletal Radiology* provides a useful practical approach to diagnosing dwarfisms.

CLEIDOCRANIAL DYSPLASIA

Cleidocranial dysplasia (cleidocranial dysostosis, pelvicocleidocranial dysplasia) results from abnormal development of membranous bones. This condition is due to a known genetic mutation and is inherited in an autosomal dominant pattern, with about one third of cases due to spontaneous mutations. Expression varies. Clinical and radiographic manifestations are usually evident at birth, and may be detected prenatally.

Clinical manifestations include a small face, wide head with hypertelorism, and generalized joint laxity. After the newborn period, dental dysplasia (too many or too few teeth, abnormal teeth), drooping shoulders, and an abnormal gait may become evident. Radiographic findings reflect the abnormal development of membranous bone (Fig. 46-1). These may include delayed closure of the cranial sutures and fontanelles, including a persistent metopic suture, wormian bones (sutural ossicles, Fig. 46-1D), and partial or complete absence of the clavicle with occasional apparent pseudarthroses due to discontinuous ossification. The middle or lateral thirds of the clavicle are most likely to be absent, probably because these portions are formed by intramembranous ossification (Fig. 46-1A). When the lateral third of the clavicle is absent, this finding may simulate other causes of an absent distal clavicle (Table 46-1). Coxa vara due to dysplasia of the femoral neck also may occur (Fig. 46-1C), perhaps reflecting the fact that portions of the long bones are partially formed by intramembranous ossification. Cleidocranial dysplasia is also in the differential diagnoses of a wide symphysis pubis (Fig. 46-1B and C, Table 46-2), and wormian bones (Table 46-3).

OSTEOGENESIS IMPERFECTA

Osteogenesis imperfecta refers to a group of disorders of collagen synthesis that result in abnormal bone formation with radiolucent bones that are easily fractured (Figs. 42-4 and 46-2, Table 46-4). The severity of skeletal manifestations varies. Severe forms result in multiple fractures in utero and are incompatible with life. Mild forms have only relatively mild bone fragility that may not be diagnosed until adulthood. Intermediate forms result in multiple fractures that can cause deformity manifesting as short-limbed dwarfism. Healing fractures often exhibit exuberant callus formation (Table 46-5). Hearing loss due to otic bone fractures, gray teeth (dentinogenesis imperfecta), and blue sclerae are seen in 90% of cases. Basilar invagination with brainstem compression may occur.

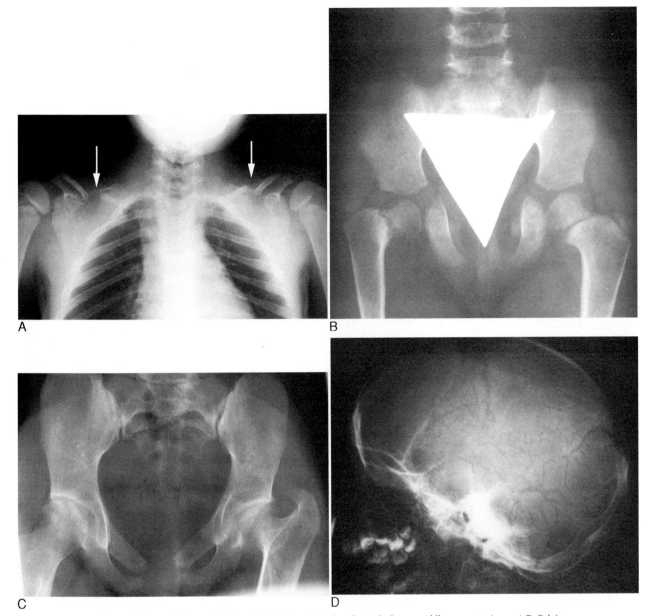

Figure 46-1   Cleidocranial dysplasia. **A,** Dysplastic clavicles with absent middle segments *(arrows).* **B,** Pelvis in a child shows no pubis ossification, and unusually shaped capital femoral epiphyses. **C,** Pelvis in an adult shows absence of ossification around the symphysis pubis and bilateral hip dysplasia with early secondary osteoarthritis. **D,** Wormian bones (sutural ossicles).

Table 46-1   Absent Distal Clavicle
Trauma: post-traumatic osteolysis (weightlifters)
Metastases/myeloma
Infection
Surgery
Rheumatoid arthritis
Hyperparathyroidism
Cleidocranial dysplasia

Table 46-2   Wide Symphysis Pubis
Trauma
Metastases/myeloma
Infection
Surgery
Hyperparathyroidism
Cleidocranial dysplasia
Epispadius/bladder exstrophy/prune belly syndrome spectrum

Key Concepts	Osteogenesis Imperfecta

A group of heritable, debilitating conditions characterized by weak bones with frequent fractures that often result in severe deformity.

Blue sclerae, osteoporosis, and wormian bones are frequently present.

Table 46-3   Wormian Bones (Sutural Bones)

Hypothyroidism
Hypophosphatasia
Cleidocranial dysplasia
Pyknodysostosis
Osteogenesis imperfecta
Zellweger syndrome (autosomal recessive, seizures, mental retardation, microcystic renal disease, death in infancy)
Menkes syndrome (males, fragile bones, abnormal copper metabolism)

Many genetic defects have been identified that cause abnormal collagen synthesis leading to osteogenesis imperfecta. Most forms are heritable in an autosomal dominant pattern, but autosomal recessive patterns are seen. Spontaneous mutations account for many cases. Sillence and colleagues have developed a widely accepted classification system that organizes osteogenesis imperfecta into four major groups based on clinical and genetic features (see Table 46-4). Some authors add a type V, which is very similar to type IV. Type I is the most frequent form of osteogenesis imperfecta (1 in 30,000). Types I and IV

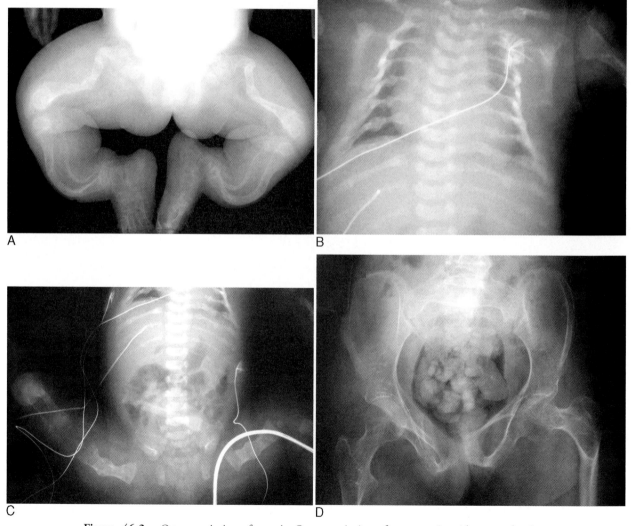

Figure 46-2   Osteogenesis imperfecta. **A,** Osteogenesis imperfecta type 3, with severe bowing. **B,** Osteogenesis imperfecta type 2 in a newborn, with multiple rib fractures. **C,** Lower body in same patient as in part B. There are numerous fractures but the bones are not bowed. **D,** Pelvis in an older child shows osteopenia, deformity due to prior fractures, and gracile and deformed proximal femurs.

(Continued)

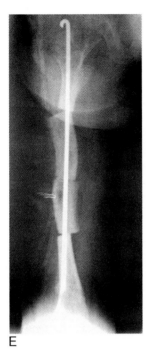

E

Figure 46-2—(Cont'd)   E, Surgical intervention for a bowed femur. Multiple osteotomies were performed with intramedullary pin fixation. (Part E courtesy of Stephanie Spottswood, MD.)

may be subtyped by the absence (subtype A) or presence (subtype B) of dentinogenesis imperfecta. Type II, the most severe form, is fatal in the neonatal period owing to extensive rib fractures and associated pulmonary hypoplasia and pulmonary infections. Type II may be divided into three subtypes, A to C, based on specific features of the osseous abnormalities. The distinction is important for genetic counseling of the parents. Type A has broad, crumpled long bones likened to an accordion, as

well as rib fractures so numerous that the ribs have a beaded appearance. Type B has similar appearance of the long bones, but with less severe rib involvement. Type C has thin long bones and ribs, with multiple fractures.

The main differential diagnosis in an infant or child with multiple fractures is child abuse or osteogenesis imperfecta. (Several very rare conditions, such as Caffey's disease and Menkes syndrome, also may resemble child abuse.) Note that child abuse is much more frequent than all forms of osteogenesis imperfecta combined. Osteogenesis imperfecta can usually be diagnosed or excluded by a combination of clinical and radiographic findings. Note that a very small subset of children with osteogenesis imperfecta does not have blue sclerae, abnormal dentition, or juvenile hearing loss. The correct diagnosis of osteogenesis imperfecta can occasionally be difficult to establish in this very rare situation. The pattern and extensiveness of fractures in osteogenesis imperfecta tend to differ from child abuse. Certain fracture patterns are highly specific for child abuse, including posterior rib fractures and metaphyseal corner fractures. Fractures in osteogenesis imperfecta more typically involve the shafts of long bones and result in deformity. Biochemical and genetic assessment for osteogenesis imperfecta also can assist in establishing this diagnosis in unusual cases.

Treatment is supportive, and includes fracture casting and internal fixation. Bisphosphonate therapy can improve bone density and strength, reducing the frequency of fractures.

SCLEROSING BONE DYSPLASIAS

A large and heterogeneous group of conditions have radiographically dense bones as a cardinal feature. Several dozen are listed in the dysplasia and syndrome textbooks. Many of these conditions result from a failure of osteoclasts to resorb

Table 46-4	Osteogenesis Imperfecta						
Type	Relative Bone Fragility	Bone Deformity	Stature	Blue Sclerae	Dentinogenesis Imperfecta	Hearing Loss	Inheritance
I	+	+ → ++	Normal or short	+	IA: − IB: +	+ +	AD
II	++++ (crumbled)	++++ (accordion)	No long-term survival	+	−	−	AD (new mutation) AR (rare)
III	+++	+++ → ++++ (bowing)	Very short	birth: + adolescence: −	−	−	AD (new mutation) AR (rare)
IV	+ → +++	+ → ++	Short	birth: ± adolescence: −	IV A: − IV B: +	− −	AD

From Sillence DO, Senn A, Danks DM: Genetic heterogeneity in osteogenesis imperfecta. J Med Genetics 16:101–116;1979; Laor T, Jarmillo D, Oestereich AE: Musculoskeletal system. In Kirks DR, Griscom NT, eds. *Practical pediatric imaging* ed 3. Philadelphia: Lippincott-Raven, 1998; Goldman AB. Heritable diseases of connective tissue, epiphyseal dysplasias, and related conditions. In Resnick D, *Bone and Joint Disorders* 3rd ed. Philadelphia: W. B. Saunders, 1995.

Table 46-5   Excessive Callus Formation

Corticosteroids (exogenous, Cushing's)
Neuropathic joint
Congenital insensitivity to pain
Paralysis
Osteogenesis imperfecta
Renal osteodystrophy
Burn patients
Subperiosteal bleed in scurvy

bone during remodeling. Several of the most common or distinctive sclerosing bone dysplasias are discussed in this section. Other potential causes of diffusely increased bone density that are not reviewed in this section include renal osteodystrophy, and, less commonly, myelofibrosis, hypothyroidism, chronic infections (including intrauterine infections, notably rubella and syphilis), and heavy metal poisoning (see Fig. 26-5). *Caffey's disease* (infantile cortical hyperostosis) is an unusual condition that causes exuberant periosteal new bone in infants, especially around the mandible (Fig. 46-3). Both sporadic (possibly infectious) and familial forms have been described.

Key Concepts   Sclerosing Bone Dysplasias

A varied group of conditions that have in common various patterns of increased bone density. Some are incidental and asymptomatic, whereas others have fragile bones that are easily fractured.

Osteopetrosis is a group of conditions characterized by diffusely very dense but brittle bones, caused by diminished osteoclast function. The osteoclast dysfunction is theorized to be variable over time, with periods of more normal function alternating with periods of diminished function. This pattern results in broad, dense metaphyseal bands or a bone-with-a-bone appearance on radiographs (Figs. 42-3A and 46-4). The metaphyses are wide owing to failure of remodeling by the impaired osteoclasts (undertubulation). Vertebral bodies tend to have dense endplates with prominent posterior vascular notches, resulting in a "sandwich" appearance on radiographs. Failure to remodel around cranial foramina during growth causes stenosis with blindness and hearing loss in the more severe forms. Dental dysplasia and infections are frequent. Long bone fractures in osteopetrosis tend to be transverse, as do many pathologic fractures.

Four clinically and radiographically distinct subtypes of osteopetrosis are recognized (Table 46-6). Radiographs of the several *infantile forms* of osteopetrosis reveal absent corticomedullary differentiation (i.e., the cortical thickening is so severe that there is almost no medullary space). This has profound consequences because normal marrow components are displaced and diminished. The resulting pancytopenia is fatal in the neonatal period, infancy, or early childhood. Hepatosplenomegaly is usually present. The *delayed* or *adult types* (including *Albers-Schönberg disease*) are clinically much less severe, and may not be discovered until later in life owing to a fracture or mild anemia, or as an incidental finding on a chest radiograph. Radiographs reveal dense bones with markedly thickened cortices. Corticomedullary differentiation is preserved, in contrast with the precocious form. A rare *intermediate autosomal recessive type* with clinical and radiographic features intermediate between the precocious and adult types is recognized. *Osteopetrosis associated with renal tubular acidosis* is a fourth distinct subtype. These patients develop cerebral calcifications and are often mentally retarded. The skeletal abnormalities tend to improve during the patient's life, in contrast with the other forms of osteopetrosis.

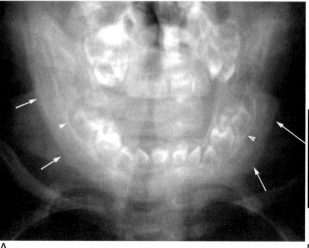
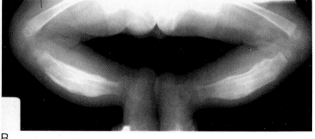

A   B

Figure 46-3   Caffey's disease (infantile cortical hyperostosis). **A,** Mandible shows prominent expansion of the mandible due to periosteal new bone formation *(arrows)*. Note the underlying mandible cortex *(arrowheads)*. **B,** Legs show bilateral prominent periosteal new bone formation in the tibias. (Part B courtesy of L. Das Narla, MD.)

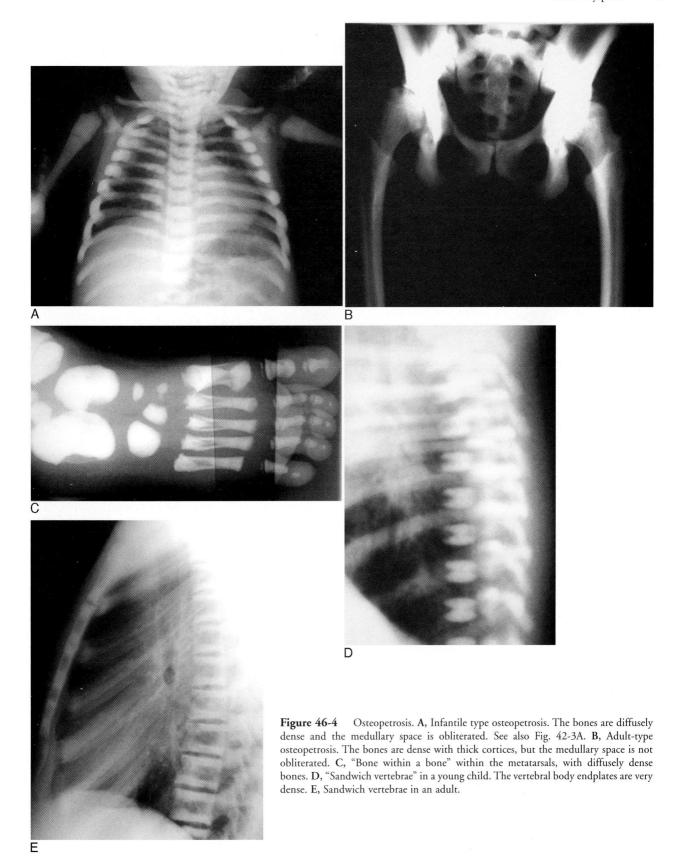

Figure 46-4   Osteopetrosis. **A,** Infantile type osteopetrosis. The bones are diffusely dense and the medullary space is obliterated. See also Fig. 42-3A. **B,** Adult-type osteopetrosis. The bones are dense with thick cortices, but the medullary space is not obliterated. **C,** "Bone within a bone" within the metatarsals, with diffusely dense bones. **D,** "Sandwich vertebrae" in a young child. The vertebral body endplates are very dense. **E,** Sandwich vertebrae in an adult.

Table 46-6   Osteopetrosis

Type	Clinical Severity	Inheritance	Comments
Precocious (infantile)	++++	AR (Rarely AD)	Often lethal early in life due to infections and anemia
Delayed (adult, Albers-Schonberg disease)	+	AD	Mild anemia Cranial nerve palsies
Intermediate	++ → +++	AR	Short stature Hip AVN
OP with renal tubular acidosis	++ → +++	AR	Cerebral calcification, mental retardation, hypotonia, long survival

OP, Osteopetrosis.

The radiographic finding of "bone within a bone" is not specific to osteopetrosis, and may be seen as a transient normal finding during periods of rapid growth, especially in very young children (Fig. 46-5).

Pyknodysostosis (Fig. 46-6) is a rare autosomal recessive type of short-limbed dwarfism with diffuse osteosclerosis, frequent transverse fractures, wormian bones (sutural ossicles, Table 46-3), preservation of the anterior fontanelle into adulthood, and progressive resorption and occasionally fragmentation of the distal phalanges. The distal clavicles also may be resorbed (see Table 46-1). The long bone findings can resemble the adult form of osteopetrosis, and some authors consider pyknodysostosis a type of osteopetrosis. The French painter Toulouse-Lautrec is believed to have had pyknodysostosis.

Progressive diaphyseal dysplasia (diaphyseal dysplasia Englemann type, Camurati-Englemann disease) is an autosomal dominant condition that results in symmetric endosteal and periosteal cortical thickening and expansion of long bone diaphyses, especially in the legs (Fig. 46-7). The epiphyses are spared. The ribs and pelvis may rarely be involved. Clinical features appear during childhood and include an abnormal gait, muscle weakness, and leg pain. Clinical and radiographic penetrance is highly variable. The condition is treated with corticosteroids.

Ribbing disease II (hereditary multiple diaphyseal sclerosis) is most likely a variant form of progressive diaphyseal dysplasia. This condition is named in honor of the person who first described it; it has nothing specifically to do with the ribs. The radiographic findings are similar to progressive diaphyseal dysplasia except that the abnormalities are asymmetric and are less widely distributed, and clinical manifestations do not appear until the third or fourth decade of life. The tibia is the most frequently involved bone. This condition also is painful and familial. (Ribbing disease I, or simply Ribbing disease, is a form of multiple epiphyseal dysplasia.)

Osteopoikilosis is a generally benign familial condition consisting of multiple bone islands clustered around joints (Fig. 46-8). A minority of patients also has small subcutaneous fibrous nodules or plaques. Rarely, there is diminished joint mobility with contractures. Osteopoikilosis in adults is easily distinguished from multiple blastic metastases by the distribution of the lesions: metastases tend to spare the epiphyses, whereas the bone islands of osteopoikilosis are most densely concentrated in the epiphyses. In addition, the individual "lesions" of osteopoikilosis are bone islands, which have characteristic findings of uniform density, continuity with the surrounding bony trabeculae, and orientation parallel to the alignment of the surrounding bony trabeculae. The number of bone islands may increase during childhood, but tends to stabilize after skeletal maturity is reached.

Osteopathia striata (Voorhoeve's disease) refers to a finding of uniform, dense linear striations in the metaphyses of the long bones. The striations are oriented parallel to the long axis of the long bones (Fig. 46-9). If the striations occur in the ilium, they radiate from the acetabulum in a "sunburst" pattern. This condition is benign.

Melorheostosis is an unusual, sporadic condition with highly distinctive radiographic findings. Dense bone is deposited along the cortex of otherwise normal bones, usually along a single extremity, in an irregular, elongate, wavy pattern that is likened to dripping candle wax (Fig. 46-10). The pattern of distribution

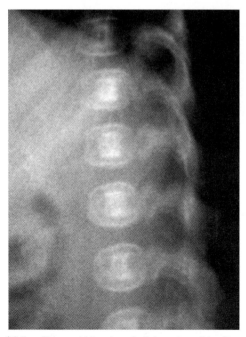

Figure 46-5   "Bone within a bone" of thoracic and lumbar vertebral bodies as a normal finding in a former premature infant. Nutritional and metabolic factors associated with prematurity often lead to this appearance, which will eventually remodel to a normal appearance.

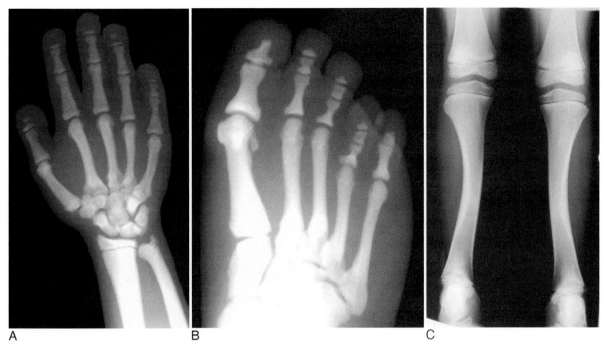

Figure 46-6 Pyknodysostosis. **A**, Hand. **B**, Foot. **C**, Legs. Note the diffuse osteosclerosis; short, tapered distal phalanges with acro-osteolysis; and mild bowing deformity of the tibias due to prior insufficiency fractures.

tends to follow a sclerotome (i.e., a portion of the skeleton innervated by a single spinal nerve). The added bone is usually periosteal but may be endosteal. It is histologically similar to cortical (compact) bone. Although life expectancy is not shortened in patients with melorheostosis, significant morbidity can occur, especially when the condition presents in childhood. Clinical features include pain, contractures, overlying skin changes (erythema, tense, shiny), and limited joint mobility. Severe cases may simulate arthrogryposis multiplex. Premature physeal closure can occur in an affected limb, resulting in growth disturbance and limb-length discrepancy. Orthopedic intervention may be required to manage these complications.

Melorheostosis, osteopathia striata, and/or osteopoikilosis have been observed to occur simultaneously in some patients. This observation probably provides a clue to the cause of these curious conditions, although each remains incompletely understood. The term *mixed sclerosing bone dysplasia* refers specifically to the simultaneous occurrence of these three conditions, acknowledging the possible association between them.

DWARFISM

Dwarfisms are skeletal dysplasias with disproportionate limb or spine shortening that results in short stature. Several types of dwarfism have been identified, many of which are extraordinarily rare. The role of the radiologist has diminished

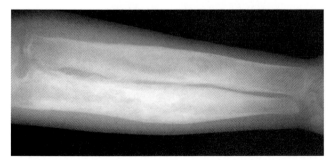

Figure 46-7 Progressive diaphyseal dysplasia. Forearm shows expansion and cortical thickening of the diaphyses of both bones. The opposite forearm and lower extremities had an identical appearance (not shown).

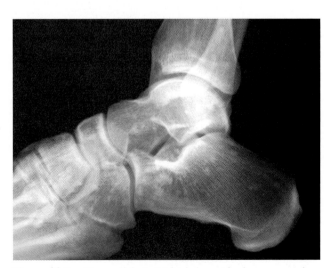

Figure 46-8 Osteopoikilosis. Multiple bone islands are centered on the joints.

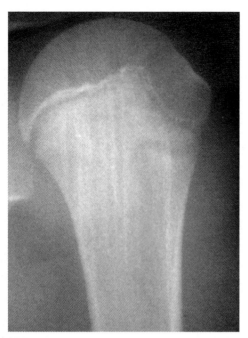

Figure 46-9 Osteopathia striata. Note the longitudinally oriented dense striations in the metaphysis of the proximal humerus.

ment of the child and genetic counseling of the parents. This is an intimidating prospect for most radiologists, as dwarfisms are complex to describe and are seen infrequently outside of specialized centers. But don't despair. An organized approach and a good reference book are invaluable, and even if you can't reach a definite diagnosis, you may be able to limit the possibilities. This section will provide a brief overview of the terminology used to describe dwarfisms, and review a few of the more common forms. Some of the many excellent reference textbooks are listed at the beginning of this chapter.

Key Concepts	Dwarfism

Dwarfisms are a large and very heterogeneous group of skeletal dysplasias with short stature and disproportionate limb or spine shortening.
Classification is based on clinical, genetic, laboratory, and radiologic features.
Achondroplasia is the most common dwarfism.
Radiologic features of achondroplasia include a large cranium; short, squat long bones; spinal stenosis; and horizontal acetabular roofs.

with the advancement of understanding of the genetic and pathophysiologic features of the dwarfisms. However, all dwarfisms have radiologic manifestations, and the radiologist may be called upon to assist in the diagnosis of these cases. Establishing the correct diagnosis is important for manage-

A dwarfism may affect all or only parts of the skeleton. Try to identify which of the following categories of bones are abnormal: skull, spine, thorax, pelvis, and limbs. If the spine is abnormal, the syndrome's name may contain the prefix "spondylo" (Table 46-7). If the limbs are abnormal, try to

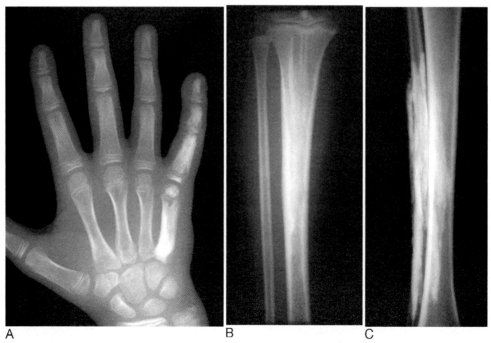

Figure 46-10 Melorheostosis. **A,** Hand. **B and C,** Tibias (all different patients). Note the dense new bone formation in a pattern similar to "candle wax dripping" of the fifth ray of the hand in part A and the tibias in parts B and C.

Table 46-7   Dwarfism with Major Spine Involvement (Partial Listing)

Normal spine length
Chondrodysplasia punctata

Short spine
Achondroplasia
Campomelic dysplasia
Diastrophic dysplasia
Metatrophic dysplasia
Spondyloepiphyseal dysplasia
Spondylometaphyseal dysplasia
Thanatophoric dysplasia

Table 46-9   Dwarfism with Short Ribs (Partial Listing)

Achondroplasia
Achondrogenesis
Asphyxiating thoracic dysplasia (Jeune syndrome)
Chondroectodermal dysplasia (Ellis-van Creveld syndrome)
Campomelic dysplasia
Metatrophic dysplasia
Spondyloepiphyseal dysplasia congenita

Table 46-10   Dwarfism with Horizontal Acetabular Roofs*

Achondroplasia
Metatrophic dysplasia
Thanatophoric dysplasia
Spondyloepiphyseal dysplasia
Chondroectodermal dysplasia
Asphyxiating thoracic dysplasia

*Horizontal acetabular roofs also seen in Down syndrome and Cleidocranial dysplasia.

localize the findings to the epiphyses, metaphyses, or diaphyses. If the limbs are short, identify whether the shortening is most severe in the humeri and femurs (rhizomelic shortening; *rhizo,* root), forearms and legs (mesomelic shortening), or hands and feet (acromelic shortening) (Table 46-8). Are the abnormal bones narrow or wide? Are the epiphyses fragmented into small "punctate" or irregular ossicles? Are the ribs short (Table 46-9)? Are the acetabular roofs horizontal or nearly horizontally oriented (Table 46-10)?

Screening radiography in a child with a dwarfism should include the following views: lateral skull, anteroposterior (AP) and lateral thoracolumbar spine, frontal chest (including the shoulders), AP pelvis and hips, AP view of a single upper extremity, AP view of a single lower extremity, and a PA hand detail view. The radiographic findings can be correlated with a series of gamuts listed in Tables 46-7 to 46-10. The following paragraphs briefly review the major clinical and radiographic findings in the dwarfisms listed in the gamuts. Neither the conditions covered nor the descriptions are exhaustive

(although you may find this topic to be *exhausting!*), but the information provided extends well beyond material routinely covered in the board examinations.

Achondroplasia and Clinical Mimickers

Achondroplasia is an autosomal dominant, rhizomelic short-limbed dwarfism (Fig. 46-11). Most cases are due to spontaneous mutations. Intelligence and life span are normal. Achondroplasia is one of the most common dwarfisms (1 in 26,000 live births). Clinical features include a protuberant forehead, normal intelligence, lumbar kyphosis in infancy that progresses to exaggerated lordosis in adulthood, and limited elbow extension. The skull is enlarged with narrowing of the foramen magnum and the jugular foramina. The vertebral bodies are bullet-shaped in infancy, and become mildly flattened in adulthood. The interpediculate distance narrows in the lumbar spine, and the pedicles are short. The ribs are shortened. The pelvis has squared iliac wings, horizontal acetabular roofs, and a narrow pelvic inlet that has been likened to a champagne glass (Fig. 46-11D). The long bones are short and wide, with flared metaphyses (see Fig. 42-3B). The hands have a "trident" configuration due to equal length of the second, third and fourth fingers. The major cause of morbidity is neurologic impingement caused by the spinal and cranial stenosis.

Hypochondroplasia is similar to achondroplasia in clinical and radiographic features except that the skull and pelvis are relatively spared in hypochondroplasia (Fig. 46-11E).

Pseudoachondroplasia is an autosomal dominant dwarfism that shares a few clinical features with achondroplasia, but is a distinct

Table 46-8   Dwarfism with Short Extremities (Partial Listing)

Rhizomelic shortening
Achondroplasia
Pseudoachondroplasia
Achondrogenesis
Thanatophoric dwarfism
Chondrodysplasia punctata
Diastrophic dwarfism

Mesomelic shortening
Dyschondrosteosis
Mesomelic dysplasia (numerous subtypes)

Acromelic shortening
Chondroectodermal dysplasia (Ellis-van Creveld syndrome)
Asphyxiating thoracic dysplasia (Jeune syndrome)

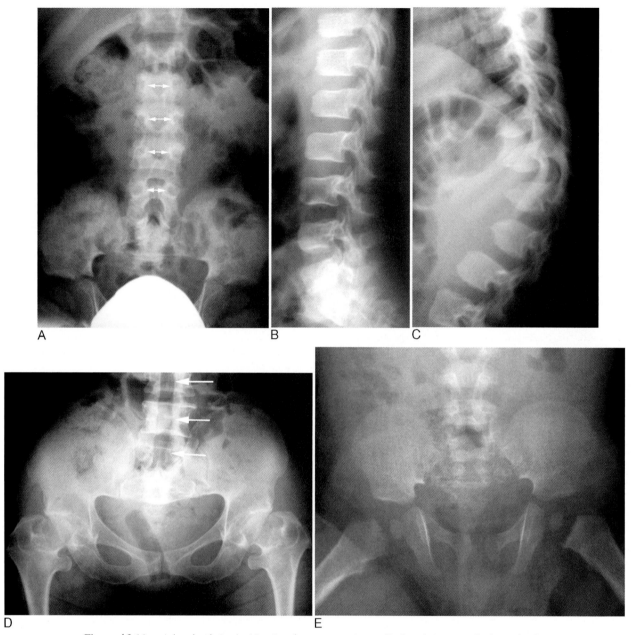

Figure 46-11   Achondroplasia. **A,** AP spine shows narrow interpediculate distance in the lower lumbar spine *(arrows).* **B,** Lateral lumbar spine. Note the posterior vertebral body scalloping, mild anterior beaking, and short pedicles. **C,** Lateral spine, more severe dysplasia. Note the thoracolumbar kyphosis with prominent anterior beaking. **D,** Pelvis in an adult. Note the prior lumbar laminectomy *(arrows)* performed to relieve spinal stenosis. See also Fig. 42-3B. **E,** Pelvis in an infant with hypochondroplasia also shows narrow interpediculate distance, but pelvis is relatively spared, as the iliac wings are less "squared" and the champagne glass configuration is less apparent. (Part B courtesy of Stephanie Spottswood, MD.)

condition. It is usually not detected until the second to fourth years of life. Clinical features include short limbs *and* a short trunk, short hands and feet, and a normal facial appearance. The skull is normal. The spine is variably affected. The vertebral bodies may be flattened and irregular with anterior beaking, or may be normal. The ribs are broad and flat, and may be likened to a spatula. The acetabular roofs are irregular and horizontal. The epiphyses are markedly abnormal, with fragmentation and deformity. The metaphyses are widened. The proximal ends of the

metacarpal bones are rounded. The carpal and tarsal bones are hypoplastic. Life expectancy in pseudoachondroplasia is normal, but early osteoarthritis can be disabling.

Dwarfisms That Are Uniformly Fatal at Birth

Achondrogenesis types I and II are fatal autosomal recessive dwarfisms associated with extremely short limbs and a large head (Fig. 46-12). The vertebral bodies are unossified or only

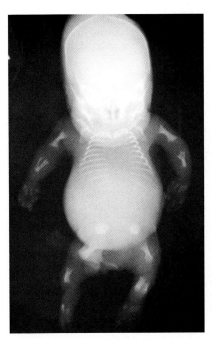

Figure 46-12   Achondrogenesis. The spine is not mineralized. Also note the shortened limbs and ribs, and the large head. (Courtesy of Stephanie Spottswood, MD.)

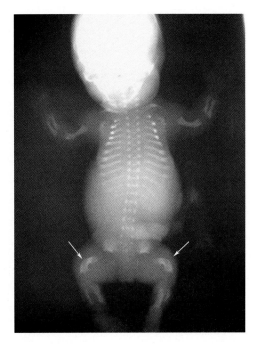

Figure 46-13   Thanatophoric dwarfism. Note the short, bowed femurs *(arrows)* and the flat, U-shaped vertebral bodies with wide disk spaces. The rhizomelic dwarfisms achondroplasia, achondrogenesis, and thanatophoric dwarfism share many morphologic and radiologic features, and can be considered as a spectrum, with achondroplasia on the mild end and thanatophoric on the severe end.

minimally ossified. The ribs are short and may be fractured. The pelvis is poorly ossified. Type II achondrogenesis has similar but less severe radiographic findings, but also is fatal.

Thanatophoric dwarfism is a fatal rhizomelic short-limbed dwarfism that may be diagnosed by prenatal ultrasonography (US). The heritance pattern is uncertain. The skull has a cloverleaf deformity due to global synostosis. The ribs are severely shortened and the chest is small. The spine has platyspondyly (flat vertebral bodies) with U-shaped vertebral bodies, and narrow interpediculate distance (Fig. 46-13). Overall spine length is normal because the disk spaces are wide. The iliac wings are squared and the acetabular roofs are horizontal. The limbs are severely shortened and the femurs are characteristically curved ("telephone-receiver femurs").

The abnormalities in achondrogenesis bear some similarity to achondroplasia but are much more severe. Thanatophoric dwarfism is a further exaggeration of these abnormalities.

Dwarfisms with Short Ribs as a Main Finding

Asphyxiating thoracic dysplasia (Jeune's syndrome) is an autosomal recessive dwarfism with a small thorax and short ribs with bulbous ends (Fig. 46-14A, B). This leads to pulmonary hypoplasia and poor ventilation that is most prominent during the first year of life. The clavicles project far above the ribs on an AP chest radiograph. The pelvis has inferiorly oriented spur-like excrescences at the triradiate cartilage ("trident pelvis," Fig. 46-14C) and often at the lateral margins of the acetabular roof as well. Ossification of the capital femoral epiphyses may be seen at birth. These centers do not normally

begin to ossify until about age 3 months or later. The limbs are shortened, usually in an acromelic pattern, with irregular metaphyses. The hands have short middle and distal phalanges with cone-shaped epiphyses. If the child survives the pulmonary complications of the first year, many of the clinical and osseous abnormalities improve with age. However, progressive renal disease develops during childhood and consequently the lifespan is shortened.

Chondroectodermal dysplasia (Ellis-van Creveld syndrome) is an autosomal recessive dwarfism that occurs most frequently in the Amish (Fig. 46-15). Clinical features include sparse hair, polydactyly with an ulnar-sided supernumerary finger, abnormal teeth and hypoplastic nails, and frequent congenital heart disease (usually atrial septal defect or common atrium). The skull and spine are generally spared. The ribs usually are short and the thorax long and narrow in infancy. These abnormalities resolve during growth. The pelvis has flat acetabular roofs with medial spur-like projections ("trident pelvis") and hypoplastic iliac wings. The capital femoral epiphyses are ossified at birth. The limbs are shortened, especially distally, and the metaphyses are wide and irregular. The distal ulna and the proximal radius are especially widened. The hamate and capitate may be fused. The proximal tibial epiphyses are hypoplastic, resulting in genu valgum. Prognosis depends on the presence and severity of congenital heart disease, and pulmonary complications due to the small thorax. Overall mortality during infancy is 50%. Chondroectodermal dysplasia

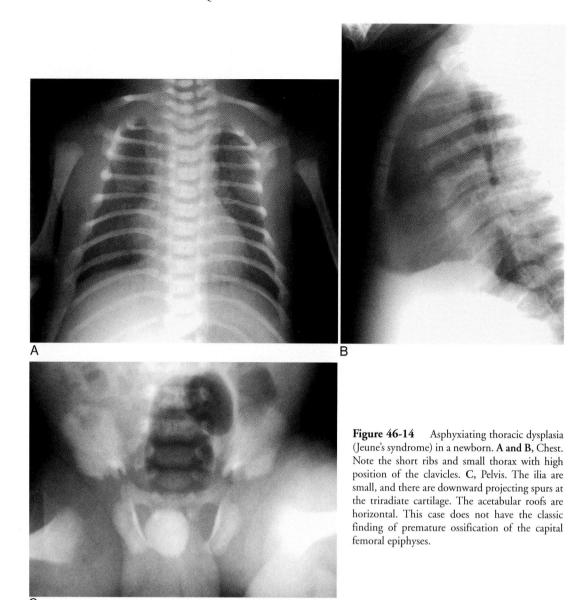

Figure 46-14 Asphyxiating thoracic dysplasia (Jeune's syndrome) in a newborn. **A and B,** Chest. Note the short ribs and small thorax with high position of the clavicles. **C,** Pelvis. The ilia are small, and there are downward projecting spurs at the triradiate cartilage. The acetabular roofs are horizontal. This case does not have the classic finding of premature ossification of the capital femoral epiphyses.

shares many features with asphyxiating thoracic dystrophy in the newborn period, but asphyxiating thoracic dystrophy does not have nail hypoplasia.

Camptomelic (camptomelic) dysplasia (camptomelic, "bent limb") is a dwarfism that often is associated with ambiguous genitalia or sex reversal (female phenotype with XY karyotype). Cleft palate is frequently present. The cervical spine and the posterior elements of the thoracic spine are poorly mineralized. The thoracic cage is small and has 11 rib pairs, and the scapulae are hypoplastic. The pelvis is dysplastic and poorly mineralized. The long bones of the lower extremity have characteristic anterior and lateral bowing. Skin dimples are present over the shins. Neonatal death due to pulmonary insufficiency and infection is common.

Metatrophic dysplasia is a rare dwarfism with *a distinctive tail-like appendage* or cutaneous fold over the sacrococcygeal region. Inheritance is heterogeneous, with fatal and nonfatal types. The skull is spared. The spine is relatively normal in length at birth, but platyspondyly and development of kyphoscoliosis lead to spine shortening as the child grows. C1–C2 instability due to dens hypoplasia may occur. The ribs are short. The pelvis has horizontal, irregular acetabular roofs. The long bones are disproportionately short at birth, but with subsequent growth the limbs attain a more normal length whereas the spine becomes markedly shortened. (The term *metatrophic* means "changing.") The long bones have wide, club-shaped metaphyses.

Dwarfism with Stippled Epiphyses as a Main Finding

Chondrodysplasia punctata is a short-limbed dwarfism, usually rhizomelic, with stippled epiphyses (Fig. 46-16). Several subtypes are recognized, but the two main subtypes are an

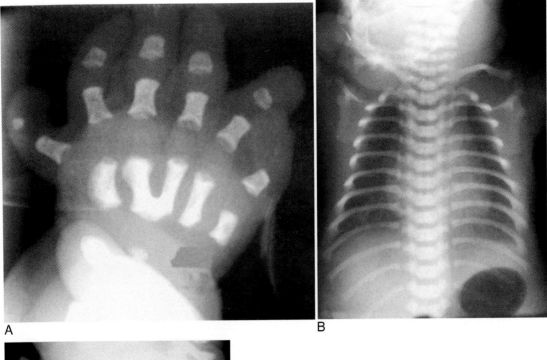

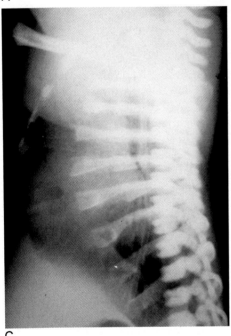

Figure 46-15   Chondroectodermal dysplasia (Ellis-van Creveld syndrome). **A,** Hand. Note the polydactyly (extra digit in the hand) and the fused metacarpals. **B and C,** Chest. The findings are essentially identical to asphyxiating thoracic dysplasia with short ribs, small thorax, and high clavicles. The hand findings and other clinical features of these syndromes allow them to be differentiated. (Courtesy of Stephanie Spottswood, MD.)

autosomal dominant form also known as *Conradi's disease,* and a rhizomelic recessive form. Clinical features include cataracts, joint contractures, and ichthyosiform (fishscale-like) skin rash. The long bone epiphyses and the spine ossify in a punctate pattern during childhood. The epiphyses in adults are no longer stippled, but they are not normally shaped. The long bones are shortened, usually unilaterally in the dominant form, and symmetrically and severely in the recessive form. The ribs and pelvis are spared. The dominant form also may have coronal vertebral body clefts. Severe cases of the dominant type are fatal in the first week of life, but milder cases may survive for years. The recessive type is fatal in infancy.

In addition to chondrodysplasia punctata, stippled epiphyses also occur in spondyloepiphyseal dysplasia and diastrophic dysplasia (both described in the following section), and in children of mothers who used Coumadin or excessive alcohol during pregnancy.

Miscellaneous Other Dwarfisms

Pyknodysostosis (Fig. 46-6) was discussed earlier with the sclerosing bone dysplasias.

Diastrophic dysplasia (*diastrophic,* "twisted") is an autosomal recessive dwarfism that may resemble arthrogryposis in severe

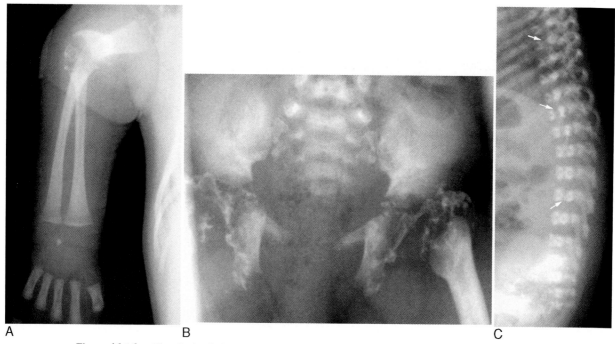

Figure 46-16   Chondrodysplasia punctata. **A,** Upper extremity. Note the short humerus (rhizomelic dwarf) and stippled epiphyses. **B,** Pelvis. **C,** Lateral spine shows coronal vertebral body clefts *(arrows).*

cases. The skull and pelvis are normal. The spine has narrowing of the lumbar interpediculate distance (potentially simulating achondroplasia), and may also have scoliosis, cervical kyphosis, or vertebral body posterior scalloping. The long bones of the extremities are short and club-shaped, and the epiphyses may be stippled or crescent-shaped. The hand has a distinctive "hitchhiker's thumb" deformity with a short first metacarpal. Clubfeet are a typical feature. The earlobes are swollen.

Mesomelic dysplasias are a group of dwarfisms characterized by mesomelic limb shortening. Over 20 types are recognized. *Dyschondrosteosis* (Leri-Weill disease) presents in late childhood with Madelung deformity (Fig. 46-17) as the primary finding. The Madelung deformity results in diminished forearm mobility and may be painful. The tibias and fibulas may be mildly shortened. Dyschondrosteosis is inherited in an autosomal dominant pattern, although the defect is located on a pseudoautosomal portion of the X or Y chromosomes. Women are more severely affected than men. Distinction from Turner syndrome, which also may have Madelung deformity, is easily made by the other clinical findings in Turner syndrome. The numerous other mesomelic dysplasias do not have Madelung deformity, but share shortening of the forearm and leg bones as a distinguishing feature. The mesomelic dysplasias are otherwise a heterogeneous group of conditions, with varying severity of skeletal dysplasia and abnormalities of other organ systems. Enumeration of these conditions is beyond the scope of this discussion.

Spondyloepiphyseal dysplasia congenita (SEDC) is an autosomal dominant dwarfism with marked abnormalities of the spine and epiphyses. Clinical features include a short spine, C1–C2 instability, muscular hypotonia, and a waddling gait. The face is flat and cleft palate may be present. The ribs are normal in length, but the chest is barrel-shaped with pectus carinatum ("bird chest," protruding sternum). Spinal manifestations at birth include ovoid or pear-shaped vertebral bodies and dens hypoplasia (Fig. 46-18). In childhood and later life, the vertebral bodies become flattened (platyspondyly) and irregular. Scoliosis is frequent. The long bones are mildly shortened. Ossification of the pelvis and the epiphyses of the long bones is delayed, and the epiphyses often are irregular and fragmented. These abnormalities consistently lead to early osteoarthritis, especially of the hips. Note that the term *spondyloepiphyseal dysplasia* is also applied to many other, less frequent skeletal dysplasias that have different clinical and radiologic manifestations. Spondyloepiphyseal dysplasia *congenita* refers to the specific condition described here.

OTHER SKELETAL DYSPLASIAS WITH SHORT STATURE

The following conditions are distinguished from the dwarfisms because they do not become clinically apparent until late childhood or adolescence, and loss of stature is milder than in the dwarfisms.

Spondyloepiphyseal dysplasia tarda (SED-tarda) is an X-linked recessive form of SED that presents in adolescence with back and hip pain, limited joint motion, and short stature due to a short spine. The radiographic findings include

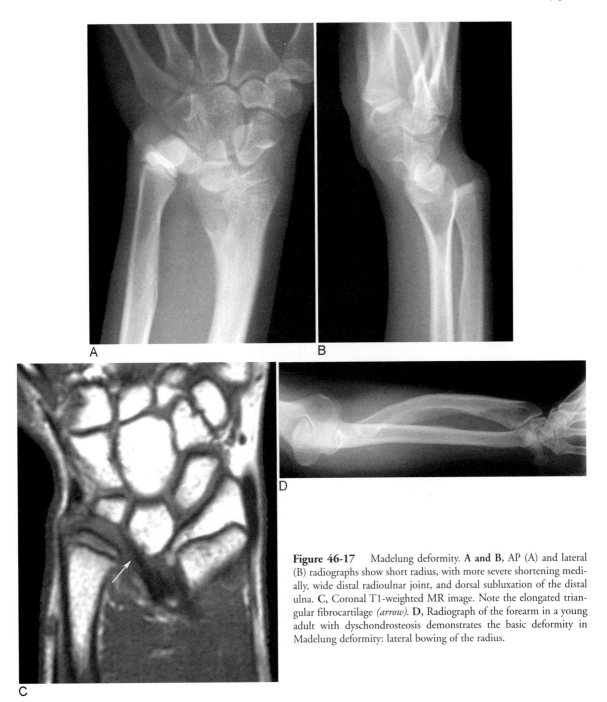

Figure 46-17 Madelung deformity. **A and B,** AP (A) and lateral (B) radiographs show short radius, with more severe shortening medially, wide distal radioulnar joint, and dorsal subluxation of the distal ulna. **C,** Coronal T1-weighted MR image. Note the elongated triangular fibrocartilage *(arrow)*. **D,** Radiograph of the forearm in a young adult with dyschondrosteosis demonstrates the basic deformity in Madelung deformity: lateral bowing of the radius.

platyspondyly with anterior disk space widening but central and posterior disk space narrowing (Fig. 46-19). The epiphyses are small and irregular, and early osteoarthritis is a typical feature.

Multiple epiphyseal dysplasia (MED, *Fairbank disease*) is an autosomal dominant skeletal dysplasia with variable expression that does not manifest clinically until late childhood or adolescence with joint pain and limp, and a mildly short limbed dysplasia (Fig. 46-20). The primary abnormality is defective secondary growth centers. The abnormalities are greatest in the secondary ossification centers of the tubular bones and the bones of the wrists and ankles, which have delayed ossification and are small and fragmented. The endplates of the spine may also be affected, with Schmorl's nodes and mild vertebral body flattening. Osteoarthritis before the fourth decade is characteristic. Clinically silent avascular necrosis occurs frequently in MED, but does not appear to accelerate the secondary degenerative changes. *Ribbing-type MED* (not to be confused with

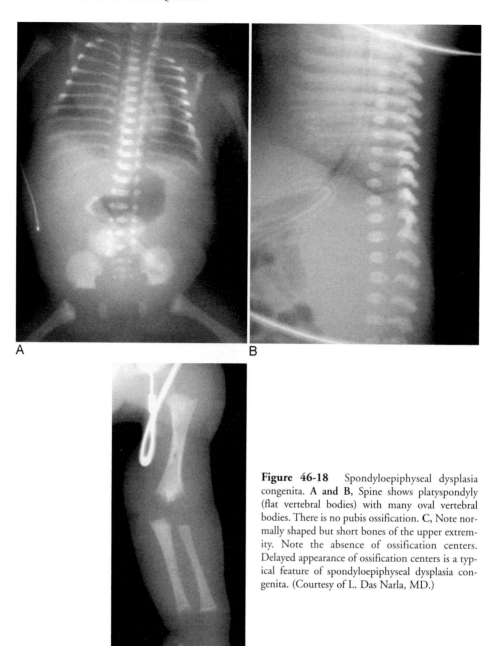

Figure 46-18 Spondyloepiphyseal dysplasia congenita. **A and B,** Spine shows platyspondyly (flat vertebral bodies) with many oval vertebral bodies. There is no pubis ossification. **C,** Note normally shaped but short bones of the upper extremity. Note the absence of ossification centers. Delayed appearance of ossification centers is a typical feature of spondyloepiphyseal dysplasia congenita. (Courtesy of L. Das Narla, MD.)

Ribbing 2 disease, discussed earlier) is a clinically and radiographically milder variant of MED than the Fairbank type. Involvement may be limited to the spine or hips, or may be more diffuse. As with Fairbank-type MED, early osteoarthritis is the main complication.

The differential diagnosis of MED is SED, early dysostosis multiplex (discussed later in this chapter), extensive osteonecrosis, juvenile rheumatoid arthritis, and hypothyroidism.

Metaphyseal chondrodysplasia (MChD) is a collection of dysplasias with metaphyseal deformity as a primary abnormality. All are characterized by short stature. The most common type is the autosomal dominant *Schmid type*, which presents during the second year with short stature, bowed legs, and a waddling gait. Radiographs reveal findings suggestive of rickets, with metaphyseal flaring, physeal widening and irregularity, and wide, cupped anterior rib ends (Fig. 46-21). However, the zone of provisional calcification

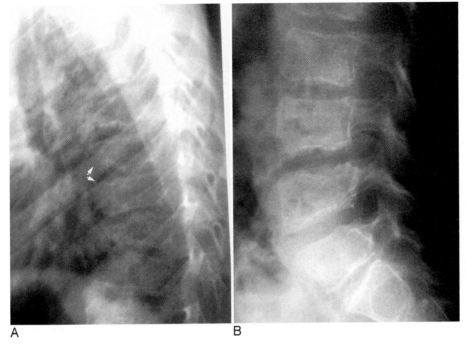

Figure 46-19 Spondyloepiphyseal dysplasia tarda. **A and B,** Lateral thoracic and lumbar spine. Note the irregular endplates with widened disk spaces anteriorly (*arrows* in part A).

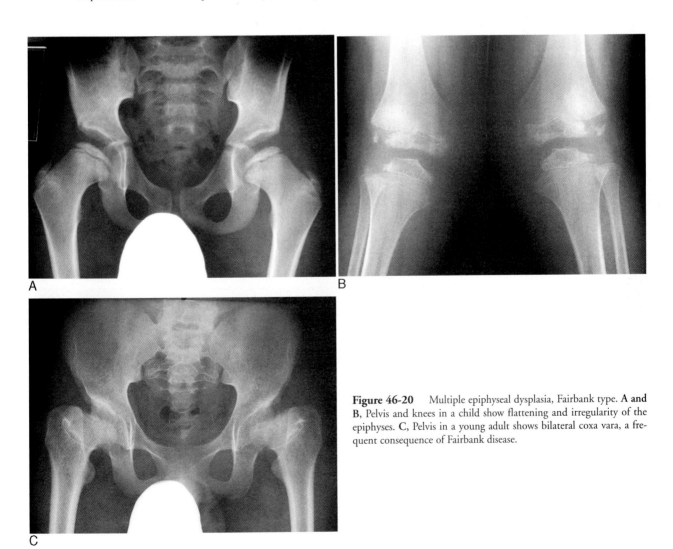

Figure 46-20 Multiple epiphyseal dysplasia, Fairbank type. **A and B,** Pelvis and knees in a child show flattening and irregularity of the epiphyses. **C,** Pelvis in a young adult shows bilateral coxa vara, a frequent consequence of Fairbank disease.

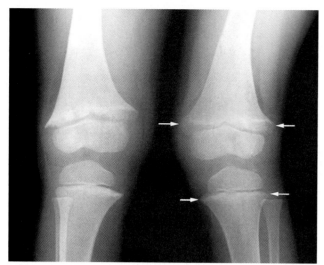

Figure 46-21 Schmid-type metaphyseal chondrodysplasia. Physeal widening and metaphyseal fraying suggest rickets, but the density of the zone of provisional calcification *(arrows)* is not diminished.

has normal density, in contrast with rickets, in which this region is radiolucent. The radiographic findings of Schmid dysplasia in the extremities can be confused with child abuse. The autosomal recessive *McKusick-type* MChD has more pronounced metaphyseal abnormalities, resulting in cone-shaped epiphyses, especially in the hands. Children with McKusick-type MChD have sparse hair, and this condition is also known as cartilage hair syndrome. Like chondroectodermal dysplasia, this condition is more common in the Amish. The autosomal recessive *Shwachman-type* MChD (Shwachman-Diamond syndrome) combines metaphyseal dysplasia with exocrine pancreatic insufficiency and lymphocyte dysfunction. The rare autosomal dominant *Jansen-type* MChD causes severe short stature.

MUCOPOLYSACCHARIDOSES AND OTHER STORAGE DISEASES

The mucopolysaccharidoses (MPS) are a group of conditions caused by inborn errors of mucopolysaccharide metabolism that result in accumulation of mucopolysaccharides in the bone marrow, brain, liver, and other organs. The MPS are distinguished by differences in clinical manifestations, biochemistry, and inheritance, outlined in Table 46-11. (*Do not* memorize this table. Your friends will worry about you.)

Key Concepts	Mucopolysaccharidoses

Inborn errors of mucopolysaccharide metabolism.
Accumulation of mucopolysaccharides in marrow, brain, liver, and other organs.
Dwarfism.
Distinctive set of skeletal abnormalities: Dysostosis multiplex.

The mucopolysaccharidoses have in common a group of skeletal manifestations that are collectively termed *dysostosis multiplex* (Fig. 46-22). Short stature is universal, and the long bones are shortened with wide metaphyses and diaphyses. The bridge of the nose is flattened. There is focal kyphosis at the thoracolumbar junction, with an L1 or adjacent vertebral body that is small, retrolisthesed, and oval in shape with an inferior or central anterior beak. Several vertebral bodies may have this finding. The hands have short wide metacarpals, with narrowed proximal ends resulting in a fan-like configuration of the hands. The pelvis has constricted (narrow) inferior iliac bones with flared iliac wings, and femoral heads are dysplastic. Additional features of dysostosis

Table 46-11   Classification of the Mucopolysaccharidoses

Type	Eponym	Heritance	MPS Stored and Excreted	Features
1 H	Hurler	AR	DS, HS	DO (severe), C1-C2 subluxation, MR, HSM, corneal clouding
1 S	Scheie	AR	DS, HS	DO, stiff joints, cardiac disease, corneal clouding
II	Hunter	XR	DS, HS	DO, often MR, HSM
III	San Filipo	AR	HS	DO, neurologic impairment
IV	Morquio	AR	KS	DO, C1–C2 subluxation, organomegaly, corneal clouding, no MR
V	none (formerly Scheie)			
VI	Maroteaux-Lamy	AR	DS	Very rare, Variable expression. DO, C1–C2 subluxation, organomegaly, corneal clouding, no MR
VII	Sly	AR	CS, DS, HS	Very rare. Variable expression. DO, MR, corneal clouding

AR, autosomal recessive; XR, X-linked recessive; DS, dermatan sulfate; KS, keratan sulfate; HS, heparan sulfate; CS, chondroitin sulfate; DO, dysostosis multiplex; MR, mental retardation; HSM, hepatosplenomegaly.
Taybi H, Lachman RS. *Radiology of Syndromes, Metabolic Disorders, and Skeletal Dysplasias.* 4th ed. St. Louis, Mosby, 1996.

multiplex include osteopenia with coarse trabeculae, macrocranium with a J-shaped sella turcica, and "oar-shaped" ribs with focal constriction at the costovertebral junction (Fig. 46-22C).

Key Concepts	Dysostosis Multiplex

Mucopolysaccharidoses
Oar-shaped ribs
Fan-like metacarpals
Macrocranium with a J shaped sella turcica
Wide iliac wings, narrow inferior iliac bones
Long bones are short with wide metaphyses and diaphyses
Focal kyphosis at the thoracolumbar junction, vertebral body
   or bodies with an anterior beak
Osteopenia with coarse trabeculae
Short stature

The MPS are unusual conditions. Hurler syndrome (MPS IH) and Morquio syndrome are the most common mucopolysaccharidoses (both 1 per 100,000 at birth). Hurler syndrome deserves special mention because it causes early and severe appearance of dysostosis multiplex beginning by about 1 year of age. Morquio's syndrome (MPS IV) deserves special mention because it is the only (relatively) common type of MPS that does not cause mental retardation. Radiographic findings of Morquio's syndrome include those of dysostosis multiplex, as well as several important or distinctive additional findings. These include dens hypoplasia with atlantoaxial instability, expansion of C2, and displacement of the posterior arch of C1 into the foramen magnum that can cause spinal cord compression. Surgical stabilization may be required. The vertebral bodies have midanterior beaking. The vertebral bodies can flatten ("platyspondyly"), especially in the lumbar spine, in contrast to Hurler syndrome, in which this finding is not present. Delayed appearance of the epiphyses, with fragmented epiphyses, may be seen.

Dysostosis multiplex is also caused by other storage diseases, such as the mucolipidoses and Gaucher disease. As with the MPS, the clinical and radiographic changes caused by these conditions are not present at birth, but rather take years to develop as the abnormal metabolites accumulate. Also as seen with the mucopolysaccharidoses, diagnosis of these conditions is based primarily on clinical and laboratory findings.

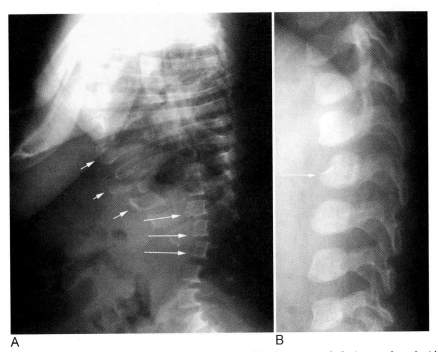

A   B

Figure 46-22 Dysostosis multiplex. **A**, Lateral thoracic and lumbar spine and ribs (mucopolysaccharidosis [MPS] VI). Note the broad "oar-like" ribs *(short arrows)* and the thoracolumbar kyphosis with small inferior beaks *(long arrows)*. **B**, Lateral thoracolumbar spine (MPS 1H). The vertebral bodies are shaped differently than MPS VI in part A, but also have a short AP size and an inferior beak in a thoracolumbar junction vertebral body *(arrow)*.

(Continued)

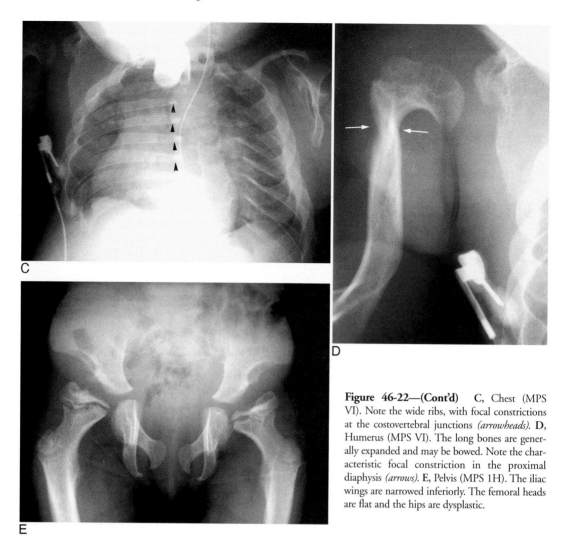

Figure 46-22—(Cont'd)   C, Chest (MPS VI). Note the wide ribs, with focal constrictions at the costovertebral junctions *(arrowheads).* **D,** Humerus (MPS VI). The long bones are generally expanded and may be bowed. Note the characteristic focal constriction in the proximal diaphysis *(arrows).* **E,** Pelvis (MPS 1H). The iliac wings are narrowed inferiorly. The femoral heads are flat and the hips are dysplastic.

Miscellaneous Congenital and Developmental Conditions

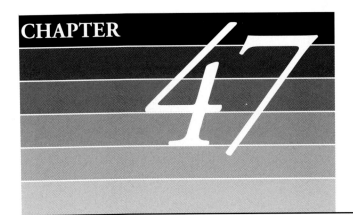

CONNECTIVE TISSUE DISORDERS
NEUROFIBROMATOSIS
CHROMOSOMAL ABNORMALITIES
RADIAL DYSPLASIAS
SYMPHALANGISM
AMNIOTIC BAND SYNDROME
ARTHROGRYPOSIS MULTIPLEX CONGENITA
GIGANTISM AND HYPOPLASIA
FIBROMATOSIS COLI
TORSION OF THE FEMUR AND TIBIA
OSTEO-ONYCHODYSOSTOSIS

CONNECTIVE TISSUE DISORDERS

Marfan syndrome is an autosomal dominant connective tissue disorder with high penetrance but variable expression. A genetic defect results in a collagen abnormality. Most cases are inherited, some occur as spontaneous mutations. Patients with Marfan syndrome are tall and have disproportionate lengthening of the distal aspects of the extremities (arachnodactyly; Fig. 47-1A). Skeletal manifestations include kyphoscoliosis, joint hypermobility, early osteoarthritis, protrusio acetabuli (Fig. 47-1B), spondylolysis of L5, posterior scalloping of the vertebral bodies due to dural ectasia (especially prominent at L5 and S1 compared with normal), and pectus excavatum. Bone mineral density is normal. Important extraosseous complications include ocular lens dislocation and cystic medial necrosis of the proximal ascending aorta and pulmonary artery. The cardiovascular lesions may lead to aortic dissection or rupture, or to aortic or pulmonic valve insufficiency.

Homocystinuria is an autosomal recessive condition caused by an inborn error of metabolism, cystathionine synthetase deficiency, that leads to accumulation of homocystine in the serum and urine and causes defective collagen synthesis. Many of the morphologic and radiographic features of homocystinuria resemble those seen in Marfan syndrome. Both conditions are associated with scoliosis, posterior vertebral body scallop-

Key Concepts	Connective Tissue Disorders

Marfan syndrome: Autosomal dominant collagen defect with variable expression, arachnodactyly, scoliosis, posterior vertebral body scalloping, lens dislocations, ascending aorta dissection, aortic and pulmonic valve insufficiency.
Homocystinuria: Autosomal recessive inborn error of metabolism that causes abnormal collagen. Findings similar to those in Marfan syndrome, but also with osteoporosis and fractures.
Ehlers-Danlos syndrome: Family of clinically similar, mostly autosomal dominant conditions with marked skin and joint laxity, and easy bleeding. Shares many features with Marfan syndrome and homocystinuria, but also with phlebolith-like subcutaneous calcifications, especially in the shins and forearms, due to subcutaneous hemorrhages.

ing, pectus excavatum, and arachnodactyly (uniformly present in Marfan syndrome, variably present in homocystinuria). However, patients with homocystinuria have osteopenia with associated vertebral compression fractures, which are not typical features of Marfan syndrome. In addition, patients with homocystinuria also have mental retardation, seizures, and joint contractures, which are not usual clinical features of Marfan syndrome.

Ehlers-Danlos Syndrome is a spectrum of mostly autosomal dominant familial conditions, each caused by a defect in collagen synthesis, that have in common exceptionally lax skin that is easily injured and heals poorly, hypermobile joints that are prone to contractures in old age, and easy bleeding due to fragile blood vessels. Musculoskeletal features overlap with those seen in Marfan syndrome and homocystinuria. Kyphoscoliosis, posterior vertebral scalloping, arachnodactyly, and spondylolysis are seen, as well as marked joint hypermobility leading to dislocations, flat feet, and early osteoarthritis. Hemarthroses may occur after minimal trauma. The great vessels are prone to aneurysm, dissection, and tortuosity. Angiography is dangerous

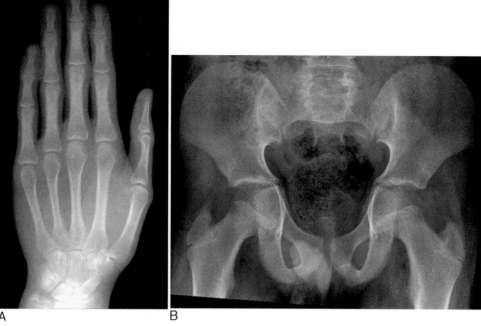

Figure 47-1   Marfan syndrome. **A,** Hand. Note the long, slender fingers (arachnodactyly). **B,** Pelvis. Note the mild bilateral protrusio acetabuli.

owing to the fragility of the vessels. Patients with Ehlers-Danlos syndrome are vulnerable to subcutaneous bleeding and fat necrosis from minimal trauma, resulting in phlebolith-like subcutaneous calcifications, especially in the forearms and shins. The presence of such calcifications combined with a history of skin hyperelasticity help to make the diagnosis of Ehlers-Danlos syndrome.

NEUROFIBROMATOSIS

Most patients with neurofibromatosis type 1 (NF1, von Recklinghausen disease) have skeletal involvement (Fig. 47-2) in addition to the characteristic central and peripheral neurologic findings. The skeletal findings are largely due to a diffuse mesodermal dysplasia, although extrinsic compression by a n eurofibroma may also cause bone deformity. Multiple nonossifying fibromas also may be seen (see Chapter 33). Perhaps the most important skeletal manifestation of NF1 is scoliosis (see Fig. 43-6). Scoliosis in NF1 may resemble idiopathic scoliosis, but may also present as a short-segment, sharply angulated thoracic kyphoscoliosis most frequently centered at T3–T7. These focal thoracic curves are prone to rapid progression and instability that can result in paralysis. Thus, scoliosis in a patient with NF1 should be closely monitored. Other spinal osseous abnormalities seen in NF1 include enlarged neural foramina and posterior vertebral body scalloping due to dural ectasia (Fig. 47-2C). Cranial osseous abnormalities include hypoplastic or absent cranial bones (sphenoid wing, posterosuperior orbital wall, mastoid), macrocranium, and enlarged cranial neural foramina due to neu-

rofibromas. Anterior distal tibial bowing, often with pseudarthrosis that may develop characteristic tapered margins, may be seen at birth or develop during childhood (Fig. 47-2, Tables 47-1 and 47-2). These pseudarthroses are frequently resistant to healing despite orthopedic fixation, and a short leg can result (Fig. 43-1). As noted earlier, multiple nonossifying fibromas may be present. In fact, a finding of multiple nonossifying fibromas in any patient should suggest the diagnosis of neurofibromatosis. Twisted, narrow, irregular "ribbon ribs" reflect the mesodermal dysplasia more frequently than extrinsic compression from adjacent neurofibromas. The plexiform neurofibromas found in NF 1 often reveal a "target sign" appearance on T2-weighted magnetic resonance imaging (MRI), with low signal intensity centrally and high signal intensity peripherally (Fig. 36-1).

Skeletal manifestations are prominent in phakomatoses other than NF1. The findings of Klippel-Trenaunay-Weber syndrome are discussed in the section on focal gigantism. Tuberous sclerosis causes patchy bone sclerosis and cyst-like changes in the bones of the hands and feet (Fig. 47-3). Gorlin syndrome (basal cell nevus syndrome) of basal cell carcinomas and palmar skin pits also causes mandible cysts, patchy and bone-island-like bone sclerosis, and scoliosis.

CHROMOSOMAL ABNORMALITIES

Skeletal manifestations of *trisomy 21* (Down syndrome, Fig. 47-4) include numerous cervical spine anomalies, most important atlantoaxial subluxation in 10% to 20% of cases. The posterior arch of C1 is often hypoplastic. Other skeletal

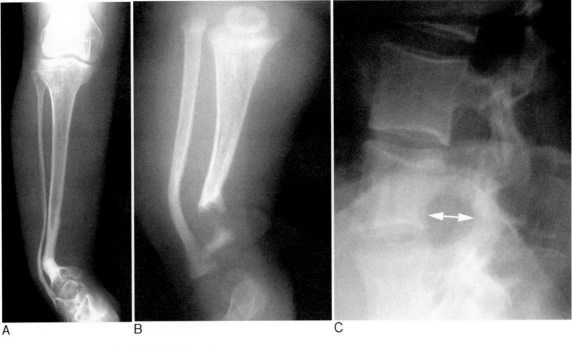

A   B   C

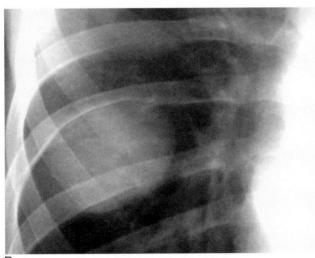

D

Figure 47-2   Neurofibromatosis type 1 (NF1), skeletal findings. **A,** Tibial bowing. Note the characteristic antero-lateral curve of the distal tibia and fibula. **B,** Distal tibial pseudarthrosis. **C,** Dural ectasia with posterior vertebral body scalloping and wide neural foramina *(arrow).* **D,** Pressure erosion of a rib due to a neurofibroma. (Most rib deformities in NF1 are due to the skeletal dysplasia, not pressure erosion.) See also Figs. 43-1, 43-6, and Chapter 33.

abnormalities may include 11 rib pairs, two manubrial ossification centers rather than the normal single ossification center, short tubular bones of the hands and fingers with fifth-finger *clinodactyly* (abnormal angulation of a finger in the coronal plane) due to a short and broad fifth-finger middle phalanx, flared iliac wings with nearly horizontal acetabular roofs, hip dysplasia, patellar dislocations, and a variety of foot anomalies.

Trisomy 18 results in abnormalities of multiple organ systems, notably severe congenital heart disease. Characteristic skeletal manifestations that may be detected on prenatal ultrasonography (US) include "rocker bottom feet" and a clenched hand with an adducted thumb and a short first metacarpal. Postnatal radiographic findings also include hypoplasia of the mandible and maxilla, and 11 rib pairs with thin, hypoplastic ribs. The fingers are in ulnar deviation. Stippled epiphyses may be seen. Survival beyond 1 year is unusual.

Turner syndrome (45X0, deletion of one X chromosome) is associated with short stature, webbed neck, and abnormalities of many organ systems, including congenital heart disease, horseshoe kidney, and streak ovaries. Aortic root dilation and dissection is an uncommon but potentially catastrophic association. The most characteristic skeletal findings are short fourth metacarpals (a finding that is also seen in pseudohypoparathyroidism and pseudo-pseudohypoparathyroidism), depression of the medial tibial plateau, tarsal coalitions, diffuse osteopenia, and Madelung deformity.

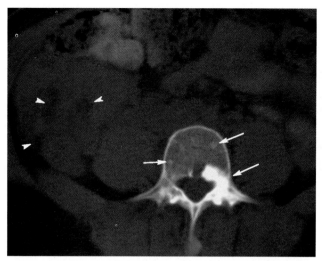

Figure 47-3 Tuberous sclerosis. Unenhanced axial CT image shows sclerotic regions in the lumbar spine *(arrows)*. Numerous fat attenuation angiomyolipomas can be seen in the lower pole of the enlarged right kidney *(arrowheads)*.

RADIAL DYSPLASIAS

Congenital absence, partial aplasia, or hypoplasia of the radius occurs in association with numerous syndromes and as part of the VACTERL spectrum (vertebral, anorectal, cardiac, tracheoesophageal fistula, renal, and limb anomalies).

Madelung deformity (Fig. 46-7) is caused by distal radius bowing that displaces the distal radius in a volar and ulnar direction. The radial curvature effectively shortens the radius when compared to the ulna, and the articular surface of the radius is oriented abnormally medially. The ulna is often dorsally dislocated. Madelung deformity can be seen as a consequence of previous trauma or growth disturbance caused by multiple osteochondromas or enchondromas, as part of the rare skeletal dysplasia dyschondrosteosis (Leri-Weill disease, Chapter 46), or as a sporadic finding.

Holt-Oram syndrome is an association of congenital heart disease (classically atrial septal defect) and thumb or radius abnormalities. The classic osseous finding is triphalangeal thumbs (Fig. 47-5A), but a spectrum of thumb abnormalities can occur, ranging from absence to hypoplasia to bifid. The radius may be absent, hypoplastic, or normal. Inheritance is autosomal dominant.

The *TAR syndrome* (thrombocytopenia-absent radius) is an association of congenital radial anomalies and severe thrombocytopenia. The classic skeletal findings are absence of the radius and shortening of the ulna with the hand held at a 90-degree angle to the forearm (Fig. 47-5B). The radii are often absent bilaterally, but the thumbs are typically present. There is evidence for autosomal recessive inheritance.

Radial club hand is similar to the deformity just described in the TAR syndrome, but the term usually also implies that the thumb and scaphoid are also absent (Fig. 47-5C).

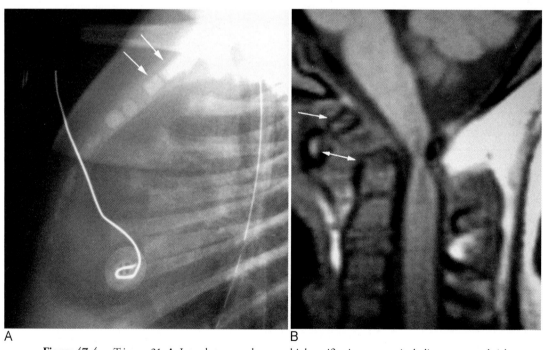

A   B

Figure 47-4 Trisomy 21. **A,** Lateral sternum shows multiple ossification centers, including two manubrial ossification centers *(arrows)*. **B,** Atlantoaxial subluxation. Sagittal T1-weighted MR image obtained with voluntary neck flexion shows severe cord compression. Note the ununited ossiculum terminale *(arrow)* and the wide interval between the anterior arch of C1 and C2 *(double arrow)*. Atlantoaxial instability is present in 10% to 20% of children with trisomy 21.

(Continued)

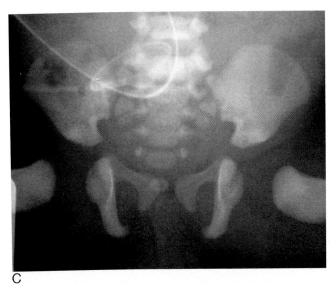

C

Figure 47-4—(Cont'd)   C, Pelvis in an infant shows low acetabular angles, rounded iliac wings, and inferior tapering of the ischia.

Fanconi anemia is an association of brown pigmentation of the skin and late childhood pancytopenia. Congenital radial ray and thumb anomalies are present in about half of cases, classically a hypoplastic thumb. A variety of congenital renal anomalies may occur as well.

Congenital radioulnar synostosis is caused by failure of segmentation of the proximal radius and ulna (Fig. 47-6). The proximal radius is often posteriorly displaced, and the radius is often bowed laterally. Radioulnar synostosis can occur as an isolated abnormality, as a familial condition, or in association with a variety of rare syndromes, such as abnormal karyotypes (XXXY, XXYY). Acquired radioulnar synostosis can occur after infection or Caffey's disease (infantile cortical hyperostosis).

Congenital radial head dislocation is discussed in Chapter 6 (see Figs. 6-21, 6-22).

SYMPHALANGISM

Symphalangism is congential coalition of metacarpals and phalanges (Fig. 47-7). The condition is variable and frequently is familial.

AMNIOTIC BAND SYNDROME

Amniotic band syndrome (Fig. 47-8) refers to congenital amputations and soft tissue defects caused by entanglement of the fetus by aberrant bands of amniotic membrane that traverse

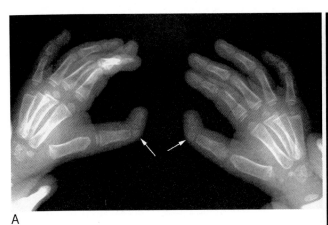

A

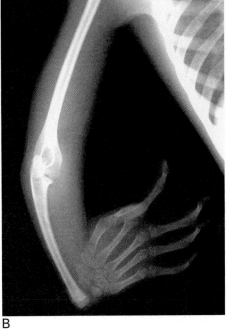

B

Figure 47-5   Radial ray dysplasias. **A,** Holt-Oram syndrome. Note the triphalangeal thumbs *(arrows)*. **B,** TAR syndrome (thrombocytopenia absent radius). The radius is absent, but the thumb and scaphoid are present.

(Continued)

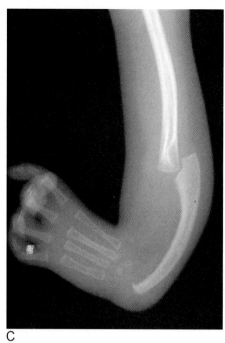

C

Figure 47-5—(Cont'd) **C,** Radial club hand. In contrast with part B, the thumb is absent.

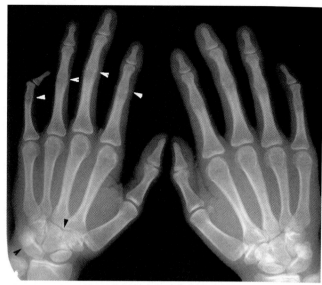

Figure 47-7 Symphalangism. This mild case involves only the PIP joints *(white arrowheads)*. Also note the lunotriquetral and trapezoid-capitate carpal coalitions *(black arrowheads)*.

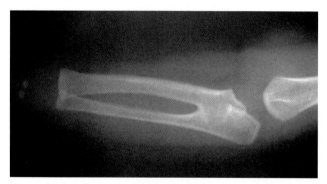

Figure 47-6 Congenital radioulnar synostosis. The proximal fusion is typical.

the gestational sac. Abnormalities range from minimal amputations or focal syndactyly to major cranial or body wall defects. Focal soft tissue constrictions may occur that may result in chronic lymphedema. Surgery is often required to minimize loss of function and to improve appearance.

ARTHROGRYPOSIS MULTIPLEX CONGENITA

Arthrogryposis multiplex congenita (Fig. 47-9) is a rare, sporadic condition characterized by severe joint abnormalities that include fixed flexion deformities, dislocations, radi-

ographically dense joint capsules, long scoliosis (neuromuscular pattern), muscle and soft tissue atrophy, and osteoporotic bones (from disuse) that are prone to insufficiency fracture. Clubfeet and hands may be present. Soft tissue webs may fix joints in flexion. The lower extremities are almost always involved, particularly the distal limbs; the distribution varies, however, and the upper extremities may be involved. Intelligence is normal. The cause is unknown, but severely restricted fetal motion as can result from chronic oligohydramnios is suspected.

GIGANTISM AND HYPOPLASIA

Abnormalities of size and shape may affect only a small portion of the body (focal gigantism), an entire extremity (macromelia), or half of the body (hemihypertrophy). Only one or two organ systems may be affected (e.g., the lymphatics or the blood vessels) or every tissue may be involved. *Hemihypertrophy* is overgrowth of half (or nearly half) of the body. A variety of syndromes and malignancies are associated with hemihypertrophy, most notably the Beckwith-Wiedemann syndrome and Wilms' tumor. *Hemiatrophy* is usually an acquired condition caused by asymmetric neurologic and neuromuscular conditions that cause severe unilateral muscle atrophy. *Hemihypotrophy* may be considered congenital hemiatrophy. This rare condition is associated with intrauterine growth retardation and chromosomal abnormalities. A leg-length discrepancy resulting from any of these conditions may require orthopedic intervention.

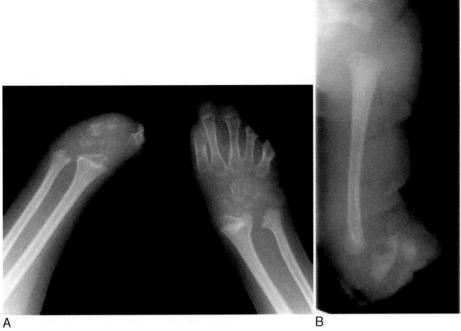

A   B

Figure 47-8   **A and B,** Amniotic band syndrome. Note the amputations of the extremities.

Macrodystrophia lipomatosa is a distinctive form of localized gigantism of unknown cause characterized histologically by overgrowth of adipose and periosteal osteoblasts (see Fig. 34-5). Fingers and toes are most frequently involved with this condition.

Klippel-Trenaunay-Weber syndrome is macromelia associated with a cutaneous capillary hemangioma (port wine nevus) and dilated and tortuous superficial veins. A lower extremity is the usual site of involvement (Fig. 47-10). Occasionally, hemangiomas also occur in the liver, spleen, bowel, and bladder wall. The limb overgrowth becomes most apparent during the growth spurt at puberty. It is speculated that the vascular abnormalities are due to failure of primitive superficial vascular channels to regress during gestation, resulting in or from failure of development of a normal deep venous system of the affected extremity. The resulting vascular abnormalities cause chronically increased blood flow that is the cause of the limb overgrowth. Remember that chronically increased blood flow results in accelerated growth in adjacent physes, regardless of the cause. Examples

---

Key Concepts   **Focal Gigantism**

Chronically increased blood flow, regardless of the cause, causes accelerated growth at adjacent physes.

Potential causes include vascular malformation, chronic synovial inflammation (as in juvenile rheumatoid arthritis), or hemophilia.

Macrodystrophia lipomatosa is idiopathic overgrowth of fingers or toes with fibrofatty proliferation.

Klippel-Trenaunay-Weber syndrome: Overgrowth of a limb, usually a lower extremity, related to congenital absence of a normal deep venous system and increased flow through an abnormal subcutaneous venous system.

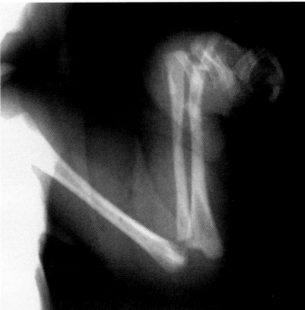

Figure 47-9   Arthrogryposis multiplex congenita. The upper extremity was fixed in this position.

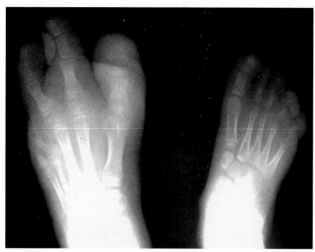

Figure 47-10 Klippel-Trenaunay-Weber syndrome. In addition to the foot overgrowth evident on this image, most of the right lower extremity was overgrown (not shown).

include vascular malformation, chronic inflammation (as in juvenile rheumatoid arthritis), and chronic low-grade infection.

FIBROMATOSIS COLI

Fibromatosis coli (Fig. 47-11) refers to a nonneoplastic, mass-like, focal or diffuse enlargement of a sternocleidomastoid muscle in an infant. This condition probably results from birth injury to the sternocleidomastoid muscle and, not surprisingly, is associated with forceps delivery. The affected sternocleidomastoid muscle often shortens, which may result in torticollis. Imaging studies reveal nonspecific enlargement of the affected muscle but are especially useful in excluding another cause of a neck mass, such as adenopathy, neoplasm, branchial cleft cyst, or cystic hygroma. Fibromatosis coli typically presents at about 2 weeks of age and may enlarge before spontaneously resolving over a period of months. Most cases respond to physical therapy with passive stretching of the shortened sternocleidomastoid muscle. Surgery is occasionally required for refractory torticollis.

TORSION OF THE FEMUR AND TIBIA

Torsion is rotation around the long axis of a bone. The term is most frequently applied to describe abnormal twisting along the long axis of the femur or tibia. Imagine that you are looking down the long axis of a lower extremity. Femoral alignment is determined by the angle formed by a line through the femoral neck and a line drawn across the posterior margins of the femoral condyles. If the femoral head projects anterior to the plane containing the femoral condyles, then *antetorsion* is present. The synonymous term *anteversion* is more frequently used. If the femoral head projects posterior to this plane, then *retrotorsion* or *retroversion* is present. The terminology used to characterize tibial torsion is slightly different, but less confusing. *Medial* or *internal tibial torsion* results in internal rotation-like twisting of the distal tibia (pigeon-toed). *Lateral* or *external tibial torsion* is the opposite (penguin-footed). Femoral anteversion is best assessed by limited computed tomography (CT). A few 10-mm, low-dose slices are obtained through the femoral neck and the femoral condyles, and their relative angle is determined (Fig. 47-12). Radiographs can easily estimate tibial torsion, but CT is occasionally used when a high degree of precision is needed.

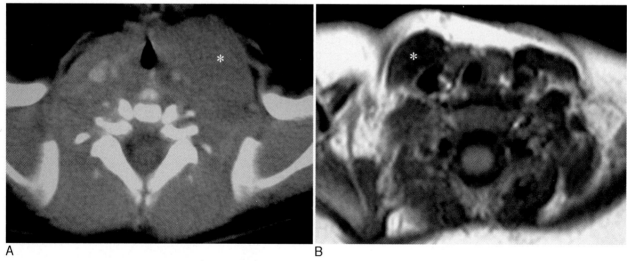

A   B

Figure 47-11 Fibromatosis coli. CT image in one patient (A) and axial T1-weighted MR image in another patient (B) show unilateral enlargement of a sternocleidomastoid muscle *(asterisks)*. No CT attenuation or MR signal intensity alterations are present. (Courtesy of Fred Laine, MD.)

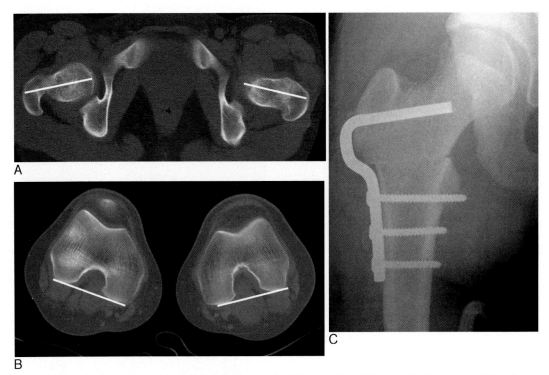

Figure 47-12   Femoral anteversion. **A and B,** Axial CT images obtained through the femoral necks (A) and condyles (B) without change in position of the patient changed allow accurate measurement of femoral anteversion. In this 13-year-old girl femoral anteversion is 33 degrees on the right and 26 degrees on the left. Bilateral proximal femoral derotation osteotomies were performed. **C,** Postoperative appearance of the right hip. Note the blade plate and the osteotomy *(arrows)*. See also Fig. 11-16.

Normal femoral torsion is 30+ degree anteversion at birth, decreasing to about 16 degrees by age 16, and to 10 degrees by adulthood. Excessive femoral anteversion causes gait and hindfoot abnormalities and contributes to hip dysplasia. Excessive anteversion occurs in developmental dysplasia of the hip, Legg-Calvé-Perthes disease, and neurologic and neuromuscular conditions. Excessive anteversion frequently resolves spontaneously during growth, but surgery may be needed. Surgical treatment is accomplished by femoral osteotomy: The femur is transversely divided into two pieces, alignment is improved, and the fragments are fixed with orthopedic hardware and allowed to heal with casting (Fig 47-12). A proximal varus osteotomy is employed when excessive valgus or hip instability and dysplasia are present to correct both problems with a single osteotomy, termed a varus derotation osteotomy (Fig. 44-9). A distal femoral osteotomy is preferred when genu valgum or varum is also present to simultaneously correct the abnormal knee alignment (Fig. 47-13).

Abnormal tibial torsion usually resolves during growth. Excessive internal torsion frequently occurs in association with congenital foot deformities or genu varum. Toddlers with excessive internal tibial torsion will have bowlegs and a pigeon-toed gait. Excessive lateral torsion causes a penguin-footed gait.

OSTEO-ONYCHODYSOSTOSIS

Osteo-onychodysostosis (nail-patella syndrome, Fong syndrome) is a rare autosomal dominant condition with multiple skeletal abnormalities. The most distinctive feature is posterior iliac horns, a pathognomonic finding that is present in most cases (Fig. 47-14A). The knees are dysplastic with absent or hypoplastic patellae (Fig. 47-14B), hypoplastic lateral femoral condyles, and associated valgus alignment (genu valgum). The elbows also are dysplastic, with a hypoplastic capitellum and associated radial head dislocation. The fifth metacarpals may be short. Clinical features include dysplastic fingernails, especially of the thumb and index fingers, clinodactyly, and renal disease.

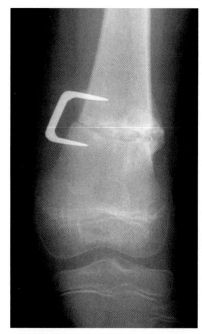

Figure 47-13 Distal femoral osteotomy performed to correct excessive anteversion in a child.

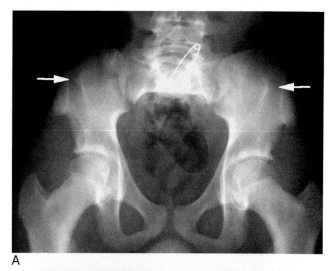

A

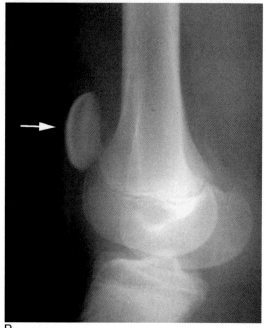

B

Figure 47-14 Osteo-onychodysostosis (Fong syndrome). **A,** Pelvis shows characteristic laterally oriented posterior iliac horns *(arrows)*. **B,** Lateral knee shows hypoplastic patella *(arrow)*.

Part VIII Sources and Suggested Readings

Elgenmark O: Normal development of the ossific centers during infancy and childhood: Clinical, roentgenologic and statistical study. Acta Pediatr 33(suppl):1–79, 1946.

Gerscovich EO: Practical approach to ultrasound of the hip in developmental dysplasia. Radiologist 5:23–33, 1998.

Graf R: Guide to Sonography of the Infant Hip. New York, Thieme, 1987.

Greenspan A: Sclerosing bone dysplasias: A target sign approach. Skel Radiol 20:561–583, 1991.

Greulich WW, Pyle SI: Radiographic Atlas of Skeletal Development of the Hand and Wrist, ed 2. Stanford, Stanford University Press, 1959.

Habermann CR, Weiss F, Shoder V, et al: MR evaluation of dural ectasia in Marfan syndrome: Reassessment of the established criteria in children, adolescents and young adults. Radiology 234:535–541, 2005.

Harcke HT: Screening newborns for developmental dysplasia of the hip: The role of sonography. AJR 162:395–397, 1994.

Harcke HT, Grisson LE: Performing dynamic sonography of the infant hip. AJR 155:834–844, 1990.

Keats TE: Atlas of Roentgenographic Measurement, ed 6. St. Louis, Mosby-Yearbook, 1990.

Keats TE, Anderson MW: An Atlas of Normal Roentgen Variants That May Simulate Disease, ed 5. St. Louis, Mosby, 1992.

Keats TE, Smith TH: An Atlas of Normal Developmental Roentgen Anatomy, ed 2. Chicago, Year Book Medical Publishers, 1988.

Kilcoyne R, Rych S, Gloch H: Radiological measurement of congenital and acquired foot deformities. Appl Radiol December:35–41, 1993.

Kleinman P: Diagnostic Imaging of Child Abuse. St. Louis, Mosby, 1998.

Laor T, Jarmillo D, Oestereich AE: Musculoskeletal system. In Kirks DR, Griscom NT (eds): Practical Pediatric Imaging, ed 3. Philadelphia: Lippincott-Raven, 1998.

Manaster BJ: Handbook of Skeletal Radiology. St. Louis, Mosby, 1997.

McAlister WH, Heman TE: Osteochondrodysplasias, dysostoses, chromosonal abberations, mucopolysaccharidoses, and mucolipidoses. In Resnick D (ed): Diagnosis of Bone and Joint Disorders, ed 3. Philadelphia, WB Saunders, 1995, pp 4163–4244.

Ozonoff MB: Pediatric Orthopaedic Radiology, ed 2. Philadelphia, W.B. Saunders, 1992.

Reimers J: The stability of the hip in children. A radiological study of the results of muscle surgery in cerebral palsy. Acta Orthop Scand Suppl 184:1–100, 1980.

Resnick D (ed): Diagnosis of Bone and Joint Disorders, ed 4. Philadelphia, W.B. Saunders, 2002.

Sontag LW, Snell D, Anderson M: Rate of appearance of ossification centers from birth to the age of five years. Am J Dis Child 58:949–956, 1939.

Spranger JW, Brill PW, Poznanski A: Bone Dysplasias, ed 2. Philadelphia, W.B. Saunders, 2002.

Swischuk LE, John SD: Differential Diagnosis in Pediatric Radiology, ed 2. Baltimore, Williams & Wilkins, 1995.

Taybi H, Lachman RS: Radiology of Syndromes, Metabolic Disorders, and Skeletal Dysplasias, ed 4. St. Louis, Mosby, 1996.

Teele RL, Share JC: Ultrasonography of Infants and Children. Philadelphia, W.B. Saunders, 1991.

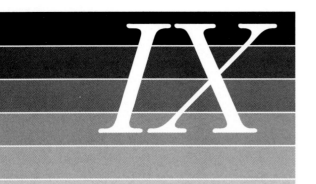

IX

TECHNIQUES

GENERAL APPROACH
NEEDLE PLACEMENT
    Shoulder Injection
    Elbow Injection
        Option 1: Posterior Approach
        Option 2: Lateral "Straight Down" Approach
    Wrist, Radiocarpal Joint Injection
    Wrist, Midcarpal Joint Injection
    Wrist, Distal Radioulnar Joint Injection
    Hip Injection
    Knee Injection
    Ankle (Tibiotalar) Injection

Arthrography is commonly used to distend joints before magnetic resonance imaging (MRI) or computed tomography (CT) in order to assess the intrinsic soft tissues of the joint or detect loose bodies or chondral lesions. The general approach is identical for all joints and is outlined in this chapter, followed by suggestions of standard approaches to specific joints.

GENERAL APPROACH

1. Informed Consent
   a. Be certain that the patient understands the reason his or her clinician has requested the examination, and describe the procedure step-by-step.
   b. Check the MR arthrography form; be certain that the patient has no contraindications to MR arthrography. Ask if there is any chance that a female patient may be pregnant. Confirm the patient's identity and which joint is to be injected.
   c. You can confidently tell the patient that the only major risk to arthrography is that of introducing an infection. The risk of this complication is 1 in 2000.
   d. You can tell the patient that, in most patients, the most painful portion of the examination is the initial

introduction of local anesthesia. In large joints, the distention of the joint itself is usually not painful (or even noticed by the patient). The major exception to this generalization is injection of wrist joints, where distention to full capacity can be painful. Mixing lidocaine with contrast medium reduces such discomfort. After wrist injection, especially if you use ionic contrast medium, it is wise to give the patient an icepack and suggest that it be used for the duration of the day.
   e. Unless the patient has unusual anatomy (e.g., significant hip protrusio), none of the standard approaches to joints places the needle close to a neurovascular bundle, so these structures are not at risk in the procedure.

2. Patient Prep Generalizations
   a. Mark the ideal needle placement on the skin.
   b. Administer standard local sterile prep.
   c. Use local anesthesia: 1% to 2% lidocaine, buffered with sodium bicarbonate (10:1 ratio lidocaine to bicarbonate) along the expected path of the arthrography needle. Lidocaine is not routinely injected intra-articularly. Although theoretically intra-articular lidocaine may enhance patient comfort, the intra-articular injection is in fact rarely painful. Furthermore, intra-articular lidocaine can rapidly enter the bloodstream, with potential for seizure or arrhythmia in some patients if a large amount is injected. However, there are two circumstances in which intra-articular anesthesia might be considered. First, we do routinely add a small amount of lidocaine to the solution injected in wrist or other small compartments, where the procedure is indeed fairly painful. Second, the clinician may request injection of anesthetic to help determine whether the cause of the patient's pain is intra-articular rather than extra-articular, often in the hip joint.

3. Contrast Mixture for MR Arthrography
   a. MR arthrography can be performed after saline injection, using T2-weighted sequences, or dilute

gadolinium, emphasizing T1-weighted images. (But do include at least one fat-suppressed, T2-weighted sequence to assess for marrow and soft tissue edema or other fluid collections.) We prefer gadolinium MR arthrography because of its superior resolution. If the patient is allergic to gadolinium, use saline.

b. Adopt a standard procedure for making the gadolinium mixture, which can be used in any joint. T1 shortening (greatest signal intensity) is maximized with a gadolinium dilution of 1:250. However, many musculoskeletal radiologists choose a higher concentration of 1:100 or 1:200 for injection. The reasons for this choice are several. First, these concentrations have only *slightly* lower signal intensity than 1:250, and the difference is almost imperceptible. Second, any pre-existing joint fluid will dilute the injected contrast medium, so the final gadolinium concentration very often is lower than the injected concentration. This is most likely to occur in a large joint, but could occur in any joint. Moreover, a popular technique is to confirm intra-articular needle tip position by injection of a small amount of lidocaine or iodinated contrast medium, then switch to a gadolinium and saline mixture. Signal intensity drops off perceptibly as the gadolinium concentration is diluted below 1:250.

c. Iodinated contrast medium shortens T2, causing lower signal intensity on all sequences, even T1-*weighted* sequences, which are affected to some degree by T2. Thus, minimizing the amount of iodinated contrast medium improves image quality. Thus, we recommend either adding the gadolinium to *dilute* iodinated contrast medium (about 80 mg iodine/mL), which is still easily seen with quality fluoroscopic equipment, or injecting only a small amount of full-strength iodinated contrast medium to confirm intra-articular needle tip position and then switching to a gadolinium-saline mixture.

d. Contrast reactions during arthrography are extremely rare. However, if the patient is allergic to iodinated contrast and you are confident of your technique, inject only dilute gadolinium in saline, or simply saline (and use T2-weighted sequences). Ultrasonographic (US) guidance is another alternative.

e. There is usually no need to add epinephrine. Intra-articular epinephrine causes local vasoconstriction, delaying imbibition of the injected fluid into the synovium, and theoretically may improve conspicuity of structures. However, especially if nonionic contrast medium is used and MR arthrography is performed within 2 to 3 hours of injection, there is no adverse effect on image quality.

4. Injection
   a. Needle placement is specific to each joint and is discussed below. In most joints, a "straight down" approach is used with fluoroscopy. Ultrasonographic guidance is more flexible but is less commonly used.

b. Avoid injection of air bubbles because they may simulate or obscure small intra-articular bodies on MR arthrography.

c. The possible techniques are many. Here is one used by one of the authors: Draw up the gadolinium-saline solution into a 20-mL syringe. Attach a flexible connector tube to the syringe. Forward flush the tubing from the syringe to eliminate all air bubbles and fill the tubing with the dilute gadolinium solution. Attach a needle, and draw full-strength iodinated radiographic contrast medium *only into the tubing*. Only 1 or 2 mL should be drawn up. There is a distinct advantage in this system over that of mixing the radiographic contrast medium into the gadolinium/saline mixture. First, when the needle is placed into the joint and you do the test injection, the radiographic contrast medium is concentrated enough that you will easily be able to see whether your placement is intra-articular. Second, if the needle placement is extra-articular, the injected radiographic contrast medium will not be seen on the T1-weighted MR arthrograms because no gadolinium was injected with it; therefore it will not potentially confuse interpretation. There is mild signal loss due to T2 shortening when iodinated contrast medium is mixed with gadolinium, but it is minimal when the radiographic contrast medium is this dilute. If, for whatever reason, the patient cannot tolerate MR arthrography after the joint is injected, the 2 to 3 mL of radiographic contrast medium injected from the tubing is often sufficient to outline intra-articular structures on CT, and the procedure can be salvaged.

d. Place the needle. Confirm placement by injecting a small amount of radiographic contrast medium. If the placement is intra-articular, the contrast medium will flow away from the needle, often in a particular pattern that is unique to the joint. If the placement is extra-articular, the contrast medium will pool around the needle tip. Once the needle is in proper position, inject the recommended amount (see below for amounts, which vary by joint). Do not overdistend the joint (e.g., if you feel resistance) because doing so will probably decompress into adjacent soft tissues and partially collapse the joint, thereby possibly confusing interpretation. Remove the needle.

5. Contrast Mixture for CT Arthrography
   a. Although MR arthrography is generally preferred to CT arthrography, there are circumstances such as contraindications, patient size, and presence of orthopedic hardware that dictate the need for CT arthrography. The resulting images can be excellent, particularly when obtained on a multichannel scanner with reformatted images in optimum planes.

b. Full-strength or diluted iodinated contrast medium can be used (especially if medium is ionic). Full-strength nonionic contrast medium and high scanner technique provide excellent images. If ionic contrast medium is used, one of the authors strongly recommends including 0.5 mL epinephrine in the contrast mixture.

   c. A double-contrast technique that involves iodinated contrast medium and room air can be used, but we prefer single contrast. Avoid injecting air bubbles with single contrast because they are unaesthetic, although not as potentially confusing as in MR arthrography.

6. Assessment for Vasovagal Reactions

   a. Before the patient sits up, take the time to be certain they do not have vasovagal symptoms.

   b. For whatever the reason, vasovagal symptoms are common with arthrography, and in our experience are most frequently seen in large or young athletic men. It is easier to recover patients on the table than after they try to stand.

NEEDLE PLACEMENTS

Shoulder Injection

1. Patient position: supine with palm up (external rotation of the shoulder) at patient's side, sandbag on hand (which otherwise drifts into internal rotation).

2. Approach: The shoulder joint is large and the needle could theoretically be placed anywhere within it, medial to the anatomic neck of the humerus (the capsular insertion). One does not need to place the needle into what appears to be "joint space," but only within the capsule. The most redundant portion of the joint lies over the inner and lower quadrant of the humeral head. Dropping the needle onto this spot, perpendicular to the table top, until it touches the humeral head, is an easy approach (Fig. 48-1). Another approach is to angle the needle medially into the "joint space." This is perfectly acceptable; the choice largely depends on operator training and comfort. A posterior approach has been suggested, to avoid injection into the anterior structures; however, if the syringe and tubing are set up as described previously, even with an initially malpositioned needle, only radiographic contrast medium flows into these anterior structures, and the T1-weighted arthrographic images will not be confusing. It is these authors' opinion that the posterior approach is not necessary.

3. Needle: 20- or 22-gauge spinal.

4. Intra-articular flow: away from the needle, often into one of the anterior bursae. You may not see contrast medium flow immediately into the "joint space" between the humeral head and the glenoid since this is a more restricted space than are the bursae.

5. Volume: 10 to 15 mL.

6. Hints

   a. The subscapularis tendon is somewhat firm and unyielding. The inexperienced operator may mistake

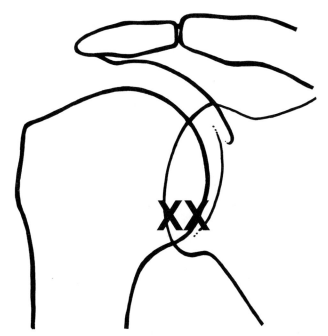

Figure 48-1   Shoulder. The "X"s mark two of the several acceptable injection sites. Two of the authors prefer the medial site. Do not place the needle further medially, as the needle will touch the labrum, which is very painful.

the tendon for the firm humeral head, resulting in an extra-articular injection. The mistake may be confounded by the fact that occasionally contrast medium from the test injection flows easily away from the needle in this position into the subcoracoid recess, not giving the tell-tale pooling that usually indicates extra-articular needle positioning.

   b. If the angled anterior approach is used, remember that the anterior labrum overlies the "joint space," and the needle must slip behind the labrum into the joint. Under fluoroscopy, it may not be possible to tell whether the needle is within the joint or on top of the anterior labrum. If you are uncertain, simply internally rotate the shoulder and watch the path of the tip of the needle. If it is intra-articular, the needle tip will stay within the "joint space"; if it is extra-articular, the needle tip will stray medially and be quite obviously outside the joint.

Elbow Injection

Option 1: Posterior Approach

1. Patient position: supine, with hand on abdomen and elbow flexed

2. Approach: palpate the lateral epicondyle, olecranon process, and radial head. These landmarks form a triangle on the posterolateral region of the elbow. Place the needle in the center of the triangle and advance toward the joint.

3. Needle: 1.5-inch, 25-gauge.

4. Intra-articular flow: away from needle, usually flows into the recesses anterior and posterior to the distal humerus, or around the radial neck.
5. Volume: 6 to 8 mL.
6. Hints: the authors feel that this is an easy approach, with the patient position being quite comfortable, and which does not disturb the structures of interest.

Option 2: Lateral "Straight Down" Approach

1. Patient position: prone with arm above head and elbow flexed 90 degrees; thumb up.
2. Approach: Perpendicular to table, entering the radio-capitellar portion of the joint (Fig. 48-2).
3. Needle: same as for option 1.
4. Intra-articular flow: same as for option 1.
5. Volume: same as for option 1.
6. Hints: this approach should be avoided if the clinical question involves the lateral supporting structures of the elbow.

Wrist, Radiocarpal Joint Injection

1. Patient position: prone with arm above the head, wrist mildly flexed over a towel. Wrist should be in mild ulnar deviation. A patient who cannot tolerate this position may remain supine, with the wrist at the side, palm down and mildly flexed.
2. Approach: marker should be placed over the scaphoid, approximately 0.5 cm distal to the radiocarpal "joint space" (Fig. 48-3). The needle is then directed at approx-

imately a 45-degree angle to slip between the scaphoid and dorsal lip of the radius.
3. Needle: 1.5-inch, 25-gauge.
4. Intra-articular flow: contrast medium may flow into the "joint space," but alternately may initially fill dorsal or volar bursae.
5. Volume: 4 to 6 mL.
6. Hints:
   a. If you are uncertain as to whether the needle is intra-articular, or need to determine whether it is "hung up" on the dorsal radial lip or the scaphoid, have the patient carefully turn the wrist into a lateral position so the tip position can be directly observed. Be sure to have the patient keep the wrist flexed; if it is extended, this thin needle will bend.
   b. Watch for flow from the radiocarpal joint into the distal radioulnar joint (DRUJ), indicating a triangular fibrocartilage complex tear, or flow into the midcarpal joint, which would indicate a scapholunate or lunotriquetral ligament tear.
   c. Although the single radiocarpal injection is usually sufficient for diagnosis, particularly when MR arthrography is being performed, there will be occasional requests for injection into the midcarpal or distal radioulnar joints. These injections may be

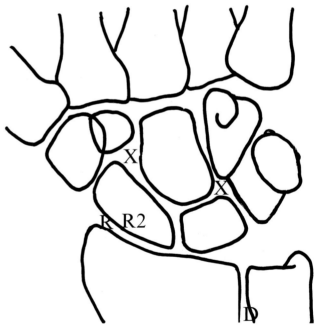

Figure 48-3   Wrist. There are three synovial compartments of the wrist. All are injected using a posterior approach. Each "X" marks an acceptable injection site for the midcarpal compartment. "D" marks an injection site for the distal radioulnar joint. One of the authors prefers a slightly more distal and lateral injection site for this compartment. "R" and "R2" mark injections sites for the radiocarpal joint. If using "R," the wrist should be elevated and slightly palmar-flexed to expose the distal radioulnar joint. This position can be accomplished by placing a rolled towel or small pad under the distal radius. If using "R2," the wrist is in neutral alignment (flat on the table), and the needle is angled proximally by 45 degrees to allow it to slip between the scaphoid and the dorsal lip of the radius.

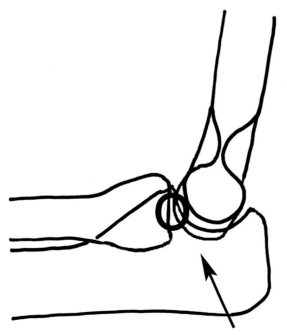

Figure 48-2   Elbow. Inject at the center of the "O" if using a lateral approach. See text regarding the easier posterior approach, which is marked by the *arrow.*

requested if a tiny "one-way" perforation is suspected, or if intra-articular details of those joints are desired (such as evaluation of the undersurface of the triangular fibrocartilage complex). Techniques for these injections are outlined in the next sections.

d. If the clinician is concerned about a dynamic carpal instability, it is important to perform several provocative maneuvers before arthrography. They are outlined as follows:

   i. Scapholunate dissociation: widening of the scapholunate interval greater than 2 to 3 mm, generally provoked with a clenched fist or ulnar deviation. The scaphoid may also angle volarly independently of the lunate, as seen in a lateral position.

   ii. Watson ("scaphoid shift") test for scapholunate dissociation. The patient's wrist is held in neutral alignment with the examiner's thumb pressed against the palmar distal pole of the scaphoid. The wrist is then moved into radial deviation while maintaining this pressure. The scaphoid will rotate further palmar in a normal wrist, but will not if scapholunate dissociation is present. This test is clinically positive if painful.

   iii. Capitolunate instability (CLIP [capitolunate instability pattern] maneuver): in the lateral projection, stabilize the patient's forearm with the wrist in slight ulnar deviation. With your other hand, grasp the patient's hand at the metacarpals and apply alternating dorsal and volar oriented force while observing for subluxation at the capitolunate articulation.

   iv. Triquetrum-hamate instability: during radial to ulnar deviation, the proximal carpal row abruptly shifts from palmar flexion to dorsi flexion just before extreme ulnar flexion is achieved. The hamate may be seen to slide against the triquetrum. Watch for this in both the frontal and lateral projections.

Wrist, Midcarpal Joint Injection

1. Patient position: prone, with arm above head, wrist flat with palm down. A patient who cannot tolerate this position may lie supine, with the wrist at the side, flat and palm down.
2. Approach: perpendicular to the table, direct the needle into the space at the "four corners" (junction of the lunate, capitate, hamate, and triquetrum), or into the space at the junction of the scaphoid, capitate, and trapezium (see Fig. 48-3). The needle should be inserted only about 1 cm; it will not be against bone.
3. Needle: 1.5-inch, 25-gauge.
4. Intra-articular flow: away from the needle, often into dorsal or volar bursae; expect flow to extend proximally between the scaphoid and lunate as well as between the

lunate and triquetrum; it will also flow approximately 1 cm between the bases of the second through fifth metacarpals.
5. Volume: 6 mL.

Wrist, Distal Radioulnar Joint Injection

1. Patient position: prone, with arm above head, wrist flat with palm down. Or, the patient may lie supine, with the wrist at the side, flat and palm down.
2. Approach: perpendicular to the table, direct the needle to the edge of the ulna at the DRUJ and gently "walk" it into the joint (see Fig. 48-3). The needle tip will not be on bone.
3. Needle: 1.5-inch, 25-gauge.
4. Intra-articular flow: directly into the small joint, centered over the distal ulna.
5. Volume: 1 mL.

Hip Injection

1. Patient position: supine, hip straight (although it may be slightly flexed if patient comfort requires it), internally rotated.
2. Approach: The hip capsule extends distally nearly to the intertrochanteric line. However, the hip joint is fairly constricted. The most redundant portion is directly over the thinnest portion of the femoral neck; it is easy to enter the joint by dropping the needle perpendicular to the table directly onto the center of the femoral neck (Fig. 48-4). Alternatively, the needle may be placed at the lateral head–neck junction. The needle tip should be on bone.

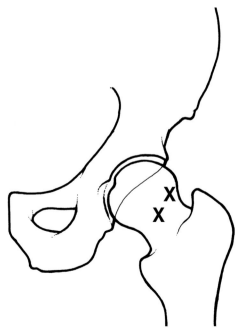

Figure 48-4   Hip. The "X"s mark two acceptable injection sites. The medial site is preferred for iliopsoas bursography (see text).

3. Needle: 20- or 22-gauge spinal. (Note: if joint *aspiration* is requested, consider using an 18-gauge needle because thick joint fluid may not return through a small needle.)

4. Intra-articular flow: into the redundant portion of the joint, usually "ringing" the femoral neck; specifically, it should *not* flow in a linear pattern outlining the angled superoinferior path of the iliopsoas bursa.

5. Volume: 10 to 15 mL.

6. Hints:

   a. If an iliopsoas bursagram is desired, use the same needle placement, but withdraw −0.5 to 1 cm from the femoral head/neck; flow will be linear and angled, outlining the iliopsoas bursa.

   b. If placing a needle for *aspiration* of suspected infection in a hip arthroplasty, use a large-gauge needle (18-gauge). Either a direct anterior approach to the femoral head/neck or an anterolateral approach to the femoral head/neck junction (advancing from above the greater trochanter) will work (Fig. 48-5). There will be a distinct "metal-on-metal" feel of the needle scraping the prosthesis. If no fluid is aspirated in this position, proof of intra-articular placement is made by injection of a small amount of radiographic contrast medium (this is only weakly bacteriostatic), followed by lavage of the joint with 10 mL of non-bacteriostatic saline and attempted aspiration. This

lavage is repeated until fluid can be aspirated. Since the fluid in the hip may be in a dependent position (behind the prosthesis), moving the hip into internal rotation or massaging the posterior part of the joint while aspirating may allow return of fluid in a difficult case.

Knee Injection

1. Patient position: supine, with the knee slightly flexed over a pillow, quadriceps relaxed.

2. Approach: push the lateral aspect of the patella medially, which "opens" the medial patellofemoral joint space; place the needle from a medial anterior position between the medial patellar facet and the anteromedial femoral condyle. This does not require fluoroscopy. Depending on patient size, the depth of the needle may be between 1.5 cm and up to its hub.

3. Needle: 1.5 inch, 20- or 22-gauge.

4. Intra-articular flow: away from the needle, generally into the suprapatellar bursa.

5. Volume: 20 to 30 mL.

6. Hints:

   a. The authors believe that the medial approach is easier, because of the angle of the medial patellar facet rather than the flatter angle of the lateral facet. However, if desired, a lateral approach is certainly reasonable.

   b. The suprapatellar bursa is potentially very large (easily holding 40 to 60 mL); therefore, it is important to aspirate as much effusion from the knee before injection of contrast medium to avoid dilution. "Milking" the suprapatellar bursa while aspirating can be helpful. If a large effusion is suspected, consider using an 18-gauge needle for the procedure since it makes the aspiration much easier.

   c. There is a fat pad located behind the patella, in its superior half. It is possible to bury the needle in this fat pad, resulting in a fat pad injection rather than intra-articular fluid. To avoid this, place the needle below the "equator" of the patella.

Ankle (Tibiotalar) Injection

1. Patient position: lying on side.

2. Approach: palpate dorsalis pedis artery and anterior tendons (to avoid them); ankle is in lateral position; using fluoroscopy, advance needle from anterior approach (Fig. 48-6).

3. Needle: 1.5-inch, 25-gauge.

4. Intra-articular flow: directly into joint.

5. Volume: 4 to 8 mL.

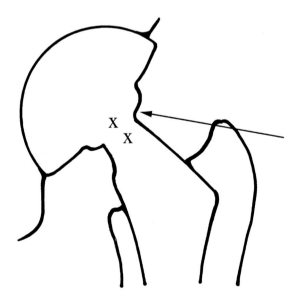

Figure 48-5 Hip arthroplasty. The "X"s mark acceptable needle placement sites if an anterior approach is used. *Arrow* marks the needle tract using an anterolateral approach, aiming for the prosthetic femoral head.

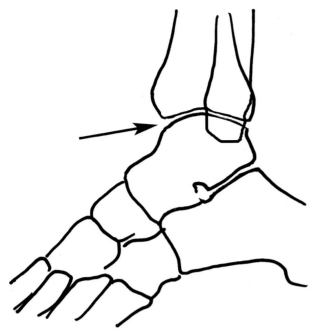

Figure 48-6   Ankle. *Arrow* marks the needle tract using an anterior approach with lateral fluoroscopy.

GUIDING PRINCIPLES
BIOPSY OF METASTASES
BIOPSY OF PRIMARY BONE TUMOR
SOFT TISSUE BIOPSY
SITE-SPECIFIC HINTS
NEEDLES
IMAGING GUIDANCE

7. *Magnetic resonance imaging (MRI) for site evaluation is recommended before biopsy*. Biopsy may result in hemorrhage, which may obscure the true extent of tumor.

BIOPSY OF METASTASES

1. Bone scan should be obtained before biopsy; there may be other sites that are more amenable to the procedure.
2. If the lesion is a metastasis or plasmacytoma, then the principles of protecting tissue planes that may be used for limb salvage surgery are not applicable.
3. Consider screening the patient's chest and abdomen with computed tomography (CT) for a primary tumor. Renal cell and thyroid carcinomas have a greater propensity for bleeding after biopsy. One may choose a smaller biopsy needle, less aggressive biopsy technique, or prebiopsy embolization when such primary lesions are suspected.
4. Fine-needle aspiration often is adequate for diagnosis of metastases or myeloma; it is useful to perform this initially and have the pathologist examine the material before moving forward with core biopsy. This will save the patient discomfort, decrease scanner time, and reduce complication risk.

BIOPSY OF PRIMARY BONE TUMOR

1. If there is a soft tissue mass, it may be easier to obtain tissue from that site than the osseous site.
2. Observe the general principles described previously in choosing the biopsy approach.
3. Infiltrate the periosteum liberally with local anesthetic.
4. If the osseous lesion is entirely lytic, it is worth placing the core needle, and then obtaining several fine-needle aspirates initially since it may be impossible to obtain a core.

GUIDING PRINCIPLES

1. *The sample must be representative*. Prior imaging should suggest which are the active portions of the tumor (e.g., part of the mass that enhances with contrast administration), and which are neither reparative nor necrotic. It is crucial to biopsy the most active portion of the tumor. In some cases of transformation of a benign process to a malignant tumor (such as enchondroma to chondrosarcoma or bone infarct to malignant fibrous histiocytoma), the imaging may demonstrate both the less aggressive benign process and the more aggressive malignant process (usually an area of bone destruction); biopsy must be of the latter site.
2. *The approach must avoid tissue that is needed for reconstruction*. This is critical for primary tumors if limb salvage surgery is contemplated. Since the entire needle track must be resected as part of sarcoma curative surgery, the biopsy plan must include consideration of which tissue will be needed for reconstruction. Thus, before biopsy it is crucial that the case be discussed in detail with the surgeon, and the biopsy approach agreed upon. Coaxial technique, in which the outer needle remains outside of the tumor, reduces but does not eliminate the possibility of needle track seeding with tumor.
3. *The needle track should cross only one compartment*.
4. *Neurovascular bundles must be avoided*.
5. *Joints must be avoided if at all possible*.
6. *Avoid contamination of the physis*.

5. If the lesion is sclerotic, or you must core through dense cortex to get to the lesion, it may take a great deal of strength. It can help to stand on a stool over the patient to use your full force while pushing the needle.

6. To obtain the core, use a bone-cutting needle, remove the stylet once the tip is at the lesion, and core for 2 cm if possible. It can be difficult to retain the core within the needle tip; to do so, keep the needle in place and wiggle the needle to break the core from the adjacent bone. Place a syringe on the coring needle and aspirate while pulling it straight out.

7. Treat the core carefully; use the obturator to back it out of the coring needle in order to reduce crush artifact.

8. Consider carefully whether or not to perform a percutaneous biopsy on a cartilage lesion. Many orthopedic oncologic teams choose to not biopsy cartilage lesions percutaneously for two reasons. First, chondrosarcoma is the most likely of all osseous tumors to recur in a biopsy track since it does not need to establish a blood supply to grow. Second, and perhaps more important, it is extremely difficult to distinguish enchondroma from an atypical enchondroma, from a low-grade chondrosarcoma pathologically. Very large amounts of tissue (often the entire lesion) are often needed before a secure diagnosis is reached. Therefore, percutaneous needle biopsy of a cartilage lesion is not likely to yield enough representative tissue to be reliable.

SOFT TISSUE BIOPSY

1. Obtain several (we recommend six) cores using a biopsy gun; these cores should be from several different sites within the tumor, allowing for the best chance of obtaining representative tissue.

2. Observe the general principles described previously in choosing the biopsy approach.

3. Neural lesions can be exquisitely tender. Consider a regional anesthetic block rather than local anesthesia when prebiopsy imaging suggests such a diagnosis.

SITE-SPECIFIC HINTS

1. *Shoulder:* If at all possible, the biopsy approach should be through the anterior third of the deltoid. The deltopectoral groove should be avoided so as to not compromise the use of the pectoralis for reconstruction. The posterior deltoid should be avoided since its resection leaves the anterior deltoid denervated and therefore functionless.

2. *Humeral shaft:* Anterolateral approach avoids the major nerves.

3. *Pelvis:* Avoid the gluteal muscle mass, as well as the rectus. These structures are most often used for reconstruction. Therefore, the best approach to a pelvic primary musculoskeletal tumor is obliquely through the anterior or posterior iliac crest.

4. *Thigh:* Avoid the rectus or quadriceps tendon since they are required for functional limb-sparing surgery.

5. *Knee:* Avoid the joint; remember that the suprapatellar bursa is large, and reaches far both proximally and laterally. Additionally, if the patient has a complex posterior mass, consider ultrasonography (US) to make certain that it is not highly vascular.

6. *Tibia:* Best approach is through the anteromedial cortex; there is no significant soft tissue to contaminate through this approach.

NEEDLES

Needle choice is to some degree a matter of personal preference. Vertebroplasty needles with a beveled diamond tip are preferred by some for ease of control and rapid access through cortex. Very dense cortex or very dense lesions may require a trephined needle, which has a crown-shaped cylindrical tip that grinds a cylindrical defect around a core specimen.

An interesting comparison of bone biopsy needles may be found in Roberts CC, Morrison WB, Leslie KO, et al: Assessment of bone biopsy needles for sample size, specimen quality and ease of use. Skeletal Radiol 34:329–335, 2005.

IMAGING GUIDANCE

Computed tomography, US, fluoroscopy, and even MRI in some centers are used to localize the tumor, the vital structures to be avoided, and the needle. User preference and "whatever works" usually make this determination. Ultrasonography allows for real-time imaging of the advancing needle. In some cases, combining US and CT can assist in avoiding vascular structures.

GENERALIZATIONS
LANDMARKS
IMAGES

GENERALIZATIONS

This chapter briefly reviews how to obtain ultrasonographic (US) images of the infant hip. The pathophysiology and interpretation of US findings of hip dysplasia are reviewed in Chapter 44. Review of that section is suggested before one reads this chapter. The US technique emphasized here is based on a popular and widely accepted approach to infant hip US. It must be emphasized that this is not the only way to reliably detect and follow developmental dysplasia of the hip. Many experienced ultrasonographers have developed slightly or even widely different approaches that have stood the test of time. For example, the Graf system (Table 50-1) of careful measurements of static coronal images is popular in many centers, at least as part of a hybrid approach. If your institution does it differently, this description is not intended as a criticism of your technique.

Scans are easiest to obtain when the child is relaxed and quiet. The temperature and lighting should be comfortable for an infant, and the gel should be warmed. Feeding the child before or during the examination helps the child to relax. Glucose water will suffice if no milk or formula is available. Enlist the parent's help in feeding, calming, and positioning the baby. Beware of male infants, as they will invariably urinate on your shoes. An appropriately placed towel or washcloth can avoid this problem. Stress maneuvers are best left until the end of the examination, as the infant may become irritated by this forceful handling.

A high-frequency linear array transducer, at least 5 MHz, is used. Occasionally, a curved transducer is used to obtain the "big picture" of a dislocated hip, and can better show the relationship of the dislocated femoral head and acetabulum. If the child is in a cast placed to maintain reduction of a previously dislocated

hip, the available window may be too small for anything other than a small footprint sector array transducer. Be creative.

If the child is in a Pavlik harness, do not remove it. The harness will not impede the examination. Do not perform stress maneuvers on an infant in a harness unless specifically requested to do so by the referring orthopedic surgeon. Stress maneuvers may redislocate a hip that was difficult for the surgeon to reduce.

A routine examination includes both hips. The examination is often easiest to perform from a lateral approach with the child in a decubitus or oblique decubitus position, scanning the upside hip. The hips may be flexed or extended, but infants usually prefer keeping their hips flexed.

LANDMARKS

Major landmarks of hip US include the femoral head, triradiate cartilage, lateral ilium, and acetabular roof (Figs. 44-3, 44-4).

The *cartilaginous femoral head* is round and hypoechoic and contains speckled internal echoes. Ossification of the femoral head begins as early as the third month as a central small, round hyperechoic focus with posterior acoustic shadowing (Figs. 50-1, 50-2). Such ossification provides a convenient landmark for localizing the center of the femoral head. In younger infants, adjust the transducer position to maximize the diameter of the femoral head on each image. This technique guarantees that the center of the femoral head is in the image.

The hypoechoic *triradiate cartilage* is located just anterior to the center of the acetabulum. It is a reasonable technique to place the triradiate cartilage at the center of the images. A few echoes will project medially to the triradiate cartilage, assisting in locating this landmark (see Fig. 50-1). On axial images, the triradiate cartilage is located between the pubic bone anteriorly and the slightly longer ischium posteriorly.

The *lateral cortex of the ilium*, like the other ossified bones, is seen as a well-defined hyperechoic line with dense posterior acoustic shadowing. The lateral ilium is continuous with the osseous *acetabular roof*. The angle formed by the lateral ilium

Table 50-1   The Graf Classification of Infant Hip Dysplasia

Hip type	Bony roof*	Angle†	Alpha angle (degrees)	Beta angle (degrees)
Ia: Mature hip	Good	Sharp	≥60	<55
Ib: Transitional form	Good	Blunt	≤60	>55
IIa: Physiologically immature (<3 months of age)	Sufficient	Round	50–59	>55
IIb: Delayed ossification (>3 months of age)	Deficient	Round	50–59	>55
IIc: Critical range (any age, normal labrum)	Deficient	Round or flat	43–49	70–77
IId: Subluxed hip	Severely def.	Round or flat	43–49	>77
IIIa: Dislocated hip (no structural alteration)	Poor	Flat	<43	>77
IIIb: Dislocated hip (with structural alteration)	Poor	Flat	<43	>77
IV: Severely dislocated hip	Poor	Flat	<43	>77

*Bony roof, coverage of femoral head. Good is ≥50%.
†Junction of osseous ilium and osseous acetabular roof.
Modified from Graf R, Wilson B: Sonography of the Infant Hip and Its Therapeutic Implications. London: Chapman and Hall, 1995, and Laor T, Jarmillo D, Oestereich AE: Musculoskeletal system. In Kirks DR, Griscom NT (eds): Practical Pediatric Imaging, ed 3. Philadelphia, Lippincott-Raven, 1998.

and the acetabular roof is the *alpha angle* not to be confused with the alpha angle used in femoroacetabular impingement (see Fig. 44-3).

The *acetabular labrum* forms an echogenic triangle lateral to the acetabular roof (Fig. 44-3C).

IMAGES

Scans are obtained in the coronal and transverse planes. The hips may be flexed or extended.

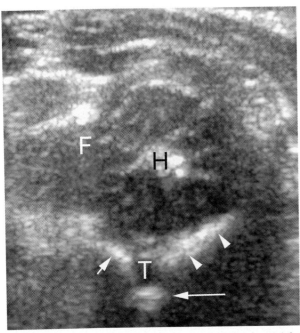

Figure 50-1   Transverse US image, with anterior to the viewer's left, in a 10-week-old girl. Note the triradiate cartilage with echoes medial to the cartilage *(long arrow)*. Also note the early ossification at the center of the femoral head, ischium *(arrowheads)*, and pubis *(short arrow)*. The pubis is partially shadowed by the femoral shaft anteriorly. F, femoral shaft; H, femoral head; T, triradiate cartilage.

Optimal coronal images have the following features (see Figs. 44-3, 50-2):

1. The lateral cortex of the ilium is displayed as a straight line parallel to the transducer.
2. The acetabular roof is clearly displayed. The alpha angle is formed by the lateral ilium and the acetabular roof (see Fig. 44-3).
3. The femoral head is on the right side of the image (inferiorly). The center of the femoral head is in the image.
4. The triradiate cartilage is in the image. The triradiate cartilage is so-named because it includes portions of all three pelvic bones: the ilium, the ischium, and the pubis. It is located just anterior at the center of the acetabulum. In a normally aligned hip, the femoral head is centered slightly posterior to the triradiate cartilage. A reasonable approach to US is to obtain images with the femoral head centered over the triradiate cartilage for reproducibility.
5. The labrum is seen as an echogenic triangle lateral to the acetabular roof.

An image with these qualities is termed "the standard plane" in the Graf system, and is the only image that this system requires.

Displaying the lateral ilium as a straight line parallel to the transducer is usually straightforward. If the lateral ilium has a concave contour, then the transducer is too far posterior (see Fig. 50-2). If the lateral ilium flares laterally toward the transducer, then the transducer is too far anterior (see Fig. 50-2). Angling the transducer slightly is often needed to fine-tune the image.

Including both the center of the femoral head and the center of the triradiate cartilage in the image requires some dexterity. One approach is to first find the lateral ilium, then, while keeping the ilium in proper alignment, find the center of the femoral head. Next is the hard part: while keeping the ilium *and* femoral head in proper alignment, find the hypoechoic triradiate cartilage to complete the image. These maneuvers require sliding the

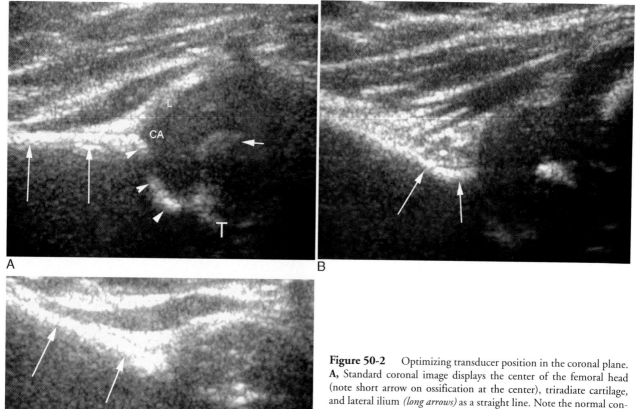

Figure 50-2   Optimizing transducer position in the coronal plane. **A,** Standard coronal image displays the center of the femoral head (note short arrow on ossification at the center), triradiate cartilage, and lateral ilium *(long arrows)* as a straight line. Note the normal concave contour of the osseous acetabular roof. Also note the hypoechoic cartilaginous acetabulum and hyperechoic labrum. **B,** Transducer too far posterior. The lateral ilium has a concave contour *(arrows).* **C,** Transducer too far anterior. The lateral ilium flares toward the transducer *(arrows).* CA, cartilaginous acetabulum; L, labrum; T, triradiate cartilage.

transducer over the hip while constantly adjusting the angle. Slight rotation off of true coronal is often helpful.

Obtain the coronal image at least twice to document that the alpha angle is reproducible.

Transverse scans are obtained with and without posterior subluxing stress. The acetabulum is demarcated by the echogenic pubic bone anteriorly, the slightly longer, echogenic ischium posteriorly and the hypoechoic triradiate cartilage between them. An optimal axial image in a normal hip will extend through both the center of the femoral head and the center of the triradiate cartilage. If the hip is flexed and the scan is obtained parallel to the femur, the ossified femoral shaft will obscure some of the pubis (see Figs. 44-4, 50-1). The greater trochanter and sometimes the femoral shaft will be included on routine transverse views with the hip in flexion. Obtaining axial scans with the hip flexed and extended also can be performed. A modified Barlow maneuver is performed with the hip flexed and adducted. Posterior

force is applied to the femur and the relationship of the femoral head and acetabulum is observed. A subluxable hip is displaced posteriorly and laterally by this maneuver. When performing this stress maneuver, you may find it helpful to hold the transducer between your thumb and index and middle fingers while placing your remaining fingers against the infant's sacrum. This allows force to be directed to the hip joint, rather than simply displacing the entire infant posteriorly. Start gently and observe closely. If no subluxation is evident during application of light force, push a little more firmly. A millimeter or two of subluxation with firm pressure is normal in neonates. (How much force is enough? The amount of force to apply is somewhat subjective, and experience is helpful. Several experienced ultrasonographers have demonstrated to one of the authors the amount of pressure they apply. Most apply a force in the range of 2 to 5 kg, but sometimes more. Practice on your bathroom scale.)

A minimum set of images obtained in a routine screening examination will include at least two coronal images that document reproducible measurement of the alpha angle (and the beta angle if you use the Graf system), and axial images with and without stress. Remember to scan both hips. Compare the hips to each other, and with any prior studies. A complete examination will document the size and symmetry of the cartilaginous femoral heads and the ossific femoral nuclei (if present), the shape of the acetabular roof (concave is normal, straight is a gray zone between normal and abnormal, wavy is abnormal), the femoral head coverage by the osseous acetabular roof (should be at least 50% covered), the position of the femoral head (should be centered over the triradiate cartilage), the position of the labrum (should not be flipped medially), and hip stability if stress views were obtained.

Scans of a dislocated hip are different. If the femoral head is subluxed or frankly dislocated, it is important to document whether alignment is improved by altering the position of the femur. This can be assessed by moving the femur through a range of motion under direct US observation. Note what you see, as this information will assist the orthopedic surgeon. Chronically subluxed or dislocated hips may demonstrate an inverted limbus (i.e., medial displacement of the hyperechoic superior labrum between the laterally and superiorly displaced femoral head and the acetabulum) (see Fig. 44-3).

Interpretation of properly obtained images is relatively straightforward, except in the most dysplastic hips. In contrast, performing the study has a slow learning curve. There is no substitute for experience. Advice to residents: take advantage of any opportunity offered to obtain the scan yourself, particularly under the direction of an experienced ultrasonographer who can assist and guide you toward obtaining reproducible and accurate images.

Index

Note: Page numbers followed by f refer to figures; page numbers followed by t refer to tables; page number followed by b refer to boxes.

A

ABC. *See* Aneurysmal bone cyst
Abduction and external rotation (ABER) position, 108f
ABER position. *See* Abduction and external rotation
Abnormal limb length, 362f
Abscess, 36t
Absent distal clavicle, 623f
Absent segmentation, 595f
AC joint. *See* Acromioclavicular
Accessory navicular, 263
Accessory ossicles, 271
Acetabular component
  anteversion of, 361f
  failed, 363f
Acetabular dysplasia, 598
Acetabular fractures, 189–193
  transverse, 190f
Acetabular labrum, 666
  tear, 204f
Acetabular osteotomy, 606f
Acetabular roof, 666
Acetabulum, primary protrusio of, 295, 608–609
Achilles peritendinitis, 260f
Achilles tendon, 250, 252
  causes of, 260–262
  rupture, 262f
  tendinosis of, 261f
  xanthomatosis of, 263f
Achondrogenesis, 632–633, 633f
Achondroplasia, 631–632
ACL. *See* Anterior cruciate ligament
Acne, 326, 559–560
Acquired Immunodeficiency Syndrome. *See* AIDS
Acromegaly, 359
Acromial spur, 89f
Acromial undersurface morphology, 85t
Acromioclavicular (AC) joint, 68, 76–77, 305, 376f
  injuries, 76b, 77f
  radiographs of, 76

Acromioclavicular osteophytes, 89f
Acromion process, 73, 88
Acromioplasty, 92f
Acro-osteolysis, 330, 331t
  leprosy, 333f
  thermal injuries, 332f
Acute chondrolysis, 45
Adamantinoma, 427, 527–529
Adenocarcinoma, 496f
Adhesive capsulitis, 85f
Adolescent tibia vara disease, 357
Adult Still's disease, 298
AIDS, 562
Ainhum, 279
Albers-Schönberg disease, 626
Alcaptonuria, 343
Algorithms, tumor work-up, 530
  osseous lesion, 532f
  soft tissue musculoskeletal lesions, 532f
Alignment, fracture, 8–11
ALL. *See* Anterior longitudinal ligament
Alpha angles, 601, 602f, 666
ALPSA lesion, 104f
Ameloblastoma, 529
Amniotic band syndrome, 647–648
Amyloidosis, 343, 343b, 344f
  spine, 345f
Anatomy
  bone, 3–6
  femur, 194
  foot, 271–272
  hip, 194
  knee, 209–212
  shoulder, 68, 112–117
  wrist, 135f, 136f
Anemia, 402
Aneurysmal bone cyst (ABC), 514, 514–519
  foot, 518f
  geographic lesion, 518
  of great toe, 518f
  key concepts of, 517b
  pathogenesis of, 518

Aneurysmal bone cyst (ABC) *(Continued)*
  secondary, 521f
  of spine, 520f
Angiography, 25
Angiosarcoma, 480, 488f
Angular deformity, 9
Anisotropic ultrastructure, 28
Ankle
  anatomy of, 249–252
  arthroplasty, 368f
  injection, 661
  instability of, 27f, 256–257
  juvenile rheumatoid arthritis of, 303f
  lateral ligaments at, 251f
  ligament injury, 268
  ligament sprain, 27f
  ligaments, 249b
  trauma patterns, 252–258
Ankle impingement, 268–269
Ankle radiographic anatomy, 250f
Ankle tendon injury, 258–268
Ankylosing spondylitis, 289, 318–321
  extraspinal complications of, 322f
  of hip, 321f
  key concepts of, 319f
  pseudarthrosis, 321f
  of SI joints, 319f
  of spine, 320f
Ankylosis, 287, 291
Anlage, 581
Annular ligament, 126
Anterior bundle, 125
Anterior capsule insertion variation, 85
Anterior column, 164, 190
Anterior column fracture, 193f
Anterior cruciate ligament (ACL), 219f
  ganglion, 246f
  graft failure, 238f
  injury to, 233–239
  normal, 233f
  reconstruction of, 237
  tear, 235f, 236f

Anterior fat pad sign, 115
Anterior humeral line, 113f
Anterior instability, 106
Anterior longitudinal ligament (ALL), 314
Anterior soft tissue injuries, 104f
Anterior talofibular ligament, 249, 268
Anterior tibiotalar ligament, 250
Anterolateral gutter impingement, 268
Anterolateral impingement, 268
Anteroposterior compression, 185, 187f
Anteversion, 194, 606
    of acetabular component, 361f
    femoral, 651f
AP position. *See* Anteroposterior
Apophyseal avulsion injuries, 189
Apophysis, spinal ring, 588f
Apposition, 9
Arthritis, 30t. *See also specific types*
    alignment and, 286–287
    bone and, 287
    cross-sectional imaging in, 288b
    distribution of, 287–288
    erosions in, 288
    fungal, 563f
    future directions in imaging, 288–289
    monoarticular, 287
    oligoarticular, 287
    polyarticular, 287
    with preserved cartilage space, 287t
    radiographic assessment of, 285, 286–288
    septic, 560–562
    soft tissues in, 288
Arthrography, 67, 656–662
    contrast mixture for, 656–657
    of elbow, 127f
    general approach, 656–658
    informed consent, 656
    injection, 657
    patient prep generalizations, 656
Arthrogryposis multiplex congenita, 648, 649f
Arthroscopic subacromial decompression, 92
Arthroscopy, of articular cartilage, 42–43
Arthrosis, 76
Articular cartilage, 40–46
    arthroscopy of, 42–43
    defects, 43b, 44f, 158f
    imaging, 42b
    normal, 42f
    properties of, 41
Asphyxiating thoracic dysplasia, 633
Atlantoaxial distance, 165
Atlantoaxial rotary displacement, 169
Atrophic nonunion, 21
Atrophy, 36t
Atypical spinal hemangioma, 484f
Autologous chondrocyte transplantation, 45f
Avascular necrosis (AVN), 21, 24f, 196, 272, 274, 328, 333, 355, 393, 541–542
    clinician knowledge in, 349f
    common sites of, 349–350
    CT of, 351f
    demographics of, 346–347
    etiology of, 346–347
    hip, 348f
    imaging of, 347–349

Avascular necrosis (AVN) *(Continued)*
    key concepts, 346
    of lunate, 349
    mimics, 353–354
    MRI of, 350f
    radiographic evaluation of, 349f
    sickle cell and, 571f
    of spine, 352f
    talar dome, 275
    treatment of, 349–351
Avian spur. *See* Supracondylar process
AVN. *See* Avascular necrosis
Avulsion fracture, 4, 10
    greater tuberosity, 97b
    of joint capsule from dorsal triquetrum, 144
    of knee, 217–219
    of tibial insertion of anterior cruciate ligament, 219f
Avulsion injuries, knee, 217–219
Axillary nerve, 87

B

Baker's cysts, 243, 244f, 245f
Bankart lesion, 100, 101, 102f
    bony, 109
    repair, 111f
    reverse, 109
    soft tissue, 103f
Barlow maneuver, 600
Bartonella henselae, 562
Barton's fracture, 139
Baseball finger, 162
Baastrup's disease, 310
Baumann's angle, 117
    measurement of, 115f
Bending-type fractures, 4
Benign fibrous cortical defect, 467–470
    key concepts of, 469b
Benign fibrous histiocytoma, 470
Bennett lesion, 107
Beta angles, 602f
Beta thalassemia, 567
Biceps, 83
Biceps labral complex, 83
Biceps tendon, 94
    insertion, 130f
    long head tendinosis, 98
    tear, 130f
Bicondylar fractures, 213
Bigliani classification, 86
Bilateral locked facets, 172, 174f
Biomechanics, bone, 3–6
Biopsy, tumor, 530–531
Bisphosphonates, 402
Blastic metastasis, 420
Blastic prostate metastases, 497f
Blount disease, 357
BMD. *See* Bone mineral density
Boehler's angle, 273, 274f
Bone
    anatomy, 3
    arthritis and, 287
    biomechanics, 3–6
    bridges, 50

Bone *(Continued)*
    drug-induced changes in, 392b
    island, 419–420, 419b, 421f
Bone biopsy
    guiding principles, 663
    imaging guidance in, 664
    of metastases, 663
    needle choice in, 664
    primary bone tumor, 663–664
    Site-specific hints, 664
Bone lesions, locations for, 413t
Bone marrow imaging, 539–542
    MRI, 540f
    normal distribution, 540f
Bone mineral density (BMD), 391, 392
Bone scanning, 421f
Bone-forming tumors
    benign, 419–428
    malignant, 429–441
Bony Bankart injury, 109
Both bones fracture, 131, 133f
Boutonnière deformity, 162, 163f, 292
Bowing fractures, 5f
Boxer's fracture, 159, 160f
Brodie's abscess, 554
Brown tumors, 376
    of hyperparathyroidism, 378f, 523
Brucellosis, 30t
Bubbly lytic metastasis, 497f
Bucket handle fracture, 59
Burns, 30t
Bursa, 28, 239–244
    gastrocnemius-semimembranosus, 243
Bursitis, 28, 29f, 97b
    pes anserinus, 244f
    trochanteric, 208
Burst fracture, 169f, 175, 177f
Butterfly-shaped comminuted fracture, 4

C

Caffey's disease, 62, 625f, 626
Calcaneal tuberosity, 273
Calcaneofibular ligament, 249b
Calcaneonavicular coalition, 616, 617f
Calcaneus, 271
    edema in, 619f
    rheumatoid arthritis of, 295f
    stress fractures of, 14f, 273
Calcaneus fracture, 272–274
Calcific bursitis, 28, 90
Calcific tendinitis, 32, 33, 34f, 90, 91f
Calcinosis cutis, 30t
Calcitonin, 373, 374, 402
Calcium homeostasis, key concepts of, 373b
Calcium hydroxyapatite, 90
Calcium pyrophosphate deposition (CPPD), 30t, 287, 307, 339–342
    terminology, 339b
Callus, 17, 60
    excessive, 626t
Camptomelic dysplasia, 634
Campylobacter, 325
Capital femoral epiphysis, slipped, 200–201

Capitellum
  OCD of, 131, 132f
  pseudodefect of, 115f
Capitolunate instability, 156
Capsular ligaments, 151b
Carpal arcs, 142
Carpal bone alignment, 134b
Carpal bone dislocations, 143–147
Carpal bone fractures, 143–147
  on coronal magnetic imaging, 146f
Carpal bones, 142–143
  miscellaneous conditions of, 156–158
  motion of, 143f
Carpal instability, 147–156
  static, 150
Carpal ligaments, 151b
  anatomy of, 153f
Carpal translocation, 156
Carpal tunnel syndrome, 46t, 157, 158f
Carpal tunnel view, 147f
Carpometacarpal dislocation, 157b
Carpometacarpal (CMC) joints, 134b, 159
Cartilage-forming tumors, 442–459
Cartilaginous anlage, 581
Cartilaginous femoral head, 665
Cartilaginous joints, 26
Caudal regression syndrome, 595
Central chondrosarcoma, 456–458
Cervical alignment, 165
Cervical spine, 164–165
  instability, 166f
  juvenile rheumatoid arthritis of, 303f
  normal variants, 166
  radiographic assessment of, 164
  rheumatoid arthritis of, 298f
Cervical spine fractures, 167–174
Chance fractures, 176, 177f
Charcot-Marie-Tooth disease, 46, 311
Charcot's arthropathy. *See* Neuropathic
  arthropathy
Chauffeur's fracture, 139
Chemotherapy, 433
Cherubism, 463
Child abuse, 58–62
  radiographic sites for, 58t
  radiologic findings for, 60t
  skeletal findings, 61f
Childhood buckle fracture, 8f
Childhood fractures, 49–52
Chip fractures, 10
Chlamydia trachomatis, 325
Chondroblastoma, 452–453, 455f, 556
  key concepts, 453b
Chondrocalcinosis, 339
Chondrodysplasia punctata, 636f
Chondroectodermal dysplasia, 633, 635f
Chondroid matrix, 410t, 411f
Chondroid tumor, in distal femur, 444f
Chondroma, juxtacortical, 450–452, 454f
Chondromalacia, 44
Chondromyxoid fibroma, 456
Chondrosarcoma, 458b
  central, 456–458
  clear cell, 459
  dedifferentiated, 459
  enchondroma v., 444b

Chondrosarcoma *(Continued)*
  intramedullary, 456f, 457f
  mesenchymal, 459
  peripheral, 458
Chordoma, 526–527, 527b
Chromosomal abnormalities, 644–6646
Chronic recurrent multifocal osteomyelitis
  (CRMO), 559–560
Class I fracture, 188f, 189
Class II fracture, 189
Class III fracture, 189
Classic metaphyseal lesion, 58–59, 61f
Clavicle, 68
  absent distal, 623f
  fracture, 68f
Clay shoveler's fracture, 173
Clear cell chondrosarcoma, 459
Cleavage fractures, 213
Cleidocranial dysplasia, 77, 622, 623f
Clinodactyly, 645
Closed fractures, open fractures v., 6–7
Closed reduction, 14
Clostridium, 545
Clubfoot, 613
CMC joints. *See* Carpometacarpal joints
Coalitions, tarsal, 615–618, 621f
  osseous, 620f
Cobb method, 586
Coccidioidomycosis, 30t
Codman's triangle pattern, 430, 437
Codman's tumor. *See* Chondroblastoma
Collagen vascular diseases, 30t
Collateral ligament injury, 239, 241f
Colles fracture, 16, 138
Comminuted fractures, 5f, 7–8
  butterfly, 8
Comminuted intercondylar fracture distal
  femur, 213f
Compartment syndrome, 39, 131
Complete fractures, incomplete fractures
  v., 7–8
Complete tears, 34f
  of posterior tibialis tendon, 265
Component loosening, 360b
Compression, 3, 4, 175
  anteroposterior, 185, 187f
  lateral, 185
  of lumbar vertebral bodies, 4f
Compression fractures, 175
Computed tomography (CT), 6, 67, 112, 134,
  164, 184, 194, 212, 213, 289, 318, 407,
  430, 435, 479
  arthrography, 42b
  of article disease, 366f
  of AVN, 351f
  contrast mixture for, arthrography, 657–658
  of foreign bodies, 48
  for fracture union, 22f
  of fractures, 10b
  of hip relocation, 191f
  in hyperparathyroidism, 377f
  in osteomyelitis, 547
  sagittal, 171f
  of scapula, 73–74
  in soft tissue infection, 545
  of transverse fracture line, 191f

Computed tomography (CT) *(Continued)*
  in tumor follow-up, 533
  in tumor work—up, 530
  of tumors, 417
Condylar sulcus, 209
Congenital foot deformities, 610–615
Congenital generalized fibromatosis, 465
Congenital radial head dislocation, 647
Congenital radioulnar synostosis, 647, 648f
Congenital scoliosis, 583
Congenital syphilis osteomyelitis, 556,
  557f
Congenital vertical talus, 613, 615f
Congruence angles, 217
Connective tissue disorders, 328–334, 583,
  643–644
Conradi's disease, 635
Contrast medium, 257, 657–660, 662
Contusion, intramuscular, 37f
Conventional osteosarcoma, 429–433
Cooley's anemia, 567
Coracoacromial arch, 85–86
Coracoacromial ligament, 86
Coracohumeral impingement, 97f
Coracoid process, 73
Cortical breakthrough, 413
Cortical desmoid, 242, 243f
Cortical tumors, 414t
Cortical tunnels, 392
Coxa valga, 194, 448, 607–608
  bilateral, 608f
Coxa vara, 607–608
  congenital, 608f
CPPD. *See* Calcium pyrophosphate
  deposition
Creeping substitution, 347
CREST syndrome, 30t, 329
Critical zone, 95
CRMO. *See* Chronic recurrent multifocal
  osteomyelitis
Crohn's disease, 376
Crossover sign, 207f
Cruciate ligament injury, 233–239
CT. *See* Computed tomography
Cubital tunnel syndrome, 46t, 130
Cuboid, 271
Cuneiforms, 271
Cyclops lesion, 237, 238f
Cysticercosis, 30t

D

Dactylitis, 568
  sickle cell, 570f
DDH. *See* Developmental dysplasia of hip
De Quervain's disease, 156
Dedifferentiated chondrosarcoma, 459
Degenerative disk disease, 165
Delamination, 43, 44
Delayed union, 21
  nonunion v., 21b
Deltoid complex, 249b
Deltoid tuberosity, 71, 72f
Denervation
  acute muscle, 38f
  chronic muscle, 39f

Dense metaphyseal bands, differential diagnosis of, 323b
Depressed fractures, 213
Dermatomyositis, 30t, 39, 331–333, 332b, 333f
Derotation osteotomy, 606
Desmoid tumor, 465
Desmoplastic fibroma, 467
Developmental dysplasia of hip (DDH), 598–606
  after reduction and casting, 604f
  imaging of, 598–604
  key concepts, 597b
  management of, 605–606
  radiography of, 599f, 600
  risk factors for, 598t
  ultrasonography of, 600–604, 603f
  untreated, 600f
DEXA. *See* Dual x-ray absorptiometry
Diabetic myonecrosis, 39, 40f
Diabetic neuropathy, osteomyelitis and, 552f
Diastasis, 26b, 27
Diastrophic dysplasia, 635
Die punch, 10, 12f
Diffuse idiopathic skeletal hyperostosis (DISH), 287, 314–315, 315f, 320
  spine fracture in, 316f
Diffuse increased bone density, 386t
  differential diagnosis of, 324b
DIP. *See* Distal interphalangeal
Discitis, 557, 558f, 559f
Discoid meniscus, 230, 231f
DISH. *See* Diffuse idiopathic skeletal hyperostosis
DISI. *See* Dorsal intercalated segment instability
Disk degeneration, 309f
Dislocation, 26b, 27
  anterior hip, 196f
  carpometacarpal, 157b
  elbow, 123
  Essex-Lopresti fracture, 124f
  finger, 161f
  glenohumeral joint, 98–109
  hip, 194–196, 196f, 668
  knee, 223
  Lisfranc's, 275–277, 278f
  midcarpal, 147
  Monteggia's fracture, 121f
  patellar, 216–217
  radial head, 117b, 122f
  of SC joint, 76
  shoulder, 104f, 105f, 106f
  teratogenic, 597
  unilateral interfacetal, 172
Displacement, 8–9
  atlantoaxial rotary, 169
  of humeral fractures, 72f
  meniscal tears, 228f, 229f
  vertical, 186
Dissociation, 148
  lunotriquetral, 156
  occipital atlas, 169f
  occipital vertebral, 167

Distal biceps tendon, 129
Distal clavicle, 77
Distal femoral osteotomy, 652f
Distal femur, chondroid tumor of, 444f
Distal fibular physis, 259f
Distal fibular stress fractures, 260f
Distal forearm, 137–138
Distal forearm fractures, 138–140
  by age, 138b
Distal humeral physis, fracture-separation of, 121
Distal humerus fractures, 123
Distal interphalangeal (DIP), 162, 291, 322
Distal radioulnar joint, 137–138
  injection, 660
Distal radius, 134b
Distal radius fracture, 139f
Distal tibia-fibula syndesmosis, 249b
  tear, 269f
Distal tibial stress fractures, 259f
Distal ulna, 134b
Distraction, 9
Divergent subluxation, 276
Don Juan fractures. *See* Calcaneus fracture
Dorsal intercalated segment instability (DISI), 150, 154f, 155
Dorsal triquetrum, avulsion fracture of joint capsule from, 144
Dorsiflexor, 113
Down syndrome, 644
Dual x-ray absorptiometry (DEXA), 391, 392
Dupuytren's contracture, 156, 465
Dwarfism, 629–636
  fatal, 632–633
  with horizontal acetabular roofs, 631t
  key concepts, 630b
  with short extremities, 631t
  with short ribs, 631t, 633–634
  with spine involvement, 631t
  with stippled epiphyses, 634–635
Dynamic carpal instability, 150
Dynamic fixation, 15
Dynamic stabilizers, 83
Dynamized intramedullary nail, 19f
Dyschondrosteosis, 636
Dysostosis multiplex, 640b, 641, 642f
Dysplasia
  acetabular, 598
  asphyxiating thoracic, 633
  camptomelic, 634
  chondroectodermal, 633, 635f
  cleidocranial, 622, 623f
  developmental, of hip, 597–606
  diastrophic, 635
  glenoid, 75f
  infant hip, 666t
  metatrophic, 634
  multiple epiphyseal, 637
  progressive diaphyseal, 628
  scapular neck, 75f
  sclerosing bone, 625–629
  spondyloepiphyseal, 636–637
Dysplasia epiphysealis hemimelica, 450, 453f
Dystrophic calcifications, 30t

E
Edema, 36t
  in calcaneus, 619f
  marrow, 541
Ehlers-Danlos disease, 30t, 643
Elbow
  anatomy, 112–117
  hemophilia in, 567f
  imaging techniques, 112
  injection, 658–659, 659f
  miscellaneous injuries, 130–131
  normal arthrographic anatomy of, 127f
  normal MR anatomy of, 127f
  radiography, 113f
  rheumatoid arthritis of, 292, 293f, 294
Elbow dislocation, 123
  soft tissue calcification after, 124f
Elbow fractures
  in adults, 122–125
  in children, 117–122
  key concepts in, 123b
Elbow ligaments, 125–130
  lateral, 126f
  medial, 126f
Elbow tendons, 125–130
Elgenmark method, 580
Enchondral ossification, 49, 577
Enchondroma, 442–445
  appearance of, 443
  chondrosarcoma v., 444b
  in hand, 443f–444f
  with malignant transformation, 445f
Enchondromatosis, multiple, 445
Endocrinopathy, 495
Endosteal scalloping, 409
Endplate spurs, 311f
Enthesis, 26
Eosinophilic granuloma, 520, 556
Epicondylitis
  lateral, 126
  medial, 126
Epiphyseal growth plate, 49, 577
Epiphyseal marrow signal, abnormal, 581t
Epiphyseal ossification, 57
Epiphyseal osteomyelitis, 555f
Epiphysiodesis, 584f
Equinus, evaluation of, 611f
Erb's palsy, 75
Erdheim-Chester disease, 523
Erlenmeyer flask deformity, 579
Erosion, in arthritis, 288
Erosive osteoarthritis, 325–326
Escherichia coli, 549
Essex-Lopresti fracture, 123, 124f, 131
Ewing's sarcoma, 431, 489–491, 490
  key concepts of, 489b
  sclerotic, 491f
Exertional compartment syndrome, 40
Exostosis, 445–447, 445b, 446, 448f
  benign complications of, 450f
  complications of, 446
  hereditary, 452f
  malignant transformation of, 447, 451f

Exostosis *(Continued)*
   MRI of, 449f
   multiple, 452f
   pedunculated, 445
   sessile, 445, 449f
Extension injuries, 172–173
Extensor carpi ulnaris, 156f
Extensor digitorum longus, 252
Extensor hallucis longus, 252
Extensor mechanisms, 211
Extensor tendon avulsions, 162f
Extensor tendon tear, 129f
External fixation, 15, 19f
Extrinsic wrist ligaments, 151

F

Fabella, 211
Facet joints, osteoarthritis of, 308
Fairbanks' disease. *See* Multiple epiphyseal dysplasia
Fallen fragment sign, 514
Fanconi anemia, 647
Fascicles, 46
Fasciitis
   infectious, 547f
   necrotizing, 545
   plantar, 279
Fat, normal, 35f
Fat pad signs, 115, 123b
   with radial head fracture, 116f
Fat-fluid levels, 10
Fatigue fractures, 12
   at ankle, 256
Fat-suppressed spoiled three-dimensional
      gradient echo, 42b
Fatty marrow, 539–540
Fatty tumors, 475–478
Femoral component, 362
   failed, 363f, 364f
   fractured, 363f
Femoral condyle subchondral insufficiency
      fracture, 246f
Femoral impingement, 205
Femoral neck fractures, 196–198
Femoral shaft fractures, 201–202
Femoral stress fractures, 202–203, 204f
Femoral torsion, 202f
Femoral trochlea, 212
Femoroacetabular impingement, 204–207
Femorotibial articulations, 209
Femur
   anatomy, 194
   anteversion of, 651f
   torsion of, 650–651
Fibrolipoma, neural, 505f
Fibrolipomatous hematoma, 503
Fibroma
   desmoplastic, 467
   nonossifying, 467–470
Fibromatosis, 465–467
   aggressive, 465, 466f
   congenital generalized, 465
   infantile dermal, 465
   juvenile aponeurotic, 465
   palmar, 465
   plantar, 466, 468f, 469f

Fibromatosis coli, 650
Fibrosarcoma, 30t, 472–473
Fibrous dysplasia, 427, 460–465, 462f
   bubbly lytic pattern, 465f
   craniofacial involvement in, 462
   key concepts, 460b
   of pelvis, 463f
   of skull, 461f
   of tubular bones, 463f–464f
Fibrous joints, 26
Fibroxanthoma, 467–470
   key concepts of, 469b
Fingers, dislocations, 161f
Fissures, 43
Flexible flatfoot deformity, 613–615
Flexion injuries, 172, 175
Flexion teardrop, 172
Flexor annular pulleys, 162
Flexor digitorum longus, 250
Flexor hallucis longus, 250, 257
   tear, 266f
Fluid-fluid levels, 418t
Fluorosis, 316, 386
Focal gigantism, 649b
Follow-up, tumor, 533–534
Foot
   anatomy, 271–272
   aneurysmal bone cyst of, 518f
   congenital deformities, 610–615
   neuropathic arthropathy in, 312f
   osteomyelitis in diabetic neuropathic, 552f
   rheumatoid arthritis of, 295
   soft tissue injury, 277–279
Footprint, 95
Forearm, 131–132
   fractures, 131–132
Forefoot, evaluation of, 614f
Forefoot fractures, 277
Forefoot valgus, 613
Forefoot varus, 613
Foreign body imaging, 47–48
Four spin-echo intermediate-T2, 42b
Fractures, 3b, 121, 365
   acetabular, 189–193
   alignment, 8–11
   anterior column, 193f
   avulsion, 4, 10
      of knee, 217–219
      of lesser trochanter, 200
   Barton's, 139
   bending-type, 4
   bicondylar, 213
   biomechanical classification of pelvic, 185–187
   both bones, 131, 133f
   bowing, 5f
   Boxer's, 159, 160f
   bucket handle, 59
   burst, 169f, 175, 177f
   butterfly-shaped comminuted, 4
   chance, 176, 177f
   chauffeur's, 139
   childhood, 49–52
   childhood buckle, 8f
   chip, 10
   Class I, 188f, 189
   Class II, 189

Fractures *(Continued)*
   Class III, 189
   clavicle, 68f
   clay shoveler's, 173
   cleavage, 213
   closed, 6–7
   Colles, 16, 138
   comminuted, 5f, 7–8
   complete, 7–8
   complications, 17–25
   compression, 175
   CT of, 10b
   depressed, 213
   description terminology, 6–11
   distal femur, 213
   distal forearm, 138–140
   distal humerus, 123
   distal radius, 139f
   elbow, 117–122
   fatigue, 12
      ankle, 256
   femoral condyle subchondral insufficiency,
      246f
   femoral neck, 196–198
   femoral shaft, 201–202
   follow-up radiographs, 17b
   forearm, 131–132
   forefoot, 277
   Galeazzi's, 131, 133f
   Garden stage I, 197f
   Garden stage IV, 197f
   greater tuberosity, 97b, 98f
   greenstick, 5f, 7
   Hangman's, 170, 171f
   healing, 14–16, 17–25
      in child, 20f, 21f
   Hill-Sachs, 99, 101f, 102, 105
   horizontal, 185
   humeral shaft, 72, 73f
   Hutchinson's, 139
   hyperextension teardrop, 171f
   incomplete, 7–8, 9f
   insufficiency, of sacrum, 16f
   intertrochanteric, 199–200
   intra-articular, 9f, 10
   Jefferson, 167
   Jones, 277
   lateral compression, 176
   lateral condylar, 117b, 119f
   lateral humeral condylar, 118f
   Lisfranc's, 275–277, 278f
   location, 8–11
   lumbar, 175–177
   Malgaigne, 186
   march, 12–13
   medial epicondylar, 119f
   medial epicondylar avulsion, 117b
   navicular bone, 274–275
   nightstick, 131
   nonunion, 21
   oblique, 7
      of fourth toe proximal phalanx, 4f
   occipital condyle, 167, 169f
   odontoid, 169, 170f
   open, 6–7
      of tibia, 7f

Fractures *(Continued)*
  osteochondral, 11, 12f
  patellar, 213–215
  pathologic, 14, 17f
  Pelkin's, 388f
  pelvic ring classification of pelvic, 187–189
  periprosthetic, 367f
  pilon, 256, 258f
  pisiform, 150
  position, 8–11
  posterior wall, 190
  proximal humerus, 69f, 70f
  radiographically occult, 7f, 198f
  reduction of, 14–16
  Rolando's, 159, 160f
  Saber-Harris I, 49, 52, 53f, 71, 72f, 121, 223f
  Saber-Harris II, 49, 59, 138, 220
  Saber-Harris III, 49, 220, 256, 257f
  sacral, 185
  scaphoid, 144f
  scaphoid waist, 157b
  Schatzker I, 213, 215f
  Schatzker II, 213
  Schatzker III, 213
  Schatzker IV, 213
  Schatzker V, 213
  Schatzker VI, 213
  seat belt, 176
  Segond, 220f, 236
  Smith's, 139
  spiral, 6f, 7
  straddle, 186
  stress, 12–14, 259f, 260f
    calcaneus, 14f
    femoral, 202–203, 204f
    knee, 222–223
    metatarsal, 277
    MRI of, 14f
    navicular, 277f
    of proximal tibia, 13f
  supracondylar, 117b, 118f
  talus, 274
  teardrop burst, 173f
  terminology, 6b
  thoracic, 175–177
  threshold, 4–5
  tibial plateau, 212–213, 214f
  Tillaux, 256, 256f
  toddler's, 8f
  trans-scaphoid perilunate, 146
  transverse, 4f, 7, 190f, 497
    of patella, 4f
  transverse process, 177
  transverse-posterior wall, 191f
  triplane, 257
  triquetrum, 157b
  T-shaped, 192f
  volar plate, 161, 161f
Freiberg's disease, 349, 351f
Frenkel's line, 388f
Frostbite, 30t
Full-thickness tears, supraspinatus, 94f
Fungal arthritis, 563f
Fungal osteomyelitis, 558–559
Fusiform swelling, 288

G

Gadolinium, 423, 563
Galeazzi's fracture, 131, 133f
Gallium-67, 547
Ganglion cysts, 157, 244, 529
Garden classification, 196
Garden stage I subcapital fracture, 197f
Garden stage III subcapital fracture, 197f
Garden stage IV fracture, 197f
Gastrocnemius, 240
Gastrocnemius-semimembranosus bursa, 243
Gaucher's disease, 346, 544f
  MRI of, 543
GCT. *See* Giant cell tumor
Generalized osteoporosis, 391–393
  key concepts of, 391b
GHLs. *See* Glenohumeral ligaments
Giant cell reparative granuloma, 514
Giant cell tumor (GCT)
  aggressive, 510f
  benign, 513
  of bone, 509–514
  growth of, 511f
  key concepts of, 509b
  metaphyseal, 511f
  MRI of, 511, 515f
  radiographic appearance of, 509
  recurring, 513
  of tendon sheath, 506, 507f
Gigantism, 648–650
  focal, 649b
Gilula's arcs, 142, 145
Glenohumeral joint, 68, 77–85
  anatomy, 78f
  anterior instability, 99b
  capsule, 84
  dislocation, 98–109
    posterior, 105
  instability, 98–109
  key concepts, 83b
  MRI of, 79f–82f
  multidirectional instability, 99b
  normal arthrographic anatomy, 78f
  posterior instability, 99b
Glenohumeral ligaments (GHLs), 84–85
  tears, 100
Glenoid, 73
Glenoid dysplasia, 75f
Glenoid fossa, 78f
Glenoid hypoplasia, 75
Gout, 30t, 335–339
  key concepts, 335b
  MRI of, 337f
  oblique hand radiograph of, 337f
  presentation of, 338f
  rheumatoid arthritis and, 337f
Gouty tophi, 336
Graf system, 600, 601, 666t
Granuloma
  eosinophilic, 520, 556
  giant cell reparative, 514
Great toe
  aneurysmal bone cyst of, 518f
  osteomyelitis in, 557f

Greater arc, 146, 147f
  injuries, 148f
Greater tuberosity, 83, 89
  avulsion fracture, 97b
  fracture, 98f
Greenstick fractures, 5f, 7
Greulich and Pyle technique, 589
Growth arrest, 50, 51f, 52f
  after distal tibial physeal injury, 52f
  after meningococcemia, 53f
Growth cartilage, 581
Growth hormone, 359
Growth plate, 49, 577
Growth recovery lines, 578, 579f
Guyon's canal syndrome, 46t, 157, 158f

H

HADD. *See* Hydroxyapatite deposition disease
HAGL lesion, 100, 104f
Haglund's disease, 262, 263f
Hair-on-end periosteal reaction, 413
Hamate hook fracture, 147f, 157b
Hamstring avulsion, 207f
Hand
  enchondroma in, 443f–444f
  juvenile rheumatoid arthritis of, 302f
  rheumatoid arthritis of, 291–292
Hand-foot syndrome, 568
Hand-Schüller-Christian disease, 519
Hangman's fracture, 170, 171f
Hardware loosening, 24f
Harrington rod, 589f
Harris lines, 578
Heavy metal poisoning, 387
Heel spurs, 279
Hemangioendothelioma, 479
Hemangioma, 479b
  atypical spinal, 484f
  spine, 485f
  vertebral body, 483f
Hemangiopericytoma, 479
Hemarthrosis, 211, 565
Hematoma, 16, 35, 36t, 37f
Hemiarthroplasty, 360
Hemiatrophy, 648
Hemihypertrophy, 648
Hemihypotrophy, 648
Hemivertebrae, 585f
Hemochromatosis arthropathy, 342
Hemophilia, 565–566
  in elbow, 567f
  key concepts of, 565b
  MRI in, 566
  pseudotumor of, 565–566, 568f
Hemorrhage, 186–187
Hemosiderin deposition, 542
Hernia, sports, 208
Herniation pit, 205–206, 206b
Heterotropic ossification, 36
  post-traumatic, 38f
High tibial osteotomy, 307, 308f
High-grade intramedullary osteosarcoma, 429–433
High-grade surface osteosarcoma, 439
Hilgenreiner's line, 600

Hill-Sachs fractures, 99, 101f, 102, 105
Hindfoot, evaluation of, 611f, 612f
Hindfoot equinus, 610
Hindfoot valgus, 610
Hindfoot varus, 610
Hinge joints, 249
Hip, 305, 320
    anatomy, 194
    ankylosing spondylitis of, 321f
    arthroplasty, 361f, 362f, 364f, 661f
    AVN of, 348f
    developmental dysplasia of, 597–606
    fracture, 196–198
    groin lateral radiographic view of, 195f
    injection, 660
    OA of, 305, 306f
    psoriatic arthritis of, 324f
    pyrophosphate arthropathy of, 341f
    relocation, 191f
    rheumatoid arthritis of, 295–296, 297f
    screws, 199f
    septic arthritis of, 560–562
    snapping, 203–204
    transient osteoporosis of, 354
Hip dislocation, 194–196, 668
    anterior, 195
    posterior, 195f
Histiocytoma, benign fibrous, 470
Hodgkin's disease, 493
Hoffa's disease, 247
Hoffa's fat pad, 211, 247
    trauma, 248f
Holt-Oram syndrome, 646
Homocystinuria, 643–644
Homolateral subluxation, 275–276
Horizontal fractures, 185
Humeral capitellum, 112
Humeral shaft, 68–73
    displacement of fractures, 72f
    fractures of, 72, 73f
Humeral trochlea, 112
Humerus, AP view of, 377f
Humpback deformity, 144
Hurler syndrome, 641
Hutchinson's fracture, 139
Hyaline cartilage injury, 244–247
Hydroxyapatite deposition disease (HADD),
    30t, 342–343
    key concepts of, 342b
Hyperemia, 395, 565
Hyperextension injuries, 176
Hyperextension teardrop fracture, 171f
Hyperflexion injury, 172
Hyperostosis, 326
Hyperparathyroidism, 30t, 77, 374–376,
    512
    bone sclerosis and, 379f
    Brown tumors of, 378f, 523
    CT in, 377f
    key concepts, 374b
    primary, 374
    radiographic features of, 375f, 376f
    secondary, 374
    tendon rupture in, 379f
    tertiary, 374
Hypertrophic nonunion, 21

Hypertrophic osteoarthropathy, 358–359
    secondary, 359f
Hypervitaminosis A, 386, 387f
Hypervitaminosis D, 386
Hypochondroplasia, 631
Hypoparathyroidism, 30t, 389
    key concepts of, 389b
Hypoplasia, 648–650
Hypothyroidism, 388–389
    congenital, 388f

I

IGHL. *See* Inferior glenohumeral
    ligament
Ilioischial line, 183, 184f
Iliopectineal line, 183
Ilium, lateral cortex of, 665
Imaging techniques
    elbow, 112
    shoulder, 67
    wrist, 134
Impingement, 27–28
    ankle, 268–269
    anterolateral, 268
    anterolateral gutter, 268
    chronic, 89
    coracohumeral, 97f
    femoral, 205
    femoroacetabular, 204–207
    rotator cuff, 88–92
Incomplete fractures, 9f
    complete fractures v., 7–8
Infantile cortical hyperostosis. *See* Caffey's disease.
Infantile dermal fibromatosis, 465
Infectious fasciitis, 547f
Infectious myositis, 39f
Inferior glenohumeral ligament (IGHL), 84
Inflammatory bowel disease, spondylitis
    of, 318–321
Informed consent, in arthrography, 656
Infrapatellar plicae, 246
Infraspinatus, 78, 86
Inserted limbus, 598
Instability
    ankle, 256–257
    anterior, 106
    capitolunate, 156
    cervical spine, 166f
    dynamic, 150
    glenohumeral joint, 98–109
    multidirectional, 107
    triquetrohamate, 156
Insufficiency fracture, of sacrum, 16f
Intercalated segments, 150
Intercarpal joint, 137b
Intercondylar fractures, 212
Internal fixation, 15, 17f
    cerclage wires and pins, 18f
    with intramedullary nail, 18f
Internal impingement, 88
Interstitial tears, 32
Intertrochanteric fractures, 199–200
Intra-articular bodies, 27, 28f
Intra-articular fractures, 9f, 10
Intracortical lucencies, 392, 393f

Intramedullary chondrosarcoma, 456f, 457f
Intramedullary nail, 18f
    dynamized, 19f
Intramembranous ossification, 577
Intramuscular lipoma, 477f
Intraosseous osteosarcoma, low-grade,
    439–440
Intrasubstance tear, 32
Intrinsic ligaments, 150
Involucrum, 550
Ischemic necrosis. *See* Avascular necrosis

J

Jaffe-Campanacci syndrome, 470
Jansen-type metaphyseal chondrodysplasia,
    640
Jefferson fracture, 167
Jerked elbow, 122
Joint arthroplasty, 360–369
    failed, 362f
    hip, 361f, 362f, 364f
    infection in, 365
    joint, 360–369
    shoulder, 109, 367f
    silastic, 367, 368f
    total, 360
Joints, 26–28
    alignment, 26b
    cartilaginous, 26
    fibrous, 26
    pain, 41
    synovial, 26
Jones fracture, 277
Judet views, 190, 191
Jumper's knee, 240–241, 241f
Juvenile aponeurotic fibroma, 366f, 465
Juvenile kyphosis, 589
Juvenile rheumatoid arthritis, 299–302
    of ankle, 303f
    of cervical spine, 303f
    of hand, 302f
    of wrist, 302f
Juxtacortical chondroma, 450–452, 454f
Juxtacortical tumors, 414t

K

Kienböck's disease, 137, 145, 349, 351f,
    357
Kite's angle, 612
Klebsiella, 550
Kleinmann, Paul, 58
Klippel-Feil syndrome, 591–594
Klippel-Trenaunay-Weber syndrome, 644,
    649, 650f
Knee
    anatomy, 209–212
    avulsion injuries, 217–219
    injection, 661
    neuropathic arthropathy of, 313
    OA of, 307
    pain causes, 247t
    partial arthroplasty, 368f
    physeal injury of, 220–222

Knee *(Continued)*
  pyrophosphate arthropathy of, 341f
  radiographic anatomy of, 209–212
  rheumatoid arthritis of, 295
  stress fractures, 222–223
  tendons of, 239–244
Knee dislocations, 223
  anterior, 223
Kümmell's disease, 349
Kump's bump, 255
Kyphoplasty, 175
Kyphosis, 589

L

Labral tears, 107–109. *See also* Superior labral anterior and posterior tears
  imaging diagnosis, 107
  posterior, 109f
Labrum, 83
Lamellated periosteal reaction, 413
Laminar tears, 32
Langer type spondyloepiphyseal dysplasia, 62
Langerhans cell histiocytosis, 491, 514, 519–523
  aggressive, 522
  key concepts of, 519b
  vertebra plana, 523f
Lateral angulation, 9
Lateral collateral ligament (LCL), 125
  complex, 251f
  injury to, 239
Lateral compression, 185, 186f
Lateral compression fractures, 176
Lateral condylar fracture, 117b, 119f
Lateral cortex of ilium, 665
Lateral epicondylitis, 126, 128f
Lateral humeral condylar fractures, 118f
Lateral ligament complex, 240f
Lateral malleolus, 249
Lateral meniscus retinacula, 226f
Lateral radiographs, 134
Lateral ulnar collateral ligament, 125
Latissimus dorsi, 68
Lauge-Hansen classification, 253
LCL. *See* Lateral collateral ligament
Lead arthropathy, 359
Lead poisoning, 387f
Leg lengthening, surgical, 584f
Legg-Calvé-Perthes disease, 205, 351–353, 597, 651
  key concepts of, 353b
Leg-length discrepancy, 582–583
Leprosy, 30t, 333f
Lesion density, 410–411
Lesser arc, 146–147, 147f
  injuries, 149f
Lesser trochanter
  avulsion fracture of, 200
  metastasis, 499f
Letournel views, 190
Letterer-Siwe disease, 519

Leukemia, 569–570
Leukemic lines, 570, 572f
Ligament of Humphrey, 224
Ligament of Struthers, 46t, 116–117
Ligament of Wrisberg, 224
Ligamentous ossification, differential diagnosis of, 320b
Ligaments, 26–28
  ankle, 249b, 267
  capsular, 151b
  carpal, 151b, 153f
  chronic lateral collateral tears, 27f
  collateral, 239
  degeneration of, 529
  elbow, 125–130
  extrinsic wrist, 151
  intrinsic, 150
  Lisfranc's, 272, 273f
  lunotriquetral, 150
  meniscofemoral, 224
  MRI of, 28
  scapholunate, 150, 151f
Limbus vertebrae, 175, 176f, 310, 311f
Lipoblastoma, 476
Lipoma, 475–477
  atypical, 475
  intramuscular, 477f
  low-grade liposarcoma v., 475f
  osseous, 476, 481f
  parosteal, 481f
Lipoma arborescens, 477
Lipomatosis, 475
Liposarcoma, 30t, 477–478, 482f
  lipoma v., 475f
Liposclerosing myxofibrous tumor (LSMFT), 470–471, 472f
Lisfranc's fracture-dislocation, 275–277, 278f
Lisfranc's ligament, 272, 273f
Little leaguer's elbow, 120, 121f
Long bone infarcts, 570f
Long bone lysis, 397
Looser's zones, 378
Lover's fractures. *See* Calcaneus fracture
Low-grade intraosseous osteosarcoma, 439–440
Lumbar fractures, 175–177
Lumbar spine, 174–175
Lumbar vertebral bodies, compression of, 4f
Lunate, 142
  AVN of, 349
  fractures, 145
  rotary subluxation of, 146
Lunate fossa, 137
Lunotriquetral dissociation, 156
Lunotriquetral ligaments, 150, 152f
Luxatio erecta, 105, 107f
Lymphoma
  non-Hodgkin's
  primary, of bone, 491–492
Lytic lesions, 428f

M

Macrodystrophia lipomatosa, 475, 480f, 649
Madelung deformity, 637f, 645, 646

Maffucci's syndrome, 445, 447f
Magic angle effect, 30, 31f, 107b
Magnetic resonance arthrograms, 102, 206
  contrast mixture for, 656–657
Magnetic resonance imaging (MRI), 6, 30b, 67, 88, 92, 134, 164, 184, 194, 212, 249, 289, 318, 322, 328, 347, 355, 393, 407, 435, 443, 479
  arthrography, 42b
  of AVN, 350f
  of bone marrow, 540f
  of bursitis, 29f
  chemical shift, 542f
  of elbow, 127f
  of exostosis, 449f
  of foreign bodies, 47f
  of Gaucher's disease, 543
  of giant cell tumors, 511, 515f
  of glenohumeral joint, 79f–82f
  of hemophilia, 566
  of ligaments and tendons, 28
  in meniscal tear diagnosis, 232b
  of muscles, 33b
  of myositis ossificans, 524
  for OCD, 56
  of osteoid osteoma, 425f
  osteomyelitis in, 547–548
  of patellar dislocation, 217f
  in radiographically occult hip fractures, 198f
  of stress fracture, 14f
  of synovitis, 29f
  of tendons, 31f, 33b
  in tumor follow-up, 533
  in tumor work—up, 530
  of tumors, 417
Maisonneuve fracture, 253, 254f
Malgaigne fracture, 186
Malignant fibrous histiocytoma (MFH), 472–473, 473b, 474f
  secondary osseous, 474f
Mallet finger, 162
Malunion, 21
March fractures, 12–13
Marfan syndrome, 643
Marginal erosions, 286f, 288
Marginal syndesmophytes, 319
Marrow edema, 541
Marrow infiltration, 540
Marrow reconversion, 540, 541f
Marrow space expansion, 569f
Mastocytosis, 568–569, 572f
Mazabraud syndrome, 465
McCune-Albright syndrome, 463
MChD. *See* Metaphyseal chondrodysplasia
McKusick-type metaphyseal chondrodysplasia, 640
MCL. *See* Medial collateral ligament
MCP joints. *See* Metacarpophalangeal
MCTD. *See* Mixed connective tissue disease
MED. *See* Multiple epiphyseal dysplasia
Medial collateral ligament (MCL), 125, 237, 249–250
  injury to, 239
  normal, 239f

Medial epicondylar avulsion fracture, 117b
Medial epicondylar fractures, in children, 119f
Medial epicondylar ossification center, avulsion of, 118
Medial epicondyle entrapment, 118, 120f
Medial epicondylitis, 126
Medial row, 143
Medial talar tilt, 257
Median nerve, 131
Mediopatellar plicae, 246, 248f
Melorheostosis, 628
MEN. *See* Multiple endocrine neoplasia
Meningoceles, 595
Meningococcemia, growth arrest after, 53f
Meniscal cyst, 232f
Meniscal homologue, 140
Meniscal root avulsion, 228, 230f
Meniscal tears, 224–232, 227f
    bucket-handle, 225, 230
    displaced, 228f, 229f
    horizontal cleavage, 225
    MRI of, 232b
    parrot-beak, 225
    vertical-longitudinal, 225
    vertical-radial, 225
Menisci
    anatomy of, 225f
    functions of, 224
    postoperative, 232f
    signal alterations, 229–230
Meniscocapsular separation, 228, 230f
Meniscofemoral ligaments, 224, 226f
Meralgia paresthetica, 46t
Mesenchymal chondrosarcoma, 459
Mesomelic dysplasia, 636
Metacarpophalangeal (MCP) joints, 159, 291, 305f, 322
    cortical thickness in, 393f
    dislocation of, 160f
    rheumatoid arthritis of, 293f
Metaphyseal chondrodysplasia (MChD), 638
    Jansen-type, 640
    McKusick-type, 640
    Schmid type, 62, 638
    Shwachman type, 640
Metaphyseal giant cell tumor, 511f
Metaphyseal lesion, 58–59, 61f
Metaphysis, 578
Metastatic disease of bone, 495–497
    blastic, 497b
    lesser trochanter, 499f
    mixed density, 498f
    mixed lytic and blastic, 497b
    purely lytic, 497b
    spinal, 498f
    therapy for, 497b
    unusual size of, 499f
Metatarsals, 271
    cortical thickness in, 393f
    stress fractures, 277

Metatarsophalangeal (MTP) joints, 295f, 323, 337
Metatarsus adductus, 615, 616f
Metatrophic dysplasia, 634
Method of Sontag, Snell, and Anderson, 579
Methyl methacrylate beads, 22f
Meyer's dysplasia, 353
MFH. *See* Malignant fibrous histiocytoma
MGHL. *See* Middle glenohumeral ligament
Midcarpal dislocation, 147
Midcarpal joint, 143
    injection, 660
Middle column, 164
Middle glenohumeral ligament (MGHL), 85
Mixed connective tissue disease (MCTD), 330
Mixed sclerosing bone dysplasia, 629
Modic changes, 309
Monarticular arthritis, 287
Monteggia's fracture, 121, 131
    dislocation, 121f
Morquio syndrome, 641
Morton's neuroma, 502–503, 505f
MRI. *See* Magnetic resonance imaging
MTP joints. *See* Metatarsophalangeal joints
Mucopolysaccharidoses, 640–641
    classification of, 640t
    key concepts of, 641f
Multidirectional instability, 107
Multiple endocrine neoplasia (MEN), 374
    ribbing-type, 637
Multiple epiphyseal dysplasia (MED), 637, 639f
Multiple myeloma, 493–495
    key concepts of, 493b
Muscle, 33–40
    calcification, 36t
    denervation, 38f, 39f
    infections of, 39
    injury patterns, 36t
    MRI of, 33b
    normal, 35f
Muscle strain, 33, 36
Musculoskeletal masses, differential diagnosis for, 417t, 418t
Mycobacterium tuberculosis, 355
Myelofibrosis, 542–543
    presentation of, 543f
Myeloid depletion, 541, 543f
Myeloma, multiple, 493–495
Myofascial defect, 40, 41f
Myonecrosis, 36t
Myositis ossificans, 30t, 35, 37f, 437, 523–525, 524f, 526f
    differential diagnosis of, 524
    MRI of, 524
Myositis ossificans progressiva, 525, 526f
Myxoma, 465

N

Navicular bone, 271
Navicular bone fracture, 274–275

Navicular stress fractures, 277f
Necrotizing fasciitis, 545
Needle placements, arthrography, 658–661
Neer system, 69
Nerves, 46–47
    normal, 46f
Neural fibrolipoma, 503, 505f
Neuritis, 97
Neurofibromas, 500
    fascicular signs, 501f
Neurofibromatosis, 644, 645f
    scoliosis associated with, 583, 586f
    type 2, 501
    type I, 470, 500, 501
Neuromuscular conditions, 39, 583
Neuropathic arthropathy, 311–314
    areas affected by, 312
    description of, 312
    in foot, 312f
    of hindfoot, 312f
    key concepts, 312b
    of knee, 313
    of shoulder, 313f
Neuropathic spine, 314f
Neurovascular bundles, 46
Nidus, 420, 423
Niemann-Pick disease, 543
Nightstick fracture, 131
NOF. *See* Nonossifying fibroma
Non-Hodgkin's lymphoma, 492
    metastatic, 493f
Nonmarginal erosion, 288
Nonmarginal syndesmophytes, 319
Nonossifying fibroma (NOF), 467–470
    healed, 470f
    key concepts of, 469b
    multiple, 471f
Nonunion, 21
    delayed union v., 21b
Notch view, 211–212
Nursemaid's elbow, 122

O

OATS. *See* Osteochondral autologous transplantation
Oblique band, 125
Oblique fractures, 7
    of fourth toe proximal phalanx, 4f
Occipital atlas dissociation, 169f
Occipital condyle fracture, 167, 169f
Occipital vertebral dissociation, 167
Occipitalization of atlas, 166, 167f
OCD. *See* Osteochondritis dissecans
Ochronosis, 343
O'Donoghue's terrible triad, 236
Odontoid fractures, 169, 170f
Odontoid process, 165
OI. *See* Osteogenesis imperfecta
Olecranon, 120
Olecranon avulsion, 125f
Olecranon bursitis, 115f
Olecranon fossa, 115
Olecranon osteotomy, 125f

Oligoarticular arthritis, 287
Ollier's disease, 445, 446f
Open fractures, closed fractures v., 6–7
Open reduction, 14
Open reduction and internal fraction (ORIF),
  159
OPLL. *See* Ossification of posterior longitudinal
  ligament
Optimizing transducers, 667f
Organomegaly, 495
ORIF. *See* Open reduction and internal fraction
Orthopedic hardware failure, 22
Os acromiale, 74, 88
Os odontoideum, 166, 168f
Os terminale, 166
Osgood-Schlatter disease, 219, 221, 222f,
  242, 357
Osseous lesions
  algorithm for, work-up, 532f
  categorizing, 407b
Osseous lipoma, 476, 481f
Osseous subtalar coalition, 620f
Osseous tumors, 30t
  age as criterion for, 416t
  aggressive, 407
  differential diagnosis for, 417t, 418t
  nonaggressive, 407
  transverse locations of, 413
Ossification centers, 119, 120
  foot, 272
  radiographic appearance of, 121f
  tibial tubercle, 221f
Ossification of posterior longitudinal
  ligament (OPLL), 314, 317f
Ossifying fibroma, 425–427
Osteitis, 326, 545
Osteoarthritis (OA), 285, 304–310, 339, 360
  cervical spine uncinate, 309f
  erosive, 325–326, 326f, 327f
  facet, 308f
  of hip, 306f
  of knee, 307
  locations of, 304b
  primary, 304
  productive changes in, 304b
  purely productive arthritic, 286f
  sacroiliac, 308f
  secondary, 304
Osteoblastoma, 423, 424–425,
  426f
Osteochondral autologous transplantation
  (OATS), 45
Osteochondral defects, 45f, 56b
Osteochondral fractures, 11, 12f
Osteochondral fragments, 44
Osteochondral injury, 257–258
Osteochondritis dissecans (OCD), 53–58, 357
  of capitellum, 131, 132f
  disorders mimicking, 60f
  with displaced fragments, 59f
  early, 54f, 55f
  in femoral trochlea, 57f
  with intact overlying articular cartilage, 56f
  key concepts of, 53b
  with loose *in situ* fragment, 57f
  management of, 57

Osteochondritis dissecans (OCD) *(Continued)*
  MRI for, 56
  patellar, 215
  sites of, 56t
Osteochondromas
  multiple hereditary, 447–450
  sessile, 448
Osteochondrosis, 357–358
Osteoclasts, 397
Osteodystrophy, renal. *See* Renal
  osteodystrophy
Osteofibrous dysplasia. *See* Ossifying fibroma
Osteogenesis imperfecta (OI), 61–62,
  622–625, 624f, 625t
Osteoid matrix, 410t, 411, 412f
Osteoid osteoma, 420–424, 422f, 584
  cortical, 424
  differential diagnosis of, 424
  with growth deformities, 425f
  intra-articular, 424
  intracapsular, 424f
  management, 426f
  mimics, 423f
  MRI of, 425f
  in spine, 422
  subperiosteal, 422
Osteoma, 419
Osteomalacia, 376–379
  key concepts, 380b
Osteomyelitis, 22, 545–560
  acute, 549b
  chronic, 550, 551f, 554b
  chronic recurrent multifocal,
    559–560
  complications of, 550f
  congenital syphilis, 556, 557f
  CT in, 547
  in diabetic neuropathic foot, 552f
  differential diagnosis of, 556
  early acute, 548f
  epiphyseal, 555f
  fungal, 558–559
  in infants, 553f
  mimicking aggressive neoplasm, 550f
  MRI in, 547–548
  in older children, 554f
  serpiginous intraosseous track of, 551f
  in stubbed great toe, 557f
  terminology, 547
  vertebral, 557, 559f
Osteonecrosis. *See* Avascular necrosis
Osteo-onychodysostosis, 651–652
Osteopathia striata, 628, 630f
Osteopetrosis, 626, 627f, 628t
  delayed, 626
  infantile forms of, 626
  with renal tubular acidosis, 626
Osteopoikilosis, 420, 628, 629f
Osteoporosis, 373. *See also* Generalized
    osteoporosis
  aggressive, 396f
  in children, 392b
  postmenopausal, 391
  primary, 391
  regional, 393–395
  senile, 391

Osteosarcoma
  central, 430f, 431f, 432f, 433f, 434f
  clinician knowledge in, 433
  high-grade intramedullary, 429–433
  high-grade surface, 439
  key concepts, 437b
  low-grade intraosseous, 439–440
  in older age group, 440–441
  parosteal, 435–437, 438f
  secondary, 440f
  soft tissue, 30t, 440
  telangiectatic, 433–435, 435f
Osteosarcomatosis, 440
Osteotomy
  acetabular, 606f
  derotation, 606
  distal femoral, 652f
  varus, 605
  varus derotation, 606
Otto pelvis. *See* Protrusio acetabuli deformity
Outlet view, 69
Overhanging edge, 335
Overtubulation, 579, 580f
  causes of, 581f

P

Pachydermoperiostitis, 358
Paget's disease, 373, 379, 397–403
  complications in, 398, 401f
  features of, 400f
  key concepts of, 397b
  lytic phase, 399f, 400f
  mixed phase, 399f, 400f
  radiographs in, 403f
  sclerotic phase, 399f
Paget's sarcoma, 402f
Painful scoliosis, 584
Palmar fibromatosis, 156, 465
Panner's disease, 358
Pannus, 285
Parameniscal cysts, 232
Paraplegia, 30t
Parasyndesmophytes, 319
Parathyroid hormone, 373
Park lines, 578
Parosteal lipoma, 481f
Parosteal osteosarcoma, 435–437
  diagnosis of, 437
  recurrent, 439f
  tumor calcification, 438f
Parsonage-Turner syndrome, 97, 99f
Partial-thickness tears, 94f, 129f
  rotator cuff, 93f
Particle disease, 365f
  CT of, 366f
Patella
  OCD of, 215
  tracking abnormalities, 216
  transverse fracture of, 4f
Patella alta, 216, 217f
Patella baja, 216
Patellar component, failure, 366f
Patellar dislocation, 216–217
  MRI of, 217f
  transient, 216

Patellar fractures, 213–215
  bipartite, 215
  multipartite, 215
Patellofemoral articulation, 209, 216, 218f
Pathologic fracture, 14, 17f
Patient prep generalizations, 656
Pavlik harness, 605f
PCL. *See* Posterior cruciate ligament
Pectoralis major, 68
Pedicle
  congenital absence of, 593f
  screws, 589
Peduncular exostosis, 445
Pelkin's fracture, 388f
Pellegrini-Stieda disease, 239
Pelvic fractures
  biomechanical classification of,
    185–187
  pelvic ring classification, 187–189
Pelvis
  anatomy, 183–185
  anteroposterior, 183f
  fibrous dysplasia of, 463f
  soft tissue conditions, 207–208
Periosteal elevation, 62
Periosteal new bone formation,
    62t, 414t
Periosteal osteosarcoma, 437–439
Periosteal reaction, 412–414, 414t
  aggressive, 415f
  hair-on-end, 413
  interrupted, 413
  lamellated, 413
  nonaggressive, 415f
  sunburst, 413
  uninterrupted, 413
Periosteum, 3
Periostitis, 545
Peripheral chondrosarcomas, 458
Peripheral nerve entrapment syndromes,
    46t
Peripheral nerve sheath tumors (PNST),
    500–502
  benign, 500b
  malignant, 501–501, 504f
Peripheral ossification, 35
Periprosthetic fracture, 367f
Peroneal tendons, 265
Peroneus brevis, 252
  split, 265
  subluxation, 267f
  tendon tears, 266f
Peroneus longus, 252
Peroneus quartus, 267
Persistent lucent synchondrosis, 166
Pes anserinus, 243
  bursitis, 244f
Pes cavus, 615
Pes planovalgus. *See* Flexible flatfoot
    deformity
PET. *See* Positron emission tomography
PFFD. *See* Proximal focal femoral
    deficiency
Phalanges, 271
Phalanxes, fractures of, 4f
Phleboliths, 30t

Physeal injury, 50–53, 578
  knee, 220–222
Physis, 49, 50, 577, 578f
Pigmented villonodular synovitis (PVNS),
    503b, 504, 506f, 507f
Pilon fractures, 256, 258f
PIP. *See* Proximal interphalangeal
Piriformis syndrome, 46t
Pisiform fracture, 150f
Pisiformis syndrome, 207
Pisotriquetral joint, 137b
Pitt's pit, 206
Plafond, 249
Plantar calcaneonavicular ligament,
    268
Plantar fascia, 279, 280f
Plantar fasciitis, 279
Plantar fibromatosis, 466, 468f
  ultrasonography of, 469f
Plantaris tendon tear, 262f
Plasmacytoma, 494f, 495
Plastic deformity, 7
Plicae, 246
  normal, 247f
PNST. *See* Peripheral nerve sheath tumors
POEMS syndrome, 495
Polyarticular arthritis, 287
Polyethylene, 364
Polymorphic fibroosseous lesion of bone,
    470–471
Polymyositis, 39, 331–333, 332b
Polyneuropathy, 495
Polyostotic disease, 461
Popliteal artery entrapment, 245
Popliteal fossa, 240, 241
Popliteus tendon, 231–232
Position, fracture, 8–11
Positron emission tomography (PET),
    407
Posterior bundle, 125
Posterior calcaneus, 250
Posterior column, 164, 190
Posterior cruciate ligament (PCL), 234
  avulsion fracture of, 239f
  normal, 234f
  reconstruction of, 237f
  ruptures of, 237–239
  tears, 238f
Posterior fat pad sign, 115
Posterior glenohumeral dislocation, 105
Posterior interosseous nerve syndrome, 46t
Posterior tibial tendinopathy (PTT), 263
Posterior tibialis tendon
  complete tear of, 265f
  tendinosis of, 264f
Posterior tibiotalar ligament, 250
Posterior wall fractures, 190
  transverse, 191f
Posteroanterior radiographs, 134
Posterolateral corner injury, 236–237
Postmenopausal osteoporosis, 391
Postoperative shoulder, 109
Post-traumatic radioulnar synostosis, 131
Pott's disease, 558
Preoperative therapy, 531–532
Prevertebral soft tissues, 165

Primary lymphoma of bone, 491–492
  metastatic, 492
Primary protrusio of acetabulum, 295,
    608–609
Progeria, 30t
Progressive diaphyseal dysplasia, 628, 629f
Pronation, 137, 254, 255
Pronation-external rotation, 255
Pronator syndrome, 46t
Protrusio acetabuli deformity, 295, 608–609
  reference line for, 608f
Proximal focal femoral deficiency (PFFD),
    607
  spectrum of abnormalities in, 607f
Proximal humerus, 68–73
  fractures, 69f, 70f
Proximal interphalangeal (PIP), 160, 291, 322
Proximal radioulnar joint, 112
Proximal radius, pseudolesion of, 114f
Proximal ulna, 112
Pseudarthrosis, ankylosing spondylitis,
    321f
Pseudoacetabulum, 598
Pseudoachondroplasia, 631–632
Pseudofractures, 380f
Pseudogout, 339
Pseudohypoparathyroidism, 30t, 389b
  characteristics of, 389f, 390f
Pseudolesions, of proximal radius, 114f
Pseudomonas, 550
Pseudo-pseudohypoparathyroidism,
    389b
Pseudotumor, of hemophilia, 565–566,
    568f
Psoriatic arthritis, 289, 321–324, 323f
  of hips, 324f
  key concepts of, 322b
  oligoarticular pattern, 324f
Pulled elbow, 122
Pulley injury, 163f
Pulvinar, 598
Pure plastic bowing deformity, 7
Pustulosis, 326
PVNS. *See* Pigmented villonodular
    synovitis
Pyknodysostosis, 628, 629t, 635
Pyle's disease, 543
Pyrophosphate arthropathy, 339–342
  of hip, 341f
  key concepts, 340
  of knee, 341f

Q

Quadriceps, 240
  tendon tears, 242f
Quadrilateral space, 87
Quadrilateral space syndrome, 46t
Quadriplegia, 30t

R

Radial club hand, 646
Radial dysplasias, 646–647
Radial head dislocation, 117b
  congenital, 122f

Radial head fracture, radiographically occult, 123f
Radial head subluxation, 122
Radial nerve, 131
 entrapment, 131
Radiation therapy, 39, 40f, 433, 584
 complications of, 533t
Radiocapitellar line, 113f
Radiocarpal joint, 137b, 141–142
 injection, 659–660
Radiographically occult fractures, 7f, 198f
Radiography, 12f, 41, 67, 134, 271
 of cervical spine, 164–165
 of DDH, 599f, 600
 elbow, 113f
 of foreign bodies, 47f
 in hyperparathyroidism, 375f, 376f
 in OCD, 57
 in Paget's disease, 403f
 scoliosis, 583b
 shoulder anatomy on, 68f
 for suspected child abuse, 58t
Radionuclide scanning, 6, 12f, 199f, 347
 of tumors, 417
Radioulnar ligaments, 140
Radius, pseudolesion of, 114f
Raynaud's phenomenon, 329, 330
Reactive arthritis, 289, 324–325
 key concepts, 325f
Rectus femoris, 240
Red marrow distribution, 539
Reflex sympathetic dystrophy, 22, 394–395, 395f
Regional osteoporosis, 393–395
Reimer's migration index, 600
Reiter syndrome. *See* Reactive arthritis
Renal dialysis sequela, 30t
Renal osteodystrophy, 381–383
 AP radiograph of, 383f
 key concepts of, 382b
Renal tubular acidosis, osteopetrosis, 626
Retinoid arthropathy, 314, 387f
Reverse Bankart injury, 109
Revision arthroplasty, 363
RF. *See* Rheumatoid factor
Rheumatoid arthritis, 77, 285, 290–303
 of calcaneus, 295f
 of cervical spine, 298f
 differential diagnosis of, 299
 of elbow, 292, 293f, 294
 extra-articular manifestations of, 291b
 of foot, 295
 gout, 337f
 hand and wrist, 291–292
 of hip, 295–296, 297f
 instability, 293f
 key concepts, 290b
 of knee, 295
 of MCP joints, 293f
 of MTP joints, 295f
 of shoulder girdle, 292–294
 of spine, 296–298

Rheumatoid factor (RF), 285
Rhomboid fossa, 68
Ribbing disease II, 628
Rickets, 380–381
 key concepts, 380b, 381b
 radiographic features of, 382f
 treatment for, 383f
Rim rent, 95
Risser classification, 581f
Risser technique, 580
Robust rheumatoid arthritis, 298
Rocker bottom feet. *See* Congenital vertical talus
Rolando's fracture, 159, 160f
Rotary subluxation
 of C1 on C2, 170f
 of lunate, 146
Rotation, 10
Rotational injuries, 4
Rotator cuff, 78
 degeneration, 92–96
 impingement, 88–92
 partial-thickness tear, 93f
 pathology mimickers, 96–98
 repairs, 111f
 tear, 92–96, 97b, 98f
 tendinosis, 93f
Rotator interval, 83
Rowe classification, 272

S

Saber-Harris I fractures, 49, 52, 53f, 71, 72f, 121, 223f
Saber-Harris II fractures, 49, 59, 138, 220
Saber-Harris III fractures, 49, 220, 256, 257f
Saber-Harris IV fractures, 49
Saber-Harris V fractures, 49
Sacral fractures, 185
Sacroiliac (SI) joint
 ankylosing spondylitis of, 319f
 osteoarthritis of, 308f
Sacroiliitis
Sacrum, insufficiency fracture of, 16f
Salmonella, 321, 325, 568
SAPHO (synovitis, acne pustulosis, hyperostosis, osteitis), 326, 327f, 559–560
Sarcoidosis, 562–563
 marrow disease, 564f
 muscular, 563, 564f
Sarcoma
 Ewing's, 431, 489–491
 soft tissue, 530, 531t
 staging, 530, 531
SBC. *See* Solitary bone cyst
Scaphoid, 142
Scaphoid fossa, 137
Scaphoid fractures, 144f
 complications, 145f
Scaphoid waist fracture, 157b
Scaphoid-trapezium-trapezoid complex (STT), 305
Scapholunate advanced collapse (SLAC), 155, 340

Scapholunate dissociation, 148, 152, 154f
Scapholunate ligaments, 150
 tear, 151f
Scapula, 73–75
 CT of, 73–74
 development of, 73–74
 fractures, 73f
Scapular foramen, 74
Scapular neck, 73
Scapular neck dysplasia, 75
Scapulothoracic joint, 68
SCFE. *See* Slipped capital femoral epiphysis
Schatzker I fracture, 213, 215f
Schatzker II fracture, 213
Schatzker III fracture, 213
Schatzker IV fracture, 213
Schatzker V fracture, 213
Schatzker VI fracture, 213
Scheuermann's disease, 357, 589, 590f
Schmid-type metaphyseal chondrodysplasia, 62
Schmorl's node, 310
Schwann cells, 500
Schwannoma, 500–501
 peripheral, 503f
Scleroderma, 30t, 329–330
 key concepts of, 330b
Sclerosing bone dysplasias, 625–629, 626b
Scoliosis, 582–589, 582b
 causes of, 582t
 idiopathic, 584–585, 586f, 587f
 long C-shaped, 586f
 neurofibromatosis and, 583, 586f
 non-idiopathic, 582t
 radiographs, 583b
Screws, 18f
Scurvy, 388
Seat belt fractures, 176
SEDC. *See* Spondyloepiphyseal dysplasia congenita
SED-tarda. *See* Spondyloepiphyseal dysplasia tarda
Segond fracture, 220f, 236
Senile osteoporosis, 391
Septic arthritis, 560–562
 of hip, 560–562
Septic joints, 561f–562f
Sequestrum, 550
Seronegative, 285
Seronegative spondyloarthropathy, 325f
Sessile exostosis, 445, 449f
Sessile osteochondromas, 448
Sever's disease, 357
SGHL. *See* Superior glenohumeral ligament
Sharpey's fibers, 26
Shear, 3, 4
Shigella, 321, 325
Shin splints, 12, 222
Shoulder
 anatomy, 68, 112–117
 arthroplasty, 109, 367f
 dislocation, 104f, 105f, 106f

Shoulder *(Continued)*
  imaging techniques, 67
  injection, 658
  miscellaneous conditions, 109
  neuropathic, 313f
  postoperative, 109
  radiography of, 68f
  rheumatoid arthritis of, 292–294
Shwachman-type metaphyseal chondrodysplasia,
  640
SI joint. *See* Sacroiliac joint
Sickle cell anemia, 567–568, 567–569
  AVN and, 571f
  key concepts of, 568b
  in spine, 572f
Sickle cell dactylitis, 570f
Sickle cell disease, 349
Signal alterations, meniscal,
  229–230
Silastic arthroplasty, 367, 368f
  failure, 369f
Sinding-Larsen-Johansson disease, 219,
  222f, 242
Single photon emission CT (SPECT),
  591
Sinus tarsi syndrome, 278
Sirenomelia, 595
Skeletal age, 581t
  Guerlich Pyle technique, 589
  Method of Sontag, Snell, and Anderson, 579
  Risser classification, 581f
  Risser technique, 580
Skeletal growth and development,
  577–581
  key concepts of, 577–581
Skier's thumb, 161f
Skull, fibrous dysplasia of, 461f
SLAC. *See* Scapholunate advanced collapse
SLAP tears. *See* Superior labral anterior and
  posterior
Sleep palsy, 46t
Slipped capital femoral epiphysis (SCFE),
  200–201, 597
  bilateral, 201f
Smith's fracture, 139
Snapping hip, 203–204
Soft tissue biopsy, 664
Soft tissue calcifications, 30t, 331t
  after elbow dislocation, 124f
Soft tissue gas, 546f
Soft tissue infection, 545, 546f
Soft tissue injury
  in arthritis, 288
  foot, 277–279
Soft tissue osteosarcoma, 30t, 440
Soft tissue sarcomas, surgical staging of,
  530, 531t
Soft tissue vascular malformations,
  485f–486f, 487f
Solitary bone cyst (SBC), 514–516
  adult, 517f
  key concepts of, 514b
Solitary bone tumors, surgical staging of,
  530, 531t
SONK. *See* Spontaneous osteonecrosis
  of the knee

SPECT. *See* Single photon emission CT
Spina bifida, 595
Spinal instrumentation, 590f
Spinal ring apophyses, 588f
Spinal rods, 589
Spinal stenosis, 595
Spine
  amyloid, 345f
  aneurysmal bone cyst of, 520f
  ankylosing spondylitis of, 320f
  AVN of, 352f
  curvature of, 586
  fracture, 172, 316f, 584
  metastasis, 498f
  osteoid osteoma in, 422
  rheumatoid arthritis of, 296–298
  segmentation anomalies, 585f, 591, 595f
  sickle cell, 572f
  tuberculosis of, 558, 560, 561f
Spine fracture, in DISH, 316f
Spine hemangioma, 485f
Spine trauma, 584
Spinoglenoid notch, 73
Spiral fractures, 6f, 7
Split peroneus brevis syndrome, 265
Spondylitis, of inflammatory bowel disease,
  381–321
Spondyloarthropathy, 287
  seronegative, 325f
Spondyloepiphyseal dysplasia congenita
  (SEDC), 636–637, 638
Spondyloepiphyseal dysplasia tarda
  (SED-tarda), 636–637, 639f
Spondylolisthesis, 591
Spondylolysis, 177, 591
  detection of, 591
Spondylosis deformans, 310
Spontaneous osteonecrosis of the knee
  (SONK), 244
Sports hernia, 208
Sprains, 26, 27
  ankle ligament, 27f
Sprengel's deformity, 594–595, 595f
Spring ligament, 268
Sprung pelvis, 186
Staphylococcus aureus, 398, 549,
  568
Static carpal instability, 150
Stener lesion, 160
Stenosing tenosynovitis, 33
Sternoclavicular joint, 68, 75–76
  dislocation of, 76
  pathologic conditions of, 76
Straddle fracture, 186
Streptococcus, 549
Stress fractures, 12–14, 259f
  calcaneus, 14f, 273
  distal fibular, 260f
  femoral, 202–203, 204f
  knee, 222–223
  metatarsal, 277
  MRI of, 14f
  navicular, 277f
  of proximal tibia, 13f
Stress injury, 52
Stress lines, 578

Stress risers, 6
STT. *See* Scaphoid-trapezium-trapezoid complex
Stubbed toe, 277
Subacromial bursa, 86
Subacromial bursitis, 89–90, 90f
Subacromial space, 86
Subchondral cysts, 320
Subchondral erosion, 288
Sublabral foramen, 83f, 107b
Sublabral sulcus, 84f
Sublocation, 32
Subluxation, 26b, 27
  divergent, 276
  homolateral, 275–276
  peroneus brevis, 267f
  radial head, 122
Subscapularis, 83
  tears, 96f
Subsidence, 362
Subtalar facets, 272f
Sulcus angle, 217
Sunburst periosteal reaction, 413
Superior glenohumeral ligament
  (SGHL), 85
Superior labral anterior and posterior
  (SLAP) tears, 107–108
Supination, 137, 254, 255
Supination-external rotation, 255
Supracondylar fracture, 117, 117b
  displaced, 118
Supracondylar process, 116
Suprapatellar plicae, 246
Suprascapular nerve injury, 97b
Suprascapular notch syndrome, 46t,
  73
Supraspinatus, 78, 83, 86
  complete tears, 95f
  full-thickness tears, 94f
Supratrochlear dorsale, 116
Surface osteosarcoma, high-grade, 439
Surgical staging
  of soft tissue sarcomas, 531t
  of solitary bone tumors, 530, 531t
Surgical treatment, tumor, 532–533
Suture anchors, 110f
Swan neck deformities, 292
Symphalangism, 647, 648f
Synchondroses, of C2, 167f
Syndesmophytes, 319
Syndesmosis sprain, 269f
Synovectomy, 504
Synovial cell sarcoma, 30t, 506–508
  without calcification, 508f
  with dystrophic calcification, 508f
  key concepts, 508b
Synovial chondromatosis, 30t, 355
  calcified bodies, 356f
  noncalcified bodies, 356f
Synovial joints, 26
Synovitis, 28, 29f, 326, 559–560
Syphilis, 556
Systemic lupus erythematosus (SLE), 30t,
  299, 328, 329f
  areas affected by, 328
  key concepts of, 328b
Systemic sclerosis, 329–330

T

Talar beak, 617, 621f
Talar dislocation, 275f
Talar dome, 249
  AVN and, 275
Talipes, 613
Talocalcaneal angle, 610, 612
Talocalcaneal coalitions, 616, 618
Talus, 271
Talus fracture, 274
TAR syndrome, 646
Tarsal coalition, 615–618, 621f
Tarsal plate, 277
Tarsal tunnel syndrome, 46t, 270
Tarsal-metatarsal articulations, 271
Tarsometatarsal joints, 272f
Teardrop, 183
Teardrop burst fracture, 173f
Tears
  labral, 107–109
    imaging diagnosis, 107
    posterior, 109f
  meniscal, 224–232
  rotator cuff, 92–96
  tendons, 32, 33b
    complete, 34f
    flexor hallucis longus, 266f
    peroneus brevis, 266f
Telangiectatic osteosarcoma, 433–435, 435f
Tendinitis, 33
Tendinosis, 32, 34f
  of Achilles tendon, 261f
  of posterior tibialis, 264f
Tendon sheath, giant cell tumor of,
    506, 507f
Tendons, 28–32
  distal biceps, 129
  elbow, 125–130
  injury patterns, 33t
  of knee, 239–244
  MRI of, 28, 31f, 33b
  peroneal, 265
  rotator cuff, 88
  tears, 32
Tennis elbow, 128f
Tenosynovitis, 30, 32, 32f, 33, 265, 267
  stenosing, 33
Tension, 3, 4
Teratogenic dislocation, 597
Teres major, 87
Teres minor, 78, 87
TFCC. See Triangular fibrocartilage complex
Thalassemia, 566–567
  major, 569f
Thalium-201 imaging, 532
Thanatophoric dwarfism, 633
Thoracic fractures, 175–177
Thoracic spine, 174–175
Three-column model, 164
Thyroid acropachy, 359, 386, 387f
Tibia
  growth arrest after injury to, 52f
  open fracture of, 7f
  stress fractures of, 13f
  torsion of, 650–651

Tibial articular margin, 249
Tibial component, loosening of, 366f
Tibial plateau fractures, 212–213, 214f
Tibial tubercle avulsion, 220f
Tibial tubercle ossification center, 221f
Tibialis anterior, 252
Tibialis posterior, 250
Tibiofibular syndesmosis, 257
Tillaux fracture, 256, 256f
Toddler's fracture, 8f
TOH. See Transient osteoporosis of hip
Tophi, 336
Torsion, 10
  femoral, 202f
  of femur, 650–651
  of tibia, 650–651
Trabeculae, 419
Tracking abnormalities, 216
  patellofemoral, 218f
Transient osteoporosis of hip (TOH),
    354, 393
Transient regional osteoporosis (TRO),
    354, 394
Transitional segmentation, 591–594
  lumbosacral, 594f
Translocation, 148
  carpal, 156
Trans-scaphoid perilunate fracture-dislocation,
    146
Transverse fracture, 7, 497
  of acetabulum, 190f
  of patella, 4f
Transverse humeral ligament, 83
Transverse ligament, 125
Transverse process fractures, 177
Transverse scans, 667
Traumatic joint effusions, 11f
Trevor disease. See Dysplasia epiphysealis
    hemimelica
Triangular fibrocartilage complex (TFCC),
    140–141
  key concepts, 140b
  tear, 141f
Triceps, 87
Triceps tendon, 130
Trigonum syndrome, 268
Triplane fracture, 257f
Triquetrohamate instability, 156
Triquetrum, 142
Triquetrum fracture, 157b
Triradiate cartilage, 665
Trisomy 18, 645
Trisomy 21, 644, 646f
TRO. See Transient regional osteoporosis
Trochanteric bursitis, 208
Trochlea, 120
T-shaped fracture, 192f
Tuberculosis, 30t
  fungal arthritis and, 563f
  of spine, 558, 560f, 561f
Tuberous sclerosis, 646f
Tubular bones, fibrous dysplasia of, 463f–464f
Tumor biopsy, 530–531
Tumor follow-up, 533–534
  CT in, 533
  MRI in, 533

Tumor imaging
  age of patient in, 414–416
  CT, 417
  discriminators in, 407–416
  lesion density in, 410–411
  lesion location in, 411–412
  MRI, 417
  radionuclide studies, 417
  ultrasonography, 418
Tumor margin, 407–410
  aggressive, 409f, 410f
  differential diagnosis, 408t
  nonaggressive, 408f
Tumor matrix, 410–411
  chondroid, 410t, 411f
  osteoid, 410t, 411, 412f
Tumor work-up, algorithms for, 530
Tumoral calcinosis, 30t, 384f
Tumors. See specific types
Turf toe, 277
Turner syndrome, 645

U

UBC. See Solitary bone cyst
Ulna
  pseudodefect of, 114f
  shortening, 52f
Ulna positive variance, 137
Ulnar collateral ligament, 159
  tear, 128f
Ulnar impaction syndrome, 142f
Ulnar impingement syndrome, 141
Ulnar negative variance, 137
Ulnar nerve, 112
  injury, 131f
  release, 131f
Ulnar translocation, 148
Ultrasonography, 28, 30b, 67, 112, 134, 194,
    289, 407
  of DDH, 600–604, 603f
  of foreign bodies, 47f
  tendons on, 32f
  of tumors, 418
Ultrasonography of infant hip, 665–668
  images, 666–668
  landmarks, 665–666
Undertubulation, 579, 580f
  causes of, 580t
Unilateral interfacetal dislocation, 172
Unilateral locked facet, 172, 174f

V

Valgus, 26b
Varus, 26b
Varus osteotomy, 605
  derotation, 606f
Vascular tumors, 478–480
  angiosarcoma, 480
  benign, 478–479
  intermediate for malignancy, 479–480
Vascularized fibular graft, 351f
Vasovagal reactions, 658
Vastus intermedius, 240

Vastus lateralis, 240
Vastus medialis, 240
Vertebra plana
    key concepts of, 521f
    in LCH, 523f
Vertebral body hemangioma, 483f
Vertebral osteomyelitis, 557, 559f
Vertebral segmentation anomalies, 585f
Vertebroplasty, 175
Vertical displacement, 186
Vertical shear, 186, 188f
VISI. *See* Volar intercalated segment
    instability
Vitamin A, 386
Vitamin D, 373, 386
Volar intercalated segment instability
    (VISI), 150, 155

Volar plate fracture, 161, 161f
Volkmann's contracture, 131

W

Watson's test, 155
Weber (AO) classification, 253
Wide symphysis pubis, 623f
Wilson's disease, 342
Wimberger's sign, 388f
Wolff's law, 3, 12
Wormian bones, 624t
Wrist
    alignment, 134b
    anatomy, 135f, 136f
    compartments of, 136, 137b
    distal radioulnar joint injection, 660

frequently missed injuries, 157b
imaging techniques, 134
juvenile rheumatoid arthritis of, 302f
midcarpal joint injection, 660
normal radiographic anatomy of, 135f
position of, 137f–138f
radiocarpal joint injection, 659–660
rheumatoid arthritis of, 291–292
tendon compartments, 156f

X

Xanthomatosis, of Achilles tendon, 263f

Y

Yersinia, 321, 325